TEXTBOOK OF HUMAN HISTOLOGY
VOLUME 1

FOUNDATIONS OF TISSUE STRUCTURE AND FUNCTION

Edited by
Dr. Neda Nikolovski

ALLIED HEALTH PRESS

Textbook of Human Histology Volume 1

Foundations of Tissue Structure and Function

Editor: **Dr. Neda Nikolovski**

Allied Health Press
4164 Lakeshore Road
Burlington ON L7L 1A4
Canada
www.alliedhealthpress.com
Email: orders@arclereducation.com

ISBN: 978-1-77956-776-5

Allied Health Press publishes wide variety of books and eBooks. For more information about Allied Health Press and its products, visit our website at www.alliedhealthpress.com

ABOUT THE EDITOR

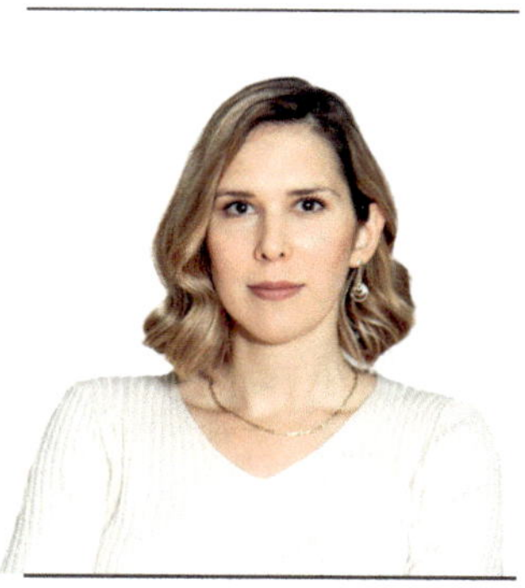

Dr. Neda Nikolovski, a Molecular Biologist and Physiologist holding a PhD in Immunology, has been dedicated to scientific research since 2015 at the Institute for Biological Research, Belgrade University, Belgrade, Serbia. Her primary areas of expertise encompass immunology, autoimmunity, neurodegenerative diseases, multiple sclerosis and its animal models, dendritic cells, and cell-based immunotherapy in autoimmune conditions. She is author of 27 research papers published in esteemed international journals and has contributed her expertise as a reviewer for numerous international publications.

Brief Table of Contents

Getting Started with This Book

Chapter Openers

A list of Chapter Outline is presented providing a brief Introduction to what will be covered in the chapter.

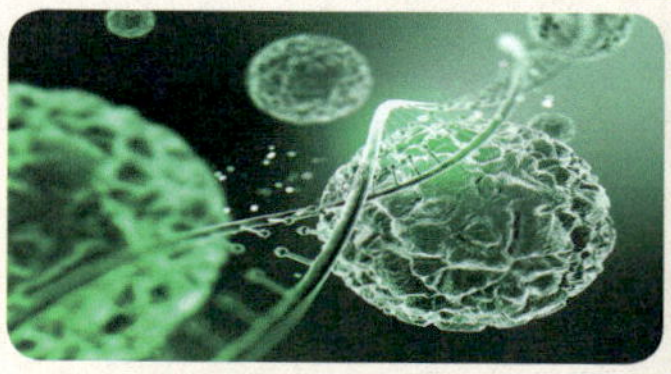

LEARNING OBJECTIVES

After studying this chapter, you will be able to:

1. Discuss the scientific method in biology;
2. Explain the cell theory;
3. Discuss the genetics and heredity;
4. Evolution and natural selection;
5. Focus on ecology and ecosystems;
6. Learn about human biology;
7. Evaluate the plant biology;
8. Explain the microbiology;
9. Focus on current trends in biology.

Introduction

Often referred to as the science of life, biology is a broad field of study aimed at comprehending the several kinds of life on Earth, from tiny creatures to sophisticated multicellular entities. Comprising several subfields, including molecular biology, ecology, and evolutionary biology, each of which advances our knowledge of living systems, this field clarifies the mechanisms controlling life events, including development, reproduction, and interaction with the surroundings, which is the central goal of biology. Moreover, biology fills in the void between the natural sciences and medicine by offering a necessary understanding of health, illness, and the interactions between organisms and their environments. Dealing with urgent global issues such as climate change, biodiversity loss, and new diseases depends on an awareness of these complex biological interactions, therefore highlighting the critical part biology plays in modern civilization. Fundamentally, biology explores and tests ideas about the living world using the scientific method. Through methodical observation and experimentation,

1.1. The Scientific Method in Biology

Learning Outcome

1. Describe the steps of the scientific method;
2. Focus on hypothesis formation;
3. Learn about experimental design.

Learning Outcomes

The beginning of each section of every chapter contains a set of Learning Outcomes that inform students of concepts they should understand. These outcomes help students understand what they should be able to do if they have mastered the material in that section.

Test Your Knowledge

Throughout each chapter, Test Your Knowledge cues you to note which topics have been covered and to self-test your understanding of the material presented.

Test Your Knowledge

1. Explain why correlation does not imply causation in scientific experiments.
2. How does the scientific method help reduce the influence of personal opinions in research?

Chapter Summary

The Summary Section appear at the end of each chapter and summarize main concepts covered throughout the chapter. These points provide key concepts in an engaging and meaningful way.

Summary

The investigation of biological principles highlights the importance of a comprehensive view of life by reflecting the intricate interactions that occur within living systems. The complexity of biology goes beyond individual species or systems, as this essay highlights; it also includes the interactions that mold ecosystems and affect biodiversity. Researchers can conduct in-depth analyses of metabolomic data using sophisticated technologies like MetaboAnalyst, which offer insights into the molecular mechanisms underlying these interactions. As demonstrated by the developments in MetaboAnalyst, for example, the integration of diverse omics data promotes a thorough understanding of metabolic pathways and helps identify important biological markers necessary for research on development and disease (Chong et al., 2018). Additionally, the phenomenon of ecological invasions is a key component of biological research and a vital field of study. The introduction of non-native species into unfamiliar habitats has significant ramifications and calls for multidisciplinary management strategies. Examining the origins and effects of these biological incursions, invasion science has become a crucial field that highlights the need to comprehend ecological dynamics and community interactions. As interest in biological invasions increases, new findings are emerging that put conventional ecological theories and practices to the test. The importance of incorporating various scientific viewpoints is shown by this developing discipline, which also highlights how invasive species shape ecosystems and advances our knowledge of ecological resilience (David et al., 2013). When taken as a whole, these discoveries from invasion science and metabolomics highlight the value of multidisciplinary biology research. Fostering cross-disciplinary collaboration and utilizing technological breakthroughs to improve our comprehension of intricate biological interactions are crucial as we look to the future of biological research. In addition to deepening our understanding of the complexities of life, this method lays the groundwork for tackling urgent environmental issues. Future studies can ensure the continued relevance of biology in a world that is constantly changing by acknowledging the interconnection of biological systems and opening the door to creative solutions that support sustainability and biodiversity conservation. We might imagine a thorough comprehension of life that serves both academia and society at large through ongoing investigation and integration of scientific knowledge.

Knowledge Assessment

The chapter includes material designed to review and reinforce each content. It includes Critical Thinking Questions to help test of your understanding of information presented in the chapter and Short answer Questions to review your understanding of the key concepts presented in the chapter.

Critical Thinking Questions

1. **Who is known as the "Father of Modern Biology"?**
   a. Aristotle
   b. Charles Darwin
   c. Gregor Mendel
   d. Louis Pasteur
2. **What is the basic unit of life?**
   a. Atom
   b. Molecule
   c. Cell
   d. Organism
3. **Which branch of biology studies the interaction of organisms with their environment?**
   a. Genetics
   b. Ecology
   c. Physiology
   d. Botany
4. **Which macromolecule is the main source of energy for living organisms?**
   a. Proteins
   b. Lipids
   c. Carbohydrates
   d. Nucleic acids
5. **DNA is primarily responsible for which function in living organisms?**
   a. Energy production
   b. Protein synthesis
   c. Storing genetic information
   d. Regulating body temperature

Short Answer Questions

1. What is biology, and why is it important to study biology?
2. What are the three main domains of life, and how are they different from one another?
3. Define homeostasis and give an example of how it works in living organisms.
4. What is the cell theory, and why is it fundamental to biology?
5. How do autotrophs and heterotrophs differ in the way they obtain energy?
6. What is the scientific method, and how is it applied in biological research?
7. Discuss how biology helps address global challenges such as climate change, disease, and food security.
8. Explain the levels of biological organization from the smallest unit to the largest. Provide examples at each level.
9. Describe the relationship between structure and function in biology, giving specific examples from cells or organs.
10. How has the discovery of genetics shaped our understanding of inheritance and variation among organisms?

Supplementary Materials

Key Terms: A list of key terms is given for quick reference

KEY TERMS FROM THIS CHAPTER

Annotation enrichment analysis	Biological structure	Cell
Cell theory	Cellular structure	Ecology
Ecosystems	Genetics	Human biology
Microbiology	Natural selection	Organism
Plant biology		

Further Resources: Recommendations for additional readings, websites, and multimedia resources.

References

1. Argelaguet, R., Velten, B., Arnol, D., Dietrich, S., Zenz, T., Marioni, J. C., Buettner, F., et al. (2018). Multi-omics factor analysis—A framework for unsupervised integration of multi-omics data sets. *Molecular Systems Biology, 14*. https://doi.org/10.15252/msb.20178124.
2. Bacher, S., Blackburn, T. M., Essl, F., & Genovesi, P. (2017). *Socio-Economic Impact Classification of Alien Taxa (SEICAT)*. https://core.ac.uk/download/286567949.pdf (accessed on 8th March 2025).
3. Barnett, R., Brace, S., Cucchi, T., & Dobney, K. (2013). *Divergent Evolutionary Processes Associated with Colonization of Offshore Islands*. https://core.ac.uk/download/20664364.pdf (accessed on 8th March 2025).

Detailed Table of Contents

CHAPTER 6

CHAPTER 7

CHAPTER 8

CHAPTER 11

Nervous Tissue 303

CHAPTER 12

Lymphatic System 337

Index 369

LIST OF FIGURES

PREFACE

In examining human tissues, there is a staggering degree of complexity and organization in the way cells work together to maintain life. In examining their microscopic make-up, where each layer, fiber, and specialized cell contributes to an organ's shape and function, it is observed how form and function are interwoven.

Where thin sections are stained to recognize distinct components, it is clear how patterns of structure control processes such as capillary nutrient transport and nerve conduction. Moreover, learning how cells adhere to each other, divide, and send chemical messages forms the groundwork for understanding disease mechanisms, guiding tissue engineering, and streamlining diagnostic processes. This understanding connects basic histology to clinical practice, illuminating directions for pathology innovation, regenerative medicine treatment, and imaging technologies.

With the growth of this science, advances in electron and light microscopy have enhanced our capacity to see ever-more minute detail. Advances in staining methods and imaging techniques have revolutionized our perspective from simple histochemical identification into three-dimensional reconstructions and dynamic cellular activity. These technological advances have not only clarified our view of human biology but have also promoted new hypotheses regarding tissue repair, developmental malformations, and the cell-mediated pathogenesis of disease. The integration of histological observations with molecular and genetic data continues to redefine our understanding, connecting microscopic appearance with clinical presentation.

This learning resource, *Textbook of Human Histology: Volume 1*, has been written to lead the student through the landscape of tissue architecture with clearness and profundity. It provides a coordinated progression from microscopic general principles on to the specialized characteristics of every tissue type. Through carefully chosen illustrations and explanatory legends, the volume is designed to serve visual as well as textual learners, providing a balanced method that bridges laboratory technique and conceptual understanding. Whether you're preparing for lab sessions or including histology in broader anatomy and physiology courses, this book is designed to be a trusted guide.

- Chapter 1 provides a history of the development of tissue research and explains the key skills of specimen preparation, staining, and imaging.
- Chapter 2 covers the principles and practice of microscopy, explaining bright-field, phase-contrast, fluorescence, and electron techniques.
- Chapter 3 covers cell structure and function, such as organelle dynamics, cytoskeletal elements, and membrane specializations.

- Chapter 4 examines epithelial tissue, its classification, surface specializations, and role in protection, absorption, and secretion.
- Chapter 5 covers connective tissue, from the loose and dense to specialized types such as reticular and elastic.
- Chapter 6 addresses adipose tissue, comparing white and brown fat according to cellular composition and metabolic significance.
- Chapter 7 is about cartilage, where structural organization of hyaline, elastic, and fibrocartilage, as well as growth and repair mechanisms, are presented.
- Chapter 8 is on bone tissue, where cellular elements, matrix mineralization, and the remodeling cycle are discussed.
- Chapter 9 is on blood and hematopoiesis, where the origin, maturation, and morphology of blood cells in bone marrow niches are described.
- Chapter 10 addresses muscular tissue, contrasting the histological features of skeletal, cardiac, and smooth muscle in terms of contractile function.
- Chapter 11 addresses nervous tissue, such as neuronal structure, synaptic structure, and supportive roles of glial cells.
- Chapter 12 finally addresses the lymphatic system, ranging from lymphatic capillaries and nodes to histology of primary and secondary lymphoid tissues.

This text is designed for undergraduate and graduate students, health-science professionals requiring a source of reference, medical and dental students, biomedical researchers, and allied health professionals who require a solid understanding of tissue architecture to inform clinical practice or laboratory research. Organizing the concepts in a clear, logical order and correlating them with excellent illustrations, the book is intended to acquaint readers with basic information that will facilitate the pursuit of further study and practice in both academic and working setups.

INTRODUCTION TO HUMAN HISTOLOGY

1

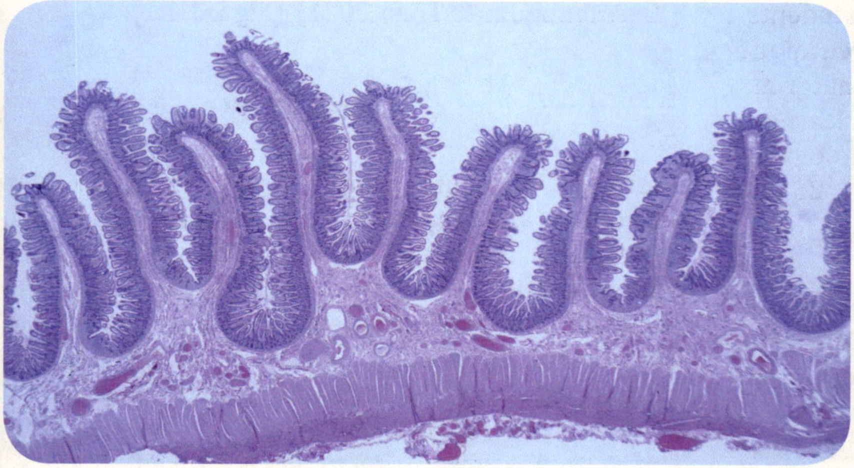

LEARNING OBJECTIVES

After studying this chapter, you will be able to:

1. Describe the four basic tissue types;
2. Describe the histological techniques and staining methods;
3. Understand the microscopy in histology;
4. Describe the histology of epithelial tissue;
5. Discuss the histology of connective tissue;
6. Describe the histology of muscle and nervous tissue.

Introduction

Human histology provides a basis for studying the intricate structure and function of human tissues and organs. By learning about microscopic tissue structure, students are exposed to cellular organization that enables them to study how these structures are involved in biological processes and mechanisms of disease. Histology integrates various scientific disciplines like biology and pathology, where the prominence of cellular and tissue properties in disease and health is given high priority. A good understanding of histology is essential for most fields of medicine since it bridges the gap between basic biology science and the complex disease presentation. This integration is shown in comprehensive materials that use full-color images and diagrams to document the finer aspects of human tissues so that it becomes conceivable for both novice students and seasoned experts (Kierszenbaum & Tres, 2021). Merging both traditional and contemporary pedagogical techniques, histology is strongly supplemented with the employment of modern teaching resources that have interactive components. Such resources not only present basic principles but also highlight clinical scenarios illustrating the relevance of histological studies in real-world medical cases. Moreover, resources can utilize adaptive learning technologies such as concept map animations and Clinical Conditions boxes that are significant to reinforce key concepts and enable learners to acquire complex concepts effectively. This pedagogical approach facilitates the better understanding of how histology is engaged with disorders, for instance, cancer and inherited diseases, thereby enriching students' competence in diagnostic and treatment situations. Generally, such learning materials not only progress learning but also arm learners with the practical knowledge of histology in clinical settings (Kierszenbaum & Tres, 2021).

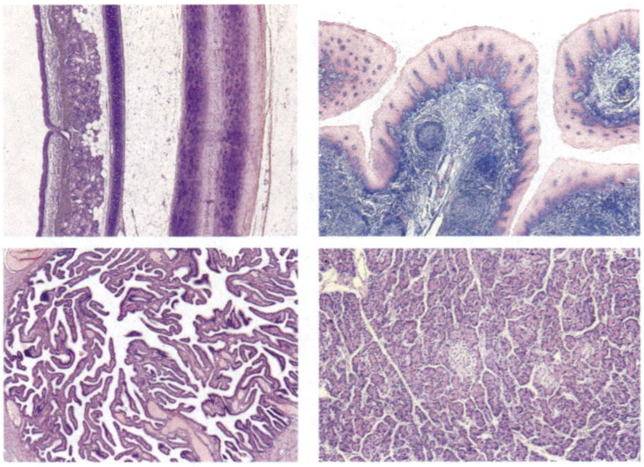

Figure 1.1. Human histology.

Source: https://www.flinnsci.com/globalassets/flinn-scientific/all-product-images-rgb-jpegs/ml1461.jpg.

Furthermore, recent advances in the histology science have contributed to the implementation of new study findings that are seminal for transforming clinical practices. For instance, research into cancer immunotherapy, angiogenesis, and mitochondrial therapies illustrates the dynamic nature of histological research and its resulting implications for therapy. Secondly, the significance of newer topics such as ciliogenesis and chromatin structure, which have impacts on numerous medical ailments, highlights why an updated approach to histology is necessary for medical professionals. By integrating this up-to-date information with foundational knowledge, learning material not only equips students with the proficiencies to interpret the subtleties of human tissue pathology but also allows for an ongoing pursuit of information required for prospective clinical advances in medicine (Kierszenbaum & Tres, 2021) (Figure 1.1).

Definition and Importance of Histology

Histology, the microscopic study of tissue structure and function, is an elementary foundation in human biology research. By studying cellular content and organizational patterns of tissues, histology provides crucial data regarding how individual cells cooperate as part of larger systems. Histology is the science that entails the study of tissues that are procured from a broad variety of organs, enabling researchers and clinicians to recognize normal anatomical patterns versus pathological alterations. These variations are vital for the detection of diseases, examination of their development, and the formulation of targeted therapy. The relevance of histology is demonstrated by its application in so many areas of study, including oncology, pathology, and regenerative medicine, rendering it even more a pillar of modern medical science. The developments in histological techniques have greatly enhanced the accuracy and efficiency of tissue analysis. Early techniques, such as fiber dissection, laid the basis for contemporary methods to allow scientists to study the sensitive layering of tissues more specifically. As implied, the history of fiber dissection depicts the evolution of histological methods over the years, particularly in neurosurgery and other specialized fields. The systematic descriptions of structures like white matter tracts illustrate how histological findings are significant in guiding surgical procedures, thus improving patient outcomes. Through its shift from descriptive to analytical in tissue observation, histology has enabled a more scientific approach to human health and disease patterns, thus its essential role in research and clinical practice (Gulsuna et al., 2025). Moreover, histology findings have profound significance in the understanding of disease processes and therapeutic intervention. By examining interactions of cellular function and form, histology unravels the pathological processes that lead to illnesses from cancer to neurodegenerative disorders. Histological examination, for instance, can reveal cellular abnormalities that indicate cancer, information which is crucial for treatment protocols. Furthermore, histology concepts extend beyond identification and encompass interactions between tissues and their role in organ systems. This dependence is of utmost significance, such as with studies on multiform complexes like the human brain, wherein the knowledge of white matter tracts composition and configuration can shed light on novel targets for intervention (Zen et al., 2024). Lastly, the definition and relevance of histology are inherently linked to its ability to provide a refined comprehension of human health (Figure 1.2).

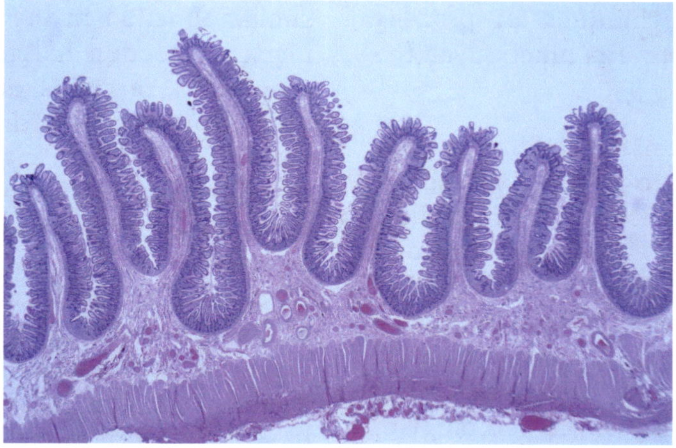

Figure 1.2. Histology.

Source: https://www.thoughtco.com/thmb/38NMxOJRhq_R3DxI8cbxF5RMd4s=/1500x0/filters:no_upscale():max_bytes(150000):strip_icc()/intestinal-lining-680800269-59a95067054ad90010f82d98.jpg.

Historical Development of Histological Techniques

The historical evolution of histological methods has been marked by spectacular developments that have worked to build on the exploration of human tissues. Initially, during the early stages of histology, samples were processed by fairly crude techniques that were not accurate or standardized. But as the field progressed during the 19th century, developments such as the invention of paraffin embedding and formaldehyde fixation were achieved. These techniques improved tissue preservation and allowed for thinner sections so that scientists could study tissues at levels of resolution never before possible. The advent of staining techniques also played a significant role in the study of cellular components, and histology became a less descriptive and more analytical science. When researchers turned to investigate complex disease, these early methods became crucial both for research application and clinical diagnosis, setting the pattern for modern histological practice.

Throughout the 20th century, histology was revolutionized technologically by the advent of electron microscopy, enabling much higher resolution in the investigation of cellular ultrastructure. This advance allowed histologists to see fine structures such as organelles and cell membranes, adding to our knowledge of normal cell architecture and disease processes. In combination with immunohistochemical techniques, which allow for the localization and visualization of specific proteins in tissue sections, researchers were able to now investigate the molecular processes of a variety of diseases. The application of molecular biology techniques to histology further expanded the discipline, providing techniques for probing gene expression and protein function at the tissue level.

Histology therefore transitioned from mere structural observation to a valuable tool in disease mechanism and action understanding, significantly influencing medical practice and research. Apart from this, emerging trends in histological research emphasize the importance of having recourse to animal models to learn more about human disease. The approach has illuminated the complexity of the pathology of disease as illustrated by studies on naturally occurring disease in animal models. For instance, research on temporomandibular joint (TMJ) ankylosis in domestic cats, showing significant intra- and extra-articular changes through histological assessment, illuminates the similar condition in humans (Arzi et al., 2020). Similarly, diabetes research in dogs offers a model of translation in the development of new treatments in human medicine, particularly utilizing methods like pancreatic islet transplantation (Adin & Gilor, 2017). These advances illustrate the dynamic interplay between histological methods and evolving biomedical research, shifting testimony to the continued utility and adaptability of histological techniques in addressing contemporary health concerns.

1.1. The Four Basic Tissue Types

Learning Outcome

1. Describe the structure and function of epithelial tissue;
2. Describe the types and characteristics of connective tissue;
3. Understand the roles of muscle and nervous tissue in the body.

Human histology verifies that the four major tissue types—epithelial, connective, muscle, and nervous tissues—each has its own specific yet similar function in the body. Epithelial tissue forms protection barriers and is involved in absorption, secretion, and sensory perception. This tissue occurs with cells that are densely packed with little extracellular matrix and therefore facilitates rapid communication and turnover. It is necessary for the integrity of structures and organs and serves as a lining for external and internal surfaces. Specialization of epithelial cells into forms like squamous, cuboidal, and columnar is related to their specific functions, allowing for multiple roles in various organ systems. Understanding the nature and function of epithelial tissue provides a foundation to understand how it interacts with the other tissue types to achieve complete homeostasis. Connective tissue, the second of the basic tissue types, binds together, supports, and protects other tissues and organs throughout the body. Compared with epithelial tissue, connective tissue contains a higher proportion of extracellular matrix, which is responsible for its extensive range of functions. This tissue is made up of fibers such as collagen and elastin, and ground substances with viscosity that ranges from liquid (such as in blood) to rigid (such as in bone). Connective tissue also acts as a reservoir for energy storage and immune defense. The sophistication of connective tissue is also brought out by the fact that it appears in various types, including loose connective tissue, dense connective tissue, cartilage, and adipose tissue. Understanding of the organization and complex functions of the connective tissue illuminates how these tissues not only provide mechanical support but also play a role in physiological processes such as inflammation and tissue repair, thus highlighting their importance in human histology. Muscle tissue, which belongs to skeletal, cardiac, and smooth muscle, constitutes the body's locomotor and involuntary systems. Skeletal muscle, as voluntary, facilitates movement through attachment to bones, striated and multinucleated. Cardiac muscle, on the other hand, is involuntary and found only in the heart, facilitating the movement of blood through rhythmic contractions.

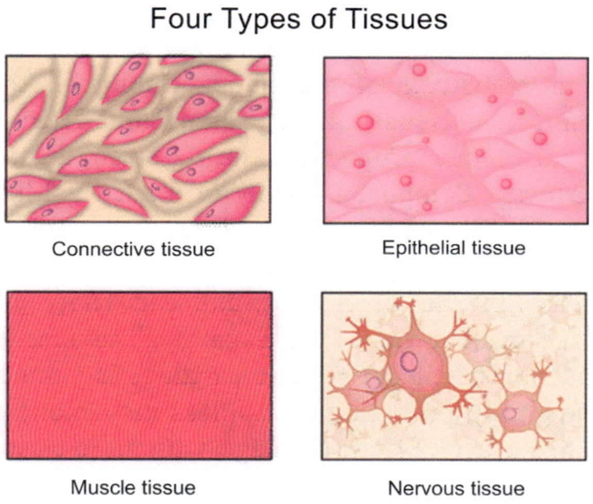

Figure 1.3. Four types of tissues.

Source: https://dr282zn36sxxg.cloudfront.net/datastreams/f-d%3A2d8ce980735ced00cf17c661eea81cbc3ab7e5054a8b27972a21ffd8%2BIMAGE_THUMB_POSTCARD_TINY%2BIMAGE_THUMB_POSTCARD_TINY.1.

Involuntary smooth muscle covers hollow organs, aiding functions such as digestion and control of blood vessels. This difference in types of muscle tissues illustrates that specialized architecture is required for specific functions, reinforcing the general physiology of the human body. The inherent properties of muscle tissues—excitability and contractility—also enable sensitive body movement and responses, showing the sophistication of human histology as it encompasses normality and sickness, particularly in scenarios where muscle function is compromised (Figure 1.3).

1.1.1. Epithelial Tissue: Structure and Function

Epithelial tissue is characterized by its specialized structure and wide variety of important functions in the human body, acting as a first line of defense and being vital to absorption, secretion, and sensation. Composed of tightly packed cells with minimal extracellular matrix, epithelial tissue is divided into several types based on cell shape and layer arrangement. Simple epithelium, which has a single layer of cells, enables absorption and filtration, whereas stratified epithelium that is formed of several layers offers wear and tear protection. The polar nature of epithelial cells, with the distinctive basal and apical surface, enables specialized functions such as selective permeability and effective transport mechanisms. Such organization is at the core of overall epithelial tissue function in all organs, highlighting the importance of their architectural organization towards maintaining bodily homeostasis. In terms of function, epithelial tissues are continuously involved in a range of physiological processes like defense of the body against external assault, secretion of vital substances, and reception of sensory stimulation. The epithelial barrier exists as a selective interface between the internal and external environment, allowing controlled material exchange. For instance, the epithelial lining of the respiratory tract traps harmful particles and pathogens while facilitating gas exchange, and the gut epithelium in the absorption of nutrients and elimination of waste. Epithelial cells also possess specialized structures such as microvilli and cilia that enhance their functional efficiency.

These adaptations enable the epithelium to dynamically adapt to physiological need and environmental stress, and thus play a role in overall health and disease process, such as inflammation and infection. More recent work has also helped elucidate the role of epithelial tissue in pathophysiological processes, commenting on its involvement in disease such as eosinophilic esophagitis (EoE). In the chronic inflammatory condition of the illness, growth factor signaling disturbances disrupt the epithelial barrier, including transforming growth factor-beta 1 (TGFβ1) signaling which is involved in tissue remodeling and affecting cellular function. Research indicates that the level of gene expression of genes involved in epithelial function and integrity in the esophagus will be influenced by differences in genotypes, including increased susceptibility to injury and dysphagia. In addition to this, understanding patterns of therapeutic drug distribution, such as antibiotics, in diseased or infected epithelial tissues is equally crucial to formulate the best treatment strategies. This also underlines the intricacy of the epithelial tissue in maintaining health and developing disease, also reinforcing its status as a research topic in human histology and pathology (Blanc et al., 2018; Duong et al., 2020) (Figure 1.4).

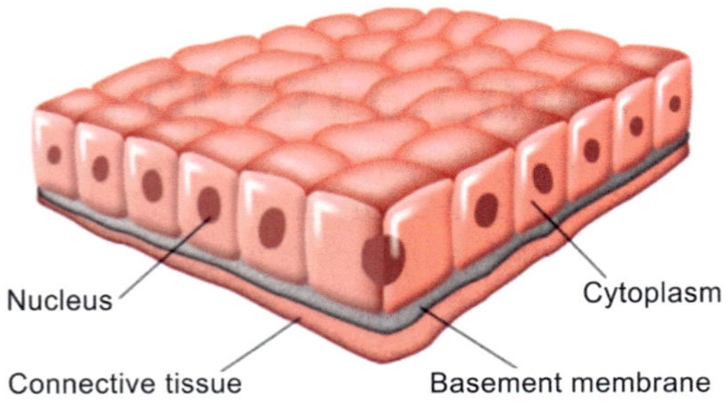

Figure 1.4. Epithelial tissue.

Source: https://www.careerpower.in/blog/wp-content/uploads/sites/2/2024/02/07164915/epithelial-tissues-1.png.

1.1.2. Connective Tissue: Types and Characteristics

Connective tissue has a vital role in the structural build of the human body, which is composed of varying forms that all have special purposes. Broadly categorized, connective tissues are made up of loose connective tissue, dense connective tissue, cartilage, bone, and blood. Loose connective tissue, for instance, serves as a protective layer to hold structures and organs, allowing flexibility and movement. On the other hand, dense connective tissue that is made of tightly packed collagen fibers is tougher and stronger and is therefore found in tendons and ligaments. The variability in composition between connective tissues is a reflection of their range of functions, from storage and support through transport and injury response and thus playing a vital function in the process of homeostasis of the body. Among all the connective tissues, cartilage stands out because of its unique properties like its strength and elasticity. Composed mainly of a hard gel-like matrix with chondrocytes lodged in it, cartilage provides rigidity while allowing flexibility in areas like the joints, ribs, and ear. There are three main forms of cartilage: hyaline, elastic, and fibrocartilage. Hyaline cartilage is smooth and glassy, providing frictionless movement at joint surfaces. Elastic cartilage, with more elastic fibers, is found where there is a requirement for elasticity, such as in the epiglottis. Fibrocartilage with dense collagenous fiber bundles is very resistant to tension and is thus essential for intervertebral discs and the pubic symphysis. Such diversity serves the special functions of cartilage in the musculoskeletal system. Recent studies underscore the prominent position of stem cells in connective tissue, including mesenchymal stem cells (MSCs), which hold immense therapeutic potential. These multipotent cells reside within numerous compartments of connective tissue and play a pivotal function in tissue restoration and regeneration since they can differentiate into numerous cell types, including chondrocytes and osteoblasts. As highlighted by studies, MSCs can remodel their microenvironment through the secretion of soluble factors, hence play an active role in the healing of a large number of tissues (Grange, 2011). The results of research into cell properties on a molecular basis reveal not just the complexity of connective tissue but also that it can regenerate, which can potentially transform the manner in which injury and degenerative disease are currently treated within clinical practice. Also, understanding the diverse functions and roles of these cells in connective tissue, including the ability for multipotency, reinforces their significance within today's medical research and treatment (Degistirici et al., 2008) (Figure 1.5).

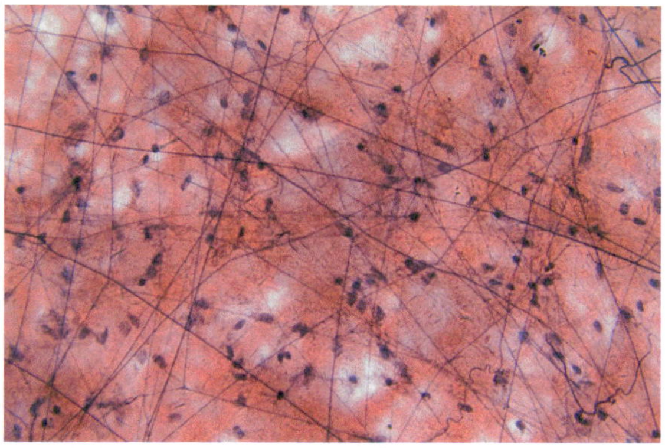

Figure 1.5. Connective tissue.

Source: https://www.verywellhealth.com/thmb/puYZV6qnIq9bcMrYumTTFUdUxdg=/1500x0/filters:no_upscale():max_bytes(150000):strip_icc()/GettyImages-182436049-590a656c239643b5a4957bb2ea67ab01.jpg.

1.1.3. Muscle and Nervous Tissue: Roles in the Body

Muscle and nervous tissues are a part and parcel of the human body and possess distinctive yet parallel functions pivotal to physiological function. Muscle tissue, of three principal forms—skeletal, cardiac, and smooth—allows movement and posture by contracting. Skeletal muscle, under voluntary control, allows precise, intentional movement, while cardiac muscle, which occurs solely in the heart, operates involuntarily to pump blood through the circulatory system. Smooth muscle, also involuntary, blankets hollow organs and vessels, regulating such functions as digestion and the circulation of blood. The unique structures and roles of such muscle types illustrate how muscle tissue has adapted to meet the diverse demands of body functions, illustrating its functionally essential role in homeostasis and overall health. At the same time, nervous tissue is essential for the body's communication and coordination functions. Composed of neurons and neuroglia, the nervous system transmits impulses and processes information to permit speeded responses to internal and external stimuli.

Neurons, specialized cells, are employed to transmit electrical impulses, while neuroglia nourish, maintain, and shield neurons. This orderly system is the foundation of all body function, from reflexes to mentation. The relationship between muscle and nervous tissues is most apparent in voluntary motion, where the nervous tissue initiates muscle contraction by employing motor signals. Hence, nervous tissue coordinates movement as well as regulates muscle response in the right way so that coordination and timing of activities of daily living are aided. Additionally, the muscle and nervous tissue relationship holds importance for the understanding of many physiological and pathological conditions. For example, the efficacy of muscle contraction can be measured by nervous system functioning and health, such as in neuromuscular disease where transmission of signals is disrupted. Additionally, the ability of muscle tissue to regenerate, particularly after trauma, might be affected by adjacent nervous tissue, which can enhance or hinder restoration Study of connective tissue interactions with muscle, such as fibrosis analysis and chronic pain mechanisms, emphasizes the importance of these interactions in both health and disease processes. Investigation into the roles of muscle and nervous tissue within the context of larger human histology enables scientists to better understand how these tissues contribute to the intricate symphony of body function (Figure 1.6).

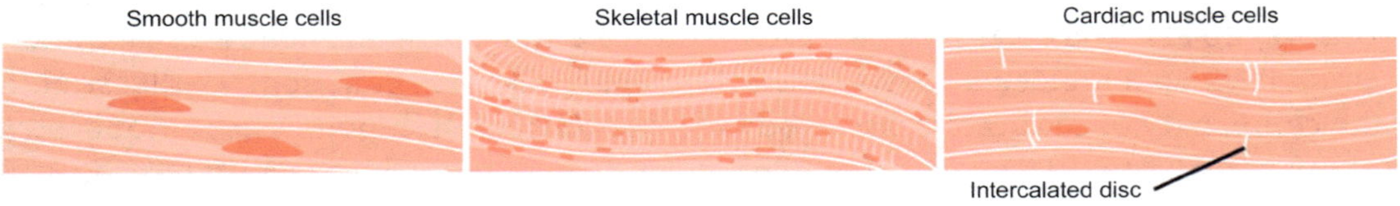

Figure 1.6. Smooth muscle cells do not have striations, while skeletal muscle cells do. Cardiac muscle cells have striations, but, unlike the multinucleate skeletal cells, they have only one nucleus. Cardiac muscle tissue also has intercalated discs, specialized regions running along the plasma membrane that join adjacent cardiac muscle cells and assist in passing an electrical impulse from cell to cell.

Source: https://s3-us-west-2.amazonaws.com/courses-images/wp-content/uploads/sites/1223/2017/01/31000817/Figure_33_02_12abc-1024x149.jpg.

Test Your Knowledge

1. What is the structure of epithelial tissue?
2. What is the nervous tissue role in the body?

1.2. Histological Techniques and Staining Methods

Learning Outcome

1. Learn about purpose and common agents of fixation;
2. Describe the techniques and equipment used for sectioning;
3. Understand the types of stains and their applications of staining.

Histological methods provide the platform for the investigation of human histology that enables the detailed examination of tissue structures at the microscopic level. These techniques commonly involve fixation of tissue samples to preserve their morphology and prevent degradation, and embedding them in solid material, such as paraffin. Tissue is cut into thin slices following the embedding of tissue, allowing observation of fine structures within cells and extracellular space. Staining methods are critical in highlighting specific portions of these sections, improving contrast and hence making observations possible under a microscope. By applying various staining protocols, such as H&E staining or immunohistochemistry, researchers can differentiate between various types of tissue and identify the presence of proteins or other biomolecules that are crucial in the analysis of both normal function and disease. The staining protocol used directly impacts the interpretation of histological samples and dictates what can be learned from the analysis. Techniques such as Alcian blue and Safranin-O are employed specifically to delineate cartilage in histology research since they possess a unique preference for binding with glycosaminoglycans present in the extracellular matrix. Such methods have been successfully utilized under conditions such as estimating postmortem interval in forensic science, where precise determination of tissue integrity can provide critical forensic information. Similarly, Masson's trichrome stain is employed to separate connective tissue from muscle fibers with a presentation of structural intricacies important in tissue pathology. The visual scoring method widely used in the assessment of staining results contains inherent biases; thus, the inclusion of semi-automatic image analysis in histological assessment is an area that is eager to enhance objectivity and reproducibility in data interpretation, as recent research comparing visual scoring with semi-automatic assessments in cartilage studies (Alibegović et al., 2024) has found.

Appreciation of the role of histological procedures and staining methodologies becomes particularly relevant when set against the background of surgical and pathologic uses. Recent evidence points towards the importance of the serosal layer in healing after anastomosis following colorectal operations, where it is implied that thorough histological examination of the layer can shed light on mechanisms of healing and guide therapeutic interventions to minimize complications such as leakage. These investigations tend to employ advanced histologic preparation and staining methodologies to visualize cellular response during repair activities in the tissue. Histological examination not only identifies structural changes but also cell movement, such as the involvement of mesothelial cells in scarring through epithelial-to-mesenchymal transition, which is relevant for healing efficacy as well as integrity (Weber et al., 2024). Accordingly, the integration of histological methods with targeted staining protocols generates a comprehensive understanding of both normal physiology and the pathological rationale which directs clinical procedures in human histology (Figure 1.7).

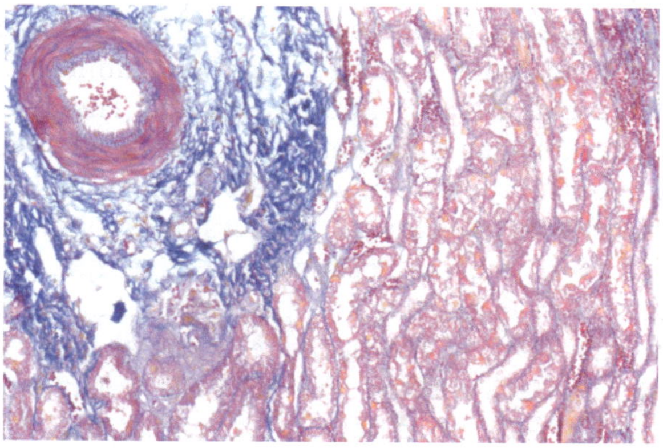

Figure 1.7. Mallory Trichrome kit.

Source: https://www.solmedialtd.com/wp-content/uploads/2021/04/Mallory-Trichrome-kit-staining-1024x683-2.jpg.

1.2.1. Fixation: Purpose and Common Agents

In human histology, fixation is a fundamental process critical to the proper preservation of tissue samples. The primary role of fixation is to halt cellular metabolism and suppress the degradation of tissue architecture, thereby preserving the structure integrity of the specimens for further analysis. Effective fixation allows pathologists to study tissues in a state that closely approximates there *in vivo* condition, which is important for precise diagnosis. Choice of fixative has a considerable impact on histological result, and this emphasizes the need to select cautiously in relation to the specific requirements of the tissue at hand. Fixation needs to be understood because it is the basis of modern histological practice, pointing the way towards enhancing imaging and diagnostic methods in medicine. Some of the most used fixatives are formaldehyde, glutaraldehyde, and alcoholic solution fixatives derived from a variety of alcohols, each of which possesses characteristics specific for fixing specific tissues and obtaining specific outcomes. Formaldehyde is the most general fixative due to its speed of penetration and retention of protein structure with cell morphology. Glutardaldehyde possesses superior electron microscope characteristics and is of great value in ultra-structure examination where detail is of prime importance. The level of fixation agents, the time of exposure, and the temperature level can all affect the histological integrity of specimens. Understanding these factors is crucial because defective fixation can result in artifacts or misrepresentation of the histology of the tissue, eventually making diagnosis less effective. Furthermore, taking into account the time factor of fixation emphasizes its importance in achieving optimum tissue preservation. As would be anticipated, the integrity of the recovered sample is often in turn reliant upon the immediate processing after excision from the patient. Delayed fixation can create cellular changes that make identification of the true pathological condition of the tissue more difficult, and it emphasizes the need for immediate handling and rapid fixation techniques within histological analysis. The specific methods applied in daily practice are varied, but all underscore the significance of fixation in histopathology. With effective application of fixation techniques, physicians and researchers enhance the quality of histopathological examination, consequently leading to improved patient outcomes and the overall advancement of medical science in disease diagnosis (Cicerone & Camp, 2017; Hilario & Alonso-Alconada, 2022).

1.2.2. Sectioning: Techniques and Equipment Used

Sectioning is a very important process in the science of human histology because it makes studying samples of tissue possible at microscopic levels. With precise cutting techniques, scientists prepare microtomes to cut thin sections, typically only a few micrometers thick. Such sections are required for finer microscopic observation. During sectioning, the tissue is generally infiltrated by paraffin wax or embedded into a cryoprotectant, which gives the structural support when the samples are being sectioned. Microtome, either rotary or sliding, is employed to provide greater control over thickness to ensure uniformity in sections. This careful preparation permits appropriate diagnosis and medical research developments, playing a significant role in our existing knowledge of various pathological conditions. As noted, optical coherence microscopy is a new frontier, expanding imaging of larger tissues past the limitations of standard slide-based methods (Min et al., 2020). There is a need for new sectioning procedures due to the limitation of standard histological methods. Standard thin-section histology often cannot record dynamic three-dimensional interactions that are found in biological tissue and are necessary to infer regarding tissue physiology (Hsueh et al., 2017). Consequently, scientists have developed advanced techniques with the ability to perform high-throughput analysis without sacrificing resolution. For example, new hydrogel-based approaches have been suggested, which preserve even the most brittle tissues' structural integrity but allow serial sectioning. This enables detailed volumetric analysis and allows studying complex tissue architectures, such as the highly ramified innervation patterns in pancreatic tissue. The developments are particularly applicable to clinical contexts, where evaluation of diseased state demands an awareness of tissue structural intricacies. Combining these new techniques, histology is converging toward improved approximation of biological substrates. As part of continued initiatives toward enhanced histological techniques, integration of automatic imaging technology is revolutionizing sectioning processes. Such systems not only allow for the precision of section cutting but also the high-throughput imaging of multiple sections in hours rather than days or weeks conventionally. Image stitching and alignment computer programs that assist in the stitching together of serial sections can recreate detailed three-dimensional structures of tissues, offering information not revealed through the sole use of pure two-dimensional sections. These technologies have been extremely useful in the domain of pathology, where minute morphological changes that are typical of disease can be detected. The convergence of these automated platforms with the principles of histology can potentially give rise to a future where examination of intricate tissue samples becomes more effective and sensitive, and therefore influences research as well as clinical diagnostics (Hsueh et al., 2017; Min et al., 2020) (Figure 1.8).

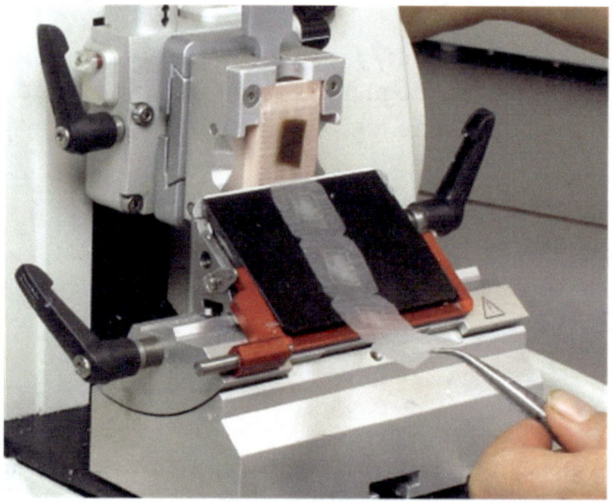

Figure 1.8. Microtomes.

Source: https://www.laboratorydeal.com/cdn/shop/articles/Microtomes_and_Staining_Manufacturer_Supplier_ff9673f8-e07e-4bc1-82d8-247cd6444b5f_1024x1024.jpg?v=1745496479.

1.2.3. Staining: Types of Stains and Their Applications

Staining is a simple human histology method that enables scientists and pathologists to visualize and differentiate between cellular and tissue structures accurately. Of the different types of staining methods, Hematoxylin and Eosin (H&E) is the most widely used due to its simplicity of application and effectiveness. H&E staining is essential for the procurement of information about tissue structure, with nuclei stained in a blue color and the cytoplasm stained pink. Contrast increases the examination of histopathological features and is important for initial diagnostic evaluations.

The disadvantages of H&E, such as low contrast and difficulties with quantitative evaluation, have yielded to improvements in staining techniques, and therefore immunohistochemistry (IHC) has emerged. The transition away from traditional techniques to newer imaging techniques is a great advancement in histopathological technique, one of a general movement toward greater accuracy of diagnosis and prediction of disease. IHC is a useful addition to standard staining techniques, and particularly to cancer diagnosis where the accurate identification of protein is most crucial.

By employing target protein-specific antibodies, IHC provides greater contrast and specificity to distinguish cellular components that are unobservable using routine H&E staining. It is a great aid in biomarker discovery that can indicate tumor behavior and type. Greater processing complexity of IHC and expenses, however, will limit its widespread application. Efforts to transcend such limitations include newer methodologies such as the conditional CycleGAN (cCGAN) model, which allows virtual IHC conversion of H&E stained images to IHC descriptions. The innovation not only makes staining easier but also leaves space for greater diagnostic accuracy in different histological environments, hence transgressing the disparities between traditional and newer staining techniques. The ongoing modernization of histopathology, with a focus on pairing quantitative methodologies, represents the dawn of a new age for tissue analysis. Tools such as Coherent Raman Imaging (CRI) allow label-free imaging, expanding the scope of histopathology. Through high-resolution, molecule-specific contrast, CRI makes the qualitative-to-quantitative transition critical for the precise characterization of disease. These innovations are most critical to bridging the gap between traditional staining techniques and facilitating robust digital image analysis and quantitative measurement of tissue components. With evolving technology, the use of various staining techniques in combination, such as the proposed cCGAN transformation and CRI, is likely to enhance diagnosis. This development mirrors a wider dedication in histopathology to adopting technological innovation, which supports enhanced patient care, paving the way for future advancements in human histology and its clinical application (Figure 1.9).

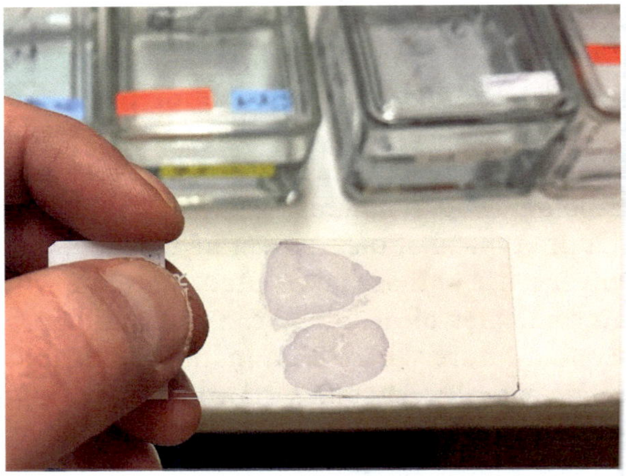

Figure 1.9. A stained histological specimen, sandwiched between a glass microscope slide.

Source: https://upload.wikimedia.org/wikipedia/commons/4/47/Stained_microscope_slide.jpg.

Test Your Knowledge

1. What is the purpose of fixation?
2. List the types of stain.

1.3. Microscopy in Histology

Learning Outcome

1. Understand the principles and limitations of light microscopy;
2. Describe the types and advantages of electron microscopy;
3. Describe the techniques and uses for fluorescence microscopy.

Microscopy is a fundamental tool employed in histology to facilitate the thorough examination of tissue structures at microscopic level. The expansion of microscopy techniques has revolutionized the ability to see cellular and extracellular elements that define various tissues structure and function. Traditional light microscopy has been the cornerstone of histological investigation; however, it is generally inadequate when dealing with three-dimensional tissue architectures. Such architectures may have complex interplays that are poorly documented by standard thin sections, leaving limited tissue physiology and pathology insights. Advances in recent times, such as computer-aided analysis programs and biphasic hydrogel methods, provide superior techniques for examining irregular and weak tissue samples, thus unlocking their dynamics inaccessible with the conventional approach. This development indicates the direction toward extensive imaging technology in histology for facilitating advances in research, as well as clinical diagnostics (Hsueh et al., 2017). The shift from the conventional single-plane imaging to advanced volumetric analysis opened up new horizons in the study of human tissues.

High-throughput technologies allow accurate assessment of both healthy and diseased tissues by opening up the potential of intact-tissue imaging modalities.

Research into pancreatic innervation and development, for instance, has been made easier through these technologies to yield a more full understanding of previously unrecognized pathologies. These advances highlight the necessity to reframe traditional histological practice, challenging a new paradigm to embrace the heterogeneity of tissue architecture. This approach integrates the beneficial elements of microscopy with numerical volumetric interrogation and has the potential to manage the issues posed by heterogeneity in clinical samples and biopsies efficiently. Improved imaging capabilities therefore provide valuable information for basic scientific research as well as practical clinical utility (Hsueh et al., 2017). Furthermore, the integration of advanced imaging techniques with magnetic resonance imaging (MRI) indicates the heightened collaboration between modalities in histological investigations. The g-ratio, an extremely crucial parameter measuring the thinness of the myelin sheaths enveloping axons, can benefit immensely from such advances because *in vivo* mapping becomes increasingly feasible. Advances in sensitive techniques to map the g-ratio can significantly improve our understanding of the functional dynamics of the central nervous system, as well as pathophysiological changes of various diseases. Though encouraging developments are being realized, efforts to strive towards accurate measurement, particularly concerning calibration and correlation between MRI-based markers and actual myelin volume, are ongoing. As noted in recent critiques, the attainment of accurate g-ratio mapping rests on high-quality *ex vivo* histological measurements to obtain a gold standard, an important milestone in histological imaging evolution (Figure 1.10).

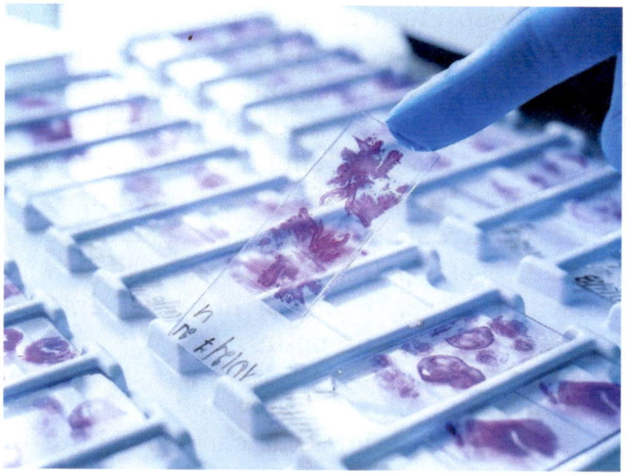

Figure 1.10. Microscopy used in histology.

Source: https://d36nqgmw98q4v5.cloudfront.net/image-handler/ts/20220323045527/ri/950/src/images/Article_Images/ImageForArticle_2183_16480257271579919.jpg.

1.3.1. Light Microscopy: Principles and Limitations

The science of light microscopy is a focal area in human histology practice, providing the opportunity to view cellular tissues and structures with maximum precision. Light microscopy takes advantage of visible light for magnification of specimens and allows scientists to pick out very small details of biological significance that play a crucial role in understanding human tissue intricacies. Focal concepts include the use of lenses to focus light, which generates magnification and specimen resolution. However, while light microscopy has revolutionized histological sample viewing and investigation, there are limitations to it. The resolution of the image that is created tends to grow progressively weaker at higher magnifications due to diffraction limits, which set a maximum on how much resolution one can obtain with standard optical configurations. This property sets a problem in attempting to see below the wavelength of visible light, with only so much detailed cellular structure being able to be examined. Recently, some of these limitations of traditional light microscopy have been overcome by new technologies such as spectral imaging and optical coherence tomography (OCT). Spectral imaging, for instance, introduces additional capabilities to analyze several parameters at the cellular and molecular levels owing to improvements in labeling reagents and optics.

This approach enables the acquisition of useful information that can contribute to both fundamental scientific knowledge and to clinical usefulness, to the credit of the inclusion of innovative imaging techniques within histological research (Levenson et al., 2012). In comparison, OCT is a groundbreaking technique of high-speed volumetric imaging, leveraging the combination of bright and dark field imaging to exploit the different scattering properties of light in an effort to acquire new tissue information. This is an aspect that favors a less obtrusive appreciation of human histology, particularly needed in the study of complex diseases such as cancer and neurodegenerative diseases (Augustin et al., 2018). Even as imaging techniques are being improved upon, the use of light microscopy has limitations within the system. An example of this limitation is the requirement for staining or labeling procedures to enhance contrast, introducing artefacts and altering the original tissue morphology. Also, while methods like spectral imaging may be capable of generating rich data, these often need sophisticated equipment, hence the technologies are not easily available for routine histological practice. Further, as researchers aim to attain higher resolution for imaging, there is a need for constant innovation, not only to improve the optical systems but also to further develop the sample preparation methods. This intricate interplay between expanding imaging capability and safeguarding against the inherent limitations is reflective of the ongoing evolution of microscopy in human histology, all aimed at enhancing our appreciation of biological complexity and disease mechanisms (Figure 1.11).

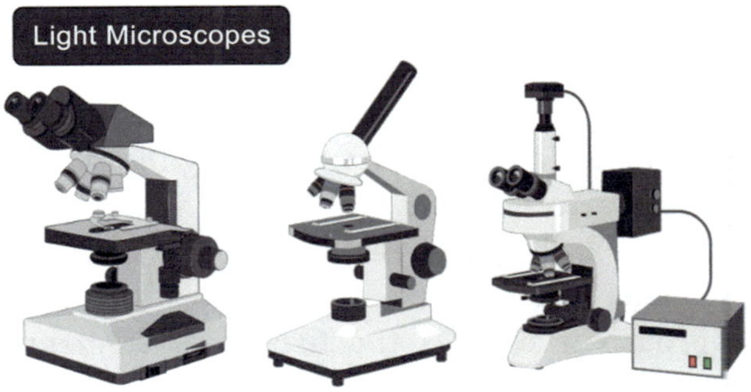

Figure 1.11. Diagram of light microscopes.

Source: https://microbenotes.com/wp-content/uploads/2020/02/Light-Microscope-diagram.jpeg.

1.3.2. Electron Microscopy (EM): Types and Advantages

EM has revolutionarily impacted biological imaging, particularly in human histology. This powerful imaging technology makes it possible to visualize structures within cells with a level of resolution not possible by traditional light microscopy, much greater in fact. Both of the main types of electron microscopy—transmission electron microscopy (TEM) and scanning electron microscopy (SEM)—are employed for differing but complementary purposes in research.

TEM delivers high-resolution sectional images of cells that reveal fine details of organelles and enable scientists to study cellular morphology and internal structure. In contrast, SEM provides three-dimensional images of surfaces, allowing detailed tissue architecture to be studied. The ability to resolve such fine detail is central to the understanding of normal cell function and the identification of abnormalities present with many diseases. The advantages of electron microscopy extend beyond resolution; they substantially enhance the quality and depth of histological analysis. For instance, the precise, high-resolution images provided by EM facilitate segmentation of structures like axons and myelin sheaths, crucial to the study of neurobiology. As already noted, AxonDeepSeg—a deep learning algorithm—exhibits high precision in segmenting axonal and myelin features from EM images with pixel-wise accuracies of 85% for rat SEM and 95% for mice TEM (Zaimi et al., 2017). This level of precision allows the determination of critical parameters such as axon density and myelin thickness that are crucial for the interpretation of the microstructure of the nervous system.

Thus, electron microscopy not only guarantees improved visualization but also provides quantitative techniques for in-depth tissue analysis. Additionally, advances in electron microscopy techniques have provided a door open to quantitative input towards the information on myelination and neuronal function. One of such developments includes the g-ratio mapping, which is most important in ascertaining the integrity of myelin sheaths around axons. This geometric invariant is of profound importance because it relates to the conduction velocity of neurons, a most important element in neural communication. The ongoing adoption of new methods has mounted the potential of *in vivo* g-ratio mapping by MRI, at the same time highlighting the necessity of gold standard measurements from histological methods, e.g., those from EM (Mohammadi & Callaghan, 2021). The integration of these new imaging technologies with modern computational techniques can enhance our knowledge of human histology, showing how disease mechanisms may be connected with structural changes of the nervous system (Figure 1.12).

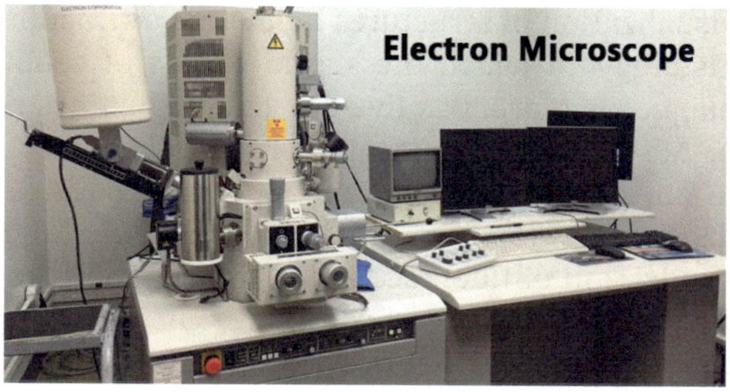

Figure 1.12. Electron microscope (EM).

Source: https://microbenotes.com/wp-content/uploads/2018/10/Electron-Microscope.jpg.

1.3.3. Fluorescence Microscopy: Techniques and Uses

Fluorescence microscopy is now an essential tool of human histology where research can view cell structure and function with unprecedented sensitivity and specificity. The technique employs the use of fluorescent dyes or proteins that bind to specific cellular components, thereby enabling the examination of tissue structure and function in detail. One of the strong points in the fluorescence microscopy is the ability to identify multiple targets simultaneously with the help of spectral multiplexing, making it highly valuable for research work that requires total understanding of cellular interaction. For instance, protein interactions and localization within tissue sections can be viewed with great meaning when it comes to understanding disease mechanism, particularly cancers where signaling mechanisms within the cell are impaired. Therefore, the application of this microscopy technique is practically redefining our vision of histological information at a molecular level. To extend the performance of fluorescence microscopy, various advanced techniques have been developed, e.g., super-resolution microscopy and live-cell imaging. The super-resolution techniques, e.g., stimulated emission depletion (STED) and photoactivated localization microscopy (PALM), enable visualization of structures below the diffraction limit of light. This is particularly relevant in human histology, in which the subtle details of cellular morphology can be diagnostic for research and diagnosis. Moreover, live-cell imaging allows researchers to observe dynamic processes occurring in tissues, offering insight into the behavior of cells with time. Such developments are crucial in unraveling the temporal aspects of pathologies, allowing for a more advanced appreciation of disease development and response to treatment. These technologies together increase the field of application of fluorescence microscopy for the investigation of histological samples. Despite all its advantages, fluorescence microscopy has some drawbacks that should be minimized for maximum efficiency in histology practice. A significant disadvantage is autofluorescence, which can complicate the interpretation of fluorescence signals.

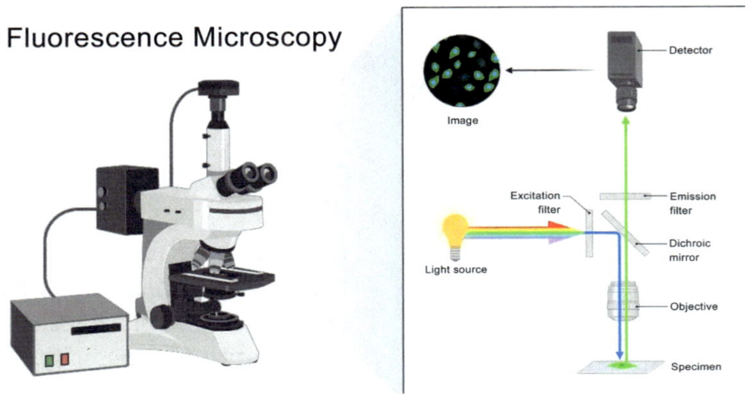

Figure 1.13. Fluorescence microscopy.

Source: https://microbenotes.com/wp-content/uploads/2022/02/Fluorescence-Microscope.webp.

This phenomenon is particularly powerful in tissues with high levels of native fluorophores, such as lipofuscin or chlorophyll, which may give rise to misleading information. Techniques such as spectral unmixing and the use of optimized fluorescent probes are being developed to counteract these limitations. The applicability of innovative methods such as microscopy with ultraviolet surface excitation (MUSE) also offers a promising outlook for the rapid high-resolution imaging without the time-consuming preparation time usually associated with traditional histological techniques. Through integration of these cutting-edge methods, researchers can enhance both precision and performance of histological assessments in the clinic and in studies with subsequent advantages to patients and enhanced scientific understanding (Fereidouni et al., 2017) (Figure 1.13).

Test Your Knowledge

1. What are the principles of light microscopy?
2. What are the types of electron microscopy?

1.4. Histology of Epithelial Tissue

Learning Outcome

1. Understand the classification of epithelial tissue;
2. Describe the functions of epithelial tissue in the body;
3. Understand the pathological changes in epithelial tissue.

Epithelial tissue is crucial to the structure and functioning of most organs of the human body. Comprised of tightly held cells with minimal extracellular matrix, epithelial tissue is protective as well as permitting selective permeability. This type of tissue is subdivided into many subtypes based on cell shape—cuboidal, columnar, or squamous—and layering, and may be simple or stratified. Each subtype is adapted to perform its specific function, e.g., secretion, absorption, and filtration. The simple squamous epithelium, e.g., consisting of a single layer of flattened cells, is efficient for diffusion processes in such locations as lungs and blood vessels. An understanding of the histology of epithelial tissue is important in diagnosing many diseases, as alterations in structure indicate secondary states of disease. Newer technology in imaging methods, such as OCT, has enhanced our ability to analyze epithelial tissue significantly. In this non-invasive method, real-time images of high-resolution tissue layers in cross-section can be observed, allowing detailed observation of structure changes on various resolution levels. In a study involving oral tissues, OCT effectively differentiated major tissue structures such as the keratin cell layer and epithelial layer with high success rates. Such data not only enable discrimination between pathological and normal tissues but also contribute to the development of diagnostic algorithms for the early diagnosis of disorders. These technological improvements in histological assessment emphasize combining improvements in new technology with traditional histological methods to achieve a wider understanding of the pathology of epithelial tissue. Light scattering techniques, including spatial frequency domain imaging (SFDI), have tremendous potential to enhance histological analysis of epithelial tissues. Through the quantification of light scatter parameters, researchers have been able to precisely predict fractions of stromal, epithelial, and adipose tissues within resected tissue samples obtained fresh, with high correlation rates with standard histology. The method enables a quantitative assessment of tissue architecture, critical for malignancy classification and determination of the microenvironment of the tumor. For example, the ratios derived from epithelial-to-stroma measurements have been highly sensitive and specific in differentiating malignant from benign specimens. As these methods like SFDI continue to mature, they will offer useful diagnostics, furthering our understanding of epithelial histology and its utility in detecting and treating disease, further developing the overall field of human histology (Figure 1.14).

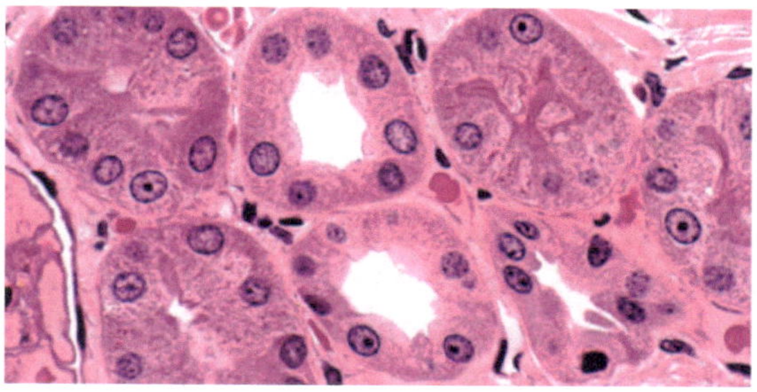

Figure 1.14. Histology of epithelial tissue.

Source: https://usmle-rx.com/wp-content/uploads/bb-plugin/cache/image-16-panorama-6a99f8a902b91066b2d70173c41e3bd6-5fad9ae55b616.png.

1.4.1. Classification of Epithelial Tissue

The classification of epithelial tissue is fundamental to the study of human histology because it acts as a means of differentiating the different shapes and functions of epithelial cells within the body. The epithelial tissues are primarily classified based on the number of cell layers and the shape of the cells within the layers. Single epithelium is made up of one layer of cells, which allows for functions like secretion, absorption, and filtration that are essential in organs such as the kidney and intestines. Stratified epithelium is made up of layers of cells that protect from mechanical stress and chemical exposure, for instance, the epidermal layer of the skin. In addition, transitional epithelium, being capable of stretching and expanding, is especially suited to those organs that experience drastic fluctuation in volume, including the urinary bladder. By this classification, not only are tissue types identified, but also our understanding of their particular function and location in the body is increased. The structural diversity of epithelial tissue is not only classification as layers and shape, but also encompassing specializations which have bearing on the functionality of epithelial cells in general. For instance, glandular epithelium is classified into exocrine and endocrine depending on secretion methods. Exocrine glands secrete their product through ducts into the exterior world, while endocrine glands secrete hormones directly into blood, thus influencing various physiological functions. These functional variations prove the essential function of epithelial tissue in systemic regulation and homeostasis. In addition, the presence of cilia and microvilli on certain epithelial cells is another instance of specialization. Ciliated epithelium is useful for transporting material across surfaces, such as in the respiratory system, while microvillous projections allow for additional surface area for increased absorption within intestines. These specialized characteristics not only facilitate critical functions but also reflect the intricate interdependence of function and structure in epithelial tissue. The investigation of specific instances of epithelial tissue can illuminate the practiced relevance of its categorization in medical practice. In dermatology, for example, the distinction between basal cell carcinoma (BCC) and squamous cell carcinoma (SCC) is largely based on the understanding of epithelial tissue types and their associated characteristics. Patterns and morphological differences seen in histological tests allow clinicians to employ advanced imaging techniques, such as optical coherence tomography, as a diagnostic tool—something advocated by Adabi et al. (2017). Similarly, odontoameloblastoma, a type of odontogenic tumor, is also studied more extensively under histological classification into epithelial tissue, for example, illustrating the relationship between other histological characteristics and clinical diagnosis as outlined in Wong et al. (2018). Therefore, the taxonomy of epithelial tissue is not merely academic but is a foundation in the diagnosis and understanding of an overwhelming majority of diseases and illnesses attacking human health (Figure 1.15).

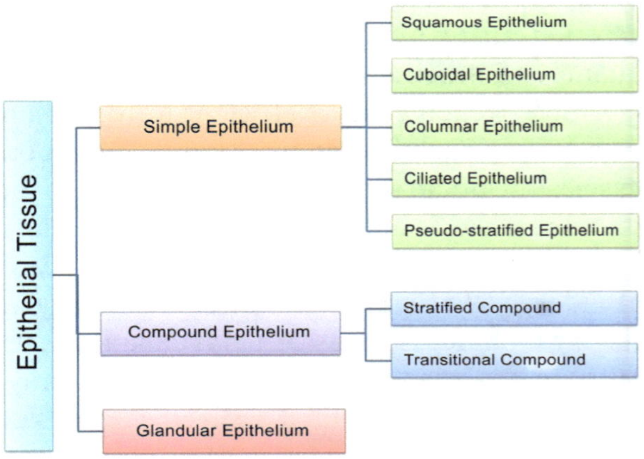

Figure 1.15. Classification of epithelial tissue.

Source: https://easybiologyclass.com/wp-content/uploads/2017/01/different-types-of-epithelial-cells.jpg.

1.4.2. Functions of Epithelial Tissue in the Body

Epithelial tissue functions several key functions in the human body, serving as a protective barrier that separates inner structures from the outside world. This tissue structure is characterized by tightly packed cells, which collectively form continuous sheets that cover surfaces and contain cavities. The primary purpose of epithelial tissue is protection, in the sense that it actually shields underlying tissues from mechanical injury, infection, and water loss. For instance, the outer layer of skin, the epidermis, is composed of stratified epithelial cells that protect against environmental intruders as well as provide sensory sensation. The importance of this protective function is underscored in a number of pathological conditions; every time epithelial integrity is breached, as in the case of chronic wounds or infection, the risk for systemic complications is dramatically increased, threatening general health and homeostasis (Bochsler et al., 2007). A second significant role of epithelial tissue is secretion and absorption, best observed in specialized forms of epithelial cells of the digestive and respiratory tracts. Simple columnar epithelium of intestines, for example, is equipped with microvilli that enhance surface area for nutrient absorption into the bloodstream. Similarly, in the respiratory tract, ciliated epithelial cells facilitate the clearance of waste and pathogens through coordinated cell motions, thus protecting the underlying tissues from infection. Glandular epithelium also consists of secretory cells that secrete various substances such as enzymes, hormones, and mucus for significant physiological functions. This dual role of absorption and secretion highlights the main roles that epithelial tissues perform, not only to absorb nutrients but also to control the body's internal environment (Brinck et al., 1998). Finally, epithelial tissue is widely utilized in the sense, serving as an important interface between the body and the external world. This function is attained by specialized epithelial cells with the ability to sense mechanical, thermal, and chemical stimuli to provide the sensory perception needed for survival. Examples of these include taste buds on the tongue, which consist of epithelial cells, providing gustatory sensations, while the olfactory epithelium in the nasal cavity plays a central part in the sense of smell. Furthermore, the presence of receptors in epithelial tissues enables a rapid response to noxious stimuli, triggering protective reflexes and signaling processes. Consequently, the sensory function of epithelial tissues confirms their intrinsic function in the body's ability to perceive and adapt its environment, balancing vital physiological reactions that ensure organism survival (Brinck et al., 1998; Bochsler et al., 2007) (Figure 1.16).

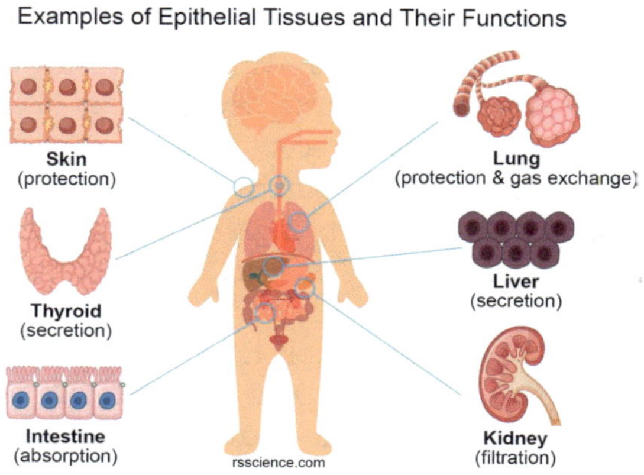

Figure 1.16. Examples of epithelial tissues and their functions.

Source: https://rsscience.com/wp-content/uploads/2022/04/epithelial-tissues-and-their-functions-1536x1056.jpg?ezimgfmt=ng:webp/ngcb1.

1.4.3. Pathological Changes in Epithelial Tissue

Pathological changes within epithelial tissue are a significant area of human histology because such changes can indicate numerous diseases and conditions. Epithelial tissues, being protective barriers and involved in secretion and absorption, are particularly susceptible to pathological changes because they experience a high turnover rate and are exposed to environmental stresses. Hyperplasia, neoplasia, and dysplasia are all normal forms of pathological change that occur in epithelial tissues. Dysplasia is a disorder of cell growth, often leading to or preceding malignant transformation, while hyperplasia is an expansion of cell number due to hormonal stimulation or irritation. Neoplasia, the uncontrolled growth of cells, may result in benign or malignant tumors, highlighting the importance of cautious histological examination to differentiate between the two and establish appropriate clinical management. Understanding the techniques utilized to identify and examine such pathological changes is necessary to build diagnostic proficiency in histology. Sophisticated techniques such as OCT provide non-invasive imaging techniques for visualizing epithelial morphology and assessing the integrity of these tissues in real time. A recent study demonstrated the capacity of OCT in differentiating normal and abnormal oral tissues, highlighting distinctive cellular architecture in various layers of the epithelium with impressive accuracy levels of 87% for the keratin cell layer and 93.5% for the epithelial layer (Al-Delayme et al., 2012). By creating a normative and pathological database with patient samples, this technology enables the possibility of earlier detection of epithelial pathologies, and thus early intervention and improved patient outcomes. The findings also highlight the importance of development in imaging techniques able to assist pathologists in evaluating epithelial changes, eventually supporting conventional histological approaches. In addition to imaging techniques, evaluation of pathological changes in epithelial tissues is complemented by a deeper understanding of the physiological processes underlying them. For instance, endometrial hyperplasia has been reported to significantly alter the morphology of the uterine epithelium in women, as indicated by studies correlating hormonal influences with uterine pathology. These studies have been used as evidence that changes in the uterine epithelium's morphology may be linked to stages of estrous cycles, and pathologies caused by hormonal regimens (Chatdarong, 2003). These findings underscore the necessity of correlating histological examination with physiological context to ensure a thorough understanding of pathological changes in epithelia that can increase the accuracy of diagnosis and therapy. Together, the partnership of advanced diagnostic techniques and strong knowledge of physiological principles are essential in unmasking the intricacies of pathologic changes within epithelial tissues.

Test Your Knowledge

1. What is the classification of epithelial tissue?
2. What are the functions of the epithelial tissue in the body?

1.5. Histology of Connective Tissue

Learning Outcome

1. Describe the types of connective tissue and their functions;
2. Understand the components and importance of extracellular matrix;
3. Understand the disorders related to connective tissue.

The histology of connective tissues is important in identifying the various roles that these tissues play in the human body. Connective tissues, characterized by their lack of cellularity and abundance of extracellular matrix, provide structural support, perform transport of nutrients, and enable immune reactions. They consist of different subtypes like loose connective tissue, dense connective tissue, adipose tissue, cartilage, bone, and blood, each tailored to perform unique functional requirements. Cellular components like fibroblasts, macrophages, and mast cells contribute to tissue homeostasis and repair. In particular, the extracellular matrix, composed of ground substance and fibers, dictates the mechanics of connective tissues and their ability to withstand forces as well as to dynamically respond to other nearby tissues, hence playing a central role in organ and system integrity. Histological analysis provides information concerning cell response profiles provoked by various foreign materials, particularly after device implantation. It has been shown that materials such as the Device for Intervertebral Assisted Motion (DIAM®) elicit a typical foreign body reaction of clusters of macrophages and foreign body giant cells showing attempts at encapsulation and sequestration by the body of the foreign material. Observations indicate that such a reaction is usually not severe as the host tissues can only be mildly to moderately chronically inflamed as graded according to accepted standards like ASTM F981-04. Such histological tests are critical in the evaluation of implant biocompatibility and the consequent impact on nearby connective tissues, contributing to improvements in materials employed for surgical devices and implants (Toth & Bric, 2019). Moreover, studies with mineral trioxide aggregate (MTA), a material which has been that much in vogue in dental applications, reveal how connective tissue responds to synthetic composites. On MTA implantation, it provokes a chronic inflammatory reaction, as evidenced by the abundant occurrence of inflammatory cells in histologic sections. Such a response is indispensable in gauging the materials compatibility and functionality in biological systems. MTA-host tissue interactions like the formation of calcium carbonate and the addition of elements like bismuth are extremely useful in explaining material behavior *in vivo* and long-term implications in accordance with tissue health. Explanation of these interactions assists in the formulation of biomaterials that better interact with human tissues, inducing few negative reactions and promoting effective recovery and healing (Camilleri et al., 2016) (Figure 1.17).

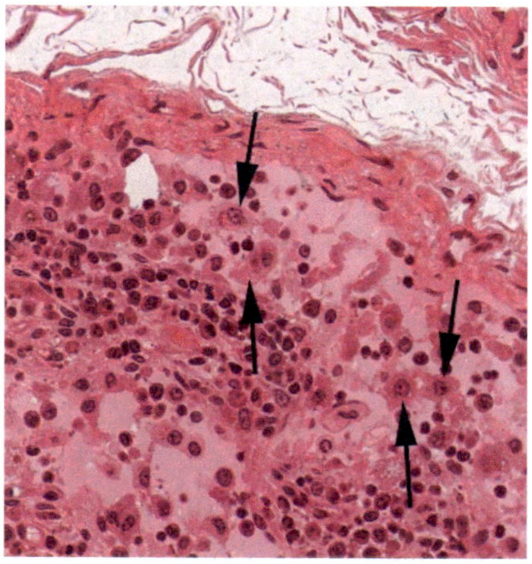

Figure 1.17. Histology of connective tissue.

Source: https://histology.medicine.umich.edu/sites/default/files/connective1.jpg.

1.5.1. Types of Connective Tissue and Their Functions

Connective tissue is a very diverse collection of tissue types that support and structure the body. The most important types of connective tissue include loose connective tissue, dense connective tissue, adipose tissue, and specialized connective tissues such as cartilage and bone. Loose connective tissue is an elastic framework supporting and connecting organs, blood vessels, and nerves. On the other hand, dense connective tissue consisting of closely packed collagen fibers provides greater tensile strength and is required in organs such as tendons and ligaments. Both possess unique properties and functions, which reveal the diversity and complexity of connective tissue in human histology (Remedios et al., 2024). Another type of significant connective tissue is adipose tissue, which serves a main function in the storage of energy, insulation, and organ padding. It consists of adipocytes, the cells that store fat and can efficiently store droplets of energy. Apart from this, adipose tissue contributes to the endocrine and metabolic control by secreting hormones such as leptin that are involved in energy utilization and appetite regulation. Adipose tissue is not just for storage purposes as it is also involved in thermoregulation and may contribute to inflammation in any kind of pathological condition. Understanding the multifaceted functions of adipose tissue underscores its importance against the backdrop of disease and health in the framework of the overall context of connective tissue (Patel et al., 2024). Specialized connective tissues like cartilage and bone provide structural support to the skeleton. Cartilage, whose matrix is hardened but elastic, provides support while permitting gliding movements of joints. It plays a very crucial role in development and growth, particularly during childhood, because it subsequently becomes hardened bone. Bone tissue, however, is a compact form of connective tissue with structural support, protecting from injury, and mineral storage. Bone tissue also has bone marrow, which is responsible for hematopoiesis. Bone and cartilage both have responsibilities for movement and general skeletal function, exemplifying the diverse functions of connective tissue in maintaining both structural and physiological homeostasis in the human body (Remedios et al., 2024).

1.5.2. Extracellular Matrix (ECM): Components and Importance

The ECM is an important scaffold for cells and tissues to rest upon, performing a multifunctional role within the composition of many organs. Composed of an intricate network of proteins, glycoproteins, and polysaccharides, the ECM is required for tissue integrity and cell-cell communication. Significant components are collagen, elastin, fibronectin, and laminin, each contributing distinct properties necessary for tissue function. Collagen provides tensile strength, and elastin allows elasticity in skin and lungs. By control of the physical and biochemical environment, the ECM not only supports the structure but also influences cellular behavior, such as proliferation, differentiation, and migration. The dynamic quality of the ECM indicates its role in normal physiology as well as response to injury or disease and, as such, is a keystone area of investigation in human histology. In human histology, the function of the ECM goes beyond mere structural support; it has a pivotal function in managing different cell processes required for homeostasis. The ECM influences tissue repair and regeneration by way of cell migration and growth signals, particularly for injury. For instance, during wound repair, ECM components change to facilitate fibroblast and endothelial cell migration to help form new tissue. Moreover, the signaling molecules incorporated in the ECM can control the cellular response to an external stimulus and play a vital role in inflammatory processes and tissue remodeling. This intricate association is responsible for the necessity of an overall view of the ECM for developmental biology as well as for its implications in regenerative medicine and treatment. Additionally, derangements within the composition or organization of the ECM have also been found to be causally involved in diseases like cancer, fibrosis, and degenerative disease. For instance, modification of ECM stiffness will influence tumor activity, promoting invasive behavior in cancer cells, as observed in research linking ECM characteristics to cancer growth. Increased levels of AKT2, observed in certain breast carcinomas, have been found to have a negative prognostic value, again pointing to the role of the ECM in disease mechanisms. Through the study of these pathological processes, researchers can identify potential targets for treatment interventions for the purposes of normalizing ECM function and composition. Appreciation of the subtle equilibrium of the ECM both in conditions of health and disease is therefore important to the advancement of the discipline of human histology as well as optimal control of several diseases, imagining the colossal role of ECM in maintenance of systemic health (Huang et al., 2016; Riggio et al., 2017) (Figure 1.18).

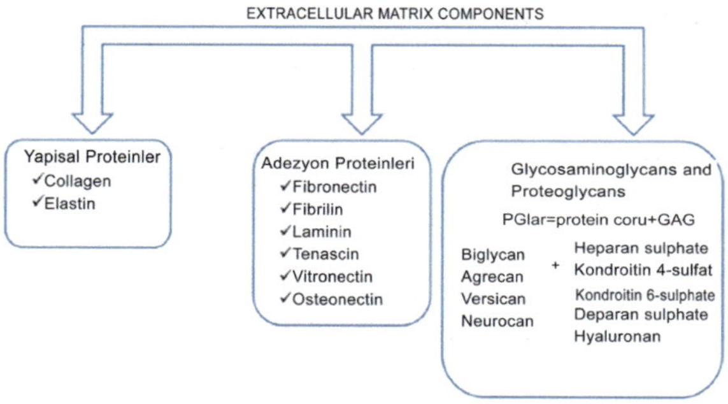

Figure 1.18. Demonstration of extracellular matrix components.

Source: https://www.researchgate.net/publication/261883030/figure/fig1/AS:296817628598281@1447778245908/Demonstration-of-extracellular-matrix-components-in-groups-These-ECM-types-consist-of-a.png.

1.5.3. Disorders Related to Connective Tissue

Connective tissue disorders consist of a wide range of pathological processes that can significantly influence the structural integrity and function of most anatomical systems. These are commonly due to changes in the extracellular matrix components, which are crucial for maintaining tissue strength and resilience.

The most prevalent category of connective tissue disorders is the inherited connective tissue disorders, such as Marfan syndrome and Ehlers-Danlos syndrome, caused by mutations disrupting collagen and elastin synthesis. The resultant defects produce clinical features of joint hypermobility, skin extensibility, and cardiovascular disease. Understanding of the histological basis of these conditions is important in illuminating the intrinsic cellular interactions as well as the molecular signaling pathways that can be engineered to generate therapeutic outcomes, thus the importance of human histology in the diagnosis and treatment of connective tissue disorders.

Mesenchymal stem cells (MSCs) have emerged as a very viable therapeutic avenue for the treatment of numerous connective tissue disorders due to their unique regenerative capacities. These cells, present in the connective tissue of most organs, are capable of differentiating into several lineage types, including bone, cartilage, and fat tissues. Their therapeutic potential is increased by the fact that they can also direct the tissue microenvironment through the secretion of soluble factors that have the potential to be involved in the repair of damaged connective tissues. There is evidence to show that MSCs possess the potential to facilitate healing processes, particularly for tendon injury. As pointed out in early studies, the first use of stem cell treatments has turned out to be effective in clinical settings where standard treatment has failed. The creation and utilization of the therapies are a significant milestone in the study of connective tissue repair and regeneration and have introduced new challenges to the field of human histology (Grange, 2011). Chronic tendon lesions demonstrate the complexity of connective tissue disease and indicate the role of growth factors in the repair of tissues. Chronic lesions are typically characterized by an inability to effectively repair or remodel the extracellular matrix following repetitive micro-damage, leading to degenerative diseases. The transforming growth factor-beta (TGF-ß) superfamily is at the center of tissue repair and remodeling processes, particularly in the tendinous biology. Studies that analyze TGF-ß isoforms in normal vs. pathological tendons illustrate a uniform pattern; whereas TGF-ß2 is consistently found in healthy and pathological tissues, the relative absence of its required receptor, TGF-ßRI, in involved tendons illustrates one reason for lesion chronicity. Without effective signaling mechanisms, the mechanisms of healing in chronic tendinopathy may be severely impaired, which emphasizes the need for new therapeutic strategies with an ability to bypass such molecular defects in connective tissue disorders (Fenwick et al., 2001).

Test Your Knowledge

1. What are the types of connective tissue and their functions?
2. What are the main components of the extracellular matrix?

1.6. Histology of Muscle and Nervous Tissue

Learning Outcome

1. Describe the structure and function of skeletal muscle;
2. Learn about cardiac and smooth muscle histology;
3. Describe the structure and function of neurons and glial cells.

The histology of muscle tissue is characterized by highly specialized cell architecture, best suited for contraction and movement. The muscle tissue has traditionally been classified into three types: skeletal, cardiac, and smooth. The skeletal muscle fibers are striated and voluntary and are made up of multi-nucleated cells that facilitate force generation during locomotion. In comparison, cardiac muscle, striated but involuntary, has intercalated discs to synchronize contractions for the heartbeats' rhythmicity. Smooth muscle, non-striated and involuntarily controlled, is found in hollow viscera and blood vessels, contributing to physiological function, such as peristalsis and vessel regulation. Muscular histology is investigated to gain insight into muscular pathologies, including muscular dystrophy and myopathy, by observing altered cellular structure using histological techniques that recognize critical components of the disease process and tissue response. Nervous tissue, constituting a basic building block of body function and control, is composed principally of neurons and glial cells. Neurons are highly specialized cells that transmit electrical impulses, while glial cells have vital supporting roles, including structural support, insulation, and the supply of nutrients. The intricately developed structure of nervous tissue allows for quick communication in the body, and this is needed for reflexes as well as for higher-order mental processes. Histological examination can reveal a variety of conditions that involve nervous tissue, such as neurodegenerative disease or traumatic injury, often by examination of tissue samples using staining techniques that highlight cellular and subcellular structure. Pathology and morphology of nervous tissue could be better appreciated by advanced imaging techniques, as traditional histological techniques cannot fully depict the complex three-dimensional tissue organization (Hsueh et al., 2017).

The interaction between muscle and nervous tissue is a significant area of study in human histology, emphasizing the physiological interaction between the two systems. Muscle contraction is regulated by nervous tissue through the transmission of signals from motor neurons to muscle fibers, illustrating the interdependence of the two tissues for function. Histological studies illustrate how the neuromuscular junction facilitates communication that is required to activate muscles. Understanding the histological properties of muscle and nervous tissue facilitates the explanation of various pathophysiological diseases, exemplified by diseases such as amyotrophic lateral sclerosis, where motor neurons are degenerated and muscle functions are impaired. Further, current advances in histological techniques, for instance, the use of hydrogel techniques for enhanced interrogation of tissues, have the potential to facilitate further study of the structural attributes of muscle and nervous systems (Fiegel et al., 2012). These evolving methods will progressively elucidate our understanding of human histology, impacting clinical practice and research (Figure 1.19).

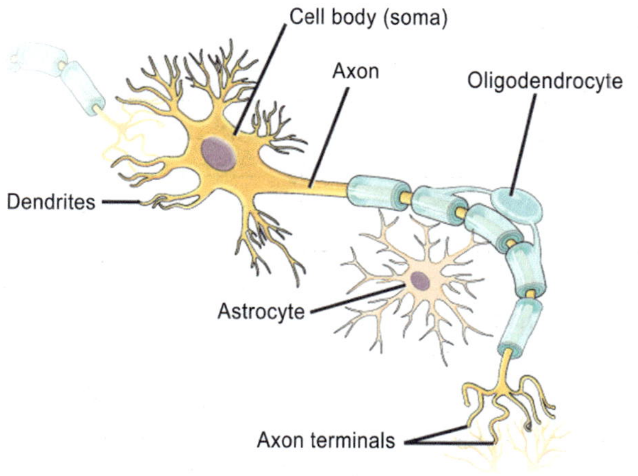

Figure 1.19. Diagram of a neuron.

Source: https://s3-us-west-2.amazonaws.com/courses-images/wp-content/uploads/sites/1223/2017/03/16155525/Figure_33_02_13.png.

1.6.1. Structure and Function of Skeletal Muscle

Skeletal muscle, a vital component of the musculoskeletal system, is primarily responsible for voluntary movements of the human body. Structurally, skeletal muscle is composed of multinucleated, elongated fibers called myofibers that are packed in bundles called fascicles. Myofibers are made up of myofibrils, intricate structures that have contractile proteins myosin and actin within them. These proteins form sarcomeres, which are the smallest units of contraction in muscles. The alignment of myofibrils in myofibers gives effective force production as well as rapid response to neural stimulation. Moreover, the muscle cell membrane, or sarcolemma, is significant in transmitting the action potential responsible for contraction, demonstrating the intricate interrelationship between skeletal muscle structure and its performance in generating movement and posture. Other than contraction, the physiological function of skeletal muscle entails regeneration and adaptation by responding to a variety of stimuli. Muscle injury initiates a complex regenerative pathway characterized by activation of satellite cells, latent stem cells located between the sarcolemma and basal lamina of the myofibers. Satellite cells proliferate and give rise to new myofibers upon activation, thereby contributing to hypertrophy and muscle repair. Muscle morphology can be better investigated by a detailed examination to enable us to understand these phenomena. QuantiMus, an emerging computer package, demonstrates this functionality through precise measurement of myofiber cross-sectional area and other morphometric variables critical for assessment of regenerative response in dystrophic conditions where muscle disease has a patchy distribution. It establishes the interface between structural evaluation and functional assessment of skeletal muscle histology, enhancing knowledge in muscle disease and health (Kastenschmidt et al., 2019).

Furthermore, the glycosylation status of proteins within skeletal muscle is crucial for the structural stability and functional competence of the tissues. Alpha-dystroglycan, which is an essential component of the dystrophin-glycoprotein complex, relies heavily upon proper glycosylation to be able to function in attaching the extracellular matrix to the underlying cytoskeleton of muscle fibers. Deficits in glycosylation can lead to muscular dystrophies, a group of degenerative disorders of progressive weakness and degeneration of muscles. Experiments have proven that the overexpression of LARGE, a glycosyltransferase, rescues normal alpha-dystroglycan glycosylation and potentially also ameliorates the phenotypes of these conditions. This is not just a demonstration of biochemical modification at the center of muscle histology but also opens up new avenues to cutting-edge therapies for sustaining skeletal muscle function in the face of genetic and pathological onslaughts (Brockington et al., 2010) (Figure 1.20).

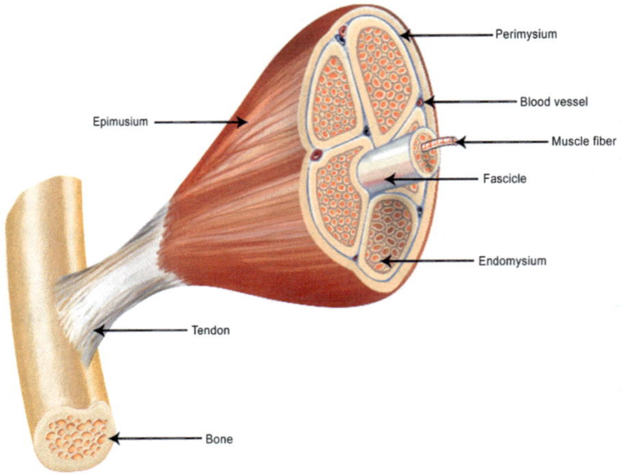

Figure 1.20. Structure of skeletal muscle.

Source: https://training.seer.cancer.gov/images/anatomy/muscular/muscle_structure.jpg.

1.6.2. Cardiac and Smooth Muscle Histology

Cardiac and smooth muscle histology depict distinctive but intricate cellular architectures that are primarily pivotal to the functioning of the human body. Striated cardiac muscle is rather specialized for rhythmic contractions required to preserve circulation. The cell structure consists of branched myocytes linked by intercalated discs, which facilitate the transmission of quick electrical impulses and mechanical coupling, hence ensuring coordinated contraction. In contrast, smooth muscle tissue is non-striated and made up of long, spindle-shaped cells. Its histological structure is such that it can contract in most involuntary organs, such as the digestive system and the blood vessels, and contributes to important autonomic functions. The difference between these architectures points to their specialized role in guaranteeing physiological homeostasis and serves to emphasize the importance of cell structure in histological analysis of human tissue. Further histology of cardiac muscle has also shown the presence of specialized conducting systems responsible for the rhythmic behavior of the heart. Structures such as the sinoatrial node and atrioventricular node possess characteristic histological features, e.g., clusters of pacemaker cells to generate spontaneous electrical activity. Cardiac myocytes also exhibit a rich supply of mitochondria and myoglobin to signify their high metabolic demands for sustained contractions. Moreover, the extracellular matrix of cardiac muscle plays a critical role in structurally stabilizing and elastic properties that enable the heart's expansion in diastole and contraction in systole. These histological features exemplify the complex inter-relationship between structure and function in cardiac tissue and provide insight into potential pathologies like heart failure and cardiomyopathies and can be unraveled by sensitive histological analysis.

Smooth muscle histology is another significant area of human tissue study characterized by its widespread occurrence inside and between organ systems. Smooth muscle cells are found primarily within the walls of hollow organs—such as the intestines, bladder, and blood vessels—and they constrict involuntarily to a variety of stimuli, including hormones and neural impulses.

The alignment of these cells in layers, often circular in orientation in some organs and longitudinal in others, facilitates the generation of coordinated patterns of contraction. Additionally, dynamic histological characteristics of smooth muscle allow for functional plasticity so that organs can adapt to changing physiological demands. Existing studies have taken into account gene and protein expression of specific genes involved in smooth muscle development and function, which is an indication of the possibility of biomarkers of diseases such as hypertension and gastrointestinal disorders and underscores the value of smooth muscle histology in the management of systemic health (Brockington et al., 2010; Snider et al., 2019) (Figure 1.21).

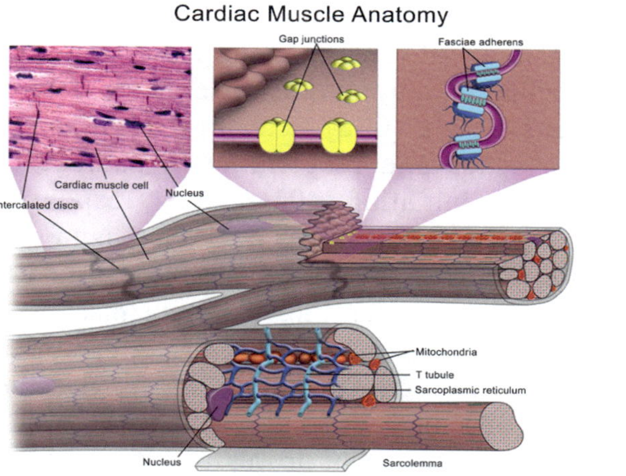

Figure 1.21. Cardiac muscle anatomy.

Source: https://books.byui.edu/content_images/bio_265_anatomy_phy_II/wIWG_2.png.

1.6.3. Neurons and Glial Cells: Structure and Function

The intricate morphology and behavior of neurons and glial cells are focal to the field of human histology. Neurons are specialized cells of the nervous system involved in sending signals, which are received by dendrites and transmitted by axons to other cells. Unlike glial cells, though, neurons are unique in their ability to generate action potentials, a critical feature required for the rapid communication along long chains throughout the brain and spinal cord. This polarization of structure—dendrites, soma, and axon terminals—allows for the integration and processing of innumerable signals from the outside world as well as within the body. The bipolar structure of neuronal elements emphasizes their vital role in maintaining communication channels required for sensory perception, reflex action, and cognitive processes. Glial cells, such as astrocytes, microglia, and oligodendrocytes, are just as vital but in support roles rather than for direct communication. Astrocytes, the star-shaped glial cells, are involved in providing neurons with structural support and nutrients and in playing a role in maintaining the blood-brain barrier, which is significant in neuroprotection. The microglia are the immune cells of the central nervous system (CNS), actively surveilling the neural space and responding to damage or disease by initiating inflammatory responses. The oligodendrocytes, on the other hand, are responsible for myelination of axons in the CNS and for accelerating the transmission of electrical impulses. This multi-faceted glial cell functionality highlights their importance not only in neuronal well-being but also in CNS homeostasis and repair processes overall, hence, their importance beyond the simple supportive role.

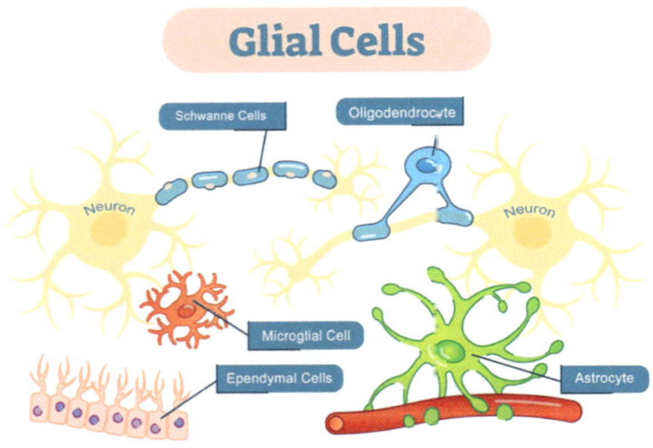

Figure 1.22. Glial cells.

Source: https://www.verywellhealth.com/thmb/KTilfCxnabrUhsp536BLMgZ_8Zk=/1500x0/filters:no_upscale():max_bytes(150000):strip_icc()/glialcellsillustration-5a94d585642dca00362568c4.jpg.

Recent work on the interaction between neural tissue and nanomaterials has also provided further insight into the fine interdependence between glial cells and neurons.

For instance, f-CNT experiments elucidate cellular uptake mechanisms by different glial cell lines and neurons and reveal differential interaction patterns within the neural tissue. Histological results demonstrate that microglia and astrocytes are actively responding to the introduction of these nanotubes with localized activation and cytokine release, which is an evidence for strong inflammatory response. Elucidation of these interactions is of the highest significance to the advancement of nanotechnology strategies for CNS therapeutics as it has the potential to guide the creation of more effective drug delivery devices.

In such a situation, understanding the fine balance between neuronal function and glial responsivity not only deepens our knowledge of human histology but also identifies the ever-present need for sophisticated methodologies to manipulate these dynamics for therapeutic aims (Bardi et al., 2013; Polanska et al., 2020) (Figure 1.22).

Test Your Knowledge

1. What is the structure and function of the skeletal muscle?
2. What are the functions of neurons and glial cells?

SUMMARY

In summarizing an inquiry into human histology is important to realize the vast importance of tissue function and structure in the general scheme of disease and health. Histology is the basic subject that connects fundamental biological sciences with pragmatic applications, offering information that is crucial for the diagnosis of disease, development of therapy, and expansion of medical knowledge. The intricate organization and cell arrangement in tissues reveal not only the physiological aspects of the human body but also illustrate pathological conditions that may arise as a result of histological alterations. Therefore, comprehensive knowledge of histology is essential for healthcare practitioners since it is the foundation for effective clinical practice and enhances the efficacy of diagnostic techniques. In addition, the development of histological methods, particularly with the introduction of digital pathology and new imaging technologies, has revolutionized our method of approaching tissue analysis. Modern histo-technological improvements enable thorough assessment on a cellular and molecular level, providing greater insight into intricate tissue mechanisms of disease. For instance, a study of chemokine (C-C motif) receptor 8 (CCR8)-expressing regulatory T cells in lung cancer shows how histological research may elucidate immune interactions that contribute to tumor behavior and patient prognosis. Such an observation underscores the significance of histology not only as a descriptive science but as a vital cog in the biomedical research spectrum towards improved patient prognosis, thereby contributing to the advancement of the discipline of human histology (Hayashi et al., 2024). Lastly, the future of human histology unquestionably lies in its intersection with other scientific disciplines such as genomics, proteomics, and bioinformatics. Multidisciplinary research will unlock more understanding regarding the dynamic relationship between tissue architecture and cellular function, especially in the context of degenerative diseases. Additionally, as seen in recent research comparing human responses with those generated by AI systems such as ChatGPT, the specificity and contextual knowledge inherent to histological interpretations emphasize the value of human expertise. The findings show that while AI is capable of assisting with the interpretation and analysis of data, human experts remain necessary to direct the use of such findings in clinical practice, particularly when analyzing complex tissues (Blacker et al., 2024). Overall, a solid understanding of human histology remains core, for individual practitioners as well as for medicine as a whole (Ly & Leveson-Gower, 2019).

Human histology, or tissue microscopy, provides important information regarding organ system structure and function. Key points in this topic highlight the need to learn about tissue arrangement, cell differentiation, and the interactions that create homeostasis. An illustration of this is the characterization of epithelial tissues, which shows that they are not only protective barriers but also active participants in absorption and secretion. Understanding the nuances of such functions is crucial in diagnosing pathologies that can be caused by dysfunctions at the cellular level. A proper grasp of human histology thus provides the foundation for furthering medical science and enhancing clinical methods. Advances in histological techniques such as immunohistochemistry and *in situ* hybridization have transformed the visual depiction of specific proteins and genetic expressions in tissues. These technologies have been beneficial in revealing the complexities of tissue repair and regeneration, particularly in orthopedic cases. For instance, research on bone graft substitutes has reflected encouraging outcomes with regard to their efficacy and compatibility with host tissue. In particular, testing involving recombinant human BMP-2 (rhBMP-2) preparations has provided unequivocal evidence for successful bone fusion, such as a 100% fusion rate under certain experimental conditions. These findings point to the importance of histology in evaluating treatment strategies and predicting patient outcomes in regenerative medicine (Toth et al., 2016). The use of digital atlasing technology in histological studies is a groundbreaking approach toward understanding organ systems compositional heterogeneity. Initiatives such as the INCF Digital Atlasing Program attempt to standardize the procedure of creating and accessing high-resolution anatomical atlases, particularly in rodent models. This project not only assists in researchers' visualization of multidimensional data but also optimizes the capacity for translational research applications. Having clear guidelines and objectives, this program also enhances collaboration among scientists and reduces the path from basic research to clinical utility. Technological advancements in histological mapping, coupled with computer systems, ensure that scientists can continue to find out more about the complexity of human anatomy and pathology (Ng et al., 2009).

KEY TERMS FROM THIS CHAPTER

- Biology
- Cellular organization
- Ciliogenesis
- Human histology
- Medical science
- Neurodegenerative disorders
- Pathology
- Cancer
- Chromatin structure
- Epithelial cells
- Malignancy
- Medicine
- Pancreatic islet transplantation
- Surgical interventions

CRITICAL THINKING QUESTIONS

1. **Histology is the study of:**
   a. Organs and their systems
   b. Cells and their structure
   c. Tissues and their microscopic structure
   d. Genetic material in cells
2. **The staining technique most commonly used in histology is:**
   a. Gram staining
   b. Hematoxylin and eosin (H&E)
   c. Periodic acid-Schiff (PAS)
   d. Wright-Giemsa
3. **The process of embedding tissues in paraffin is done to:**
   a. Preserve the tissues
   b. Dehydrate the tissues
   c. Harden the tissues for sectioning
   d. Stain the tissues
4. **Which of the following is NOT a step in preparing a histological slide?**
   a. Fixation
   b. Sectioning
   c. Incubation
   d. Staining
5. **How many basic types of tissues are there in the human body?**
   a. Two
   b. Three
   c. Four
   d. Five

Short Answer Questions

1. What is human histology?
2. Why is histology important?
3. Explain the historical development of histological techniques.
4. Name the four basic types of tissues.
5. What are the 3 types of connective tissue?

Answers to Critical Thinking Questions

1. (c); 2. (b) ; 3. (c); 4. (c); 5. (c)

REFERENCES

1. Riggio, M., Perrone, M., Polo, M. et al. AKT1 and AKT2 isoforms play distinct roles during breast cancer progression through the regulation of specific downstream proteins. Sci Rep 7, 44244 (2017). https://doi.org/10.1038/srep44244(accessed on 7th August 2025).
2. Duong, L. D., Rawson, R., Bezryadina, A., Manresa, M. C., Newbury, R. O., Dohil, R., Liu, Z., Barrett, K., Kurten, R., & Aceves, S. S. (2020). TGFβ1 single-nucleotide polymorphism C-509T alters mucosal cell function in pediatric eosinophilic esophagitis. Mucosal immunology, 13(1), 110–117. https://doi.org/10.1038/s41385-019-0214-9 (accessed on 7th August 2025).
3. Adabi, S., Clayton, A., Conforto, S., Daveluy, A., et al. (2017). Universal in vivo textural model for human skin based on optical coherence tomograms. http://arxiv.org/abs/1706.02758 (accessed on 7th August 2025).
4. Adin, C. A., & Gilor, C. (2017). The diabetic dog as a translational model for human islet transplantation. https://core.ac.uk/download/323071786.pdf (accessed on 7th August 2025).
5. Al-Delayme, R., Hamdoon, Z., Hopper, C., Jay, A., et al. (2012). Structural validation of oral mucosal tissue using optical coherence tomography. https://core.ac.uk/download/16220461.pdf (accessed on 7th August 2025).
6. Alibegović, A., Umek, N., Pušnik, L., & Martinez, I. Z. (2024). Comparison of the visual scoring method and semi-automatic image analysis for evaluating staining intensity of human cartilage sections. Image Analysis and Stereology. https://www.semanticscholar.org/paper/9f9c546fd b4054a20b20d7a776d29632c1b09509 (accessed on 7th August 2025).
7. Enrique Hilario & Daniel Alonso-Alconada (2022). Human Histology: Manual of Practicals. ISBN: 978-84-1319-425-7.. https://core.ac.uk/download/547377171.pdf (accessed on 7th August 2025).
8. Zaimi, A., Wabartha, M., Herman, V., Antonsanti, P. L., Perone, C. S., & Cohen-Adad, J. (2018). AxonDeepSeg: automatic axon and myelin segmentation from microscopy data using convolutional neural networks. Scientific reports, 8(1), 3816. https://doi.org/10.1038/s41598-018-22181-4(accessed on 7th August 2025).
9. Hsueh, B., Burns, V. M., Pauerstein, P., Holzem, K., Ye, L., Engberg, K., Wang, A. C., Gu, X., Chakravarthy, H., Arda, H. E., Charville, G., Vogel, H., Efimov, I. R., Kim, S., & Deisseroth, K. (2017). Pathways to clinical CLARITY: volumetric analysis of irregular, soft, and heterogeneous tissues in development and disease. Scientific reports, 7(1), 5899. https://doi.org/10.1038/s41598-017-05614-4(accessed on 7th August 2025).
10. Arzi, B., Garcia, T., Hatcher, D. C., Vapniarsky, N., et al. (2020). Intra- and extra-articular features of temporomandibular joint ankylosis in the cat (Felis catus). https://core.ac.uk/download/287623916.pdf (accessed on 7th August 2025).
11. Augustin, M., Baumann, B., Eugui, P., Harper, D. J., et al. (2018). Beyond Backscattering: Optical Neuroimaging by BRAD. http://arxiv.org/abs/1712.00361 (accessed on 7th August 2025).
12. Kastenschmidt, J. M., Ellefsen, K. L., Mannaa, A. H., Giebel, J. J., Yahia, R., Ayer, R. E., Pham, P., Rios, R., Vetrone, S. A., Mozaffar, T., & Villalta, S. A. (2019). QuantiMus: A Machine Learning-Based Approach for High Precision Analysis of Skeletal Muscle Morphology. Frontiers in physiology, 10, 1416. https://doi.org/10.3389/fphys.2019.01416(accessed on 7th August 2025).

13. Min, E., Ban, S., Lee, J. et al. Serial optical coherence microscopy for label-free volumetric histopathology. Sci Rep 10, 6711 (2020). https://doi.org/10.1038/s41598-020-63460-3 (accessed on 7th August 2025).

14. Levenson, R., Beechem, J., & McNamara, G. (2012). Spectral imaging in preclinical research and clinical pathology. Analytical cellular pathology (Amsterdam), 35(5-6), 339–361. https://doi.org/10.3233/ACP-2012-0062(accessed on 7th August 2025).

15. Bardi, G., Nunes, A., Gherardini, L., Bates, K., Al-Jamal, K. T., Gaillard, C., Prato, M., Bianco, A., Pizzorusso, T., & Kostarelos, K. (2013). Functionalized carbon nanotubes in the brain: cellular internalization and neuroinflammatory responses. PloS one, 8(11), e80964. https://doi.org/10.1371/journal.pone.0080964(accessed on 7th August 2025).

16. Fereidouni, F., Harmany, Z.T., Tian, M. et al. Microscopy with ultraviolet surface excitation for rapid slide-free histology. Nat Biomed Eng 1, 957–966 (2017). https://doi.org/10.1038/s41551-017-0165-y(accessed on 7th August 2025).

17. Black, C. C., Kanick, S. C., McClatchy, D. M., Paulsen, K. D., et al. (2018). Light scattering measured with spatial frequency domain imaging can predict stromal versus epithelial proportions in surgically resected breast tissue. https://core.ac.uk/download/231149102.pdf (accessed on 7th August 2025).

18. Blacker, S. N., Chen, F., Winecoff, D., Antonio, B. L., Arora, H., Hierlmeier, B. J., Kacmar, R. M., et al. (2024). An exploratory analysis of ChatGPT compared to human performance with the anesthesiology oral board examination: Initial insights and implications. Anesthesia and Analgesia. https://www.semanticscholar.org/paper/188e070b75231c962972007b670698eb9823b97b (accessed on 7th August 2025).

19. Blanc, L., Chen, P. Y., Dartois, V., Daudelin, T., et al. (2018). High-resolution mapping of fluoroquinolones in TB rabbit lesions reveals specific distribution in immune cell types. https://core.ac.uk/download/323072944.pdf (accessed on 7th August 2025).

20. Bochsler, V. S., Galloway, S. B., Harley, R. A., Kramarsky-Winters, E., et al. (2007). Coral Disease and Health Workshop: Coral Histopathology II. https://core.ac.uk/download/11017972.pdf (accessed on 7th August 2025).

21. U. Brinck, M. Korabiowska, R. Bosbach, H.-J. Gabius; Detection of Inflammation- and Neoplasia-Associated Alterations in Human Large Intestine Using Plant/Invertebrate Lectins, Galectin-1 and Neoglycoproteins. *Acta Anatomica* 1 July 1998; 161 (1-4): 219–233. https://doi.org/10.1159/000046460(accessed on 7th August 2025).

22. Bozóky, B., Moro, C. F., Xu, Z., Zhang, L., et al. (2019). GAN-based virtual re-staining: A promising solution for whole slide image analysis. http://arxiv.org/abs/1901.04059 (accessed on 7th August 2025).

23. Toth, J. M., & Bric, J. D. (2019). An evaluation of the host response to an interspinous process device based on a series of spine explants: Device for Intervertebral Assisted Motion (DIAM®). Journal of spine surgery (Hong Kong), 5(4), 483–495. https://doi.org/10.21037/jss.2019.10.13 (accessed on 7th August 2025).

24. Brockington, M., Brown, S. C., Cirak, S., Liu, K., et al. (2010). Transgenic overexpression of LARGE induces alpha-dystroglycan hyperglycosylation in skeletal and cardiac muscle. https://core.ac.uk/download/1730280.pdf (accessed on 7th August 2025).

25. Ng, L., Zaslavsky, I., Nissanov, J. et al. The INCF Digital Atlasing Program: Report on Digital Atlasing Standards in the Rodent Brain. Nat Prec (2009). https://doi.org/10.1038/npre.2009.4000.1(accessed on 7th August 2025).

26. Mohammadi, S., & Callaghan, M. F. (2021). Towards in vivo g-ratio mapping using MRI: Unifying myelin and diffusion imaging. Journal of neuroscience methods, 348, 108990. https://doi.org/10.1016/j.jneumeth.2020.108990(accessed on 7th August 2025).

27. Camilleri, J., Cappello, F., Lung, C. Y. K., Rappa, F., et al. (2016). Assessment of the interaction of Portland cement-based materials with blood and tissue fluids using an animal model. https://core.ac.uk/download/323186322.pdf (accessed on 7th August 2025).

28. Cicerone, M. T. , & Camp Jr, C. H. (2017). Histological Coherent Raman Imaging: A Prognostic Review. **Analyst**, 2018,**143**, 33-59. http://arxiv.org/abs/1709.07325 (accessed on 7th August 2025).

29. Chatdarong, K. (2003). Reproductive Physiology of the Female Cat. https://core.ac.uk/download/11694645.pdf (accessed on 7th August 2025).

30. Snider, P. L., Snider, E., Simmons, O., Lilly, B., & Conway, S. J. (2019). Analysis of Uncharacterized mKiaa1211 Expression during Mouse Development and Cardiovascular Morphogenesis. Journal of cardiovascular development and disease, 6(2), 24. https://doi.org/10.3390/jcdd6020024 (accessed on 7th August 2025).

31. Fenwick, S. A., Curry, V., Harrall, R. L., Hazleman, B. L., Hackney, R., & Riley, G. P. (2001). Expression of transforming growth factor-beta isoforms and their receptors in chronic tendinosis. Journal of anatomy, 199(Pt 3), 231–240. https://doi.org/10.1046/j.1469-7580.2001.19930231.x(accessed on 7th August 2025).

32. Degistirici, O., Götz, W., Jaquiery, C., Martin, I., et al. (2008). Defining properties of neural crest-derived progenitor cells from the apex of human developing tooth. https://core.ac.uk/download/18240097.pdf (accessed on 7th August 2025).

33. Painter, J. N., O'Mara, T. A., Batra, J., Cheng, T., Lose, F. A., Dennis, J., Michailidou, K., Tyrer, J. P., Ahmed, S., Ferguson, K., Healey, C. S., Kaufmann, S., Hillman, K. M., Walpole, C., Moya, L., Pollock, P., Jones, A., Howarth, K., Martin, L., Gorman, M., ... Spurdle, A. B. (2015). Fine-mapping of the HNF1B multicancer locus identifies candidate variants that mediate endometrial cancer risk. Human molecular genetics, 24(5), 1478–1492. https://doi.org/10.1093/hmg/ddu552 (accessed on 7th August 2025).

34. Polanska, M. A., Kirchhoff, T., Dircksen, H., Hansson, B. S., & Harzsch, S. (2020). Functional morphology of the primary olfactory centers in the brain of the hermit crab Coenobita clypeatus (Anomala, Coenobitidae). Cell and tissue research, 380(3), 449–467. https://doi.org/10.1007/s00441-020-03199-5Fiegel, H. C., Gfrörer, S., Metzger, R., Ramachandran, P., et al. (2012). Changes of smooth muscle contractile filaments in small bowel atresia. https://core.ac.uk/download/14530388.pdf (accessed on 7th August 2025).

35. Grange S. (2012). Current issues and regulations in tendon regeneration and musculoskeletal repair with mesenchymal stem cells. Current stem cell research & therapy, 7(2), 110–114. https://doi.org/10.2174/157488812799218983Gulsuna, B., Gungor, A., Borcek, A., & Ture, U. (2025). 1127 Revealing the confusion of the evolution of the term sagittal stratum: Historical overview and systematic literature review. Neurosurgery. https://www.semanticscholar.org/paper/85454d1b579126b0cabf5cf51983db675a8d6b2c (accessed on 7th August 2025).

36. Hayashi, Y., Ueyama, A., Funaki, S., Jinushi, K., Higuchi, N., Morihara, H., Hirata, M., et al. (2024). In situ analysis of CCR8+ regulatory T cells in lung cancer: Suppression of GzmB+ CD8+ T cells and prognostic marker implications. BMC Cancer, 24. https://www.semanticscholar.org/paper/0be15f4254f6ff0fc237431991491180f255c280 (accessed on 7th August 2025).

37. Wong, H. E., Hedley, J., Stapleton, N., Murphy, B., & Priestnall, S. L. (2018). Odontoameloblastoma with extensive chondroid matrix deposition in a guinea pig. Journal of veterinary diagnostic investigation : official publication of the American Association of Veterinary Laboratory Diagnosticians, Inc, 30(5), 793–797. https://doi.org/10.1177/1040638718794784(accessed on 7th August 2025).

38. Huang, A. S., Mohindroo, C., & Weinreb, R. N. (2016). Aqueous humor outflow structure and function imaging at the bench and bedside: A review. https://core.ac.uk/download/323065079.pdf (accessed on 7th August 2025).

39. Kierszenbaum, A. L., & Tres, L. (2021). Histology and cell biology: An introduction to pathology (5th ed.). Morphologia. Elsevier. ISBN : 9780443284885(accessed on 7th August 2025).

40. Diana Ly & Dennis Leveson-Gower (2019). Bion-M2 PI 1-Pagers. https://ntrs.nasa.gov/api/citations/20190033476/downloads/20190033476.pdf (accessed on 7th August 2025).

41. Toth, J. M., Schwartz, D. G., Mobasser, J. P., & Williams, J. (2016). Instrumented Lumbar Corpectomy and Spinal Reconstruction Comparing rhBMP-2/Compression-Resistant Matrix, rhBMP-2/Absorbable Collagen Sponge/Ceramic Granules Mixture, and Autograft in Two Different Devices: A Study in Sheep. Spine, 41(6), E313–E322. https://doi.org/10.1097/BRS.0000000000001256(accessed on 7th August 2025).

42. Patel, K., Yadav, S., Sahu, G., Patel, D., Sahu, R., & Sahu, T. (2024). Skin necrosis: Pathophysiology and innovations in tissue regeneration. International Journal of Science and Research Archive. https://www.semanticscholar.org/paper/71f8b7751d04efddfeda24cdb72f2779af2c9843 (accessed on 7th August 2025).

43. Remedios, L. W., Bao, S., Remedios, S. W., Lee, H. H., Cai, L., Li, T., Deng, R., et al. (2024). Data-driven nucleus subclassification on colon hematoxylin and eosin using style-transferred digital pathology. Journal of Medical Imaging, 11(6), 067501. https://www.semanticscholar.org/paper/0acbb4f557745c31a9ffa874026919b9fcd5b2dd (accessed on 7th August 2025).

44. Weber, M., Clees, Z., Buck, A., Fischer, A., Steffani, M., Wilhelm, D., Martignoni, M., et al. (2024). Role of the serosa in intestinal anastomotic healing: Insights from in-depth histological analysis of human and murine anastomoses. BJS Open, 8. https://www.semanticscholar.org/paper/8d120b21c22d50a4403182fcf2dfdb89b672356c (accessed on 7th August 2025).

MICROSCOPY IN HISTOLOGY

2

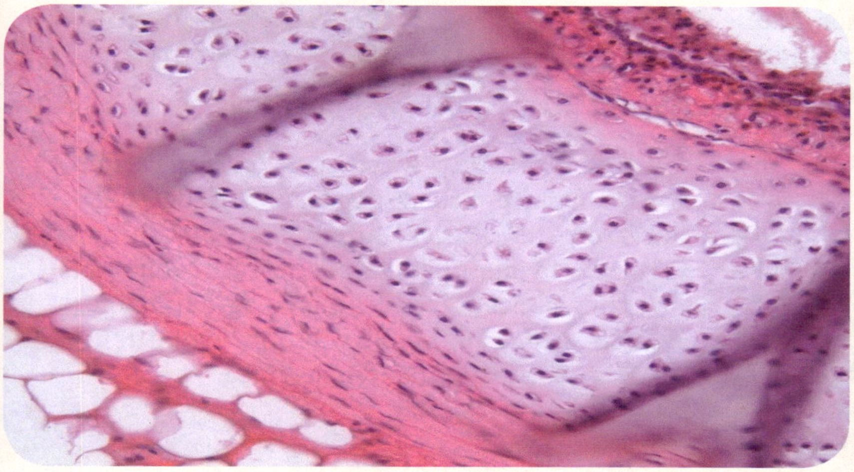

LEARNING OBJECTIVES

After studying this chapter, you will be able to:

1. Describe the types of microscopy;
2. Learn about sample preparation techniques;
3. Discuss about advances in microscopy technology;
4. Learn about applications of microscopy in medicine.

Introduction

The field of human histology, the microscopic study of tissue structure, is greatly enhanced by advances in microscopy technology. The co-existence of microscopy with histological investigation has allowed for an unprecedented visualization of the morphology of cells and interactions between cells. These advances not only allow us to better appreciate normal tissue development but also allow us to discover pathological changes that may develop as a result of disease. With the advancement in imaging technologies, histologists can now explore the complicated details of tissue morphology and learn valuable insights into conditions from infectious diseases to cancer. Due to the advancement in the field, innovative teaching techniques, such as virtual microscopy, become apparent. Those tools are needed to equip the upcoming health science professionals with the expertise needed to handle the complexity of tissue examination properly and effectively. On top of that, traditional methods used in histology cannot represent the three-dimensional arrangement of tissues, which hides valuable information about physiological and pathological conditions. New advances have led to the development of techniques that maintain tissue architecture integrity while permitting extensive analysis. This shift towards the intact tissue examination is vital, as it supports the more accurate assessment of structures that may be irregular or heterogeneous, common in the majority of clinical samples. In particular, biphasic hydrogel technologies provide a route to high-throughput volumetric investigation, centered on aspects including cell innervation and organogenesis. By adopting these methods, researchers can obtain quantitative information capable of pushing the limits of conventional thin-section histology, again expanding the uses of microscopy for research and clinical applications. This achievement is a notable milestone in histology education and practice. Under the umbrella of learning advances, virtual microscopy is transforming student learning about histological specimens. Programs such as the DMU e-Parasitology package are leading the way through the offer of digitized tissue and slide images simulating the use of traditionally employed microscopy. These teaching materials, aside from offering greater access to a diverse range of tissue samples, offer a tool with which to bridge the gap in learning, particularly concerning the understanding of pathogens and their actions on host tissue. With each technological advancement, these digital platforms are offering a twofold benefit: they are reinforcing future practitioners' diagnostic skills, and they also help in their process of training. Additionally, with the inclusion of advanced imaging techniques, such as 3D super-resolution microscopy, they will also promote an integrated comprehension of cell architecture and morphology. The convergence of these resources will be determinant of successful academic outcomes in human histology, preparing students to be competitive within the dynamic horizon of biomedical sciences (Hsueh et al., 2017; Peña-Fernández et al., 2019) (Figure 2.1).

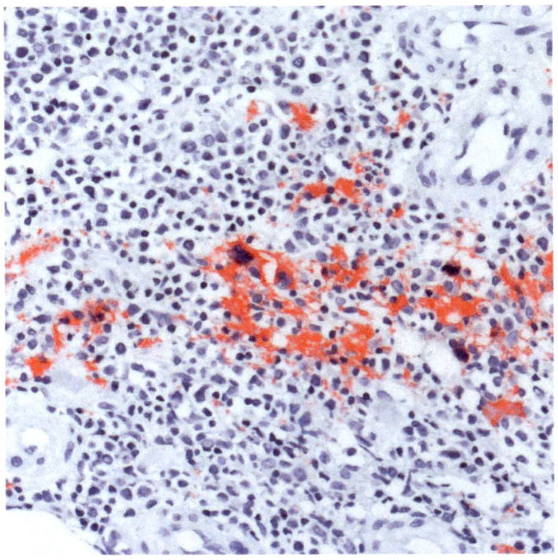

Figure 2.1. Microscopes for Histology.

Source: https://www.zeiss.com/content/dam/rms/reference-master/applications/laboratory-and-routine/clinical-laboratory/histology/brightfield_histological-section_axio-imager.jpg/_jcr_content/renditions/original.image_file.884.884.149,0,1033,884.file/brightfield_histological-section_axio-imager.jpg.

Definition of Microscopy

Microscopy is a critical histology technology through which scientists and doctors can study biological structures at magnification levels that reveal the smallest cellular structure details. Generally, microscopy is the use of various optical instruments for observing specimens that are too small to be viewed with the naked eye. This technique is required for viewing the finer details of human tissue, with the ability to visualize cell structures such as nuclei, organelles, and the extracellular matrix. In histology, there are forms of microscopy ranging from light microscopy up to specialized techniques such as electron microscopy that offer a series of resolutions and imaging characteristics. These methods extend beyond mere observation; they permit identification and analysis of tissue structure, pathology, and function, therefore facilitating informed clinical decision-making. Microscopy application in human histology helps to emphasize its role not just in research endeavors but also in diagnostics. Dermatopathology, for example, is largely reliant on the competence of the histologists analyzing tissue samples to diagnose skin cancers and other skin-related ailments. Previously, these diagnoses have been based on the trained eye's ability to recognize patterns, emphasizing the subjective component in initial determinations. Recent advances in non-invasive imaging techniques, such as optical coherence tomography (OCT), have begun to supplement conventional methodologies. They provide an avenue for the examination of skin conditions with more objectivity and accuracy. With further advancement of this technology, it facilitates systematic investigation of microstructural changes, facilitating distinction of disease, e.g., basal cell carcinoma and squamous cell carcinoma, from normal tissue, thus enhancing the reliability of diagnosis and subsequent treatment regimens (Adabi et al., 2017). The integration of sophisticated digital atlasing in microscopy also discloses the ongoing advancement of this significant research area. The INCF Digital Atlasing Program aims at standardizing methods for constructing digital atlases of complex structures such as the rodent brain in order to make multidimensional data accessible for research purposes. This initiative shows the importance of implementing uniform standards that would enhance reproducibility and usability of microscopy findings among varied scientific disciplines. Through the development of sophisticated atlases, researchers can compare pathological states to baseline information for normal tissues and thereby gain a more complete understanding of disease mechanisms. With the advancement of the field, it is evident that microscopy will play an ever more important role in bridging the gap between basic and clinical practice, establishing its necessity in human histology research developments (Ng et al., 2009) (Figure 2.2).

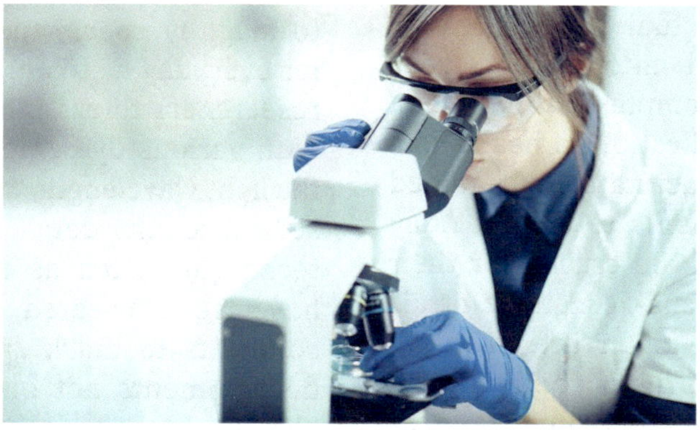

Figure 2.2. Microscopy.

Source: https://d36nqgmw98q4v5.cloudfront.net/image-handler/ts/20220323045633/ri/950/src/images/Article_Images/ImageForArticle_2183_16480257944042763.jpg.

Importance of Histology in Understanding Human Biology

Histology is a pillar of human biology research that provides important data on tissue structure and tissue function at the microscopic level. From the study of tissues, histologists can elucidate certain cellular compositions that are accountable for organ function and systemic interaction within the body. Such information turns out to be crucial in disease diagnosis, as most pathologies appear as particular histological changes. The application of contemporary microscopy techniques underpins this research, allowing it to deliver high-quality images that reveal the nuances of cell shape. Such methods ensure that anomalies can be detected at an early stage and hence are essential in medical diagnostics, treatment planning, and research of human illness. With the development of the histology field, its incorporation with modern teaching methods, such as virtual microscopy, further increases students' and professionals' appreciation of tissue biology (Peña-Fernández et al., 2019). Incorporation of the latest technology in the teaching of histology emphasizes its importance in contemporary medical education. Traditionally, the discipline has evolved from reliance upon light microscopes to newer technologies, such as immunohistochemistry and virtual microscopy. These advancements follow on from the educational trend towards student-centered materials, which assist the learning process without sacrificing academic rigor. Examples like DMU e-Parasitology demonstrate how digital resources may offer an interactive and complete comprehension of histological techniques. The possibility to control virtual slides in ways similar to conventional microscopy frees learning to navigate the complexities of human tissues and see their application to health and disease. In addition, it facilitates self-guided learning that allows students to delve deeply into the material that will be crucial for their later medical practice (Peña-Fernández et al., 2019). Lastly, histology is an intermediate science between basic science and clinical practice, emphasizing the interconnectedness of biological systems in solving human health. Through its constant inclusion of technological advances, the discipline not only remains pertinent but also essential in the context of a constantly evolving medical curriculum. The shift towards electronic materials and virtual microscopy confirms the need for multidisciplinary practice, integrating histology with clinical medicine to achieve an integrated understanding of patient care. With advances in learning processes, the role of histology in understanding human biology will continue to grow, allowing future healthcare providers to gain a better understanding of the complexities of human physiology and pathology. With such integration, histology prepares students well to handle present-day medical challenges (Hussein et al., 2015).

2.1. Types of Microscopy

Learning Outcome

1. Learn about light microscopy and its applications;
2. Describe the electron microscopy and its advantages;
3. Understand fluorescence microscopy and its uses in histology.

The learning of types of microscopy is important in enhancing our knowledge regarding human histology, particularly for efficient identification of cellular elements. Light microscopy remains a fundamental technique, relying on visible light to magnify specimens. It is extremely helpful for everyday histological examination, allowing researchers to examine tissue sections stained with various dyes. However, it is restricted by the light wavelength, which inhibits the ability to see subcellular detail. To avoid these restraints, techniques such as fluorescence microscopy have been created, employing fluorescent colorants to mark specific molecules. These developments not only enhance contrast but also enable observation of dynamic cellular processes and the provision of insights into molecular interactions that are crucial for interpreting mechanisms of disease. Electron microscopy is another revolutionary technique, with much greater resolution than light microscopy, with electron beams instead of photons. This technique allows the visualization of intricate detail at the ultrastructural level and is thus critical in the histological investigation of diseases such as cancer. Transmission electron microscopy (TEM), for instance, allows for the study of tissue architecture and cell organelles with unprecedented resolution. In cancers, for instance, basal cell carcinoma (BCC), electron microscopy has yielded critical information about cellular architecture and tissue organization. Such information regarding structure obtained with the aid of these tools is used by clinicians and researchers to understand disease causation and histopathological characteristics, and also leads to the formulation of targeted therapeutic strategies. Recent advances in microscopy have led to the integration of advanced imaging modalities, which have greatly enhanced diagnostic capability in human histology. Techniques such as two-photon microscopy and photoacoustic tomography exhibit promising results in non-invasive tissue assessment, thus overcoming the limitations of conventional histological methods. For example, ultrasound and photoacoustic modalities have been shown in research to produce highly resolved 3D images of skin lesions and correlate strongly with traditional histological Breslow thickness measurements (Kukk et al., 2024). Besides, the development of spectral- and time-resolved two-photon microscopy has allowed researchers to acquire accurate biochemical data without necessitating the use of invasive methods, thus making it possible to delineate tumor margins directly and with speed in BCC (Guo et al., 2024). Not only does this widen the diagnostic armamentarium, but it also sets the stage for personalized strategies for skin cancer, as well as other histopathological diseases

2.1.1. Light Microscopy and Its Applications

Light microscopy has seen tremendous development, changing its applications in human histology. Using this technique, cellular structures and tissue architecture can be observed and thus better understand normal and pathological states. Using variable magnifications, light microscopes can show minute details of cells required for diagnosing diseases. Recent advances, such as polarized-light methods, have brought about enhanced image quality and contrast, which have permitted the examination of complex tissues such as articular cartilage. Such advancement not only benefits histological research but also shows promise for tissue engineering applications in treating diseases such as osteoarthritis, reflective of the intersection of light microscopy and regenerative medicine (Matcher, 2009). Historically, histological analysis has relied on bright-field microscopy, which is time-consuming and requires complex tissue preparation, and can retard timely diagnostic approaches. Microscopy with ultraviolet surface excitation (MUSE) addresses these problems by providing fast, non-destructive imaging capabilities without the lengthy preparation time traditionally needed in traditional approaches. MUSE operates by using ultraviolet light, which selectively excites fluorescent markers in tissue surfaces, thus generating high-resolution diagnostic images within minutes rather than hours or days. Such efficiency not only enhances the quality of patient care but also facilitates the rapid translation of research findings to clinical use. As such, MUSE is an excellent example of how the use of light microscopy can be adapted to meet the needs of modern healthcare with high diagnostic accuracy (Fereidouni et al., 2017). The application of light microscopy is not restricted merely to visualization; it's also the key to seeking more advanced research in allied sciences and histopathology. Thanks to improved imaging technologies, researchers are now able to study cellular motion, tissue interactions, and disease mechanisms at an unprecedented resolution. The coupling of light microscopy with molecular diagnostics allows for an extensive study of the histological topography to uncover the working biology. This versatility can enable breakthroughs in the investigation of complex diseases as well as the development of targeted therapies. Moreover, through the presence of advanced methods in even low-resource settings, light microscopy serves to act as a knowledge bridge for better dissemination, enabling global health programs and guaranteeing high-quality diagnostic agents to become available in a range of healthcare environments (Figure 2.3).

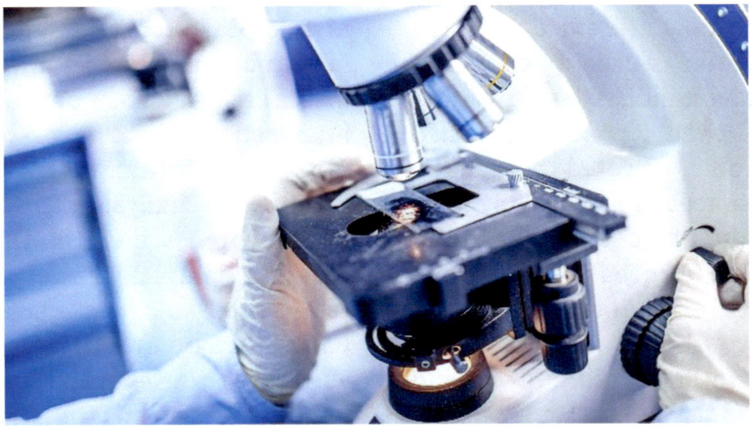

Figure 2.3. Light microscopy.

Source: https://assets.technologynetworks.com/production/dynamic/images/content/351924/an-introduction-to-the-light-microscope-light-microscopy-techniques-and-applications-351924-1280x720.webp?cb=12603659.

2.1.2. Electron Microscopy (EM) and Its Advantages

The development of EM has revolutionized human histology, providing nanoscale information on cellular and tissue structure unimaginable only a few years ago. In contrast to wavelength-limited light microscopy, electron microscopy uses electrons to achieve much greater resolution and depth of field.

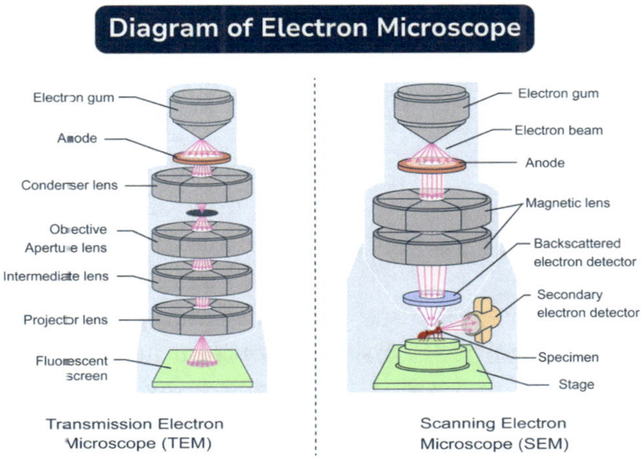

Figure 2.4. Diagram of an electron microscope.

Source: https://media.geeksforgeeks.org/wp-content/uploads/20240409132318/Diagram-of-Electron-Microscope.png.

This allows cellular components such as organelles, membranes, and cytoskeletal elements to be observed in detail. High resolution of EM enables the study of intricate cellular relationships and processes that are crucial in understanding physiology and disease pathogenesis. Electron microscopy is thus a valuable tool in research and clinical laboratory settings, facilitating the identification of properly different histopathologic conditions. One of the numerous advantages of electron microscopy is the visualization of cellular morphology with high precision. This aspect is particularly important for the investigation of complex tissues, where structural data can inform functional ability. A case in point is the segregation of myelin and axons, as demonstrated in recent publications, to provide requisite quantitative data on tissue microstructure. Approaches like AxonDeepSeg have seemed to facilitate the analysis of axonal and myelin structure from EM images by deep learning algorithms, largely simplifying data extraction and interpretation. These advancements underscore the potency of EM in performing detailed assessments of tissue integrity and function, as well as its applications for checking other imaging techniques, such as magnetic resonance imaging.

TEM is also crucial for determining cellular injury and organelle distribution, often producing detailed results that cannot be derived with routine methods. For instance, ultrastructural analysis to study embryo cytoplasmic fragmentation uses TEM as a tool to investigate the cause of developmental problems that affect fertility. This ability underscores the significance of EM in reproductive biology and other related fields because it has the potential to guide practices on how embryonic health may be improved. The establishment of protocols that would reduce damage caused to specimens during EM preparations is vital, reinforcing the necessity for continued innovation in histological methods. These advances allow for a better understanding of developmental processes and confirm the central role of electron microscopy in human histology research (Figure 2.4).

2.1.3. Fluorescence Microscopy and Its Uses in Histology

Fluorescence microscopy has transformed the field of histology, enabling one to better understand tissue architecture and the molecular etiology of several diseases. Compared to traditional bright-field microscopy, which can require extensive sample preparation and which can obscure intrinsic cellular detail, fluorescence microscopy permits visualization of discrete cellular components through utilization of fluorochrome-stained tissue. This technique enables cell structures to be investigated in high contrast and specificity by researchers and clinicians, facilitating the identification of pathological changes in tissues. With the aid of the specific fluorescent labels, it is now possible to target proteins, nucleic acids, and other biomolecules and thus reveal intricate information about cellular interactions and tissue structuring that were not readily separable prior. Such advancements are poised to improve diagnostic capabilities and patient outcomes in clinical settings, underscoring the pivotal role of fluorescence microscopy in contemporary histological methodology (Fereidouni et al., 2017). One of the superior applications of fluorescence microscopy in histology is in the detection of cancer. Through the technique, pathologists can label tumor markers to enable differentiation between malignant and benign tissue. The capacity to visualize definitive cellular features, including membrane proteins and intracellular signaling molecules, enables the identification of tumor subtypes, which is critical for the development of effective treatment strategies. In addition, fluorescence microscopy is amenable to the analysis of the tumor microenvironment, showing how adjacent tissues and different cell types engage to modulate tumor progression and treatment response. This complete approach not only assists pathologists in providing more accurate diagnoses but also opens the door to personalized medicine, where treatment regimens may be tailored to a patient's individual molecular profile of their tumor (Fereidouni et al., 2017). Fluorescence microscopy is also essential in the assessment of disease mechanisms at the level of the cell and the molecule. The use of advanced methods like fluorescence *in situ* hybridization (FISH) and immunofluorescence allows for the identification of specific patterns of gene expression and protein targeting within tissues. This is particularly useful in neurological disease research, where the visualization of neuronal populations and synaptic connections has the potential to shed light on disease pathology. The ability to monitor changes in gene expression and protein location in real-time contributes to our knowledge of dynamic biological processes along the trajectory of disease progression. However, researchers must be careful against certain limitations, such as the autofluorescence phenomenon, which may blind results whenever lower-strength promoters are used. However, the promise carried by fluorescence microscopy keeps pushing its application and advancement in histology and making it a cornerstone technique in modern-day biomedical science (Figure 2.5).

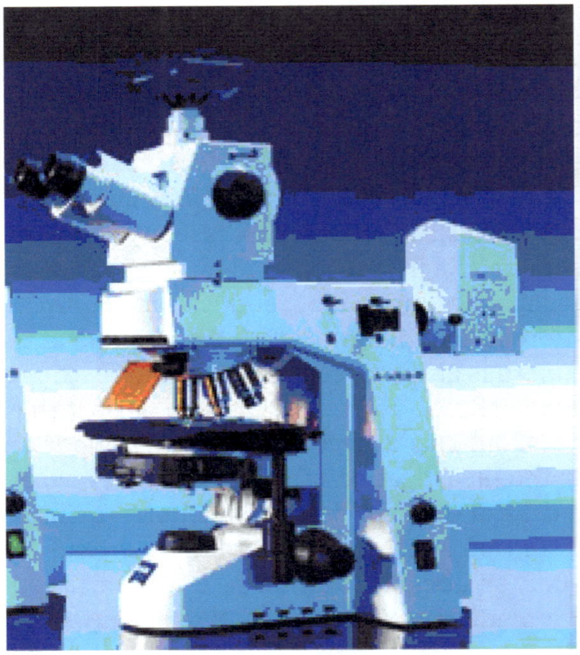

Figure 2.5. Fluorescence microscope.

Source: https://cdn.serc.carleton.edu/images/microbelife/research_methods/microscopy/fluorescent_microscope.gif.

Test Your Knowledge

1. What are the applications of light microscopy?
2. What are the advantages of electron microscopy?

2.2. Sample Preparation Techniques

Learning Outcome

1. Learn about fixation methods for preserving tissue samples;
2. Describe the embedding techniques for sectioning;
3. Understand the staining protocols to enhance the visibility of structures.

Sample preparation is the central theme in human histology to allow microscopic analysis. Traditional techniques may include meticulous processes such as fixation, embedding, sectioning, and staining to generate thin tissue slices for microscopic observation. Every process counts in preserving cellular morphology and making diagnostic information maximally visible. For instance, fixation is supposed to stabilize tissue structure by halting enzymatic activity and preserving proteins so that staining may be easier in subsequent steps. Furthermore, paraffin embedding allows for precise sectioning into micrometer-thick slices so that they can be mounted on glass slides with ease. However, such protocols have their drawbacks in that they take time and consume resources at the risk of delaying diagnosis and treatment in the clinic, particularly in high-stress situations where quick decision-making is crucial. Advances in microscopy technology have encouraged innovative solutions to sample preparation, attempting to counteract some of the inherent limitations. One of these methods is the use of microscopy with ultraviolet surface excitation (MUSE), which yields a rapid, slideless substitute for conventional histological processing. MUSE uses ultraviolet light to excite fluorescent stains on the surface that produce high-resolution images closely similar to those produced by standard histological techniques without the laborious preparation. Through offering instant access to diagnostic histological images, this technique is a far leap ahead in research and clinical practice. Interestingly, MUSE has also been shown not to have any detrimental effect on downstream molecular assays, maintaining sample integrity for further analysis while improving the tempo of histology, thus promising tremendous advances in patient care and research efficiency (Fereidouni et al., 2017). The repercussions of adequate sample preparation do not extend to mere diagnosis alone; they may deeply influence forensic science as well. In recent studies, the histological characteristics of burnt and unburnt cranial bone fragments were examined, and vital information to support forensic examination were determined. Series of cranial bone reference samples were made through standardized manual sectioning and semi-automatic grinding procedures to facilitate a scrupulous comparison of structural coherence prior to and following combustion.

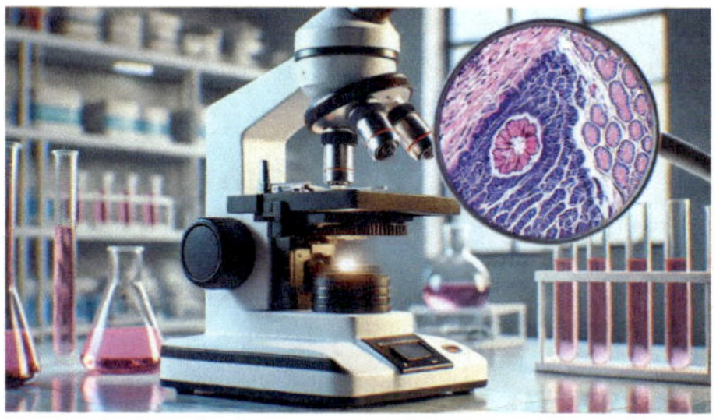

Figure 2.6. Histology sample preparation.

Source: https://wpengine-lmg-cl-blog.s3.amazonaws.com/wp-content/uploads/Histology-sample-preparation-1-980x561.jpg.

The resulting photomicrograph catalogue not only showed the histomorphologic preservation but also provided a stringent validated decision tree for the discrimination of human from non-human bone with excellent rates of accuracy. This data not only indicates the importance of accurate sample preparation in forensic use but also shows how histological techniques remain indispensable for resolving intricate identification issues in both burnt and unburnt samples, opening up a pathway towards greater reliability in forensic analysis (Simmons et al., 2016) (Figure 2.6).

2.2.1. Fixation Methods for Preserving Tissue Samples

Fixation methods are critical in the preservation of tissue samples for microscopic analysis in human histology, stabilizing cellular shape and preventing breakdown. The principal objective of fixation is to conserve the morphological and biochemical shapes of tissues for microscopic observation. Formaldehyde, glutaraldehyde, and alcohol solutions are the most commonly used fixatives, each having special advantages and disadvantages. For instance, formaldehyde is popular due to its tissue penetration and ability to cross-link proteins and thereby preserve cellular structure. However, its use may cause artifacts if applied incorrectly. As before, glutaraldehyde with greater cross-linking properties is usually used for electron microscopy, but it is too intense for certain tissues, which can be ruptured in the process. Consequently, a judicious choice of the fixation process must be exercised in relation to applications downstream as well as to the cellular features of interest. Effects of fixation processes extend beyond preservation; fixation impacts the quality of histological stain and visualization of cell material. For instance, fixation level can impact intensity and specificity of staining, crucial in delineating cell type and structural constituents in tissues. Under-fixation may result in the inability to preserve cellular morphology, which hides crucial diagnostic information. Optimal fixation, however, can enhance visualization of vital structures, such as organelles and extracellular matrix components, which can be critical in pathological assessment. It is imperative for histologists to correctly interpret results by understanding the effect of different fixation protocols on staining and microscopical outcome. This cross-talk between fixation and histology highlights the obligation to adhere meticulously to the procedure to gain consistent microscopical information. Recent advances are also being made to make tissue fixation more efficient and view complex 3D cell structures. For instance, recent advancements in optical coherence microscopy (SOCM) allow high-throughput imaging of large volumes of tissue with preserved native 3D architecture, with or without contrast agents. The method can possibly circumvent some of the drawbacks of traditional fixation and sectioning techniques, broadening the scope of tissue analysis. Furthermore, research into technologies such as 3D Bridging of Optically-clear histology with Neuroimaging Data (3D-BOND) suggests possible pathways for convergence of various imaging modalities, effectively mapping histological samples onto higher anatomical data. As such, new methods are developed, they may redefine tissue sampling and fixation benchmarks, enabling scientists to obtain more comprehensive observations of tissue microstructure and enabling clinical diagnostics and therapeutic development (Stolp et al., 2018; Min et al., 2020) (Figure 2.7).

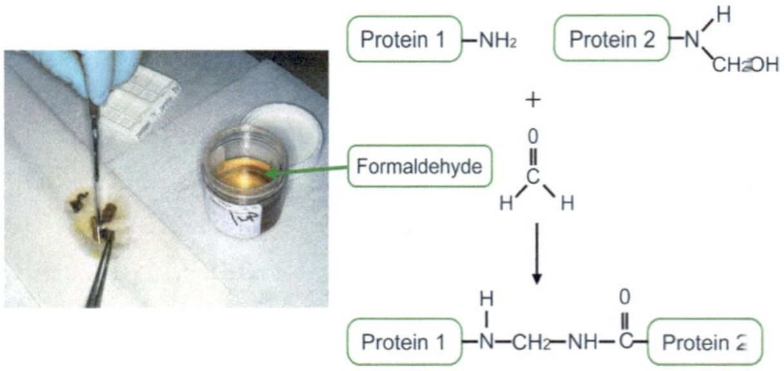

Figure 2.7. Fixation with Formaldehyde.

Source: https://s3.us-east-2.amazonaws.com/yalehistology/histological_features_of_cells/fixation_formaldehyde.jpg.

2.2.2. Embedding Techniques for Sectioning

The embedding processes applied in histology are of critical significance in managing the quality of tissue sections obtained for microscopic imaging. The primary role of embedding is to provide a rigid matrix that supports the tissue during sectioning to make sure that thin slices with accuracy are obtained, and can be imaged effectively using microscopy. Paraffin wax, being a historical embedding medium, remains in widespread use because it can be utilized with an extensive number of staining protocols and yet retains adequate preservation of tissue architecture. However, the application of paraffin does have certain shortcomings, primarily the inability to detail fine three-dimensional structure, so crucial to the proper understanding of highly intricate tissues. This limitation has led to efforts in investigating alternative embedding methods that may potentially improve visualization and analysis, as attested by advancements in imaging technologies that can bypass sampling limitations inherent in traditional sectioning methods (Min et al., 2020). Newly invented and innovative tissue embedding techniques have since been created that improve imaging capacities while maintaining the biological health of specimens to a greater degree. Techniques such as cryo-embedding, where the rapid freezing of tissues is achieved, and hydrogel-based embedding, where biocompatible materials are used to maintain structure, are some of the techniques that are prospective for histological applications. Hydrogel embedding also allows for encapsulation of soft and irregular tissues, which would be difficult to section accurately, thus allowing for more accurate volumetric analysis (Hsueh et al., 2017). These methods not only facilitate improved visualization but also enable high-throughput analysis, which enables researchers to analyze large quantities of samples with consideration of spatially complex structures. Moreover, these new methods can significantly advance the biomedical understanding of tissue pathologies through the provision of more informative datasets for assessment. The evolution of embedding methods has dramatic consequences for the science of human histology, particularly in pathophysiological states. Where conventional sectioning methods fall short in accurately reflecting the 3D tissue structure, advanced embedding procedures come to the rescue, and one may now achieve new perspectives on tissue-cellular interaction and dynamics. These methods are becoming indispensable for the examination of clinical materials, particularly for the exploration of the complex relationships in developing or diseased tissues. The ability to maintain native structures during the process of preparation enhances the prospect of accurate diagnosis and treatment planning, ultimately toward breakthroughs in personalized medicine. By applying these new approaches to the practice of histology, researchers can pave the way to improved knowledge of disease mechanisms and therapeutic targets, supporting the importance of embedding techniques as part of the overall approach of microscopy in human histology (Hsueh et al., 2017; Min et al., 2020) (Figure 2.8).

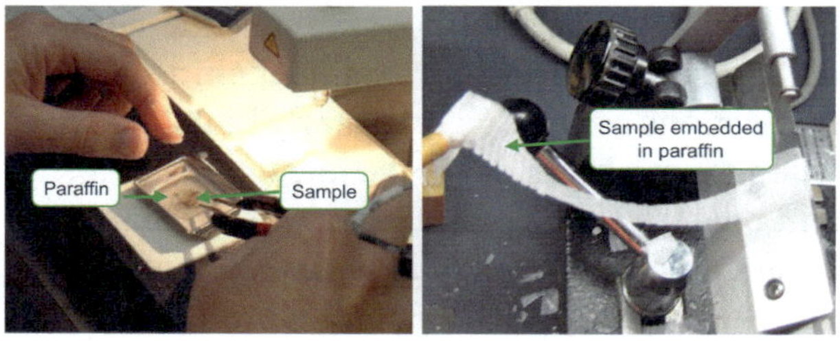

Figure 2.8. Embedding and sectioning sample.

Source: https://s3.us-east-2.amazonaws.com/yalehistology/histological_features_of_cells/embedding_sectioning_sample.jpg.

2.2.3. Staining Protocols to Enhance Visibility of Structures

The application of effective staining methods is at the core of enhancing the visibility of human histology structures critical for accurate microscopic analysis. Staining methods significantly increase tissue sample contrast, whereby pathologists and researchers can effectively identify cell morphology and organization. Traditional methods, such as hematoxylin and eosin (H&E) staining, are still extremely valuable to highlight general tissue features, but the creation of targeted contrast agents has provided new options for visualization. So, for instance, several of the most recent studies have investigated the use of iodine and tungsten-containing stains for microtomographic analysis of ovarian tissues, which are weakly radiopaque. Through the application of a variety of staining protocols, tissue structures can be emphasized to facilitate better understanding of complex biological systems, as described in research showing increased imaging capability with optimized staining methods. Additionally, which contrast agent used significantly determines what information can be gleaned from microscopy. It has been discovered through recent research that although tungsten-based agents are better at identifying larger structures, iodine-based agents possess a unique capability to reveal more minute details, which are required for acquaintance with some of the cellular constituents and their relationships. These distinctions assume a particularly important role when examining in detail the intrafollicular forms and ovarian follicle maturation, as is clear from recent advances in histological techniques. This versatility is expressed in their interaction with various energies during imaging, particularly in synchrotron radiation phase-contrast microtomography, leading to the enhanced definition of micro-anatomical structures. Hence, the proper choice and application of staining procedures are important in gaining integrated information regarding biological tissues. Keeping in mind this evolution, union of staining techniques with advanced imaging technology accounts for a significant advance in histological studies. Combining staining regimes with high-resolution images allows three-dimensional analysis of tissues, which reveals delicate details impossible to capture previously. Use of different energies in the imaging, which has been tuned to maximize contrast based on the specific metal used for staining, also increases the resolution and sensitivity of visualization. This dual-pronged strategy, besides maximizing the range of structures that can be visualized, also enhances the depth of the interpretative value of histological examinations. Therefore, the creation of staining methods, coupled with new imaging methods, is a significant advance in microscopy for human histology that provides opportunities for imaging not yet possible from biological samples (Figure 2.9).

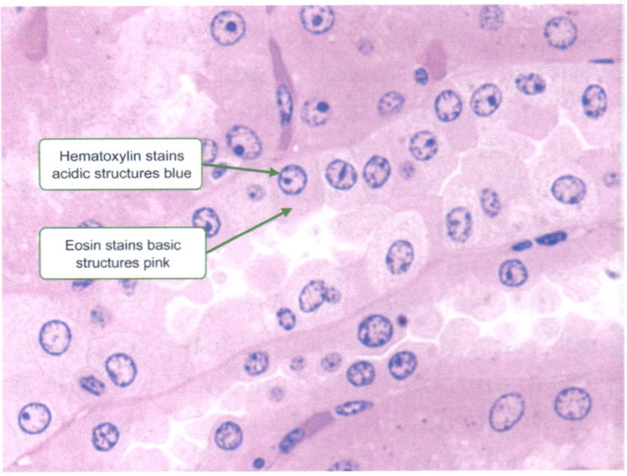

Figure 2.9. H&E-stained sample.

Source: https://s3.us-east-2.amazonaws.com/yalehistology/histological_features_of_cells/h_and_e_stained_sample.jpg.

Test Your Knowledge

1. Describe the fixation methods for preserving tissue samples.
2. What are the embedding techniques for sectioning?

2.3. Advances in Microscopy Technology

Learning Outcome

1. Understand the development of super-resolution microscopy;
2. Discuss about integration of digital imaging in histology;
3. Understand the future trends in microscopy research.

The microscopy technology has made remarkable advances that significantly enhance our understanding of human histology. One of the technological advancements is the fibered confocal fluorescence microscopy (FCFM), which has been designed to specifically observe the bronchial and alveolar mucosa in real-time during bronchoscopy. The technique involves a flexible miniprobe measuring only 1.4 mm and able to thread through the bronchial tree to provide information regarding the autofluorescence characteristics of lung tissues. Preferably, this capability of FCFM to image together with emission spectra has indicated significant structural differences in smoker and non-smoker tissues, e.g., greater autofluorescence of macrophages in the former. More developmentally advanced, FCFM's ability to investigate *in vivo* the bronchial and alveolar extracellular matrix can have profound implications for disease diagnosis and treatment of pulmonary diseases (Bourg-Heckly et al., 2008). Another significant technical breakthrough in microscopy is confocal laser endomicroscopy (CLE), which has emerged as an extremely useful tool for enhancing intraoperative precision during resections of malignant brain tumors. The imaging technique provides subcellular resolution, which enables neurosurgeons to observe tissue morphology in real time during surgery. Visualization of the fluorescence images, however, can be challenging for those who are not particularly trained. Existing efforts to bridge bioinformatics and deep learning to analyze CLE images have the promise of closing this gap. By employing advanced machine learning algorithms, researchers are developing tools that can classify images into diagnostic bins, such as glioma versus non-glioma, to provide improved decision-making and individualized treatment plans during surgery. Thus, CLE is not only revolutionizing the visual understanding of human histology but also enhancing the accuracy of surgical interventions (Izadyyazdanabadi et al., 2018). These advances in microscopy technology represent the shifting paradigms in the science of human histology from traditional static image analysis to dynamic real-time applications. The marriage of sophisticated imaging techniques such as FCFM and CLE provides a higher-resolution image of tissue microenvironments, which is essential for accurate diagnosis and treatment. The potential to image in real time also presents new horizons for scientists and clinicians to observe disease processes unfolding in real time and understand things that static histologic technologies could never reveal. As these new technologies are developed and applied to the practice of medicine, they have the potential to dramatically enhance our capacity to diagnose, treat, and understand human disease at a cellular and molecular level, ultimately to improve patient outcomes in histopathology (Bourg-Heckly et al., 2008; Izadyyazdanabadi et al., 2018).

2.3.1. Development of Super-Resolution Microscopy

The discovery of super-resolution microscopy has totally transformed the science of human histology by allowing scientists to visualize cellular structures with unforeseen detail and resolution. Light microscopy is hindered by the diffraction limit of light, restricting resolution to roughly 200 nanometers. Super-resolution imaging techniques, such as STED (Stimulated Emission Depletion) and PALM (Photo-Activated Localization Microscopy), are now powerful tools that bypass this limitation by exploiting the physics of fluorescent dyes and advanced imaging strategies. These techniques produce images that have the potential to reveal fine details of cell structures, thus enhancing the understanding of tissue architecture and disease. By overcoming classical microscopy limitations, super-resolution techniques are facilitating meaningful progress in the diagnosis and treatment of diseases like cancer and other tissue pathologies, which are significant parts of histological examination (Liue, 2024). Moreover, the incorporation of super-resolution microscopy into human histology holds profound clinical practice implications, particularly regarding wound diagnosis and therapy. Correct assessment of tissue and skin health is important, especially in the case of chronic wounds involving significant health hazards. Routine wound diagnosis often relies on subjective visual observation that may result in inconsistency in treatment methodologies. Super-resolution imaging facilitates more quantitative assessment of sample morphology with improved visualization of cellular interactions and structural integrity of tissues. These advances can aid plastic reconstructive surgery and aesthetic interventions by providing detailed information on the processes of tissue repair, which are crucial for efficient patient management. Improved understanding of cellular processes of wound healing can ultimately lead to better therapeutic strategies based on the particular demands of individual patients (Deka et al., 2016). Furthermore, the continuous evolution of super-resolution microscopy is accompanied by technological challenges and developments that widen its applicability. Researchers are currently exploring the integration of artificial intelligence, through deep learning algorithms, to enable improved data analysis and interpretation. Such vast amounts of data produced through high-resolution imaging need sophisticated computational techniques for image segmentation and processing. These technologies not only improve visualization but also streamline the diagnostic pipeline in the clinical setting. As the intersection of super-resolution microscopy and computational approaches develops, the prospect for research and clinical advances in human histology becomes increasingly evident. Ultimately, these evolving technologies will enable holistic views into cellular dynamics, disease pathology, and tissue regeneration and revolutionize our perspective on histological investigations and patient treatment (Liu, 2024) (Figure 2.10).

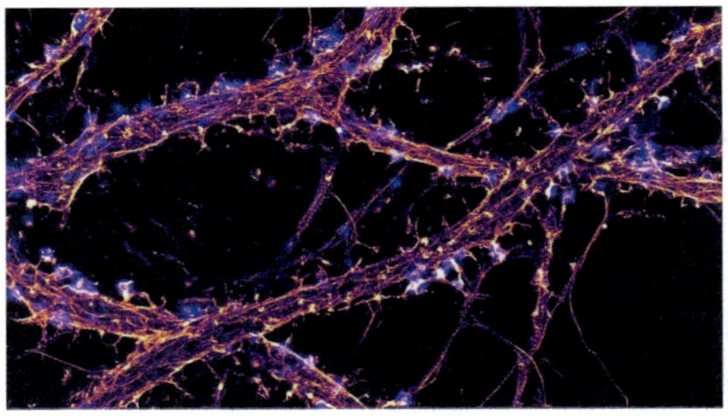

Figure 2.10. Super-resolution microscopy.

Source: https://assets.technologynetworks.com/production/dynamic/images/content/328572/what-is-super-resolution-microscopy-sted-sim-and-storm-explained-328572-1280x720.webp?cb=12153212.

2.3.2. Integration of Digital Imaging in Histology

Digital imaging integration in histology is a revolutionary innovation in the history of microscopy that has significantly enhanced the accuracy and speed of tissue analysis. Traditional techniques of histology involve long manual preparations, and hence, result in time lags as well as potential errors in analysis. The latest technologies, such as digital whole-slide imaging, allow for pathologists to capture high-resolution digital images of full tissue sections for live review and remote consultation. This shift not only enhances workflows but also diagnostic capability by enabling more precise pathological change identification. Besides, computer systems can support complex methods of image analysis that connect quantitative information and histology to provide solid findings regarding tissue structure and disease evolution, thereby consolidating digital imaging's central role in modern histopathology. Technological progress in imaging techniques also eliminates limitations associated with conventional thin-section histology. Conventional methods do not succeed in recording three-dimensional tissue-structural relationships, which form the core for understanding physiology and pathology. The finding of improved methods, such as biphasic hydrogel methods, has widened the scope of volumetric interrogation of irregular and sensitive tissue structures. The technique verifies the usefulness of non-destructive imaging, which permits quantitative analysis of normal and pathological conditions of tissue. With the help of these advanced imaging technologies, researchers can investigate a greater range of tissues, even recalcitrant tissues, which are difficult to investigate by conventional methods, and thereby pave the way for greater diagnostic accuracy and greater research potential in both clinical and academic settings (Hsueh et al., 2017). Also, modalities like microscopy with ultraviolet surface excitation (MUSE) illustrate once again the promise of digital histological imaging. This bright-field-free technique generates high-resolution images with less preparation time, providing an accessible alternative to bright-field microscopy. Besides generating diagnostic histological images in a matter of seconds, MUSE preserves tissue samples for downstream molecular assays such as fluorescence *in situ* hybridization and RNA sequencing. The ability to speed up histological evaluations enhances patient care through the provision of timely results, particularly in acute clinical situations. Also, MUSE illustrates the potential of digital imaging integration to be effective in both state-of-the-art and low-resource environments and thus avows its utility in modern-day histological practice (Fereidouni et al., 2017).

2.3.3. Future Trends in Microscopy Research

Future directions of microscopy research hold promise for revolutionizing the field of human histology by offering unprecedented insight into cellular and tissue architecture. With advances in imaging technologies such as super-resolution microscopy and cryo-electron microscopy, scientists can now see biological specimens at molecular resolutions that were previously considered unachievable. The technologies not only enhance image resolution but also facilitate real-time observation of cellular function, allowing dynamic examination of disease processes. Furthermore, new approaches such as multimodal imaging integrate various microscopy approaches, producing high-dimensional data that can be investigated in combination. Such methodological collaboration can better examine complex histological patterns, and with that, allow researchers to make useful biological conclusions that went undetected under conventional approaches. Coupled with technological advancements, automation and artificial intelligence (AI) trends are revolutionizing the practice of microscopy research. Automated imaging systems simplify the process of examining samples, significantly improving throughput while doing away with human error. The application of AI algorithms is particularly critical as it assists in image analysis through the detection of patterns and irregularities that are not readable to the naked eye. The technologies are capable of enhanced diagnostic accuracy and improved efficacy in histological assessment. Machine learning models also get better by learning through vast image databases, which results in greater analyses with time. The interaction between automation and AI portends a future in microscopy where advanced imaging methodologies can move beyond the confines of academic investigation into medical applications, solidifying microscopy's place in daily medical practice. Finally, microscopy research in simulated microscopy's future highlights the growing necessity of interdisciplinary research. By closing the gap among biology, engineering, and computational science, researchers can bring together various expertise to address intricate biological problems. For instance, the use of Ultrasound-targeted microbubble destruction (UTMD) as a new gene delivery method is a prime example of imaging and therapeutic approach convergence towards creating human histology applications. As in recent studies, UTMD has shown significant promise for enhancing transgene expression in retinal cells with little cytotoxicity (Li et al., 2009). This intersection of methods is meant to underscore the potential of microscopy to not only elucidate histological features but to actively participate in therapeutic discovery. The future of microscopy research promises to be utterly transformative for advancing significant advances in human disease and health, underscored by its central role in the scientific enterprise (Brauer et al., 2011).

Test Your Knowledge

1. Explain the development of super-resolution microscopy.
2. Describe the future trends in microscopy research.

2.4. Applications of Microscopy in Medicine

Learning Outcome

1. Describe the role of microscopy in diagnosing diseases;
2. Understand the importance of microscopy in cancer research;
3. Learn about the contribution of microscopy to regenerative medicine.

The development of microscopy technology has made a huge difference in the practice of medicine, particularly in the field of human histology. Microscopy enables the detailed examination of tissues at the cellular level to decipher an intricate landscape that underpins physiological and pathological processes. Classical methods, which most typically demand tissue cutting to thin sections for bright-field microscopy, are time-consuming and artifact-prone. This deficiency cripples timely diagnosis in the clinical laboratory. Emerging methods such as biphasic hydrogel methodology now enable high-throughput volumetric analysis of deformed tissue architecture, bridging the gap between conventional histology and current diagnostic needs. The ability to observe developing and diseased tissue in three dimensions opens doors for new opportunities to understand diseases like pancreatic disorders, eventually resulting in improved patient outcomes through increased diagnostic accuracy (Hsueh et al., 2017). Within new developments in recent years, new microscopy techniques have emerged that challenge conventional methods, with a concentration on speed and usability in diagnostics. For example, the method of microscopy with ultraviolet surface excitation (MUSE) offers a rapid, non-destructive substitute for traditional histological preparation. In comparison to traditional bright-field microscopy with time-consuming tissue preparation, MUSE can yield high-resolution images within minutes, hence accelerating the diagnostic process. In addition to maintaining the tissue integrity for additional molecular analysis, this method also provides essential histological details required for neoplasm diagnosis and other diseases. By infusing such technologies into routine practice, healthcare professionals can significantly boost the efficiency of patient care even in resource-poor settings, hence showcasing the extensive applicability of microscopy toward enhanced medical diagnosis (Fontaine et al., 2017). The far-reaching implications of high-resolution microscopy in human histology extend beyond individual prognosis to touch on the broader field of biomedical research and treatment strategies. Better imaging technologies provide better access to tissue morphology, cellular interactions, and the behavior of disease, enabling investigators to study pathophysiological processes with unprecedented confidence. Such advances facilitate the development of target therapies and personalized medicine by providing accurate histological descriptions that inform treatment decisions. Furthermore, as microscopy technology is constantly advancing and becoming increasingly standard, it will be able to bridge the gap between study and clinical practice, facilitating the easier translation of study findings into practice. Such convergence of state-of-the-art microscopy thus has the potential not just to revolutionize diagnosis but to increase our understanding of human disease and health (Fereidouni et al., 2017; Hsueh et al., 2017).

2.4.1. Role in Diagnosing Diseases

The role of microscopy in the diagnosis of disease is pivotal, particularly in human histology, where it is a crucial instrument for observing the structural lesions present in various pathological conditions. Microscopic examination allows for assessing tissue architecture, cell content, and any deviation from the normal. For example, histopathological tumor examination, where the ability to detect malignant over benign cells can drastically determine the direction of treatment. The challenge in diagnosing complex diseases like malignant mesothelioma highlights the need for accurate cytological and histological techniques. There has been established standardized diagnostic procedures to improve consistency and reliability to achieve a widely acceptable diagnostic protocol (Ascoli, 2015). Apart from tumor identification, microscopy plays a key role in infectious disease diagnosis. For instance, the characterization of pleural effusion is essential in the instance of suspected tuberculosis. Traditional diagnostic techniques are prone to yield sub-optimal results, and thus, the exploration of new approaches that are more specific and sensitive is initiated. Recent evidence shows that newer biomarkers such as IP-10 have the potential to provide valuable diagnostic information as they can differentiate between infectious and non-infectious pleural effusion (Dheda et al., 2009). In addition, the persistent attempt to apply these new tools in an integrative way with conventional practice is a step forward towards increasing diagnosis accuracy in clinical use. This is particularly in cases of high disease burden, whereby one can dramatically alter patient outcomes through early and precise diagnosis. The integration of microscopy with advanced diagnostic methods not only boosted the capability of pathologists to diagnose disease but has also facilitated the development of targeted therapeutic interventions. The holistic understanding of cellular and tissue-level changes empowers clinicians with critical information that guides therapeutic interventions. For example, the careful study of biopsy material can reveal distinctive histological patterns that direct therapeutic interventions in diseases like malignant mesothelioma and tuberculosis, ultimately leading to personalized medicine strategies. As science further refines these methods, the role of microscopy in disease diagnosis will necessarily expand, solidifying the place of microscopy as a cornerstone of medical pathology. This constant modification emphasizes the importance of continuous professional development for histotechnologists and pathologists for the acquisition of both traditional and new methods in effective disease diagnosis.

2.4.2. Importance in Cancer Research

Precision to visualize cells provided by microscopy is essential in cancer research. Standard histology procedures, while essential, are not sufficient in capturing the intricate relationships required to decipher cancers' rich biology. By utilizing advanced microscopy methodologies, researchers can inspect three-dimensional tissue structure more precisely. This allows spatial relationships in tumor microenvironments to be explored that more conventional thin-section histology can fail to detect. An example is biphasic hydrogel techniques, which have become a significant innovation enabling high-throughput volumetric tissue analysis, e.g., within cancer-affected tissues. Such methods' validation affirms their ability to reveal essential dynamics of oncogenesis and tumor growth, enabling greater insight into cancer pathology and treatment strategies (Hsueh et al., 2017). Its use in combination with digital and computational approaches also becomes more applicable in cancer research. The transition from conventional histopathology to digitized image analysis is a paradigm shift, in that machine learning algorithms can be applied for diagnosis. With tissue samples being scanned by whole slide scanners, computer-assisted diagnostic (CAD) technologies can be harnessed by pathologists and researchers to enable their diagnosis and provide more accurate disease forecasting and prognosis. These innovations not only streamline the pathologist's process but also contribute to more precise results in identifying cancer tissues. This juncture of high-tech imaging and computational diagnosis is a milestone in oncological studies that ultimately leads to more focused therapy and better patient outcomes (Gurcan et al., 2009). Additionally, the importance of microscopy in cancer research permeates into its application in therapeutic and clinical procedures. By the careful examination of tumor histology with levels of resolution previously out of reach, scientists are able to separate resistance mechanisms to existing treatments. This capability plays a key role in the design of personalized medicine strategies that rely on accurate histological information for tailoring treatment protocols to the individual patient. Visual information rendered by cutting-edge microscopy techniques can clarify numerous tumor characteristics, including heterogeneity and microenvironmental interactions, critical to the understanding of cancer behavior. Thus, the constant improvement of microscopy not only fuels research but also enhances the clinical management of cancer, backing its vigor in the fight against malignancies (Gurcan et al., 2009; Hsueh et al., 2017).

2.4.3. Contribution to Regenerative Medicine

Microscopy's contribution to regenerative medicine has played a key role in enhancing our understanding of tissue engineering and cell behavior. With the field attempting to create methods of repairing or replacing damaged tissues and organs, advanced imaging has emerged as essential. Traditional histological methods have paved the way with preliminary results, but their ineffectiveness in imaging volumetric structures holds back the development of regenerative approaches. The union of volumetric imaging techniques, most prominently those developed in microscopy, allows researchers to examine engineered tissue in its natural state. These improvements enable real-time assessment of tissue constructs, enabling scientists to image key processes like vascularization and cell distribution. By combining conventional histological principles with cutting-edge imaging modalities, the art of regenerative medicine is on the cusp of revolutionary breakthroughs, rendering engineered tissues an exact simulation of their natural counterparts. Of various imaging modalities, photoacoustic microscopy (PAM) is a sophisticated approach that amalgamates optical and ultrasound methodologies to bridge the limitations of traditional histological methods. PAM enhances the capacity to visualize the internal features of biomaterials and tissues in non-invasive manners, thereby yielding information regarding dynamic biological processes. This technology is particularly valuable in monitoring tissue breakdown and formation in engineered constructs, permitting assessment of the efficacy of regenerative strategies. By providing researchers with the ability to observe host tissue-biomaterial interactions, PAM provides more insight into engineered tissue interactions and function within the body. The ability to non-invasively delineate these interactions is a landmark in regenerative medicine, paving the way for greater interaction design and application of tissue-engineered products. With regard to the educational implications of this technology, integration of advanced microscopy in medical curricula is crucial to enabling future clinicians and scientists with the capability to handle the complexity of regenerative medicine. The shift from classical histology to modern imaging technologies follows the general trend towards more effective learning methods in medical school. The utilization of virtual microscopy and interactive imaging techniques not only improves students' understanding of the principles of histology but also emphasizes their application in clinical cases. By bringing histology course material up to date to include these advanced imaging methods, educational systems are equipping a new generation of doctors with the training and education that will be needed to cope with the complexities of regenerative therapeutic methods. This shift underscores the continued utility of histology, given that it remains pivotal in bridging the gap between basic science and clinical practice in regenerative medicine, underpinning the field's dynamic nature and potential to improve patient treatment.

Test Your Knowledge

1. What is the role of microscopy in diagnosing diseases?
2. Why is microscopy important in cancer research?

SUMMARY

In short, the application of microscopy to human histology is a basis for expanding our understanding of tissue structure and disease. Through the tool of optical imaging, sophisticated microscopy increases our ability to visualize cellular components and their interactions in the histological environment. This visualization is particularly significant in intricate tissues like the nervous system, where g-ratio, a measure of the thickness of myelin sheaths, is crucial to understand to appreciate the neuronal conduction velocity and neural function overall. The potential to measure such parameters *in vivo* with advanced imaging techniques is of central importance in grasping normal physiology as well as disease states, with attendant overreaching ramifications of the inclusion of microscopy into clinical research and diagnosis (Mohammadi & Callaghan, 2021). Further, the evolution of microscopy techniques remains to have even deeper impacts on the field of tissue engineering and regenerative medicine. For instance, advances in polarized-light methods and optical coherence tomography have been promising for articular cartilage evaluation, hence providing hints towards effective treatment modalities for diseases like osteoarthritis. Such new imaging methods are pivotal as they not only facilitate structure analyses at the minute level but also assist in tracking the efficacy of tissue engineering approaches (Matcher, 2009). The intricate relationship between microscopy and histology emphasizes the potential of developing novel therapeutic techniques, the basis of the need for ongoing research and refinement of such techniques in clinical practice. Summarily, the conclusion arrived through the convergence of microscopy in human histology realizes its revolutionary impact on scientific research and practical healthcare. As researchers move deeper into the domain of histological techniques, the convergent evolution of imaging technologies leads the way to unparalleled discovery and understanding of human tissues. The prospects for widespread disease diagnosis, monitoring, and therapeutic use are tremendous, promising future breakthroughs in medicine and biology. As we step further away from the old paradigms, the future of microscopy in human histology promises to unlock new horizons that will enrich our knowledge of human disease and health and, consequently, reveal something about the very nature of life itself.

The examination of microscopy in human histology brings forth some very critical information regarding the analysis and comprehension of cell structures. Among the key topics of debate is the digitization of atlasing, which significantly enhances research on histological specimens. The INCF Digital Atlasing Program aims to create an openly accessible database for information accumulated from rodent brains in a multidimensional presentation. Through the establishment of standards, guidelines, and policy recommendations, the program addresses the need for a coordinated recording and sharing of complex histological information. This kind of infrastructure not only supports the sustaining of knowledge gained but also research endeavors undertaken together. The emphasis placed on creating a centralized database affirms the importance of effective data management in enhancing histological study and looks toward the future where histology will benefit from novel imaging techniques to provide complete analysis (Ng et al., 2009). Also, the interaction between g-ratio mapping development and microscopy is another area of controversy in histological studies today. The g-ratio is a significant element to take into consideration when examining the function of neurons and, more specifically, conduction velocity, which is pivotal in neurological health and disease. The most recent developments in magnetic resonance imaging (MRI) technology allow for *in vivo* mapping of the g-ratio, the potential of which is a revolution in the way white matter integrity can be studied in human brains. By laying down methodological directions and some potential pitfalls in the use of MRI to quantify g-ratio, the discussion highlights the imperative for precise calibration against histological standards. The quest for valid *in vivo* biomarkers is an evolving recognition of microscopy and non-invasive imaging as intertwined sciences and our greater ability to examine and analyze human histology (Mohammadi & Callaghan, 2021). Finally, the application of digital imaging techniques to human histology has profoundly important implications for medicine and science. Advances in microscopy not only increase our ability to image detail in tissues but also make us better able to understand disease processes at the cellular level. High-resolution imaging techniques and their applications for studying myelin sheaths and neuronal features are noteworthy, most especially. Because scientists keep on innovating and experimenting with new imaging biomarkers, the relationship between basic histological study and clinical application becomes even more evident. This convergence fosters a hybrid approach that enhances diagnostics and therapeutic interventions, ultimately providing more enlightened interventions in neurodegenerative disease. By situating microscopy as a cornerstone of human histology, the discourse continues to enlighten and improve research protocols to address major healthcare challenges facing society (Ng et al., 2009; Mohammadi & Callaghan, 2021).

KEY TERMS FROM THIS CHAPTER

- Basal cell carcinoma
- Dermatopathology
- Extracellular matrix
- Histology
- Light microscopy
- Nuclei
- Organelles
- Biomedical sciences
- Electron microscopy
- Fluorescence microscopy
- Immunofluorescence
- Microscopy
- Optical coherence tomography
- Skin cancers

CRITICAL THINKING QUESTIONS

1. Which type of microscope is most commonly used in routine histological studies?

a. Electron microscope

b. Light microscope

c. Fluorescence microscope

d. Confocal microscope

2. The resolution of a light microscope is typically around:

a. 200 micrometers

b. 20 micrometers

c. 0.2 micrometers

d. 2 nanometers

3. Electron microscopy provides higher resolution because it uses:

a. X-rays

b. Shorter wavelengths of light

c. Electron beams instead of light

d. Magnetic fields

4. Electron microscopy is necessary for studying:

a. Gross organ structures

b. Intracellular structures like ribosomes

c. Blood cells

d. Tissues without staining

5. Confocal microscopy is particularly useful for:

a. Observing fixed tissue sections

b. Imaging thick specimens in 3D

c. Visualizing atomic structures

d. Studying live bacterial colonies

Short Answer Questions

1. What is microscopy in histology?
2. Why is histology important in human biology?
3. How many types of microscopy are there?
4. What are the methods of sample preparation?
5. What are the applications of microscopy in medicine?

Answers to Critical Thinking Questions

1. (b); 2. (c) ; 3. (c); 4. (b); 5. (b)

REFERENCES

1. Peña-Fernández, Antonio & Izquierdo, Fernando & Acosta, Lucrecia & Peña, María & Magnet, Angela & Evans, Mark & Torrado, Guillermo & Young, Chris. (2019). Virtual libraries of tissue and clinical samples: potential role of a 3-D microscope. 9132-9138. 10.21125/inted.2019.2269. (accessed on 7th August 2025).

2. Adabi, S., Clayton, A., Conforto, S., Daveluy, et al. (2017). *Universal in vivo textural model for human skin based on optical coherence tomograms.* http://arxiv.org/abs/1706.02758 (accessed on 7th August 2025).

3. Al-Ayyad, M. S., Al-Nabulsi, J., Owida, H. A., Turab, et al. (2024). *Available Medical Imaging Modalities for Melanoma Screening.* https://core.ac.uk/download/622481089.pdf (accessed on 7th August 2025).

4. Al-Delayme, R., Hamdoon, Z., Hopper, C., Jay, et al. (2012). *Structural Validation of Oral Mucosal Tissue Using Optical Coherence Tomography.* https://core.ac.uk/download/16220461.pdf (accessed on 7th August 2025).

5. Zaimi, A., Wabartha, M., Herman, V. *et al.* AxonDeepSeg: automatic axon and myelin segmentation from microscopy data using convolutional neural networks. *Sci Rep* **8**, 3816 (2018). https://doi.org/10.1038/s41598-018-22181-4(accessed on 7th August 2025).

6. Hsueh, B., Burns, V. M., Pauerstein, P., Holzem, K., Ye, L., Engberg, K., Wang, A. C., Gu, X., Chakravarthy, H., Arda, H. E., Charville, G., Vogel, H., Efimov, I. R., Kim, S., & Deisseroth, K. (2017). Pathways to clinical CLARITY: volumetric analysis of irregular, soft, and heterogeneous tissues in development and disease. *Scientific reports*, *7*(1), 5899. https://doi.org/10.1038/s41598-017-05614-4(accessed on 7th August 2025).

7. Ascoli, V. (2015). *Pathologic diagnosis of malignant mesothelioma: Chronological prospect and advent of recommendations and guidelines.* https://core.ac.uk/download/54521402.pdf (accessed on 7th August 2025).

8. Min, E., Ban, S., Lee, J. *et al.* Serial optical coherence microscopy for label-free volumetric histopathology. *Sci Rep* **10**, 6711 (2020). https://doi.org/10.1038/s41598-020-63460-3(accessed on 7th August 2025).

9. Dheda, K., Van-Zyl Smit, R. N., Sechi, L. A., Badri, M., Meldau, R., Symons, G., Khalfey, H., Carr, I., Maredza, A., Dawson, R., Wainright, H., Whitelaw, A., Bateman, E. D., & Zumla, A. (2009). Clinical diagnostic utility of IP-10 and LAM antigen levels for the diagnosis of tuberculous pleural effusions in a high burden setting. *PloS one*, *4*(3), e4689. https://doi.org/10.1371/journal.pone.0004689(accessed on 7th August 2025).

10. Gianoncelli A, Sena Souza G, Kourousias G, Pascotto E, Tafforeau P, Longo E, Barroso RC, Salomé M, Stebel M, Zingaro F, et al. Morphological and Chemical Investigation of Ovarian Structures in a Bovine Model by Contrast-Enhanced X-ray Imaging and Microscopy. *International Journal of Molecular Sciences.* 2023; 24(4):3545. https://doi.org/10.3390/ijms24043545(accessed on 7th August 2025).

11. Izadyyazdanabadi, M., Belykh, E., Mooney, M. A., Eschbacher, J. M., Nakaji, P., Yang, Y., & Preul, M. C. (2018). Prospects for Theranostics in Neurosurgical Imaging: Empowering Confocal Laser Endomicroscopy Diagnostics *via* Deep Learning. *Frontiers in oncology*, *8*, 240. https://doi.org/10.3389/fonc.2018.00240(accessed on 7th August 2025).

12. Fereidouni, F., Harmany, Z.T., Tian, M. *et al.* Microscopy with ultraviolet surface excitation for rapid slide-free histology. *Nat Biomed Eng* **1**, 957–966 (2017). https://doi.org/10.1038/s41551-017-0165-y(accessed on 7th August 2025).

13. Gurcan, M. N., Boucheron, L. E., Can, A., Madabhushi, A., Rajpoot, N. M., & Yener, B. (2009). Histopathological image analysis: a review. *IEEE reviews in biomedical engineering, 2*, 147–171. https://doi.org/10.1109/RBME.2009.2034865(accessed on 7th August 2025).

14. Bourg-Heckly, G., Thiberville, L., Vever-Bizet, C., Viellerobe, et al. (2008). *In vivo endoscopic autofluorescence microspectro-imaging of bronchi and alveoli.* http://arxiv.org/abs/0802.3783 (accessed on 7th August 2025).

15. Brauer, D. S., Hilton, J. F., Marshall, G. W., Marshall, et al. (2011). *Nano- and micromechanical properties of dentine: Investigation of differences with tooth side.* https://core.ac.uk/download/30695360.pdf (accessed on 7th August 2025).

16. Ng, L., Zaslavsky, I., Nissanov, J. *et al.* The INCF Digital Atlasing Program: Report on Digital Atlasing Standards in the Rodent Brain. *Nat Prec* (2009). https://doi.org/10.1038/npre.2009.4000.1(accessed on 7th August 2025).

17. Mohammadi, S., & Callaghan, M. F. (2021). Towards in vivo g-ratio mapping using MRI: Unifying myelin and diffusion imaging. *Journal of neuroscience methods, 348*, 108990. https://doi.org/10.1016/j.jneumeth.2020.108990(accessed on 7th August 2025).

18. Deka, G., Chu, S.-W., & Kao, F.-J. (2016). Skin Wound Healing Revealed by Multimodal Optical Microscopies. InTech. doi: 10.5772/64088(accessed on 7th August 2025).

19. Simmons, T., Goodburn, B., & Singhrao, S. K. (2016). Decision tree analysis as a supplementary tool to enhance histomorphological differentiation when distinguishing human from non-human cranial bone in both burnt and unburnt states: A feasibility study. *Medicine, science, and the law, 56*(1), 36–45. https://doi.org/10.1177/0025802415589776 (accessed on 7th August 2025).

20. Stolp, H.B., Ball, G., So, PW. *et al.* Voxel-wise comparisons of cellular microstructure and diffusion-MRI in mouse hippocampus using 3D Bridging of Optically-clear histology with Neuroimaging Data (3D-BOND). *Sci Rep* **8**, 4011 (2018). https://doi.org/10.1038/s41598-018-22295-9 (accessed on 7th August 2025).

21. Fedorov Kukk, A., Scheling, F., Panzer, R., Emmert, S., & Roth, B. (2024). Non-invasive 3D imaging of human melanocytic lesions by combined ultrasound and photoacoustic tomography: A pilot study. *Scientific Reports, 14.* https://www.semanticscholar.org/paper/699a8c86c337043a3fe431a1e3d695397c2b234b (accessed on 7th August 2025).

22. Guo, F., Lin, F., Shen, B., Wang, S., Li, Y., Guo, J., Chen, Y., et al. (2024). Multidimensional quantitative characterization of basal cell carcinoma by spectral- and time-resolved two-photon microscopy. *Nanophotonics, 13*, 217–227. https://www.semanticscholar.org/paper/8bd13f8e501ba6a7e78bea673912046534a41d5d (accessed on 7th August 2025).

23. Halvaei, I., Khalili, M., & Nottola, S. A. (2016). *A novel method for transmission electron microscopy study of cytoplasmic fragments from preimplantation human embryos.* https //core.ac.uk/download/54530668.pdf (accessed on 7th August 2025).

24. Korbar, B., Olofson, A. M., Miraflor, A. P., Nicka, C. M., Suriawinata, M. A., Torresani, L., Suriawinata, A. A., & Hassanpour, S. (2017). Deep Learning for Classification of Colorectal

Polyps on Whole-slide Images. *Journal of pathology informatics, 8*, 30. https://doi.org/10.4103/jpi.jpi_34_17 (accessed on 7th August 2025).

25. Hussein, I., Jurjus, A., Jurjus, R. A., Raad, et al. (2015). *Once Upon a Microscopic Slide: The Story of Histology*. https://core.ac.uk/download/230815267.pdf (accessed on 7th August 2025).

26. Kim, H. K., Cho, I. H., Hwang, E. A., Han, B. H., & Kim, B. H. (2024). Advancing river health assessments: Integrating microscopy and molecular techniques through diatom indices. *Water*. https://www.semanticscholar.org/paper/a69b342c87a8b95a8cf3b94da978dd4fca72a85e (accessed on 7th August 2025).

27. Li, F., Li, H., Wang, H., Du, L., Zheng, X., & Wu, Y. (2009). *Ultrasound-targeted microbubble destruction enhances AAV mediated gene transfection: Human RPE cells in vitro and the rat retina in vivo*. https://core.ac.uk/download/pdf/288309.pdf (accessed on 7th August 2025).

28. Liu, Y. (2024). *Computational Microscopy for Biomedical Imaging with Deep Learning Assisted Image Analysis*. https://core.ac.uk/download/622134427.pdf (accessed on 7th August 2025).

29. Matcher, S. J. (2009). *A review of some recent developments in polarization-sensitive optical imaging techniques for the study of articular cartilage*. https://core.ac.uk/download/50699.pdf (accessed on 7th August 2025).

30. Wang, H., Gong, D., Augustinack, J., & Magnain, C. (2023). Quantitative optical coherence microscopy of neuron morphology in human entorhinal cortex. *Frontiers in Neuroscience, 17*. https://www.semanticscholar.org/paper/c66ad9a9fa80886b40b0b501b04a403b597713d8 (accessed on 7th August 2025).

31. Wang, L. V., Xia, Y., & Zhang, Y. S. (2016). *Seeing through the surface: Non-invasive characterization of biomaterial-tissue interactions using photoacoustic microscopy*. https://core.ac.uk/download/77925002.pdf (accessed on 7th August 2025).

CELL STRUCTURE AND FUNCTION

3

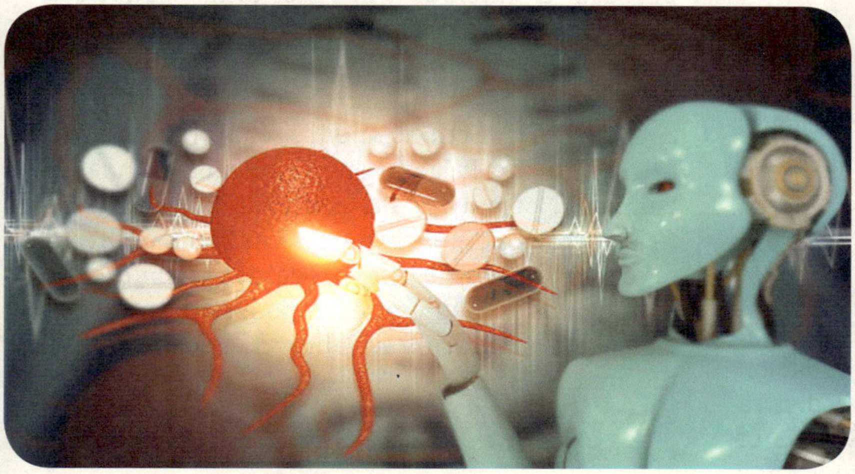

LEARNING OBJECTIVES

After studying this chapter, you will be able to:

1. Describe the basic cell structure;
2. Describe the types of human cells;
3. Learn about organelles and their functions;
4. Learn about cell division and growth;
5. Describe the cellular adaptations and responses.

Introduction

Cell structure and function play a central role in the discipline of human biology, as cells are the building blocks of life. All cell types have evolved to be specially suited to perform specific functions that are integral to health and homeostasis. For instance, muscle cells are suited for contraction, enabling movement, while nerve cells are suited for the transmission of signals throughout the body. This specialty demonstrates the principle of structure-function relationships in biology, where the morphology of a cell dictates its function within an organism. Therefore, a thorough analysis of types of cells, their morphology, and their respective functions is necessary to grasp the intricate mechanisms of human physiology. During the past few decades, breakthrough findings in cellular research have uncovered novel insights on cellular dynamics and their relationship with disease and health. Higher-order studies have employed genetic algorithms to explore how cellular automata function, isolating some rules that govern the behavior of cells in complicated biological processes (Yang & Billings,

1999). The new approach accentuates the sophisticated interdependencies between the shape and function of cells, such as the manner in which cells respond to environmental stimuli and are engaged in life-important activities such as metabolism and apoptosis. Therefore, exploring the relationship between cell structure and function not only informs us about normal physiology but also about the potential sites for therapeutic intervention across many diseases. In addition, the interaction of cellular processes can be watched with the eyes of multimodal data acquisition and increases our appreciation of how human cells function in a variety of contexts. The employment of structured memory modules in systems predicting human behavior is a classic example of such a strategy, wherein previous cellular information aids in decision-making operations (Fernando et al., 2019). By properly integrating different sources of information, researchers can model the complexity of human physiology and successfully predict cell behavior. This intersection of cell structure and predictive modeling not only deepens our knowledge of cellular function but also paves the way for innovative therapies aimed at the treatment of disease at the cellular level. Thus, the study of cell structure and function is an evolving field with significant implications for our knowledge of human health (Figure 3.1).

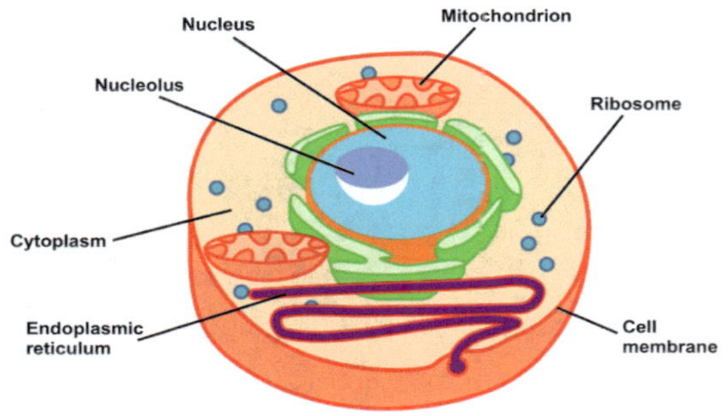

Figure 3.1. Cell Structure and Function.

Source: https://www.medicalexamprep.co.uk/wp-content/uploads/2020/04/Eukaryotic-Cell.png

Definition of Cells

Cells are the fundamental structural and functional units of life and the building blocks of all living things, including mankind. Since the smallest structural and functional units of life, cells, could be broadly classified as prokaryotic and eukaryotic cells. While there is no distinct nucleus and membrane-bound organelles in prokaryotic cells, such as bacteria, eukaryotic cells, found in higher organisms, possess a nucleus that contains genetic material. This dichotomy serves to highlight the evolutionary trend in cellular makeup that enables eukaryotic cells to undertake more specialized functions, hence enabling them to fit into the larger scheme of multicellular animals. Not only is the cell characterized by its structural complexity, but also by its ability to carry out basic life processes, including metabolism, growth, and response to stimuli, which are critical in enabling homeostasis in the human organism. The importance of cells extends beyond mere structure; they have an essential role in many of the physiological processes that keep us alive. Cells in humans also contain complex signaling machinery so that they can communicate and coordinate activity according to internal and external cues. These signaling pathways, consisting of a wide range of molecular interactions, can have profound effects on cellular behavior and are vital to overall health. Cells also possess specialized roles, as evidenced by distinct types like muscle cells and neurons, which possess unique structures and capabilities suited to their task. Moreover, the interconnectedness of various cell types reinforces the sophistication of human physiology, whereby coordination between several cells facilitates basic functions. Biomedical professionals need to realize, particularly in the knowledge that disturbances at the cellular level can lead to diseases. In addition to their structural and functional significance, cell research finds application in fields of medical research, as well as treatment.

For instance, the TCR study illustrates that similar sequences are often shared by various individuals and exhibit potential immune function accessible for utilization in therapeutic strategies in immunotherapy (Elhanati et al., 2018). Additionally, signaling pathway research has provided vital data on cellular communication and activity processes that control diverse health situations. The SignaLink database depicts the complexity of signaling interactions, which could be tissue type and human disease state dependent, supporting the need to understand cellular dynamics for the development of drug target discovery (Korcsmáros et al., 2010). As scientists learn more about cell structure and function, it is progressively clear that cells are not just the basic building blocks of life in the biological world but play a fundamental role in seeking new medical cures (Figure 3.2).

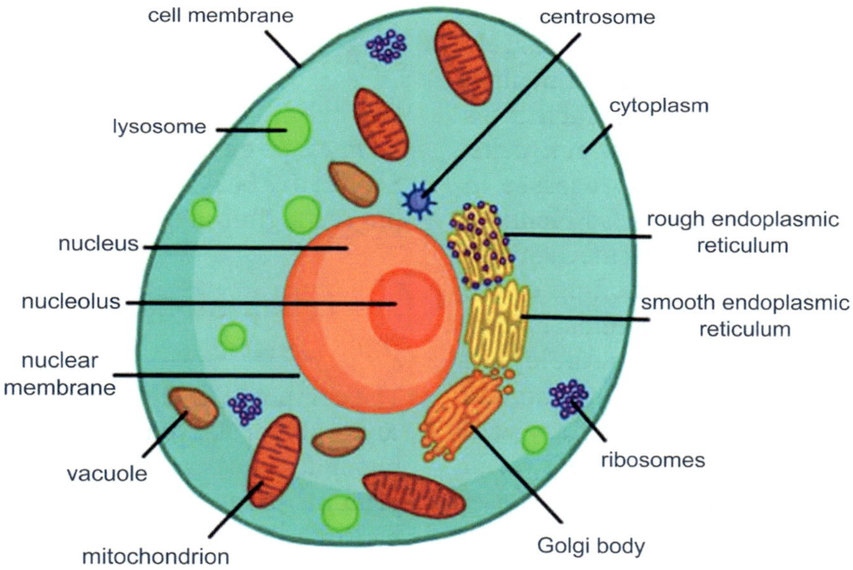

Figure 3.2. Cells in the human body.

Source: https://images.twinkl.co.uk/tw1n/image/private/t_630/u/ux/wiki-cells-1_ver_1.jpg.

3.1. Basic Cell Structure

Learning Outcome

1. Describe the cell membrane composition and function;
2. Understand the cytoplasm and its components;
3. Describe the nucleus and genetic material.

The building blocks of simple cell structure form the foundation of all forms of life, including the human organism. In the simplest form, cells consist of two simple forms: prokaryotic and eukaryotic cells. Prokaryotic cells, typically single-celled organisms like bacteria, lack a fixed nucleus and membrane-bound organelles. Eukaryotic cells in more complex organisms like humans, however, have a well-defined nucleus with genetic material. This structural disparity is paramount in cellular activities, as eukaryotic cells can isolate various metabolic processes in organelles, thereby maximizing efficiency in general. The presence of various structures, like mitochondria to produce energy and the endoplasmic reticulum for protein synthesis, is a validation of the intricacies of eukaryotic cells and to accentuate their role in sustaining life within human tissues and organs. Core to an understanding of cell structure is the concept of the plasma membrane, the essential role of which is homeostasis. The semipermeable membrane surrounds the cell and regulates the passage of substances in and out of the cell and, therefore, serves as a selective barrier to the external environment. Composed largely of a bilayer of phospholipids with embedded proteins, the plasma membrane facilitates communication and signaling between cells, which is crucial to coordinated processes in tissues. The membrane proteins also facilitate other processes, including transport mechanisms and cell identification. The functioning of the plasma membrane is crucial to human health; changes in its integrity create pathological conditions such as cancer and autoimmune disorders, illustrating how elementary cell structure plays a direct role in the overall physiological status of an organism. Closer inspection of cell structure reveals the intricate functions of cytoskeletal elements, which impart structural integrity and shape to the cell. The cytoskeleton, which consists of microfilaments, intermediate filaments, and microtubules, plays a critical role in cellular dynamism and integrity. The network not only maintains the shape of the cells but also helps in intracellular transport through the movement of vesicles and organelles in the cell. The cytoskeleton is also involved in significant processes like motility and cell division. More recent cell biology studies have further highlighted the cytoskeleton's sensitivity to mechanical stress as a marker for its involvement in signaling pathways that control how cells respond to external stress. The understanding of cytoskeletal structure is thus pivotal in appreciating how cells perceive their environment, the basic part of the broader theme of cell structure and function in humans (Figure 3.3).

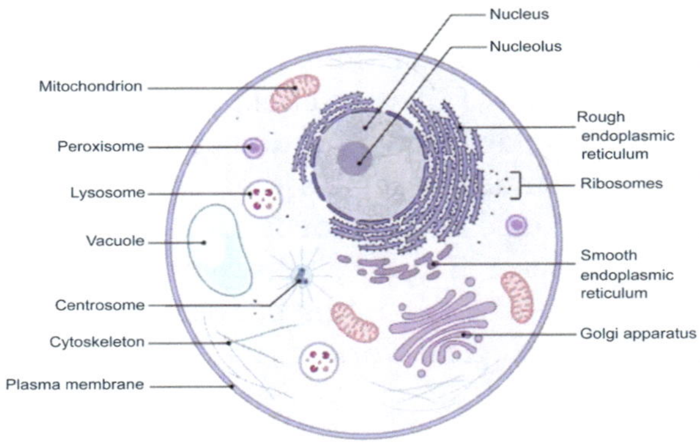

Figure 3.3. Human cell structure.

Source: https://biologynotesonline.com/wp-content/uploads/2025/03/Structural-Overview-of-an-Animal-Cell.png?ezimgfmt=ng:webp/ngcb1.

3.1.1. Cell Membrane Composition and Function

The composition of the cell membrane is crucial to its numerous functions, primarily due to its phospholipid bilayer structure with embedded proteins, cholesterol, and carbohydrates. The hydrophilic heads and hydrophobic tails of the phospholipid molecules create a semipermeable membrane that regulates materials coming in and going out and maintains the inside homeostasis. Integral and peripheral proteins play crucial roles in transport processes. For instance, transport proteins can ensure glucose uptake, in GLUT1 of erythrocytes, to support cellular metabolism and energy production. The transport represents the requirement of membrane composition in ensuring cellular functions like oxidative stress response and metabolic adaptation. Therefore, the intricate balance of lipid and protein composition of the membrane is vital to numerous physiological processes, affecting the general operation and survival of cells. In addition to its structural roles, the cell membrane is also a signaling center that picks up and transmits signals that regulate cell behavior. In the lipid bilayer, membrane proteins also serve as receptors that react with extracellular material such as hormones and neurotransmitters. This contact creates signal transduction cascades that translate extracellular stimuli into equivalent cellular responses. For instance, membrane signaling cascades can control gene expression, enzyme activity, and cell metabolism, exemplifying the cell membranes' critical role in having an organized response to external change. The dynamic interaction between lipid environments and membrane proteins also influences the efficiency and specificity of signaling, emphasizing the importance of membrane composition in determining cell-intrinsic function. Thus, a deeper investigation of such processes reveals how alterations in the composition of membranes can lead to altered signal transduction, and hence to a variety of diseases, such as mitochondrial disease. In addition, variations in cell membrane composition correlate directly with cellular metabolic function and well-being. As illustrated by GLUT1-deficient reticulocytes, alterations in membrane protein expression can significantly affect cell metabolism without affecting vital developmental processes. The absence of GLUT1, by restricting glucose importation and perturbing metabolic equilibria, does not otherwise impair red blood cell function in the promotion of oxygen transport. Instead, it initiates within the cell compensatory responses that affect antioxidant metabolism and cellular resilience in general. This finding suggests that the cell membrane is not a passive barrier but an active participant in cellular health and metabolism, which initiates adaptations to change. Thus, a comprehensive understanding of cell membrane structure and its associated functions gives valuable information regarding human physiology since it gives an insight into how cellular integrity and function sustain human life in various pathological and physiological contexts (Figure 3.4).

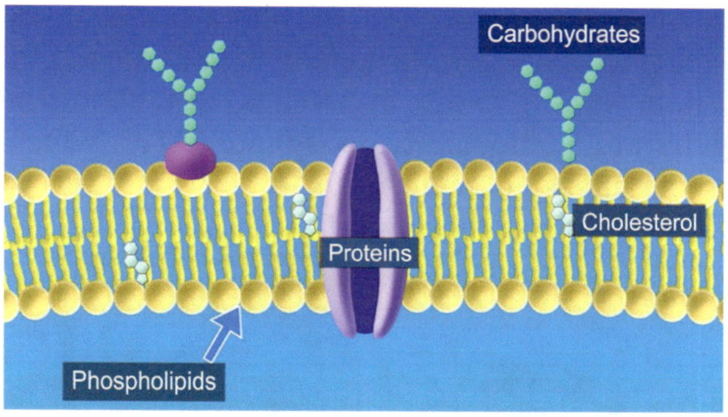

Figure 3.4. Cell membrane structure and function.

Source: https://i.ytimg.com/vi/fJfTDc3WzQ8/maxresdefault.jpg.

3.1.2. Cytoplasm and Its Components

Cytoplasm, the jelly substance that fills the interior of a human cell, is crucial in the maintenance of cellular structure and the facilitation of numerous biochemical activities. Carrying all of the organelles, the cytoplasm is also the site of such major metabolic activities as protein synthesis, cellular respiration, and cellular signaling. Within this context, the cytoskeleton, composed of microfilaments, intermediate filaments, and microtubules, functions in the structural support and intracellular transport. The cytoplasm's fluidity allows organelles to share information and collaborate, enabling required functions to go on uninterrupted. The integrity of cytoplasm therefore largely depends on the health and functionality of cells, which is the foundation for general human tissues and organ well-being. Cytoplasm comprises various organelles that each have specific activities required for cell function. The endoplasmic reticulum (ER), dividing into smooth and rough regions, is particularly responsible for lipid and protein synthesis, respectively. Once synthesized, these units are transported in vesicles to the Golgi apparatus for additional modification and sorting. Additionally, lysosomes, also referred to as the waste disposal system, play a fundamental role in cell debris breakdown and recycling. Underpinning these organelles, mitochondria generate adenosine triphosphate (ATP), which is the energy currency.

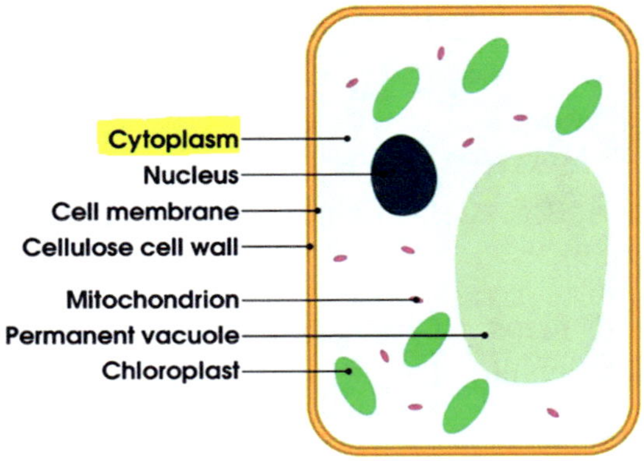

Figure 3.5. Structure of cytoplasm.

Source: https://biologynotesonline.com/wp-content/uploads/2021/11/Cytoplasm.webp?ezimgfmt=ng:webp/ngcb1.

Abnormalities within these structures of the cytoplasm can lead to impaired cellular function, which can eventually impact human health, justifying the role of the cytoplasm in supporting life. Current studies indicate intricate relationships between cytoplasmic structures and participation in disease transmission. For example, the apicomplexan parasites Toxoplasma and Plasmodium utilize special organelles within the cytoplasm to successfully invade and hijack host processes, demonstrating the adaptability of cytoplasmic structure in disease states (Tomavo et al., 2013). These processes indicate how valuable it is to understand the dynamics of the cytoplasm not only in terms of normal cellular function but within the context of infectious disease as well. Second, the dialogue between epigenetic mechanisms and cytoplasmic components puts the spotlight on the general perspective of cell function, illustrating how nuclear and cytoplasmic activities lead to cellular identity and plasticity (Costa & Frezza, 2014). Thus, grasping the complexity of the cytoplasm plays a significant role in gaining insight into cellular function and disease in humans (Figure 3.5).

3.1.3. Nucleus and Genetic Material

The nucleus is a fundamental organelle of eukaryotic cells that serves as the command center of cellular activities through the regulation of gene expression and the deposition of genetic information. Enveloped by a double lipid bilayer known as the nuclear envelope, the nucleus not only protects DNA but also facilitates the transcription and RNA processing activities. This compartmentalization allows eukaryotic cells to possess a distinct environment for DNA transcription that is fundamental to stimulating accurate and efficient gene expression. The nucleoplasm, the semi-fluid matrix of nucleoids surrounding chromatin and nucleoli, contains required components like nucleotides and enzymes that are vital for DNA and RNA synthesis. In addition, nuclear pore complexes incorporated in the nuclear envelope provide selective transportation of molecules between the cytoplasm and nucleus, thereby maintaining the integrity of cellular processes while still enabling essential communication with other cellular compartments. At the center of the nucleus is chromatin, a DNA-protein complex that packs the genetic material in an orderly manner. Chromatin is present in two states: euchromatin, which is less compacted and is actively engaged in transcription, and heterochromatin, which is more compacted and typically transcriptionally silent. Such structural plasticity is essential in facilitating the dynamic control of gene expression and enabling cells to adapt to changing environments. Chromatin arrangement is also important in genome stability maintenance and replication control. Furthermore, methylation and acetylation of histones—proteins on which DNA is wound—are involved in controlling chromatin structure and influencing gene expression directly. Therefore, the interaction between genetic regulation and chromatin dynamics shows the complexity of the nucleus as a cellular function center. Genetic material, primarily deoxyribonucleic acid (DNA), contains information necessary for the development and functioning of all living organisms. Human DNA consists of approximately 3 billion base pairs arranged into 23 pairs of chromosomes, each being a repository of genes responsible for phenotypic characters and biological processes. Accurate replication of DNA during the process of cell division is critical to maintain genetic continuity from one generation to the next, emphasizing the importance of the various repair mechanisms conserved by the nucleus to correct mistakes. Besides, the expression of specific genes through messenger RNA (mRNA) controls the development of proteins that play a significant role in the cell's functions. Present studies, such as research on the role of DISC1 in brain connectivity and genetic susceptibility to psychiatric disease, provide insight into how specific genetic factors can control complex traits and more clearly outline the intricate relationship between genetics and cellular function in human beings. Thus, the nucleus and its contents are focal not only for cellular functions but also for the total biological diversity in human beings (Rose, 1999; Dawson et al., 2015) (Figure 3.6).

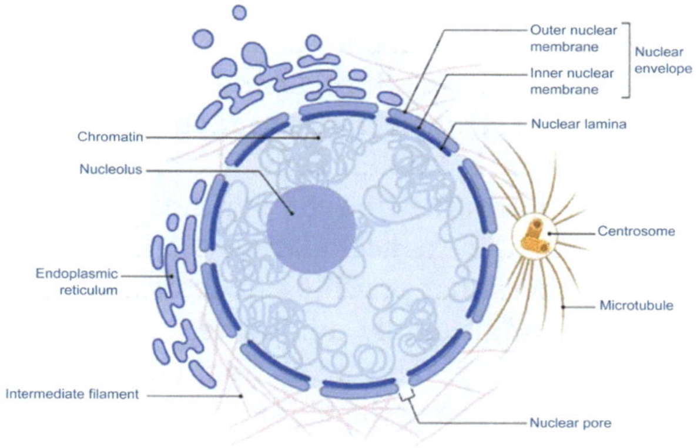

Figure 3.6. Structure of the nucleus.

Source: https://biologynotesonline.com/wp-content/uploads/2024/08/Cell-Nucleus-Structure.png?ezimgfmt=ng:webp/ngcb1.

Test Your Knowledge

1. What is the composition of the cell membrane?
2. What is cytoplasm and its components?

3.2. Types of Human Cells

Learning Outcome

1. Describe the epithelial cells and their roles;
2. Understand the muscle cells and contraction mechanisms;
3. Learn about neurons and signal transmission.

The human body holds more than 200cell types, all designed to perform specific functions for the overall physiology. Maybe the most significant types are epithelial cells, which construct barriers to protect and enable absorption and secretion. These cells line organs and body cavities, suggesting flexibility in shape and function depending on location. For instance, the lung epithelial cells are flat and thin to enable rapid gas exchange, while those of the intestines are columnar with microvilli for improved nutrient uptake. This heterogeneity demonstrates how cellular structure is closely associated with function, underpinning the body's complex systems and shedding light on the mechanisms of functioning in various organ systems in humans, as outlined in studies on human embryonic stem cells accounting for the development processes of differentiated cell types in maintenance and function (Ren et al., 2009). Yet another significant category consists of connective tissue cells, whose role is to support and attach body structures. Examples include cells such as fibroblasts and adipocytes, cells that are structurally and functionally quite distinct from epithelial cells. Fibroblasts, for example, have the job of synthesizing and maintaining the extracellular matrix, a complex array of fibers that provides structural support to tissues. Additionally, adipocytes are devoted to energy storage and insulation, emphasizing the fundamental metabolic roles that connective tissue cells undertake. Strikingly, the diversity among these cells, from cartilage-forming chondrocytes to bone-residing osteocytes, reflects their evolutionary adaptability to meet specific physiologic needs. The critical role played by these cells of connective tissue in physiology varies from healing to stress response, as indicated by the expression patterns found in studies concerned with cellular responses to disease conditions (Chen et al., 2010). The muscle cell category is another overarching one that is tasked with movement and mechanical activity in the human body. These cells are generally classified into three categories: skeletal, cardiac, and smooth muscle cells. Skeletal muscle cells enable voluntary movements and are identified by their striated character due to the ordered arrangement of myofilaments. Cardiac muscle cells, striated but involuntary, are suited for rhythmic contractions to pump blood throughout the body, while smooth muscle cells line hollow organs and enable involuntary movements. This specialization of muscle cells is needed for the maintenance of body functions such as circulation and digestion. Also, the special structural elements of such cells, e.g., the occurrence of intercalated discs in cardiac muscle, contribute to their functional efficiency, bearing witness to the close association between cellular structure and body function in humans (Ren et al., 2009) (Figure 3.7).

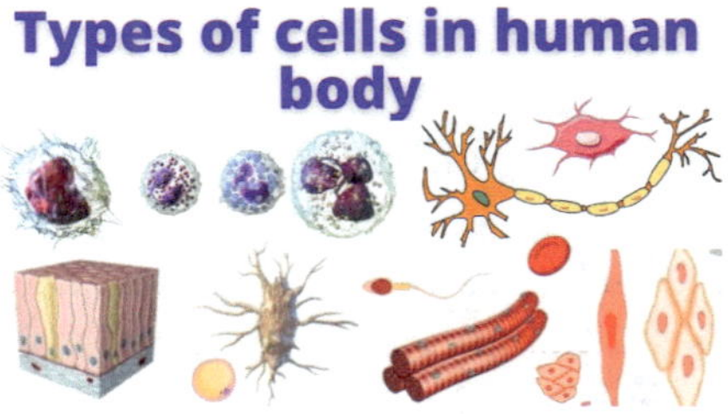

Figure 3.7. Types of cells in the human body.

Source: https://i.ytimg.com/vi/g68bAHCEv-k/maxresdefault.jpg.

3.2.1. Epithelial Cells and Their Roles

Epithelial cells are the building blocks of the human body and exhibit vital functions due to their particular structural characteristics. The cells form unbroken sheets that enclose internal as well as external surfaces such as skin, respiratory passages, and digestive passages. It facilitates selective absorption, secretion, and sensation, thus having a crucial function in homeostasis. Furthermore, epithelial cells are also important for the formation of barriers, as evidenced by the existence of tight junctions that restrict paracellular transport, pointing to their function in ion and solute transport. Components like MarvelD3 have been found in recent studies to play a role in junctional function, pointing further to the complexity and significance of epithelial cell shape in cell-to-cell contact as well as permeability properties (Steed et al., 2009). Epithelial cell activity extends beyond mechanical support; they are actively engaged in metabolic and immune functions. In the gastrointestinal tract, for instance, epithelial cells perform key functions like nutrient transport and biochemical metabolism, having specialized cells that mount immune reactions inside. The fact that they can respond to adjacent cells and the underlying immune system illustrates their two-way activity in homeostasis and defense mechanisms. Moreover, the vulnerability of such cells to pathogens results in infection, as with *Candida albicans*, which exploits epithelial cells by a molecular mimicry of host molecules like E-cadherin and N-cadherin (Phan et al., 2007). The mode of interaction suggests the dynamic interaction between the epithelial cells and pathogens, emphasizing the need for robust epithelial integrity to prevent disease. The importance of the function of epithelial cells can be highlighted by an exploration of their capacity for tissue regeneration and repair. When injury or disease occurs, epithelial cells have the apparently miraculous ability to multiply and reorganize to restore barrier functions. This is tightly regulated by several signaling mechanisms that illustrate the plasticity and robustness of epithelial tissues. Failure of these pathways can lead to pathological events, such as cancer. Epithelial cell conversion into a mesenchymal state, or epithelial-mesenchymal transition (EMT), plays a critical role in tumor development and metastasis. Understanding these processes illuminates novel therapeutic strategies to enhance tissue healing or prevent tumorigenesis, demonstrating the significance of epithelial cells in health and disease (Figure 3.8).

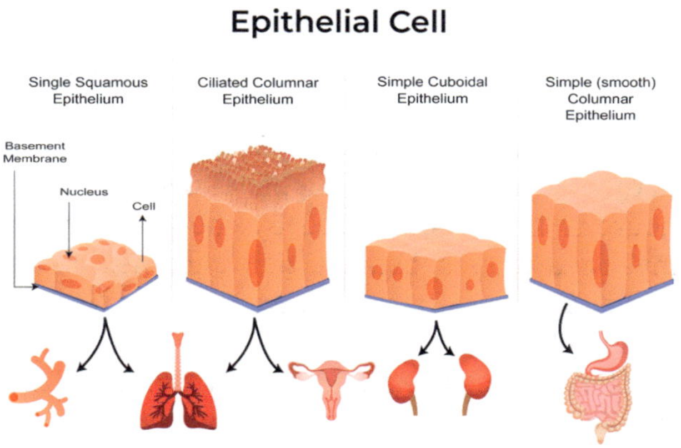

Figure 3.8. Epithelial cells.

Source: https://media.geeksforgeeks.org/wp-content/uploads/20220706123250/Epithilialcells.png.

3.2.2. Muscle Cells and Contraction Mechanisms

Muscle cells, or myocytes, are crucial to the mechanics of motion and functioning of the body, characterized primarily by their ability to contract. There are three types of muscle tissue in humans: skeletal, cardiac, and smooth muscle, each different in structure and function. Voluntarily controlled skeletal muscle consists of long, striated fibers that permit locomotion, while cardiac muscle fibers in the heart possess inherent rhythmic contractions to keep blood flowing. Involuntary smooth muscle cells appear in hollow organs such as the intestines and blood vessels and are responsible for digestion and regulating blood pressure. The exact structural make-up of a muscle type determines how it contracts and thus makes an appreciation for cell structure the key to human physiology in general. Contraction of muscle cells relies on complicated biochemical processes, primarily revolving around myofilaments—actin and myosin. Contraction of skeletal and cardiac muscle depends on the sliding filament theory, in which actin filaments are attracted to myosin heads, pulling them inwards and thus shrinking the muscle fiber. This is initiated by an intracellular increase in calcium ion concentration, which acts with troponin to result in a conformational change that reveals the actin-bound myosin-binding sites. In addition to calcium-dependent mechanisms, new evidence indicates that calcium-independent mechanisms via RhoA-Rho kinase (ROCK) and protein kinase C (PKC) are important in the control of muscle contraction, particularly in smooth muscle cells. Their comprehension not only provides information regarding the normal function of muscle tissue but also explains therapeutic practices in the case of disorders characterized by impaired muscle contraction. With other pathological situations, such as hypertension, vascular smooth muscle cell regulation is of utmost importance. Regulation of the contraction of these cells directly relates to vascular resistance and blood pressure control and therefore to severe health risks such as heart failure and stroke. Vascular smooth muscle cells are highly plastic, alternating between the contractile and proliferative phases upon pathological stimulation, which affects their function and contractile effectiveness. The increase in intracellular calcium content favors actin-myosin cross-bridge formation, but dysregulation of the signaling pathway may lead to adaptive muscle function.

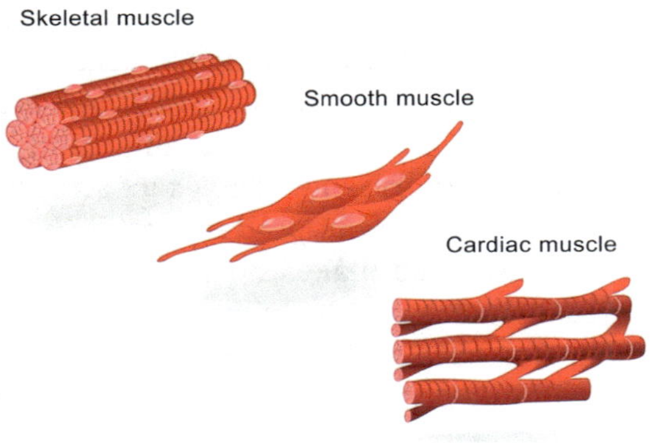

Figure 3.9. Muscle cells.

Source: https://www.sciencelearn.org.nz/_next/image?url=https%3A%2F%2Fwww.datocms-assets.com%2F117510%2F1722387917-types-of-muscle-tissue20161111-16640-1c2x74o.jpg%3Fw%3D1840%26h%3D1231.5930388219545&w=1920&q=85&dpl=dpl_4n9pVfrF4H6vbtWLHqt8okXU1ahu.

It therefore becomes imperative to examine the interaction between muscle function and disturbed signaling pathways, since they have the potential to provide greater insight into the pathophysiological pathways of vascular reactivity during disease states such as hypertension (Touyz et al., 2018). Furthermore, cell communication mechanisms like extracellular matrix contacts and growth factors also have a crucial role to play in determining muscle cell behavior during healing and repair processes, once again putting fibroblast function at the forefront of tissue structure maintenance. Awareness of collagen fiber alignment and its impact on cellular movement sheds light on fibrotic responses to muscle damage once more highlighting the intricacy of muscle cell responses to varying stimuli (Maini et al., 2005). In totality, the relationship between muscle cell structure, mechanisms of contraction, and external factors forms a network that is complex in nature and fundamental to the maintenance of overall physiological balance within the human body (Figure 3.9).

3.2.3. Neurons and Signal Transmission

Neurons, the fundamental units of the nervous system, are central to the complex processes of signal transmission in human beings. These specialized cells are designed to receive, process, and transmit information in the form of electrical and chemical messages. Structural components of a neuron, i.e., the cell body, dendrites, and axon, enable this capability. Dendrites are receptive surfaces upon which synaptic inputs from other neurons can influence the electrical status of the neuron. When a neuron reaches a level of a certain degree of excitation, it discharges an action potential, a rapid flow of ions that is propagated along its axon to tell other neurons or muscles. This rapid transfer of information is vital to coordinating physiologic responses and sensory processing, and thus illustrates the significance of neuronal anatomy in facilitating effective transmission of signals in the human body. The efficiency of signal transmission in neurons is also enhanced by the presence of myelin, a fatty substance that sheathes axons and supports saltatory conduction. Myelinated axons allow action potentials to leapfrog from node to node of Ranvier, small pores in the myelin sheath. This mechanism greatly increases the speed of conduction of electrical impulses greatly increased so that rapid communication over distances is possible within the nervous system. Moreover, it is the interplay between excitatory and inhibitory signals that maintains the fine balance necessary for optimal neuronal response. Malfunctions in this transmission of signals could lead to neurological disease, illustrating the delicacy of neuronal systems. More understanding of the mechanisms behind these two signal transduction mechanisms is imperative since it is particularly relevant to the pathogenesis of therapeutic interventions employed to manage neurodegenerative diseases, where the neurons' signaling is compromised. Recent research on the ubiquitin signaling system (USS) highlights its pivotal status in the regulation of neurobiological processes, including signal transmission by neurons. The USS is implicated in protein degradation and activity, which controls neuronal health and function. Notably, the Anaphase-Promoting Complex (APC), which has multiple subunits and is an E3 ubiquitin ligase, is linked to different developmental and signaling processes in post-mitotic neurons. Studies that investigate the APC in model systems such as *Caenorhabditis elegans* illustrate its function in chemosensory function and find that disruptions in APC function can reroute routes of neuronal communication. The significance of these studies extends beyond simple model systems since the conservation of neuronal mechanisms between *C. elegans* and humans has the potential to inform us on human sensory function and resultant disease. Such information can ultimately guide therapy to restore damaged neuronal circuits and enhance our general knowledge regarding how neuronal signal transmission plays a crucial part in human physiology (Herms et al., 2004; Wang et al., 2016).

Test Your Knowledge

1. What are the epithelial cells and their roles?
2. Name the three types of muscle tissue.

3.3. Organelles and Their Functions

Learning Outcome

1. Learn about mitochondria and energy production;
2. Describe the ribosomes and protein synthesis;
3. Discuss the endoplasmic reticulum and cellular transport.

In the colorful world of cellular biology, organelles are mandatory entities that permit an array of functions necessary to sustain life. Organelles such as mitochondria, lysosomes, and endoplasmic reticulum each possess their own distinct function that contributes to the overall homeostasis of human cells. Mitochondria, which are also known as the powerhouses of the cell, are responsible for energy production in the form of aerobic respiration that yields ATP, the energy that drives cellular functions. In addition, lysosomes are the cell's garbage collecting system, using enzymes to break down and recycle cell debris. This organelle differentiation demonstrates the intricacy and efficacy of cellular functions, enabling organisms to promote their structural integrity and adapt to shifts in metabolism. Lastly, the exploration of organelles within parasitic organisms offers valuable insights into cellular machinery that can be applied to human health. For instance, the secretory organelles in apicomplexan parasites such as *Toxoplasma gondii* provide insight into the remarkable adaptations of these parasites to infect host cells. The specialized secretory structures, including micronemes and rhoptries, play a critical role in the invasion process by binding to host cell membranes and signal pathways. The biogenesis and operation of these organelles require a complex interplay between the endoplasmic reticulum and Golgi apparatus, as evidenced by results linking the trafficking of these proteins to endosomal-like compartments (Jackson et al., 2013; Tomavo et al., 2013).

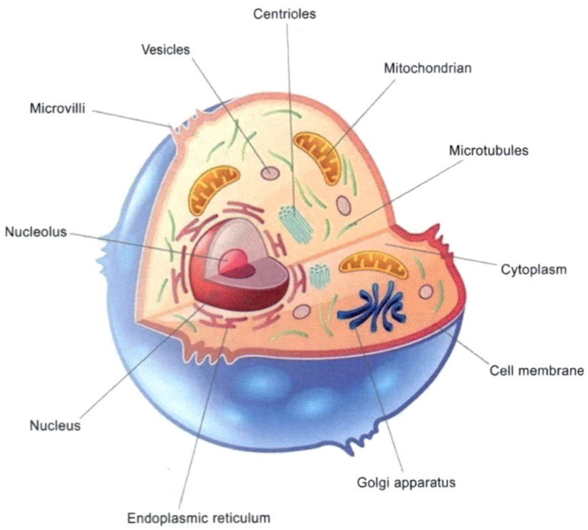

Figure 3.10. Organelles.

Source: https://d2jx2rerrg6sh3.cloudfront.net/image-handler/ts/20160602012811/ri/590/picture/2016/6/shutterstock_250674061.jpg.

This intricate system of organelle operation not only signifies the veracity of cellular functions but also suggests lines of potential therapeutic interventions intended to forestall these invasive mechanisms. Lastly, organelle analysis extends beyond structural description to encompass their functional relevance in disease and health. Each organelle performs vital functions, and the integrity of the organelle is directly involved in overall cellular function. Discoveries that are made with the observation of organelles in human cells and model systems lead to a deeper understanding of how these organelles affect metabolism, signaling, and developmental biology. As scientists increasingly break down the complexity of organelle function, it becomes increasingly clear that their interactions and relative capacities are interrelated. By continuing to study these cellular components, scientists can gain a greater understanding of cellular physiology and potentially develop targeted therapies for diseases resulting from organelle dysfunction or organelle manipulation by disease-causing pathogens (Figure 3.10).

3.3.1. Mitochondria and Energy Production

Mitochondria, which have become familiarly referred to as the cell powerhouse, are critical organelles responsible for the production of ATP, the primary energy currency in biological organisms. The production of ATP begins with the degradation of carbohydrates, lipids, and proteins, leading to the generation of acetyl-CoA, which is routed to the tricarboxylic acid (TCA) cycle. Throughout this process, energy-rich electrons are transferred to electron carriers such as NADH and FADH2. The carriers transfer the electrons to the electron transport chain (ETC) found in the inner mitochondrial membrane, where oxidative phosphorylation takes place. This very sophisticated mechanism not only highlights the essential role of mitochondria in energy production but also their control over cellular homeostasis and metabolism, thereby confirming the importance of these organelles in sustaining life. Current research has revealed the intricate relationship between mitochondrial function and intracellular signaling pathways, particularly in energy production as a reaction to cellular demands. Mitochondria also interact intensively with nuclear genomes to control cellular homeostasis, as certified through two-way communication that controls metabolic activities. Evidence suggests that mitochondrial bioenergetics is controlled through cyclin B1/CDK1 complexes in the sense that they coordinate energy production with cell cycle and other physiological demands (Jiang et al., 2019). This dynamic relationship reflects how mitochondria not only generate energy but are also fuel sensors for cellular needs, leading to cell adaptation and survival, especially under fluctuating stress conditions or disease states, e.g., cancer or metabolic disorders. Mitochondrial dysfunction has high-stakes implications, most prominently in the pathophysiology of numerous diseases, e.g., brain cancers, e.g., glioblastoma (GBM).

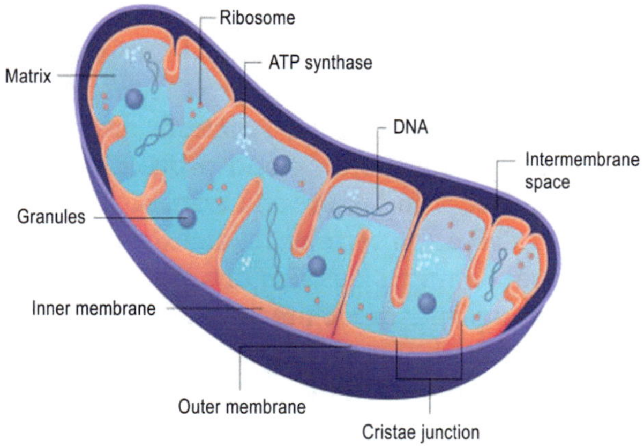

Figure 3.11. Mitochondria.

Source: https://media.istockphoto.com/id/1166599563/vector/vector-diagram-of-mitochondria-cross-section-view-medical-infographics.jpg?s=612x612&w=0&k=20&c=mc8xzwONuy6XO5CShe6elZHy4nyk3CMRznmCGNLfuRo=.

Mitochondrial protein alterations have been linked with disease onset, with a study involving 256 mitochondria-associated proteins and significant clinical alterations in 117 proteins in GBM patients (Deighton et al., 2014). Of special note is the higher abundance of proteins in the oxidative stress response pathway identified together with the reduction of respiratory chain components, pointing towards a core disruption of mitochondrial energy metabolism. The phenomenon of cristolysis, which is a mitochondrial structural change, further displays the complexity of mitochondrial dysfunction and its impact on cellular energy production. Explanation of these pathological alterations provides useful information on potential therapeutic targets in conditions complicated by mitochondrial dysfunction (Figure 3.11).

3.3.2. Ribosomes and Protein Synthesis

Ribosomes play a critical role in the synthesis of protein, necessary for cellular structure and function in humans. Such complex molecular machinery can be found in several cell locations, including the cytoplasm and attached to the endoplasmic reticulum, leading to the classification of ribosomes as bound or free. Their intricate composition consists of proteins and ribosomal RNA (rRNA) that work together in the translation of mRNA into polypeptide chains. This translation is critical because it takes the genetic information in DNA and converts it into proteins that function to perform a variety of biological activities. Thus, ribosomes not only enable the one-way transmission of genetic information but also yield the location where cellular response to environmental alteration can be invoked speedily, once more highlighting their central role in cellular adaptation and homeostasis. Protein synthesis, initiated with mRNA binding to the ribosome, proceeds through three primary phases: initiation, elongation, and termination. At the initiation stage, ribosomes engulf the strand of mRNA, and transfer RNA (tRNA) molecules deliver amino acids to the ribosome based on the codon sequence of the mRNA. This precise anticodon-mRNA codon correspondence is vital for fidelity during protein synthesis. Elongation follows initiation when ribosomes orchestrate the formation of peptide bonds between the amino acids to form longer chains of polypeptides. It consists of various elongation factors and energy in the form of guanosine triphosphate (GTP). The termination process terminates protein synthesis upon encountering a stop codon, leading to the ejection of the completed polypeptide by the ribosome and its subsequent disintegration, an activity that ultimately decides on the nature and amount of protein produced by the cell. Ribosomal protein synthesis is also closely associated with the overall function of the cell because abnormalities in the ribosomal proteins can lead to varied cellular and developmental anomalies.

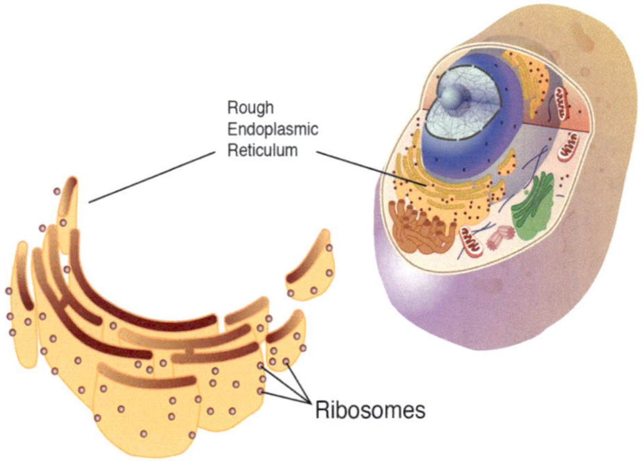

Figure 3.12. Ribosome.

Source: https://www.genome.gov/sites/default/files/tg/en/illustration/ribosome.jpg.

It has been demonstrated through experiments that mutations in genes that encode ribosomal proteins may have several phenotypic abnormalities, such as the Minute syndrome observed in organisms like *Drosophila melanogaster*. This syndrome demonstrates that ribosomal function abnormalities may lead to abnormal protein synthesis, which is required for growth and fertility. Furthermore, identification of numerous cytoplasmic ribosomal protein genes and their localization to genetic loci further demonstrates the importance of ribosomes for cellular integrity. Overall, the intricate relationship between ribosomes, protein synthesis, and human cell function highlights the importance of correct regulation of these functions to obtain proper cellular response and adaptations, as explained in recent studies (Marygold et al., 2007) (Figure 3.12).

3.3.3. Endoplasmic Reticulum (ER) and Cellular Transport

The ER plays a key role in maintaining cellular homeostasis and protein transport essential for cellular processes. The organelle exists in a tubular and sac membranous network in two forms: rough and smooth. The rough ER, which is covered with ribosomes, is primarily involved in protein synthesis and the folding of proteins that will be secreted or incorporated into the membrane. The smooth ER, in contrast, is associated with lipid synthesis as well as detoxification. Understanding ER function is important, as most cellular functions are based on correct protein folding and processing. For instance, aberration in protein transport across the ER can result in serious cellular dysfunction, which again emphasizes this organelle's role in cellular blueprints of architecture and processes (Miesbauer et al., 2010). Endoplasmic reticulum dysfunction may initiate an activity referred to as ER stress, which deforms protein folding and trafficking. These disturbances have the capability of initiating several pathological pathways, further establishing the ER's essential role not just in protein transport but also in cell signaling and stress responses. Misfolding in certain proteins has the capability of causing them to accumulate and thus be harmful, like in neurodegenerative disorders. For example, the mislocalization of prion proteins, which are vital for neuronal function, can be neurotoxic in their consequences when they are transported inappropriately into the cytosol under stress (Miesbauer et al., 2010). This complex regulation of protein biogenesis and misfolding thus reveals the multifaceted relationship between ER functioning and disease, implying that the understanding of these mechanisms could yield avenues of treatment based on targeting cellular transport mechanisms. In addition, the endoplasmic reticulum is important in cellular communication and metabolic transport functions apart from protein synthesis. The ER is a gateway to various intracellular transport pathways, regulating the admission and discharge of gigantic molecules using transport mechanisms such as caveolar uptake and retrograde transport. These pathways are particularly beneficial for therapeutic intervention aimed at enhancing drug delivery within cells. Recent studies with the entry routes of the pathogen, including the routes via prion proteins, show that the employment of such endocytic pathways may promote the efficiency of therapeutic molecules. Thus, the endoplasmic reticulum not only ensures proper protein transport but also plays a pivotal role in the grand cellular transport dynamics and therapeutic strategy planning. Multifunctional roles of ER indicate the significance of ER in cellular organization and human physiology (Figure 3.13).

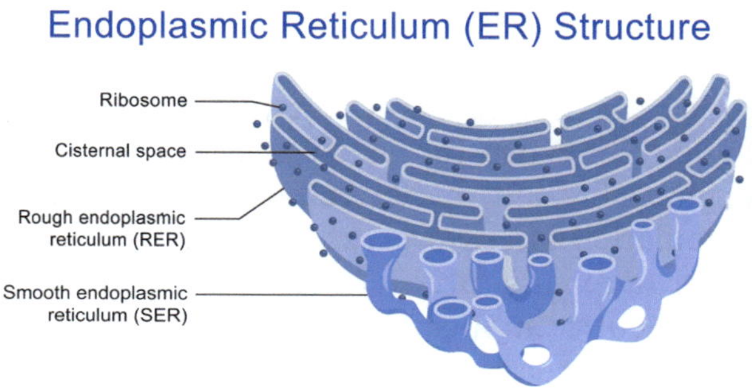

Figure 3.13. Diagram of endoplasmic reticulum (ER).

Source: https://microbenotes.com/wp-content/uploads/2024/03/Diagram-of-Endoplasmic-Reticulum-ER.jpeg.

Test Your Knowledge

1. What is the role of mitochondria in energy production?
2. What is the role of ribosomes in protein synthesis?

3.4. Cell Division and Growth

Learning Outcome

1. Describe the mitosis and its phases;
2. Understand the meiosis and genetic diversity;
3. Understand the regulation of the cell cycle.

Cell growth and division are critical processes that ensure the growth and survival of living organisms, particularly man. Cell cycle involving interphase and mitotic phases is accountable for normal cell function and cell reproduction. Interphase consists of three phases: G1, S, and G2, in which the cell increases in size, its DNA is duplicated, and it prepares to divide. Mitosis follows, resulting in two identical daughter cells with the parent cell's genetic material. Cyclins and cyclin-dependent kinases regulate this process tightly so that division is efficient and precise. Cell division abnormalities may lead to a variety of diseases, including cancer, where unchecked growth makes normal tissue growth and tissue homeostasis challenging. The symphonic orchestration of these cell processes is at the heart of understanding human cellular structure and function. Furthermore, cell division is important not only as a replication process but also in tissue repair and regeneration. For example, during injury to tissues, the ability of cells to divide and regenerate lost or damaged cells is critical for healing. Such regenerative capacity is controlled by many growth factors and signaling pathways that adjust repair processes in such tissues as skin or liver. The immune reaction also relies on skilled cell division because immune cells divide to effectively combat pathogens. The understanding of these processes is important not just for general biology but also for medical use, like tissue engineering and regenerative medicine. The modulation of cell processes that are involved in growth and proliferation has important therapeutic implications in clinical therapy and the generation of biopharmaceuticals, as highlighted in reflections in biotherapy (Gallucci & McCarthy, 1995).

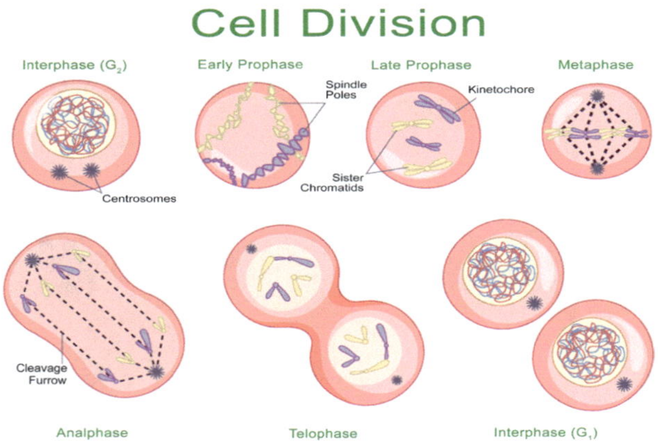

Figure 3.14. Cell division diagram.

Source: https://media.geeksforgeeks.org/wp-content/uploads/20230320155637/Cell-Division.png.

From the perspective of reflecting upon advances in cell biology, investigations of cell division pathways have revealed intricate networks of control that operate not just in growth, but differentiation, which determines the specialized function of cells in organisms. Studies have shown that specific proteins and gene regulators are the keys to dictating the fate of cells, deciding whether they will grow, differentiate, or undergo programmed cell death. The more they learn about the process, the more technologies like genetic engineering will enlighten us on how to manipulate cellular behavior for therapeutic purposes. This finding is important, especially in space life sciences, where cell division and human growth under microgravity's influence are studied to maintain astronaut health and performance (N/A, 1990). Ultimately, cell division and growth will keep shaping our focus in the treatment of human disease and human health (Figure 3.14).

3.4.1. Mitosis and Its Phases

Mitosis is a critical cell division process that ensures genetic continuity by accurately dividing chromosomes among daughter cells. Mitosis entails several different stages: prophase, metaphase, anaphase, and telophase. In prophase, the chromatin condenses to create visible chromosomes and the mitotic spindle begins to develop as microtubules project from the centrosomes. The nuclear envelope begins to dissolve to accommodate the eventual alignment of chromosomes. The precision of this phase sets the stage for the subsequent crucial step in mitosis, and this enables the cell division to take place without any issues. The complexities of these processes illustrate how meticulously regulated mechanisms play a role in maintaining genomic integrity and regular cellular functions in humans. As cells progress into metaphase, the chromosomes form an imaginary line along the metaphase plate under the regulations of the spindle apparatus. This orientation is critical as it ensures that each daughter cell receives an equal number of chromosomes. During this process, interactions between spindle microtubules and the kinetochores, which have attached to chromosomal centromeres, play a crucial role. Attachment is ensured by the spindle assembly checkpoint, which makes certain that all chromosomes are correctly attached to the spindle before advancing to anaphase. Failure of these checkpoints may cause genomic instability, as evidenced by research that has seen defective mitotic checkpoints as the primary cause of such diseases as congenital microcephaly (Alcantara & O'Driscoll, 2014), hence the importance of intense control throughout this phase of mitosis. Anaphase and telophase are the final phases of mitosis, with the separation and release of the chromosomes.

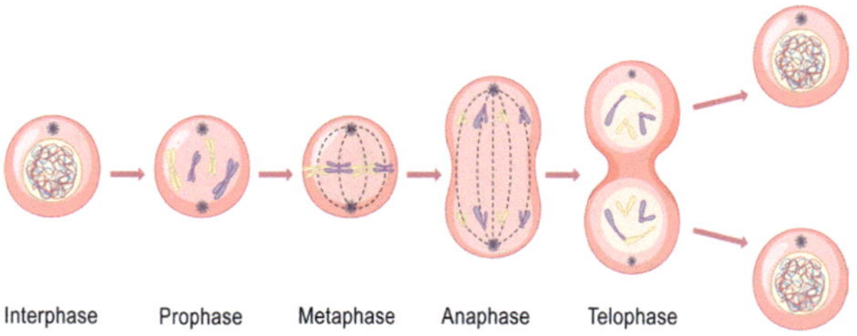

Figure 3.15. Diagram of mitosis.

Source: https://media.geeksforgeeks.org/wp-content/uploads/20220803112423/Mitosis.png.

During anaphase, sister chromatids are pushed to opposite poles of the cell, a process that is dependent on the operation of the mitotic spindle. Errors during this stage might result in unequal segregation of genetic material, resulting in aneuploidy. During the telophase, the decondensed chromatids reform into chromatin, and each set of chromosomes is wrapped in a re-established nuclear envelope, giving rise to two nuclei within the cell. Cytokinesis typically follows, completing the process of division. In cells like *Giardia intestinalis*, with unique mitotic mechanisms, there has been research showing that there is a connection between minimal mitotic checkpoint proteins and issues with chromosome alignment, proving the significance of these proteins in successful mitosis, even in more primitive eukaryotic cells (Cande et al., 2014) (Figure 3.15).

3.4.2. Meiosis and Genetic Diversity

Meiosis is the key process of sexual reproduction and is crucial in generating genetic diversity among human beings. Unlike mitosis, which produces two genetically equivalent daughter cells, meiosis has two phases of division yielding four different haploid gametes. This diploid-to-haploid reduction is necessary to promote the stability of the organism's genome from generation to generation.

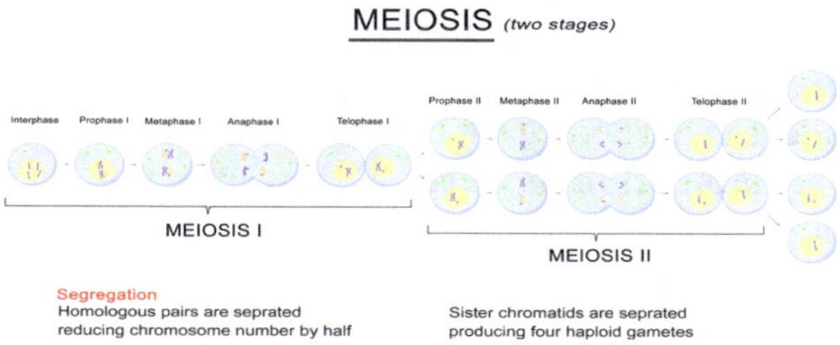

Figure 3.16. Meiosis diagram.

Source: https://media.geeksforgeeks.org/wp-content/uploads/20220720174903/C61.png.

During meiosis, in prophase I, the homologous chromosomes pair and undergo recombination by the mechanism of exchange of DNA segments among chromatids. The exchange introduces new gene combinations responsible for variability in offspring, an important consideration for evolution and adaptation to environmental change. Moreover, meiotic recombination is a sophisticated but delicately controlled process contributing to genetic diversity. Activation of homologous recombination by DNA double-strand breaks (DSBs) is crucial for ensuring correct chromosome segregation and exchange of genes. The DSBs are highly regulated such that they occur at the appropriate locations in the genome, preventing subsequent genomic instabilities due to random instances of recombination. Cooper et al. (2016) recognize the way in which spatial control and distribution of DSBs are critical to facilitating the correct formation of crossovers so that genetic diversity is generated without jeopardizing cell integrity. Such a fine-tuned coordination not only guarantees diversity in the gene pool but also adaptive evolution, and therefore, the significance of meiosis cannot be exaggerated if one takes into account the greater human biological context. Interestingly, the recombination dynamics are sexually dependent and affect genetic diversity in various ways. It has been established in studies that females have increased rates of recombination relative to males, and this leads to a greater overall map length of cross-over events. Sardell et al. (2018) state that recombination patterns are affected by both sex-specific constraints and the structure of chromosomes. In males, recombination is focused towards the end points of chromosomes, while in females, it is distributed evenly. This difference could have profound implications for evolutionary processes, such as sexually antagonistic selection, where sex-specific recombination variation can result in different evolutionary paths. It is thus crucial to comprehend the intricacies of meiosis and how it relates to genetic diversity to understand human development and evolutionary biology (Figure 3.16).

3.4.3. Regulation of the Cell Cycle

Cell cycle regulation is a cellular biology feature that is crucial for the maintenance of homeostasis and proper tissue functioning in human beings. The cell cycle has various stages—G1, S, G2, and M—each of which is strictly regulated so that cells divide and reproduce correctly. This control is achieved by a coordinated interplay of cyclins, cyclin-dependent kinases (CDKs), and a series of checkpoint proteins that monitor the integrity of DNA and the cellular environment. Cell cycle regulation anomalies may lead to uncontrolled cell division, a characteristic of neoplastic growth. The consequences of such dysregulation have been observed not only in healthy somatic cells but also in specialist cells, implying broader relevance to tissue health and development processes. Elucidation of such a regulatory system is central to advancing therapeutic approaches to restore normal cell cycle function in disease conditions such as cancer. Primary cilia are now key regulators of the cell cycle, synchronizing sensory input with cell response pathways. Primary cilia participate in a variety of signal transduction pathways, including those of growth factors, which can be direct cell cycle regulators. In most cases, the number and function of primary cilia have been shown to correlate with cell cycle stage, with cancer cells exhibiting altered expression.

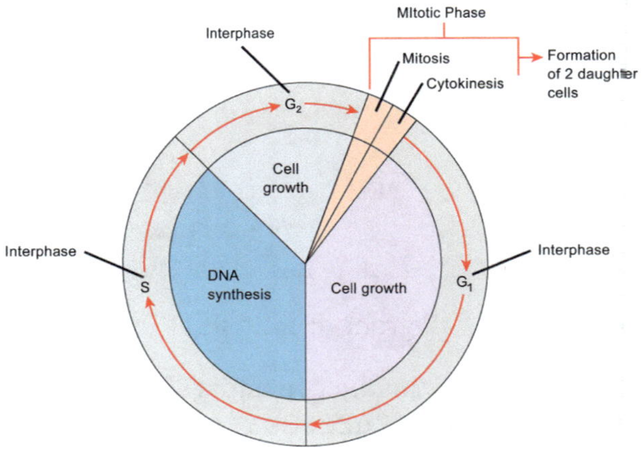

Figure 3.17. A cell moves through a series of phases in an orderly manner. During interphase, G1 involves cell growth and protein synthesis, the S phase involves DNA replication and the replication of the centrosome, and G2 involves further growth and protein synthesis.

Source: https://opentextbc.ca/biology/wp-content/uploads/sites/96/2015/02/Figure_06_02_01.jpg.

For instance, in glioblastoma cells, it has been observed that the formation of primary cilia is defective, which leads to disrupted signaling pathways that underlie malignant phenotypes. These findings are in line with the understanding that primary cilia are more than just basic sensory structures; they have a significant role in maintaining the regulatory pathways that underlie cell cycle integrity and cell fate determination in human tissue (Moser et al., 2009). Moreover, molecular intermediaries like prostaglandin E2 (PGE2) illustrate how extracellular signaling molecules can regulate cell cycle control. In granulosa cells, for example, PGE2 has been shown to coordinate the inhibition of cell division needed for ovulation. Such a regulatory mechanism illustrates the complexity of the cell cycle, wherein not just intrinsic factors like cyclins but possibly extrinsic signals may dictate the outcome of cellular processes. Inhibitors of these pathways, including celecoxib, demonstrate how inhibiting certain signaling pathways can affect cell cycle dynamics and general tissue function. The comprehension of how these types of interactions between signaling molecules and the cell cycle machinery operate is critical for understanding the complex balance of growth and division of cells in a variety of physiological and pathological situations (Lundberg et al., 2020) (Figure 3.17).

Test Your Knowledge

1. What is mitosis and the phases?
2. What is the process of meiosis?

3.5. Cellular Adaptations and Responses

Learning Outcome

1. Learn about hypertrophy and atrophy;
2. Understand apoptosis and programmed cell death;
3. Describe the stem cells and differentiation.

Cellular adaptations are crucial processes by which cells respond appropriately to environmental stresses to ensure survival and homeostasis. Such a response tends to manifest as cellular changes in structure or function and can be divided into adaptive responses in the form of hyperplasia, hypertrophy, atrophy, and metaplasia. For instance, hypertrophy is an increase in cell size, and it occurs because of enhanced workload, such as in cardiac muscle cells of athletes. Atrophy, on the other hand, is a decrease in cell size because of disuse or decreased stimulation, as could happen with bedridden patients. Understanding these adaptations reveals the delicate interaction between cellular requirements and environmental conditions, the dynamic nature of cellular function and form in the maintenance of human health and the development of pathology. One significant aspect of cellular adaptation is the role of oxidative stress in skeletal muscle homeostasis. In contrast to the perception that oxidative stress entirely causes cellular damage, more recent evidence has shown that ROS possess the capacity to serve as beneficial signaling molecules that regulate important physiological processes. Within physiological concentrations, ROS are implicated in muscle adaptation by triggering various signaling pathways tasked with driving growth and differentiation, which is essential for sustaining muscle function and integrity. However, when oxidative stress passes its threshold, it becomes a source of pathological conditions and muscle pathophysiology. Hence, the two-fold nature of oxidative stress represents the complexity of cell responses and the demand for tightly controlled redox balance for the best muscle health and function. Understanding this equilibrium is essential for developing treatment strategies against muscle-associated disorders (Musarò et al., 2010). With increasing age, one experiences multiple cellular changes directly affecting muscle quality and function, a phenomenon known as sarcopenia. The aging-induced deterioration is not just through loss of muscle mass but also through changes in muscle composition, including increased adiposity, which negatively affects muscle function. Fat infiltration into non-adipose tissues, particularly skeletal muscle, can lead to lipotoxicity and decrease the contractility of muscles as well as overall strength. Moreover, with aging, the inflammatory profile of the fat tissue is altered with the enhancement of local pathogenic effects on muscle cells. As muscle mass and quality are indispensable for maintaining physical function and preventing disability, adaptation and response processes at the cellular level due to aging must be known to promote healthy aging and devise interventions to mitigate sarcopenia effects (Carter et al., 2019) (Figure 3.18).

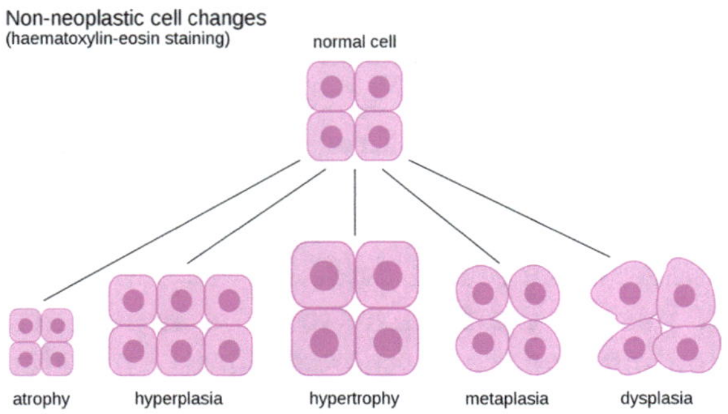

Figure 3.18. Depiction of non-neoplastic changes a cell can undergo.

Source: https://teachmephysiology.com/wp-content/uploads/2021/03/1920px-Non-neoplastic_changes.svg-1024x576.png.

3.5.1. Hypertrophy and Atrophy

The concepts of hypertrophy and atrophy are central to the understanding of the cellular dynamics that determine muscle function in the human body. Hypertrophy refers to the growth of muscle fiber size, primarily a result of external stimuli such as resistance training, resulting in augmented myofibrillar protein synthesis. This physiological reaction not only enhances strength within the muscle but also impacts metabolic function and general health. Atrophy, in contrast, is a decrease in the size of muscle fibers, often due to lack of use, illness, or age. This distinction between the two processes is significant because hypertrophy and atrophy identify a fine balance in muscle homeostasis that has implications for both functional capability and resilience to a wide array of stressors. At a cellular level, hypertrophy and atrophy control is multifactorial and under tight regulation. In hypertrophy, anabolic signaling pathways, such as the mTOR pathway, are responsible for augmenting protein synthesis and cell enlargement, thereby promoting muscle growth. In contrast, atrophy is characterized by catabolic processes via the ubiquitin-proteasome and autophagy-lysosome machinery. Enhanced protein degradation, particularly under pathological conditions, leads to muscle wasting and decreases functional reserve. It is valuable to understand these regulatory pathways because they inform us about the machinery of the formation or degeneration of muscle fibers over time. Current research reveals that not only are they activated by different stimuli, but that having independent control provokes the question of what each contributes separately to the health of muscle under different conditions (Bouchè et al., 2018). Endocrine changes also play a role in the regulation of hypertrophy and atrophy, playing a significant role in the overall function of the muscles. The morphological and functional changes, such as a reduction in the number of motor units and muscle fiber atrophy, especially type II fibers that contribute to strength and power, occur with advancing age. This loss is reinforced by diminished physical activity, leading to considerable muscle loss and a decrease in strength. Remarkably, despite all these disadvantages, regular engagement in physical exercise has emerged as an effective intervention that can not only alleviate but also reverse age-related muscle loss. Importantly, progressive resistance training can trigger counteractive adaptive processes against the effects of aging on the muscles. Therefore, it is worth learning how atrophy, hypertrophy, and exercise interact with each other for the facilitation of a healthy aging process and optimization of functional independence (Malone, 2016) (Figure 3.19).

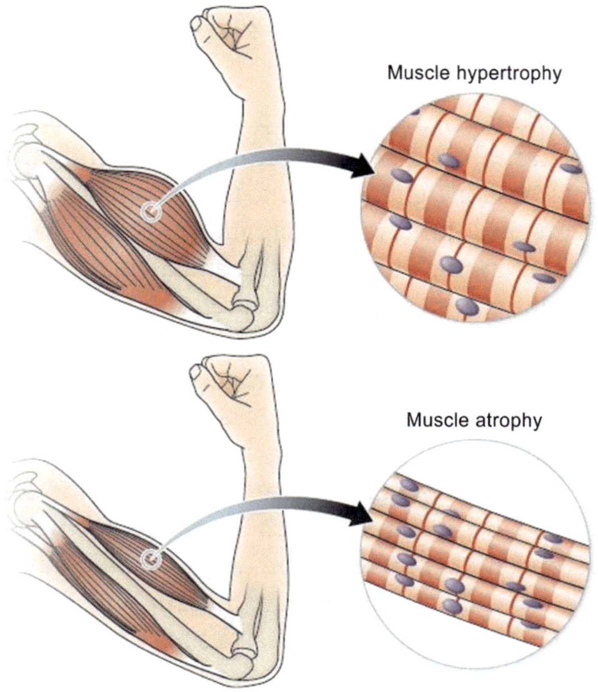

Figure 3.19. Skeletal muscle cell atrophy versus hypertrophy.

Source: https://i.pinimg.com/564x/ce/e1/a6/cee1a6c4205541cb9ad5febe92064ff3.jpg.

3.5.2. Apoptosis and Programmed Cell Death

Programmed cell death or apoptosis is an essential process to secure cellular homeostasis in the human organism. Unlike necrosis, which is a non-energy-requiring, uncontrolled process of cell death caused by external injury, apoptosis is an energy-dependent, regulated process necessary for normal tissue turnover and growth. It permits the elimination of damaged or dysfunctional cells without activating inflammation, significant in autoimmune disease prevention and chronic disease. Through activation of a caspase cascade, apoptosis leads to characteristic morphological changes, such as cell shrinkage, chromatin condensation, and DNA fragmentation. Such changes allow for sequential disassembling of cellular components, whereby cellular debris is effectively removed by phagocytes. Study of the mechanism of apoptosis not only uncovers the underlying biology but also underlies the medical study of manipulation of cell death pathways in disease. The function of apoptosis is normal physiological processes; dysregulation of apoptosis is a common aspect of many pathologies, including cancer, neurodegenerative diseases, and cardiovascular disease. In cancer, for example, cancer cells prefer to acquire mutations that enable them to evade apoptotic signals so that the cells proliferate uncontrollably and develop a tumor. In other cases, excess apoptosis has been found to be responsible for pathologies such as Alzheimer's disease, where neuronal apoptosis degrades essential neural networks. Moreover, apoptosis participates in myocardial ischemia, where prolonged lack of blood supply causes death among myocardial cells, depicting the transition from reversible to irreversible injury. As outlined in the literature, the dynamics of cell death in this instance reflect the complexity of cardiac repair mechanisms and the need for specifically targeted therapies able to modulate apoptosis effectively, which underlies its role in disease and health (Turillazzi et al., 2015). Research has gone on to study the intricacy of programmed cell death, particularly during embryonic life, early on. In bovine embryo research, extensive cell death incidence has been observed in the most important stages of cleavage, and this poses questions about the developmental and biological importance of these incidents. Incidentally, while a few transcripts that caused apoptosis were noted to be minimally expressed, the correlation with cell death suggests various mechanisms or pathways in early development. This view implies that, while apoptosis has traditionally been a caspase-mediated process, other mechanisms of programmed cell death taking place involve complexity in the sense of cell fate during development. As a result, a comprehensive study in this realm not only enhances our grasp of cell signaling and development but also highlights potential avenues for addressing developmental disorders that arise from aberrant cell death (Bettegowda et al., 2011) (Figure 3.20).

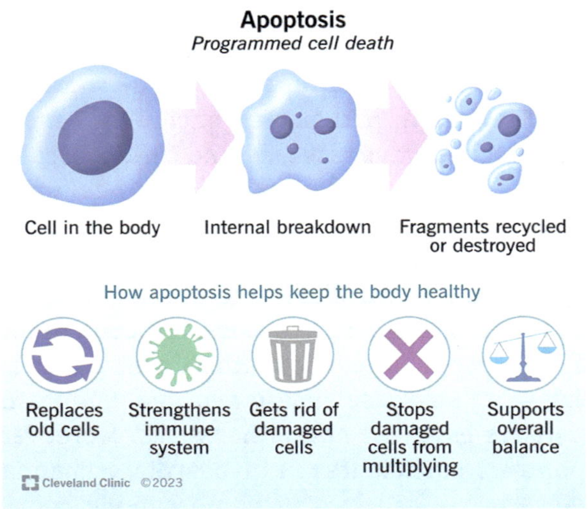

Figure 3.20. Apoptosis supports your health by breaking down cells into bits that your body recycles or destroys.

Source: https://my.clevelandclinic.org/-/scassets/images/org/health/articles/apoptosis.jpg?io=transform:fit,width:780.

3.5.3. Stem Cells and Differentiation

The mechanism of stem cell differentiation is crucial to cell structure and function studies in humans, as it shows how undifferentiated cells differentiate to form differentiated cell types required for tissue development and repair. Stem cells, particularly embryonic and adult mesenchymal stem cells, possess the intrinsic ability to self-renew and lineage commit into multilineages. This is controlled by many extrinsic factors, including biochemical signals and cellular microenvironment. Studies have unveiled the significance of physical properties of substrate materials, including surface topography and stiffness, in the control of stem cell fate. For instance, engineered surfaces with microgrooves were shown to induce osteogenic differentiation of human mesenchymal stem cells, unveiling the potential of biomaterials for tissue engineering and regenerative medicine (Funaoku et al., 2025).

These findings expose the intricate relationship between stem cells and the environment, giving clues to tissue regeneration strategies. Moreover, the creation of biomaterials closely mimicking the extracellular matrix has revolutionized stem cell research and application in regenerative medicine. One such material is peptide-based fibrillar hydrogels, which provide a permissive platform for stem cell growth and differentiation. Such hydrogels not only offer a three-dimensional niche that fosters cell viability and growth but also facilitate osteogenic differentiation when subjected to appropriate stimuli. Human mesenchymal stem cells seeded in such biomaterials have previously demonstrated the potential to secrete required bone proteins and mineralize, which are critical to effective bone regeneration (Diaz et al., 2016). This new approach of biomimetics highlights the significance of biomimetic materials in enhancing stem cell function and possibilities for their application in damaged tissue and organ repair. Implications of differentiation of stem cells extend well beyond basic biological understanding; they hold massive potential for the development of treatments for numerous degenerative diseases and injuries. By taking advantage of the ability of stem cells to differentiate, researchers are optimistic that new therapies with the potential to replace damaged or missing tissues can be created, hence addressing significant health challenges. Through ongoing research in stem cell biology, integration with advanced materials science has shown great promise in terms of streamlining differentiation methods. The regulation of stem cell fate by designed milieus not only improves our insight into cellular dynamics but also bridges the gap between research and therapy. Therefore, research into stem cell differentiation, coupled with biomaterials advances, holds a leading position among groundbreaking methods in regenerative medicine (Figure 3.21).

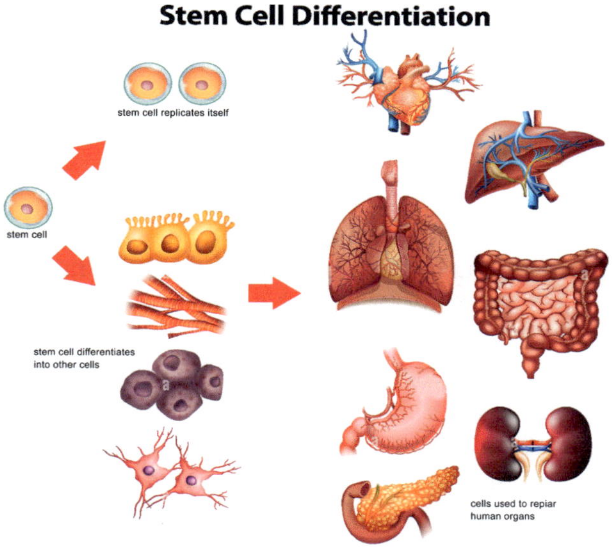

Figure 3.21. Stem cell differentiation.

Source: https://c7.alamy.com/comp/2GW189A/stem-cell-differentiation-diagram-2GW189A.jpg.

Test Your Knowledge

1. What does hypertrophy mean?
2. What is apoptosis?

SUMMARY

In synthesizing the discovery of cell structure and function in the human body, it can be seen that there is a complex interaction between cellular elements and their specific roles in overall biological functions. Every organelle, ranging from the mitochondria responsible for generating energy to the nucleus containing genetic material, plays a critical role in maintaining homeostasis and enabling development. This complex organization facilitates not only cellular integrity but also specialization in complicated organisms, highlighting cellular diversity and adaptabilityin terms of evolutionary importance. Understanding these interactions on the cellular level not only explains individual cell functions but also illustrates how their decompensation can lead to overall health effects, demonstrating the validity of continued research in cellular biology. In addition, the research findings' implications on cell structure and function transcend simple biology; they are also of central importance in medicine. Discoveries based on research on the hippocampus and corpus callosum have demonstrated essential connections between brain structure and memory processes, highlighting the need for refined approaches to treating neurological disorders. For example, research shows that certain brain areas being damaged have been found to cause specific impairments, which indicates that therapies should be tailored according to in-depth knowledge of the cellular mechanisms involved. Dealing with such complexities creates new treatment approaches that can have a vital impact on patient outcomes, highlighting the power of knowledge in transforming biological sciences. Finally, the research on neural networks as cognitive models of human processes adds another layer to cell function. Through research on how neural networks emulate human reasoning and decision-making processes, researchers are making connections between cellular processes and higher cognitive function. Research has indicated that such networks show human-like behavior, including bounded rationality and the emergence of decision heuristics, thus enhancing our comprehension of both micro-cellular-level and macro-cognition. And as research continues deeper into these interactions, an increasingly interdependent understanding of cell structure and function will certainly continue to advance cognitive science and medicine, creating new avenues to learn and for therapeutic intervention across domains of human wellness.

When considering the complexities of cellular composition and function within the human organism, one can see that cellular interaction and structure play an essential role in overall bodily health. The cell, at times referred to as the unit of life, is a highly structured entity composed of various organelles such as the nucleus, mitochondria, endoplasmic reticulum, and Golgi apparatus. All organelles possess specialized but interdependent functions—whereas the nucleus holds genetic data, the mitochondria are the energy-producing structures of cells that generate ATP through cellular respiration. This specialization allows cellular processes to function efficiently, showing how function is closely linked with structure. Moreover, cellular dynamics in cell mechanisms for communication and signaling are important in maintaining homeostasis and cell response to environmental stimuli. Cellular signaling pathways, such as those for growth factor responses, are just a few examples of cells interpreting stimuli and making the appropriate response. This level of complexity can be found in immune responses, in which cells send signals to organize defense against infections. The rational architecture of cellular elements, as the Global HIV Vaccine Enterprise argues, underscores the centrality of these interactions to the development of therapeutic interventions, bridging conceptual knowledge of cell structure with translational applications in medicine (Mascola et al., 2010). Beyond the fundamental roles played by various organelles, the knowledge of chronic diseases, including tendon disease, underscores the centrality of cell structure in disease and health. The ordered fibrillar matrix, which is made up largely of type I collagen and other structural components, defines tendons. The remodeled matrix and cellular changes in tendinopathy, a condition seen extensively, expose the fine balance for optimal tendon function. The changes, including the increased expression of type III collagen and other markers, are not only a pathological response but also an adaptive one to mechanical stressors (Riley, 2008). Hence, the study of cell structure and function not only enhances our knowledge of human physiology but also guides therapeutic intervention for many diseases, transferring basic biological science to clinical practice.

KEY TERMS FROM THIS CHAPTER

- Bacteria
- Cellular respiration
- Cytoplasm
- Eukaryotic cells
- Human cells
- Plasma membrane
- Prokaryotic cells
- Cellular automata
- Cellular signaling
- Endoplasmic reticulum
- Homeostasis
- Muscle cells
- Predictive modeling
- Protein synthesis

CRITICAL THINKING QUESTIONS

1. **The smallest unit of life capable of carrying out all life processes is:**
   a. Molecule
   b. Atom
   c. Cell
   d. Tissue
2. **Which of the following structures is found in both prokaryotic and eukaryotic cells?**
   a. Nucleus
   b. Mitochondria
   c. Ribosome
   d. Golgi apparatus
3. **The process by which a cell takes in material by engulfing it with the cell membrane is called:**
   a. Osmosis
   b. Endocytosis
   c. Exocytosis
   d. Diffusion
4. **Which organelle is known as the "powerhouse of the cell"?**
   a. Ribosome
   b. Mitochondria
   c. Endoplasmic Reticulum
   d. Golgi apparatus
5. **The primary function of the rough endoplasmic reticulum is:**
   a. Lipid synthesis
   b. Protein synthesis
   c. ATP production
   d. DNA replication

Short Answer Questions

1. What is a simple definition of a cell?
2. What is the basic structure of the cell?
3. List the types of human cells.
4. What are the organelles and their functions?
5. What is the regulation of the cell cycle?

Answers to Critical Thinking Questions

1. (c); 2. (c) ; 3. (b); 4. (b); 5. (b)

REFERENCES

1. Deighton, R. F., Le Bihan, T., Martin, S. F., Gerth, A. M. J., McCulloch, M., Edgar, J. M., Kerr, L. E., Whittle, I. R., & McCulloch, J. (2014). Interactions among mitochondrial proteins altered in glioblastoma. *Journal of neuro-oncology, 118*(2), 247–256. https://doi.org/10.1007/s11060-014-1430-5(accessed on 7th August 2025).
2. Alcantara, D., & O'Driscoll, M. (2014). Congenital microcephaly. *American journal of medical genetics. Part C, Seminars in medical genetics, 166C*(2), 124–139. https://doi.org/10.1002/ajmg.c.31397(accessed on 7th August 2025).
3. Jackson, A. J., Clucas, C., Mamczur, N. J., Ferguson, D. J., & Meissner, M. (2013). Toxoplasma gondii Syntaxin 6 is required for vesicular transport between endosomal-like compartments and the Golgi complex. *Traffic (Copenhagen, Denmark), 14*(11), 1166–1181. https://doi.org/10.1111/tra.12102 (accessed on 7th August 2025).
4. Touyz, R. M., Alves-Lopes, R., Rios, F. J., Camargo, L. L., Anagnostopoulou, A., Arner, A., & Montezano, A. C. (2018). Vascular smooth muscle contraction in hypertension. *Cardiovascular research, 114*(4), 529–539. https://doi.org/10.1093/cvr/cvy023(accessed on 7th August 2025).
5. Korcsmáros, T., Farkas, I. J., Szalay, M. S., Rovó, P., Fazekas, D., Spiró, Z., Böde, C., Lenti, K., Vellai, T., & Csermely, P. (2010). Uniformly curated signaling pathways reveal tissue-specific cross-talks and support drug target discovery. *Bioinformatics (Oxford, England), 26*(16), 2042–2050. https://doi.org/10.1093/bioinformatics/btq310(accessed on 7th August 2025).
6. Steed, E., Rodrigues, N. T., Balda, M. S., & Matter, K. (2009). Identification of MarvelD3 as a tight junction-associated transmembrane protein of the occludin family. *BMC cell biology, 10*, 95. https://doi.org/10.1186/1471-2121-10-95 (accessed on 7th August 2025).
7. Cooper, T. J., Garcia, V., & Neale, M. J. (2016). Meiotic DSB patterning: A multifaceted process. *Cell cycle (Georgetown, Tex.), 15*(1), 13–21. https://doi.org/10.1080/15384101.2015.1093709(accessed on 7th August 2025).
8. Bastidas Orihuela, J. J., & Roman Aquice, L. Y. (2009). *Learning Backward Induction: A Neural Network Agent Approach.* https://core.ac.uk/download/pdf/12021066.pdf (accessed on 7th August 2025).
9. Bellacose, C., Demirel, E., Duffy, D. M., Lundberg, et al. (2020). *Granulosa cell proliferation is inhibited by PGE2 in the primate ovulatory follicle.* https://core.ac.uk/download/346492916.pdf (accessed on 7th August 2025).
10. Turillazzi, E., Pomara, C., Bello, S., Neri, M., Riezzo, I., & Fineschi, V. (2015). The meaning of different forms of structural myocardial injury, immune response and timing of infarct necrosis and cardiac repair. *Current vascular pharmacology, 13*(1), 6–19. https://doi.org/10.2174/1570161111311999008(accessed on 7th August 2025).
11. Bettegowda, A., Jurisicova, A., Crosier, A. E., Jakobsen, A. S., Robert, C., et al. (2011). *Cell Arrest and Cell death in Mammalian Preimplantation Development.* https://core.ac.uk/download/12175482.pdf (accessed on 7th August 2025).
12. Yang, Y. X. & Billings, S. A. (1999). *Neighborhood Detection and Rule Selection from Cellular Automata Patterns.* https://core.ac.uk/download/58513.pdf (accessed on 7th August 2025).
13. Bouchè, M., Lozanoska-Ochser, B., Madaro, L., Proietti, et al. (2018). *Do neurogenic and cancer-induced muscle atrophy follow common or divergent paths?* https://core.ac.uk/download/188830432.pdf (accessed on 7th August 2025).

14. Dawson, N., Kurihara, M., Thomson, D. M., Winchester, C. L., McVie, A., Hedde, J. R., Randall, A. D., Shen, S., Seymour, P. A., Hughes, Z. A., Dunlop, J., Brown, J. T., Brandon, N. J., Morris, B. J., & Pratt, J. A. (2015). Altered functional brain network connectivity and glutamate system function in transgenic mice expressing truncated Disrupted-in-Schizophrenia 1. *Translational psychiatry, 5*(5), e569. https://doi.org/10.1038/tp.2015.60(accessed on 7th August 2025).

15. Elhanati, Y., Sethna, Z., Callan, C. G., Jr, Mora, T., & Walczak, A. M. (2018). Predicting the spectrum of TCR repertoire sharing with a data-driven model of recombination. *Immunological reviews, 284*(1), 167–179. https://doi.org/10.1111/imr.12665(accessed on 7th August 2025).

16. Cande, W. Z., & Vicente, J. J. (2014). *Mad2, Bub3, and Mps1 regulate chromosome segregation and mitotic synchrony in Giardia intestinalis, a binucleate protist lacking an anaphase-promoting complex.* https://core.ac.uk/download/323082061.pdf (accessed on 7th August 2025).

17. Carter, C. S., Justice, J. N., & Thompson, L. (2019). *Lipotoxicity, Aging, and Muscle Contractility: Does Fiber Type Matter?* https://open.bu.edu/bitstream/2144/40625/7/carter_justice_thompson_Lipotoxicity_paper_04302019.pdf (accessed on 7th August 2025).

18. Castillo Diaz, L. A., Elsawy, M., Gough, J. E., Miller, et al. (2016). *Osteogenic differentiation of human mesenchymal stem cells promotes mineralization within a biodegradable peptide hydrogel.* https://core.ac.uk/download/83948822.pdf (accessed on 7th August 2025).

19. Chen, N. T., Liao, Y. C., Lin, Y., Lo, et al. (2010). *DLC2 modulates angiogenic responses in vascular endothelial cells by regulating cell attachment and migration.* https://core.ac.uk/download/323069301.pdf (accessed on 7th August 2025).

20. Sardell, J. M., Cheng, C., Dagilis, A. J., Ishikawa, A., Kitano, J., Peichel, C. L., & Kirkpatrick, M. (2018). Sex Differences in Recombination in Sticklebacks. *G3 (Bethesda, Md.), 8*(6), 1971–1983. https://doi.org/10.1534/g3.118.200166(accessed on 7th August 2025).

21. Costa, R., & Frezza, G. (2014). CROSSOVERS BETWEEN EPIGENESIS AND EPIGENETICS. A MULTICENTER APPROACH TO THE HISTORY OF EPIGENETICS (1901-1975). *Medicina nei secoli, 26*(3), 905–942.(accessed on 7th August 2025).

22. D'Alessandro, A., Dzieciatkowska, M., Freire, C. M., King, et al. (2024). *Complete absence of GLUT1 does not impair human terminal erythroid differentiation.* https://core.ac.uk/download/599589411.pdf (accessed on 7th August 2025).

23. Maini,Philip K.; Dallon,J C; Sherratt,J A; (2005). *A Multiscale Model for Collagen Alignment in Wound Healing.* University of Oxford (2004) **J Physiol 561P, SA11** https://core.ac.uk/download/pdf/96773.pdf (accessed on 7th August 2025).

24. Djuranovic, S., Djuranovic, S. P., & Erath, J. (2019). *Adaptation of translational machinery in malaria parasites to accommodate translation of poly-adenosine stretches throughout its life cycle.* https://core.ac.uk/download/286537327.pdf (accessed on 7th August 2025).

25. Phan, Q. T., Myers, C. L., Fu, Y., Sheppard, D. C., Yeaman, M. R., Welch, W. H., Ibrahim, A. S., Edwards, J. E., Jr, & Filler, S. G. (2007). Als3 is a Candida albicans invasin that binds to cadherins and induces endocytosis by host cells. *PLoS biology, 5*(3), e64. https://doi.org/10.1371/journal.pbio.0050064(accessed on 7th August 2025).

26. Musarò, A., Fulle, S., & Fanò, G. (2010). Oxidative stress and muscle homeostasis. *Current opinion in clinical nutrition and metabolic care, 13*(3), 236–242. https://doi.org/10.1097/MCO.0b013e3283368188(accessed on 7th August 2025).

27. Tomavo, S., Slomianny, C., Meissner, M., & Carruthers, V. B. (2013). Protein trafficking through the endosomal system prepares intracellular parasites for a home invasion. *PLoS pathogens*, *9*(10), e1003629. https://doi.org/10.1371/journal.ppat.1003629(accessed on 7th August 2025).

28. Funaoku, K., Gokcekaya, O., Matsugaki, A., Matsuzaka, et al. (2025). *PBF-LB fabrication of microgrooves for induction of osteogenic differentiation of human mesenchymal stem cells*. https://core.ac.uk/download/597800091.pdf (accessed on 7th August 2025).

29. Gallucci, B. B., & McCarthy, D. O. (1995). *The Immune System*. https://core.ac.uk/download/213081395.pdf (accessed on 7th August 2025).

30. Herms, J., Kretzschmar, H. A., & Vassallo, N. (2004). *The Molecular Pathology of Prion Diseases*. https://core.ac.uk/download/46601891.pdf (accessed on 7th August 2025).

31. Wang, J., Jennings, A. K., & Kowalski, J. R. (2016). The Anaphase-Promoting Complex (APC) ubiquitin ligase affects chemosensory behavior in C. elegans. *PeerJ*, *4*, e2013. https://doi.org/10.7717/peerj.2013(accessed on 7th August 2025).

32. Jiang, N., Li, J. J., Wang, S., Xie, et al. (2019). *Cyclin B1/CDK1-regulated mitochondrial bioenergetics in cell cycle progression and tumor resistance*. https://core.ac.uk/download/286361500.pdf (accessed on 7th August 2025).

33. Ren, J., Jin, P., Wang, E., Marincola, F. M., & Stroncek, D. F. (2009). MicroRNA and gene expression patterns in the differentiation of human embryonic stem cells. *Journal of translational medicine*, *7*, 20. https://doi.org/10.1186/1479-5876-7-20(accessed on 7th August 2025).

34. Moser, J. J., Fritzler, M. J., & Rattner, J. B. (2009). Primary ciliogenesis defects are associated with human astrocytoma/glioblastoma cells. *BMC cancer*, *9*, 448. https://doi.org/10.1186/1471-2407-9-448(accessed on 7th August 2025).

35. Malone, J. K. (2016). *The EFFECTS of ageing and exercise on skeletal muscle structure and function*. https://core.ac.uk/download/228176394.pdf (accessed on 7th August 2025).

36. Mascola, J., Steinman, R., King, R. C., & the Working Group convened by the Global HIV Vaccine Enterprise. (2010). *Immunogens and antigen processing: Report from a Global HIV Vaccine Enterprise Working Group*. https://core.ac.uk/download/pdf/289325.pdf (accessed on 7th August 2025).

37. Riley G. (2008). Tendinopathy--from basic science to treatment. *Nature clinical practice. Rheumatology*, *4*(2), 82–89. https://doi.org/10.1038/ncprheum0700(accessed on 7th August 2025).

38. Miesbauer, M., Rambold, A., Tatzelt, J., Winkelhofer, et al. (2010). *Targeting of the prion protein to the cytosol: Mechanisms and consequences*.

39. N/A. (1990). *Space life Sciences: A Status Report*. https://core.ac.uk/download/pdf/10427803.pdf (accessed on 7th August 2025).

40. Marygold, S. J., Roote, J., Reuter, G., Lambertsson, A., Ashburner, M., Millburn, G. H., Harrison, P. M., Yu, Z., Kenmochi, N., Kaufman, T. C., Leevers, S. J., & Cook, K. R. (2007). The ribosomal protein genes and Minute loci of Drosophila melanogaster. *Genome biology*, *8*(10), R216. https://doi.org/10.1186/gb-2007-8-10-r216(accessed on 7th August 2025).

41. Rose, A. P. (1999). *Reproductive misconception: Why cloning is not just another assisted reproductive technology*. https://core.ac.uk/download/62549068.pdf (accessed on 7th August 2025).

42. Fernando, T., Denman, S., Sridharan, S., Fookes, C. (2019). Pedestrian Trajectory Prediction with Structured Memory Hierarchies. In: Berlingerio, M., Bonchi, F., Gärtner, T., Hurley, N., Ifrim, G. (eds) Machine Learning and Knowledge Discovery in Databases. ECML PKDD 2018. Lecture Notes in Computer Science(), vol 11051. Springer, Cham. https://doi.org/10.1007/978-3-030-10925-7_15 (accessed on 7th August 2025).

43. Scheffler, I. E. (2014). *Mitochondrial disease associated with complex I (NADH-CoQ oxidoreductase) deficiency*. https://core.ac.uk/download/323082631.pdf (accessed on 7th August 2025).

44. Zaidel, D. W. (1995). *The case for a relationship between human memory, hippocampus and corpus callosum*. https://core.ac.uk/download/pdf/84583.pdf (accessed on 7th August 2025).

EPITHELIAL TISSUE

4

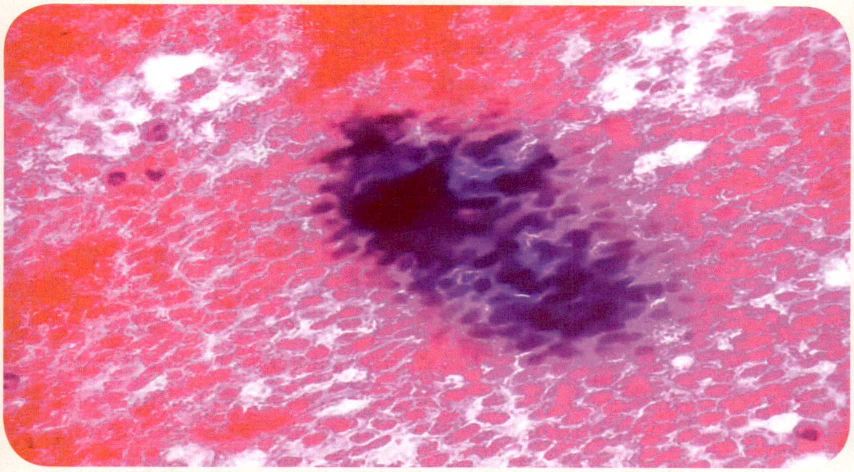

LEARNING OBJECTIVES

After studying this chapter, you will be able to:

1. Describe the types and functions of epithelial tissue;
2. Understand the structure of epithelial tissue;
3. Describe the locations of epithelial tissue in the body;
4. Learn about epithelial tissue and disease.

INTRODUCTION

Epithelial tissue is one of the four fundamental tissue types in humans and serves critical functions in protection, absorption, secretion, and sensation. It is made up of tightly packed cells that constitute continuous sheets and cover body surfaces, line cavities, and give rise to organs. The organizational pattern of the tissue can vary extensively, with simple, stratified, squamous, cuboidal, and columnar types specialized for specific functions in various organs. For instance, the presence of a single epithelium in alveoli enables gas exchange to take place in the lungs, while stratified epithelium in the skin provides a robust protective barrier against environmental damage. Familiarity with the intricate architecture and diverse functions of epithelial tissue is required for an appreciation of its pivotal roles in homeostasis and overall physiological health, hence providing a basis for subsequent discussion of its importance in disease and health. In addition to its structural significance, epithelial tissue is also key in many physiological functions, subject to several signaling mechanisms that control cell behavior and interaction. Cellular pathways of signaling, including BMP and Wnt, are reported in recent literature to have a critical function in controlling epithelial cell proliferation, differentiation, and homeostasis. For instance, fine-tuning of signal pathways can lead to tissue homeostasis in normal conditions or cancer and other pathologies upon disruption. Study of epithelial tissue has advanced our understanding of diseases such as high-grade serous ovarian cancer, which has been linked to alterations in the epithelium of the fallopian tube (Hoffmann et al., 2020).

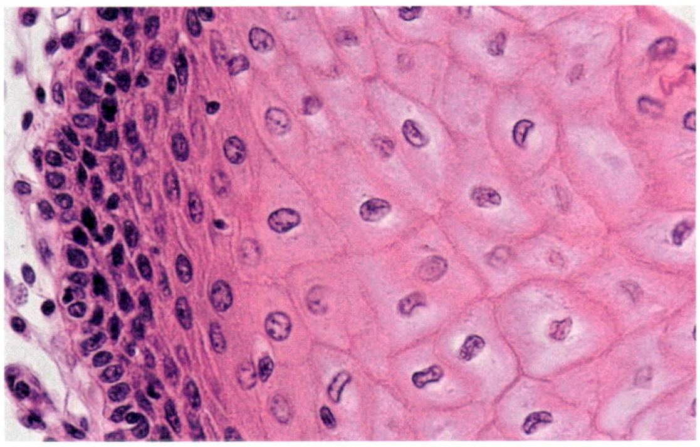

Figure 4.1. Epithelial tissues.

Source: https://www.careerpower.in/blog/wp-content/uploads/sites/2/2024/10/17145635/epithelial-tissue.png.

These results emphasize the significance of exploring the molecular foundation of epithelial tissues, both at a basic biological level and for the development of targeted treatment. Moreover, the development of organoid technology has allowed for more advanced analysis of epithelial tissues by which researchers can generate three-dimensional models closely recapitulating their *in vivo* tissue structure and function. Such advances have unveiled the complex interaction of signaling pathways and the impact of the tissue microenvironment on cell behavior. Specifically, the ability to study how changes in the niche conditions affect the fate decisions of the cell has the promise to lead to paradigm shifts in cancer studies and regenerative medicine. The ability to produce stable cultures of organoids from patient-derived samples provides the key to investigating individualized drug responses and the dissection of tumorigenesis and metastasis causes (Galluzzi et al., 2018). With further advances in technology, understanding epithelial tissue dynamics will be vital in furthering medical knowledge and improving patient care (Figure 4.1).

Definition of Epithelial Tissue

Epithelial tissue is one of the four large tissue groups of the human body, and it plays critical roles in protection, absorption, secretion, and sensation. With its cellular composition, epithelial tissue is densely packed with cells and minimal extracellular matrix, which allows it to establish effective barriers. Epithelial tissue is bound to connective tissue by a basement membrane, providing it structural strength and also serving as a selective filter. Epithelial cells are classified based on their shape—squamous, cuboidal, and columnar—and their organization—simple, stratified, and pseudostratified. Heterogeneity in epithelial structures affirms special function, such as nutrient uptake in the intestine and defense against invasion by pathogens on the outer skin layer. Understanding the definition of epithelial tissues is necessary to fully embrace their contribution to human disease and health. The roles of epithelial tissue are not just simple protection and absorption; they play roles in numerous physiological functions, such as secretion and sensation. The glandular epithelia, that is, both the endocrine and exocrine glands, play roles in synthesizing and secreting various substances such as hormones, enzymes, and mucus. Secretion is required for homeostasis and the facilitation of communication between body systems. The functional heterogeneity of epithelial tissue is evident from its specialized sensory receptors located in areas such as the skin, nose, and retina and involved in basic functions of environmental perception. The structure of epithelial tissue can also be modified to suit physiological needs, as in the instance of transitional epithelium, which adapts to varying amounts of urine in the bladder. Such functions demonstrate the responsive structure of epithelial tissue in human physiology. The study of epithelial tissue has broader applications, specifically in developmental biology and pathology. Epithelial disease has been shown to be connected with a variety of illnesses, including cancer, autoimmune conditions, and developmental defects. Epithelial cells, for instance, undergo enormous morphogenetic changes during development, emphasizing their function not just as a barrier but as an active tissue in organ and system formation. The interaction of epithelial tissue with other tissues implies a complex interaction for growth and health. Improved insight into such processes can potentially transfer findings from animal models such as mice into human disease. But caution is needed due to anatomical and developmental differences, as evidenced by studies of the impact of chemical exposure on reproductive tract development, such as the characterization of flutamide-induced hypospadias in model systems. Baskin et al. (2017, 2019) highlights the pivotal role of epithelial tissue in normal function and pathology that results when homeostasis fails (Figure 4.2).

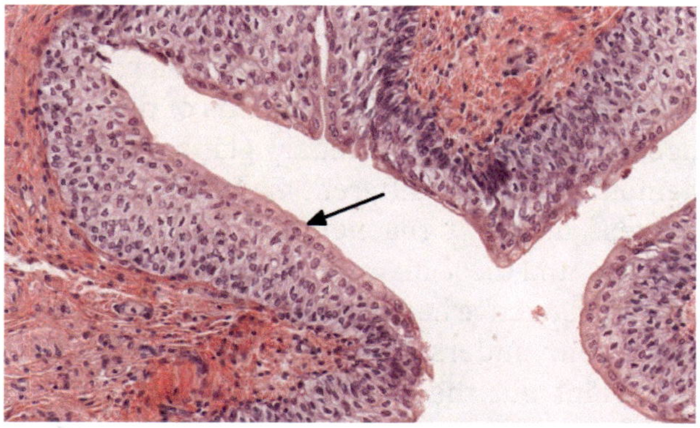

Figure 4.2. Understanding the epithelial tissues.

Source: https://histology.medicine.umich.edu/sites/default/files/Q1%20epithelial.jpg.

Importance of Epithelial Tissue in the Human Body

Epithelial tissue is an indispensable protective layer in the human body that has a function that cannot be replaced in order to provide homeostasis and guard inner components against damage. The epithelial tissue forms the outer skin layer as well as lining various cavities and organs, thereby keeping them safe from bacteria, mechanical damage, and chemicals. Interestingly, epithelial cells are tightly packed to minimize the risk of harmful materials passing through to the underlying tissues. Such functionality is not passive defense but rather involves the epithelial tissues actively engaging with the environment due to selective permeability that regulates the diffusion of wastes and nutrients. Therefore, the integrity of epithelial tissue is of crucial importance; any damage could result in serious health problems, highlighting the vital function this tissue performs in overall body function and immune protection. Aside from its protective function, epithelial tissue is also significant in absorption and secretion functions, which are essential in upholding physiological balance. Specialized epithelial cells of organs such as the intestines can absorb water and nutrients from food, which has been digested, such that the body absorbs necessary nourishment. Meanwhile, glands evolved by epithelial tissue, such as endocrine and exocrine glands, secrete hormones, enzymes, and other necessary substances. Secretions perform a variety of functions, from facilitating digestion to regulating metabolism. Moreover, the several types of epithelial tissues that vary in structure and function reflect their adaptability to meet particular requirements throughout the body. Thus, the multifaceted functions of epithelial tissue extend far beyond mere protection, encompassing vital processes that sustain life and enhance health. Epithelial tissue function also extends to immune responses, in which it not only acts as a barrier but also as an active component of the immune response. Certain epithelial cells produce antimicrobial peptides and cytokines that help eliminate infection and stimulate other immune cells during an immune response. An example is defensins, antimicrobial peptides found in most epithelial tissues. They exhibit a critical role in the neutralization of the invasion of pathogens and perform an essential role in innate immunity. Their presence emphasizes the interactive dynamics between immune defense mechanisms and epithelial tissue. This significant interaction equips the body to counteract the pathogens more effectively, reducing the likelihood of infection-related diseases. Understanding these major functionalities highlights the importance of epithelial tissue towards the upholding of health, further strengthening its standing as a central member in the grand framework of human physiology and immune resistance (Raj & Dentino, 2002; Parvy et al., 2018).

4.1. Types of Epithelial Tissue

Learning Outcome

1. Describe the simple epithelium and stratified epithelium;
2. Understand the transitional epithelium.

Epithelial tissue, a vital component of the human body, can be categorized into various types based on cellular organization and function. The two main types are simple and stratified epithelia. Simple epithelial tissue consists of a single layer of cells, which facilitates processes such as absorption, secretion, and filtration. Simple squamous epithelium, for instance, covers vessels and alveoli to facilitate the best possible exchange of gases due to its thinness. Conversely, stratified epithelial tissue is made up of over one layer of cells, which provides better protection from physical and chemical forces. A notable example is the stratified squamous epithelium found in skin, which acts as a protective measure against pathogens, dryness, and abrasion. The particular structures and characteristics of such epithelial tissues play important roles in the upkeep of homeostasis and overall body function. Several specialized epithelial tissues are adapted to meet specific physiological needs in the human body. Cuboidal and columnar epithelia, for example, are often involved in secretion and absorption. Simple cuboidal epithelium is normally found in glandular tissue and renal tubules, where it aids in the secretion and absorption of substances like hormones and ions. On the other hand, simple columnar epithelium is common in the gastrointestinal tract for promoting nutrient uptake and mucus secretion for effortless digestion. In addition, certain epithelial cells could have modifications, including cilia or microvilli, for further development of their functional ability. Ciliated epithelial tissue, common in the respiratory tract, facilitates the removal of debris and pathogens, demonstrating how epithelial tissue structure is irrevocably linked to functions and the general health of the organism. The significance of epithelial tissue also lies in its participation in the processes of regeneration, demonstrating dynamic flexibility present in different types. For example, transitional epithelium in the urinary bladder allows for the extension and expansion of the organ and the storage of different amounts of urine. This specialized type of epithelium demonstrates the capacity to adjust its structure to reflect the continuous demands of the body's needs. Additionally, mammary gland epithelium demonstrates that different mammalian species possess different regeneration and functional abilities, and these may greatly affect on lactation and reproductive health. These comparisons also enrich our understanding of epithelial biology and point out the evolutionary developments that have occurred between species, expanding our knowledge of normal function and potential states of disease (Cunha et al., 2019; Spaas et al., 2012) (Figure 4.3).

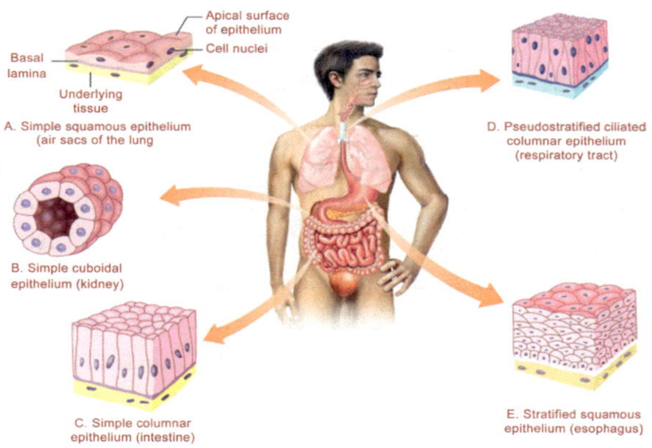

Figure 4.3. Types of epithelial tissue.

Source: https://img.brainkart.com/article/article-Epithelial-Tissue-tqv.png.

4.1.1. Simple Epithelium

Simple epithelium is a primitive component of epithelial tissue in humans, which is composed of one close-packed cell layer. Such a structural plan enables simple epithelium to carry out very important physiological functions, such as absorption, secretion, and filtration. Simple epithelium is generally classified into various types based on cell shape: squamous, cuboidal, and columnar. The most typical function of all types is to match its structure at the cellular level; e.g., simple squamous epithelium, with cells being thin and flat, is perfectly adapted for diffusion and filtration procedures. Understanding these functions is crucial, as they explain the specialized functions that simple epithelium provides in contributing to homeostasis within the human body through selective material transfer at tissue interfaces. The significance of simple epithelium extends beyond structural composition in that it serves to cover and safeguard numerous body cavities and organs. Simple cuboidal epithelium, for example, covers glandular ducts and kidney tubules, where the secretory role allows for the regulation of electrolytes and body fluids. Besides, simple columnar epithelium is also found to cover the gastrointestinal tract, which has a role to play in the secretion of mucus and absorption of nutrients, essential for digestion and maintenance of intestinal lining integrity. Proper functioning of the epithelia is central to the organism's overall health since not only do they offer important metabolic activities but also safeguard the organism against pathogens and toxic materials from the environment. Research continues to unveil the intricate interrelations of plain epithelium with other body systems, particularly of gut microbiota.

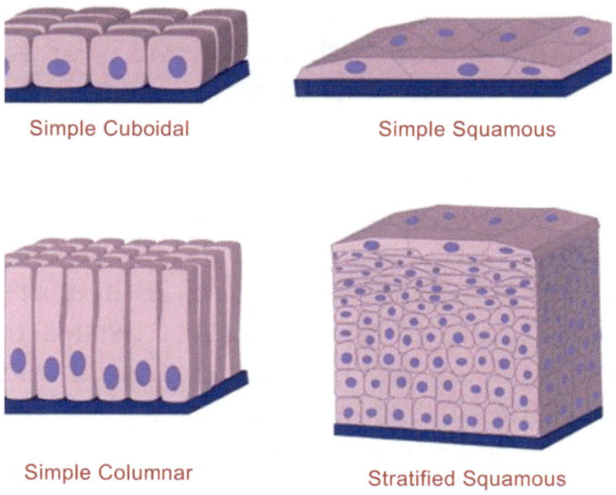

Figure 4.4. Simple epithelium.

Source: https://www.careerpower.in/blog/wp-content/uploads/sites/2/2024/10/17145637/simple-epithelial-tissue.png.

It is discovered that properties and spatial organization of the epithelial cells have significant roles in influencing microbial populations of intestines. Integrity of plain epithelium may also influence biogeography of symbiotic bacteria, which is crucial for nutrient absorption and immune protection. Furthermore, changes in the epithelial layer can lead to dysbiosis, a condition that goes along with most health illnesses, including inflammatory bowel disease and metabolic syndrome. Understanding the relationship between simple epithelium and gut microbiota not only enhances our knowledge of human health but also encourages new therapeutic approaches that strive to restore epithelial integrity and promote a normal microbiome (Donaldson et al., 2016; Tallitsch & Guastaferri, 2022) (Figure 4.4).

4.1.2. Stratified Epithelium

Among numerous types of epithelial tissue, stratified epithelium is particularly significant due to both its functional diversity and structural complexity. It is characterized by more than one cell layer, not only providing an extremely effective barrier but also enhancing tissue resistance to mechanical stress. Stratified epithelial tissues are essential where the body comes into contact with friction and wear, such as in skin, mouth, and esophagus. The layered design allows for maximum protection from environmental injuries, such as pathogens and mechanical abrasions. By creating a location for rapid cell replacement, stratified epithelium also aids in wound healing and is therefore a crucial feature in the defense of tissues that are immediately exposed to the external world. In immune interactions, stratified epithelium has been demonstrated to have an impressive capability to respond to a wide range of stimuli, particularly in the respiratory and gut. For example, research involving epithelial cells has revealed that they can act as sentinels and barriers in managing host-pathogen interactions. In research on ovine tracheal epithelial cells, some growth conditions were found to significantly impact cell differentiation and ciliation, showing the dynamic nature of stratified epithelia in response to environmental stimuli (O'Boyle et al., 2018). This plasticity not only indicates the importance of stratified epithelium in physical defense but also its role in immune surveillance. The interaction of epithelial cells with pathogens suggests a complex relationship that plays a crucial role in disease susceptibility and infection control. Furthermore, stratified epithelial pathologies provide information concerning their critical functions in health and disease. For instance, an explanation of herpes simplex virus 2 (HSV-2) infection of epithelial tissues identifies the vulnerabilities of such barrier tissues. Experiments demonstrating the histological changes in the squamous epithelium, such as ballooning degeneration and viral antigen detection, point out the manner in which stratified epithelium can be injured in infection (Burgener et al., 2019). The awareness of inflammatory response and structural alterations due to viral activity underlines both the susceptibility and importance of stratified epithelial tissues to global well-being. A study of these interactions not only adds depth to our comprehension of epithelial function but also helps towards the development of therapeutic strategies targeted at epithelial integrity in infection (Figure 4.5).

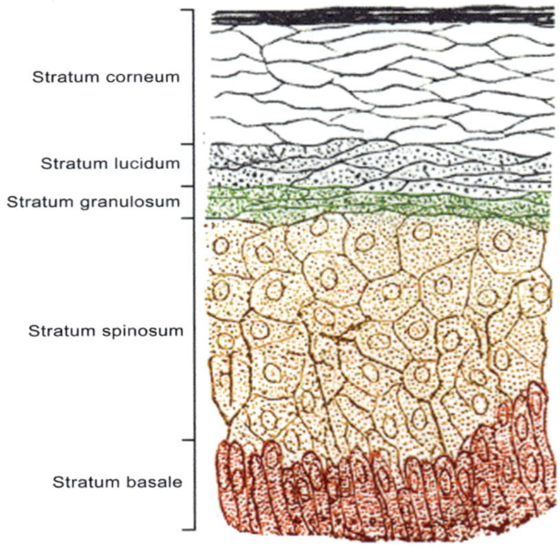

Figure 4.5. Human skin

Section of the human skin showing the stratified squamous epithelial surface, referred to as the epidermis. The layer of keratin here is named the stratum corneum.

Source: https://upload.wikimedia.org/wikipedia/commons/2/20/Skinlayers.png.

4.1.3. Transitional Epithelium

Transitional epithelium, being a unique form of epithelial tissue, plays a significant role in the human body, particularly in the urinary system. This unique epithelium is predominantly found lining the bladder, ureters, and parts of the urethra, where its specific characteristics enable extensive stretching and distension. The specialized structure of transitional epithelium, including its ability to change from cuboidal stratified to squamous, allows it to accommodate varying amounts of urine while still presenting an obstruction to leakage. This flexibility is crucial for effective urinary function, as it allows for the assurance of safe storage and transport of urine without compromising the integrity of surrounding tissues. The cellular composition of transitional epithelium is made up of many layers of cells that cooperate to provide it with full functionality. The outermost layer, or the umbrella cells, possesses a dome-shaped morphology that also assists in stretching. It is this structure that prevents permeability so that solutes and water become entrapped within the urinary system and, therefore, homeostasis is maintained. One of the most intriguing features of transitional epithelium is the mechanism it undergoes, termed desquamation, wherein the surface cells peel off as a result of tension, such that the epithelium layer can be renewed constantly. Such features pose intriguing questions regarding cell signaling and regeneration processes at the molecular level in this tissue and how these could drive developments in treatment modalities for urinary tract conditions (Basil et al., 2020). Research also examines the role of transitional epithelium beyond structural considerations. As a case in point, the work on how transitional epithelium interacts with basement tissues and reacts to pathological conditions could potentially result in a better understanding of many urological afflictions. Diseases like bladder cancer or interstitial cystitis can radically alter the functional integrity of transitional epithelium, which underscores the tissue's function within health. By employing novel research approaches to study the cellular biology and repair mechanisms of transitional epithelium, scientists can design personalized therapies aimed at restoring normal function in pathological patients. Upcoming research could provide further insights into the complexities of this form of epithelium and its role in homeostasis and potential therapeutic interventions in urinary disorders (Tallitsch & Guastaferri, 2022) (Figure 4.6).

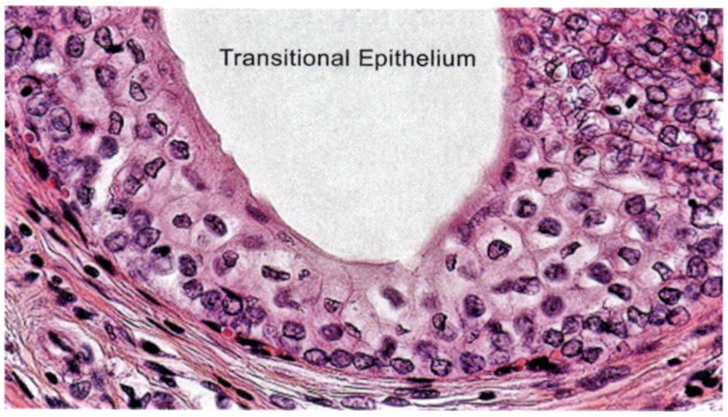

Figure 4.6. Transitional epithelium.

Source: https://study.com/cimages/multimages/16/epithelial_tissue8209859355989304 52.jpg.

Test Your Knowledge

1. What are the 3 types of simple epithelium?
2. What is transitional epithelium?

4.2. Functions of Epithelial Tissue

Learning Outcome

1. Describe the function of protection;
2. Understand the process of absorption;
3. Understand the secretion.

Epithelial tissue plays a critical role in the human body, essentially as a protective cover against physical, chemical, and biological damage. The tissue covers internal as well as external surfaces, thus protecting the structures and organs underneath. Its small cell design inhibits the free flow of harmful pathogens and toxins but enables selective adsorption of essential substances. The preservation of epithelial layer integrity is of utmost importance because loss of it will cause severe implications for health, as evidenced by infection and inflammation. The importance of epithelial barriers is also emphasized in disease states, particularly in immunocompromised hosts, where breaches in epithelial integrity can facilitate tissue invasion by opportunistic pathogens with subsequent risk of virulent systemic infections, as noted in chronic microbial colonization observations in human immunodeficiency viruses (HIV) and simian immunodeficiency virus (SIV) infection studies (Ocon et al., 2013). In addition to its defensive function, epithelial tissue is crucial in absorption and secretion processes that are vital to maintaining homeostasis. The intestinal epithelium, for instance, is particularly constructed to maximize nutrient uptake at the same time as it serves to expel waste products. Certain cells of this layer, like enterocytes, possess gigantic enlargements of surface area in the form of microvilli, which amplify their absorptive capability. The role of epithelial tissue is more than simple absorption; it is also the secretion of enzymes, hormones, and mucus that assist in digestion and lubricate and protect other underlying tissues. Strikingly, dysregulation of these secretory activities can induce gastrointestinal disease, highlighting the crucial nature of unbroken epithelial function for general metabolic health and appropriate regulation of the body (Andrews-Polymenis et al., 2010).

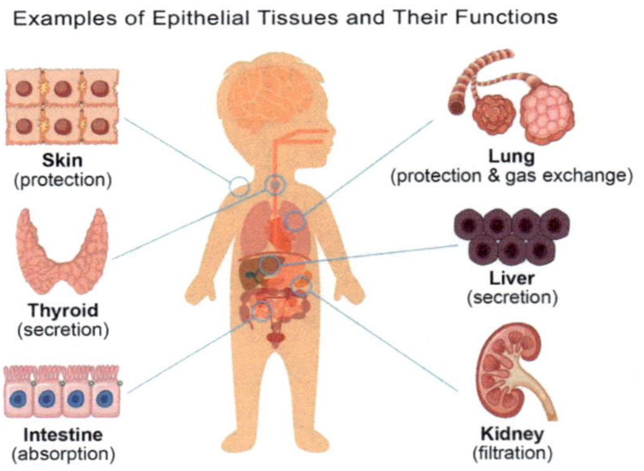

Figure 4.7. Epithelial tissues pick up specialized functions to fit the needs of different organs in our body.

Source: https://rsscience.com/wp-content/uploads/2022/04/epithelial-tissues-and-their-functions-1536x1056.jpg?ezimgfmt=ng:webp/ngcb1.

Furthermore, epithelial tissues are responsible for sensory perception as a result of their unique cell organization and special structure. Certain epithelial cells are equipped with sensory receptors, which enable them to react to stimuli from the external environment, such as touch, temperature, and pain. This function is particularly evident in the special epithelial tissues within the skin and mucous surfaces, where they are a web of sensory stimuli necessary for protective reflex and direct response to injurious stimuli. Importantly, the interaction of epithelial cells with the immune system provides for continuous dialogue required in sustaining local as well as systemic immunity, particularly by pathogen-associated molecular pattern recognition. The coordination of sensory and immunologic function within epithelial tissue emphasizes the intricate roles of epithelial tissue in the protection of human health and disease, and thus, it is a pivotal research field to understand health and wellness (Figure 4.7).

4.2.1. Protection

Epithelial tissue serves as the first defense of the body, providing critical protection from environmental elements outside of the human body. This protective purpose is vital during homeostasis because epithelial cells create a physical barrier that prevents the invasion of pathogens, toxins, and other harmful substances. The packing of cells in epithelial tissue enhances its barrier function, limiting permeability while allowing selective passage of essential nutrients and gases. The specialized junctions, for instance, the tight junctions and desmosomes, also enhance this barrier function by offering intercellular adhesion and preventing infiltration. Such a barrier role is particularly necessary in those areas subject to constant wear and tear, i.e., the skin and the gut, where the need for firm and potent barriers is greatest in protecting underlying tissue from damage and infection. In addition to physical barriers, epithelial tissue plays an essential role in immunological protection through its relationship with the immune system. Epithelial cells are not mere passive barriers but actively participate in defense mechanisms by the release of cytokines and other signaling molecules in the event of microbial or chemical attack. This activation, in addition to potentiating local immune responses, also activates the systemic immune mechanisms and hence allows for a rapid and effective response to danger. For instance, when epithelial cells detect noxious stimuli, they initiate the release of chemokines that recruit immune cells to sites of injury or infection. Such a response is a vital component of immune surveillance, deterring colonization by pathogens and facilitating healing of wounds. Epithelial cell interactions with resident immune cells show the active role of epithelial tissue in providing protection, which proves its vital role in maintaining overall human health (Beebe et al., 2016). Additionally, the protective benefits of epithelial tissues also include beyond the physical barrier and immunological reactions. Epithelial cells are involved in the production of many antimicrobial peptides and proteins that further reinforce the body's defense system. For example, in the respiratory and gastrointestinal tracts, other secretions and mucus secreted by epithelial cells capture pathogens and particulate matter, keeping them from invading the deeper tissues. Lastly, ascorbic acid (AsA), a potent antioxidant found in epithelial tissues, can detoxify reactive oxygen species (ROS) generated upon exposure to environmental stress.

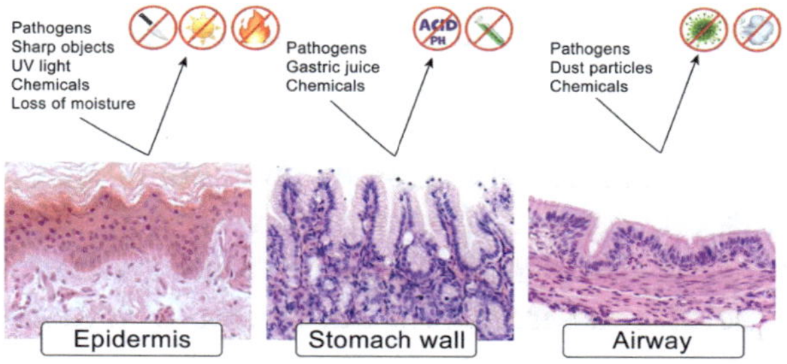

Figure 4.8. Examples of epithelial tissues that function as a protective barrier are the epidermis (skin), stomach wall epithelium, and ciliated airway epithelium.

Source: https://rsscience.com/wp-content/uploads/2022/04/epithelia-function-protection-1536x888.jpg?ezimgfmt=ng:webp/ngcb1.

The movement of AsA, which is critical to its protective roles, is made possible through specific sodium-dependent transporters in human epithelial cells, suggesting an adaptive process that enables robustness against oxidative damage (Beebe et al., 2016). Such a multidirectional approach to protection demonstrates the complexity and necessity of epithelial tissue in the preservation of human well-being and underscores its importance within the realm of tissue homeostasis and overall health (Figure 4.8).

4.2.2. Absorption

The absorption function is significant to the role of epithelial tissue in the human body, particularly in the gastrointestinal tract. Epithelial cells, through their particular structural characteristics like microvilli, greatly increase the surface area for the uptake of nutrients. This specialization allows the epithelium to transport essential nutrients from the intestinal lumen directly into the bloodstream. Operations that take place here involve a combination of active and passive transport operations, which are vital for the selective absorption of proteins, carbohydrates, and fats. In addition, the integrity and well-being of the epithelial barrier are of maximum importance as any disruption will lead to malabsorption and illness. This intricate mechanism emphasizes the important role of epithelial tissue not just in absorption, but primarily in upholding body homeostasis and general body nutrition. Furthermore, nutrient digestion is also intertwined with the epithelial tissue engagement with other bodily systems, particularly when it comes to disease. For example, studies have shown that bioactive molecules, such as Lactoferrin (Lf), can promote the absorption process and deliver therapeutic benefits in disease conditions, e.g., cancer. Lf, a glycoprotein with iron-binding capacity, is highly bioavailable after oral ingestion and can selectively target cancer cells while improving normal cellular function. This feature is of utmost significance in improving the absorption of the therapy agent as well as total nutrient intake among treated patients. Therefore, understanding the mechanisms through which the epithelial tissue facilitates absorption, particularly when nutraceuticals are involved, may illuminate new directions for enhancing treatment efficacy and patient care in clinical practice (Bonaccorsi di Patti et al., 2020). In addition, the establishment of therapeutic methods that reverse the issues of absorption can significantly impact the management of complex diseases. Recent research highlights the potential of glycosylphosphatidylinositol (GPI) modification of therapeutic proteins to enhance their oral bioavailability and target-deliver them through the epithelial barrier. The process is meant to bypass traditional hurdles that hinder the efficacy of protein-based treatment. If successful, it would be a paradigm shift in drug delivery, leveraging the natural absorption capabilities. Moreover, such sophisticated techniques can introduce personalized therapy that is more effective and accessible, particularly for patients with genetic risk of a disease. Exploring these techniques underscores the importance of epithelial function for drug absorption and general health outcomes, pointing to the intersection of basic science and clinical translation in modern medicine (Mueller, 2010) (Figure 4.9).

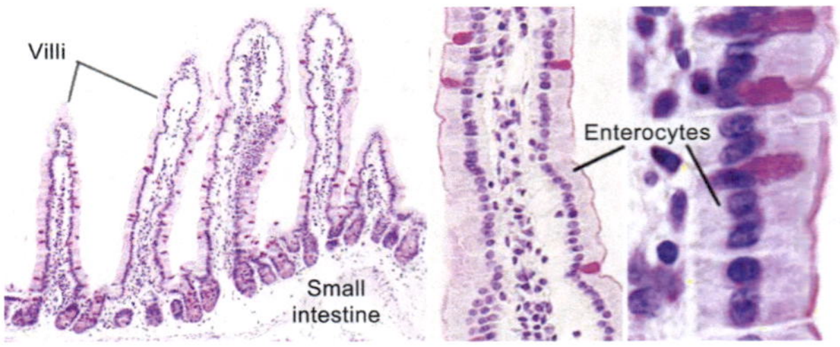

Figure 4.9. Villi arrangement of small intestine epithelium.

Source: https://rsscience.com/wp-content/uploads/2022/04/villi-small-intestine-epithelium.jpg?ezimgfmt=ng:webp/ngcb1.

4.2.3. Secretion

Secretion is the fundamental function of epithelial tissue important to the physiology of humans. Epithelial cells are adapted for the secretion of a variety of substances from enzymes and hormones to mucus and sweat, according to their location and purpose. For example, epithelial cells lining the gastrointestinal tract secrete digestive enzymes and protective mucus, which aid in breaking food down and protecting the underlying tissues, respectively. Similarly, endocrine glandular epithelial cells release hormones that regulate many functions of the body. This specialized secretion exemplifies the responsiveness of the epithelial tissues, which are capable of meeting the diverse requirements of the body in different physiological conditions, contributing significantly to homeostasis and overall health. One of the most common examples of epithelial tissue secretion is the production of mucus by goblet cells, which are characterized by their unique shape and structure within the layer of epithelium. Found primarily in the gastrointestinal and respiratory tracts, goblet cells lubricate and shield epithelial surfaces. The mucous layer generated by these cells creates an obstruction to pathogens and irritants and facilitates immune protection. Further, the ability of goblet cells to rapidly secrete mucus upon stimulation highlights the dynamic nature of epithelial tissue. The secretory process is crucial in maintaining the integrity of the epithelial surface, particularly in areas subjected to mechanical and chemical stress, thus highlighting the protective function of epithelial tissue in covering sensitive structures while ensuring proper functioning of organ systems. Apart from the protective roles of secretory epithelial cells, abnormal secretion leads to several diseases, demonstrating the delicate balance of these tissues. For instance, *Helicobacter pylori*, a virulent bacterium, infects the gastric mucosa, exploiting the epithelial barrier for persistence and inducing inflammation. This chronic inflammation can interfere with normal secretory functions to give rise to diseases like peptic ulcer disease and gastric cancer. The host epithelial cell and bacterial virulence determinant interaction demonstrates a complex relationship where the regulation of secretion is crucial to disease outcomes. The mechanisms can give insight into therapy and prevention strategies, and another value is attached to the normal secretion by epithelial tissues in disease prevention and the maintenance of human health (White et al., 2015) (Figure 4.10).

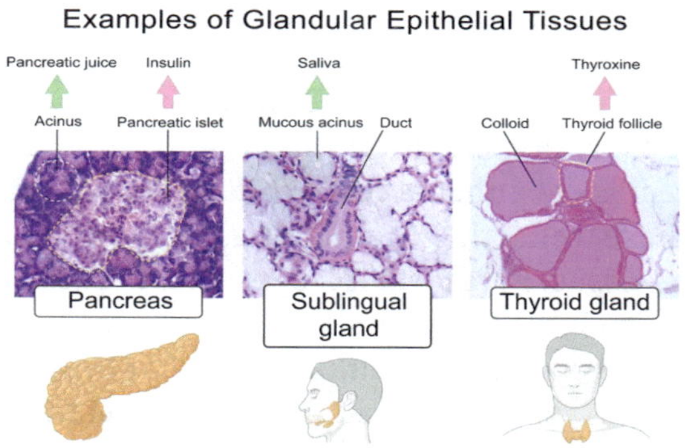

Figure 4.10. Examples of epithelial tissues that secrete essential substances for our body: pancreatic juice and insulin from the pancreas; saliva from the sublingual gland; and thyroxine from the thyroid gland.

Source: https://rsscience.com/wp-content/uploads/2022/04/glandular-epithelial-tissue-pancreas-sublingual-gland-tyroid-gland-1536x1039.jpg?ezimgfmt=ng:webp/ngcb1.

Test Your Knowledge

1. What is the process of absorption?
2. What is secretion?

4.3. Structure of Epithelial Tissue

Learning Outcome

1. Learn about cell arrangement;
2. Understand the polarity of epithelial cells;
3. Describe the basement membrane.

The structure of epithelial tissue is characteristically distinguished by tightly packed cells that form uninterrupted sheets, providing a protective cover over various body surfaces. The collective arrangement not only prevents extraneous harmful substances from penetrating interior environments but also facilitates the selective permeability required for absorption, secretion, and sensation. The nucleolus of epithelial cells typically lies near the cell base, reflecting the functional requirement of the tissue. Furthermore, epithelial tissues are classified into two general categories: simple and stratified epithelium. Simple epithelia consist of a single layer of cells and hence are effective in processes such as diffusion and filtration, while stratified epithelia, composed of multiple layers, provide more protection in areas that are subject to abrasion. This cell structure accounts for the variability of epithelial tissues in responding to their specific physiological functions. In addition to the cellular layers, tissue organization also varies depending on the specific function that it serves. For instance, squamous epithelium, consisting of flat cells, is efficient in enabling diffusion, for instance, in the alveoli of the lungs. Cuboidal and columnar epithelia are concerned with secretion and absorption due to their increased surface area and amount of cytoplasm. These shapes of cells directly affect the efficiency of organ function, such as that of the kidneys or the gastrointestinal system. Further, special epithelial forms such as cilia or microvilli may facilitate special functions, such as mucus movement in the respiratory tract or increased absorption in the intestines. Understanding these adaptations emphasizes the importance of epithelial tissue in maintaining homeostasis in the body. Epithelial tissue growth and homeostasis also rely heavily on signaling pathways and molecular determinants that regulate cell behavior. There are specialized transcription factors that are part of these processes and influence not only normal tissue formation but also disease pathogenesis. For example, changes in epithelial architecture are typically associated with disease states, such as cancers or developmental disorders. Particularly, studies into aspects like the PBX family of genes have elucidated their function in midfacial development, illustrating how the defects can lead to cleft lip and palate, revealing the sophistication of epithelial tissue functions over the simplistic structural nature. The intricate structure of epithelial tissue structures magnifies their important functions in human development and health, warranting their relevance in physiological and pathologic terms (Welsh et al., 2018; Cunha et al., 2019).

4.3.1. Cell Arrangement

Cell arrangement is central to comprehending the functioning and efficiency of various organs of the human body with regard to epithelial tissue. Epithelial cells possess a dense structure and cell shapes that range from simple to diverse, with the consequent classifications such as simple, stratified, cuboidal, columnar, and transitional epithelium. All of the arrangements are adapted to specific physiological functions; for instance, simple squamous epithelium facilitates rapid filtration and diffusion due to its thinness, but stratified epithelium protects abrasion areas. The structure of such cells not just allows for functional demands but also contributes to the overall efficiency of epithelial barriers that line surfaces and cavities, thereby impacting processes such as absorption, secretion, and sensation. The structure of epithelial cells is inherently linked to their developmental origin and cellular signaling pathways that define tissue architecture. During embryonic growth, mesenchymal-epithelial interactions shape the epithelial sheets that later develop into the organs. For example, within the bladder, epithelial structures such as the trigone (a triangular region on the floor of the bladder,) and ureterovesical (point where each ureter enters the bladder) junction develop due to complex signaling network, such as Sonic Hedgehog (Shh) signaling pathway and TGF-β, that coordinate proper cell arrangement as well as differentiation.

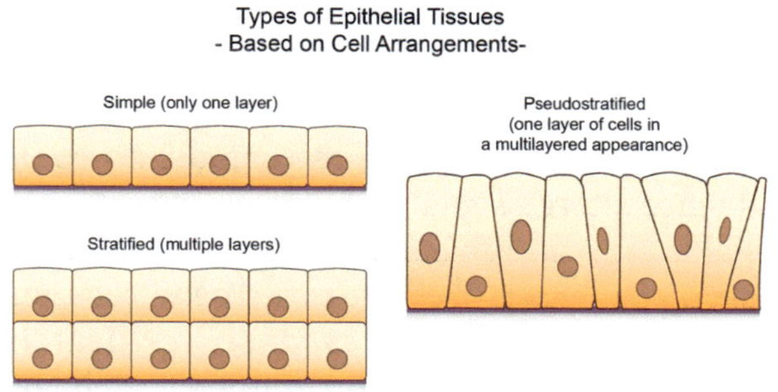

Figure 4.11. Schematics of simple, stratified, and pseudostratified arrangements of epithelial cells.

Source: https://rsscience.com/wp-content/uploads/2022/04/Simple-Stratified-Pseudostratified-epithelial.jpg?ezimgfmt=ng:webp/ngcb1.

The transitional arrangement is supportive of the bladder's ability to hold urine and manage urination effectively. Such interruptions in the process may result in malformations that weaken the structural integrity and functionality of the organ, suggesting the importance of proper cellular disposition in development as documented in existing literature on bladder development and cell signaling (Liaw et al., 2019). In addition, epithelial tissue organization also suggests the importance of adaptive responses to mechanical and environmental cues. In specific regions of the body, such as in the respiratory system, epithelial cells possess a ciliated type that is essential for mucociliary clearance. Such unique patterns serve in trapping and elimination of harmful particles, and they present evidence for the adaptive nature of epithelial tissues to their particular environments. Furthermore, studies have discerned variation in epithelial structures, such as apical versus basal layer differentiation in stratified epithelium, influencing barrier integrity and permeability. The dynamic nature of epithelial cell organization, fueled by functional demands and extrinsic stimuli, emphasizes the complexity and central roles that these tissues fulfill in homeostasis and the protection of underlying tissues (Berloco et al., 2017) (Figure 4.11).

4.3.2. Polarity of Epithelial Cells

Epithelial polarity is a fundamental property that distinguishes this tissue from others and is essential to its diverse functions in the body. Epithelial cells possess apical and basolateral surfaces, which allow them to perform specialized functions like absorption, secretion, and protection. This compartmentalization plays a significant role in maintaining homeostasis, as molecules and ions may be transported across the layers of cells selectively. Epithelial polarity dysregulation can potentially generate severe health issues, such as a broad spectrum of diseases spanning from cancer to inflammatory diseases. Understanding why and how the polarity is established and regulated is critical in the therapeutic intervention design, aiming to restore normal function in pathological states. The necessity of polarity in regulating epithelial cell stress response is highlighted in a new study. The stress-polarity pathway (SPS) is uncovered to be a significant mechanism that maintains epithelial integrity under energetic stress situations. SPS is activated by AMP-kinase, which enhances epithelial polarity, particularly in the intestinal epithelial system, and promotes barrier function. This underscores the dual role of epithelial polarity in maintaining homeostasis and resistance to environmental stressors.

Furthermore, the study of the SPS pathway describes how aging and disease mechanisms can disrupt epithelial integrity, leading to diseases such as leaky gut, which can enhance systemic inflammation. These observations emphasize the importance of epithelial polarity in disease and health, suggesting possibilities for novel therapeutic strategies. In cancer biology, disruption of epithelial cell polarity is a key mechanism that promotes tumor growth. As elaborated in recent reports, interaction between the tumor and its microenvironment can significantly impact not just tumor expansion but systemic physiology as well. As epithelial cells become non-polarized, these cells can be rewired towards a more invasive phenotype and get engaged in cancer metastasis. Experiments in organisms such as *Drosophila melanogaster* allow scientists to investigate tumor-intrinsic as well as non-tumor-derived modulation of effects on epithelial integrity. These findings have the potential to increase our appreciation of how restoration of polarity could contribute to treating cancers, thus underlining the complex interrelation between epithelial tissue polarity and disease prognosis. Knowledge of these processes offers a roadmap for the design of targeted treatments for maintaining or restoring epithelial function in cancer patients.

4.3.3. Basement Membrane

The basement membrane is a significant feature of epithelial tissue that serves as a ground layer between the epithelium and the connective tissue beneath it. Composed largely of a complicated mixture of proteins, glycoproteins, and proteoglycans, it provides structural support and influences cell behavior. Not only does this layer anchor epithelial cells, but it also acts as a selective barrier that regulates the passage of molecules between the epithelium and the underlying connective tissue. Its organization may vary quite significantly from tissue to tissue, adapting to the specific functional requirements of particular epithelial types. The addition of fibrous proteins like collagen and elastic fibers serves to contribute to the mechanical strength of the epithelial tissue, with the glycoproteins aiding cell adhesion, creating a dynamic interface that is essential for tissue well-being and regeneration. In addition to its structural role, the basement membrane also plays an essential role in signaling pathways that control cellular functions like proliferation, differentiation, and migration. Cell-basement membrane interactions are transduced via specific receptors, which are capable of activating pathways important in tissue repair and homeostasis. For example, alterations in basement membrane integrity can result in pathological mechanisms such as cancer, where basement membrane remodeling could influence altered signaling and thus unrestricted cellular growth. Further, the unique biochemical makeup enables it to create a microenvironment conducive to cellular responses critical in preserving tissue integrity. Epithelial cells are dependent on these signals for function, toward identifying the basement membranes key role in structure as well as epithelial tissue function throughout the human body. Some of the latest tissue engineering developments have revealed the importance of the basement membrane as a substrate for cell growth and healing. Progress in the application of amniotic membrane (AM) as a biological scaffold has revealed the capability of basement membranes in regenerative medicine. The thick basement membrane of AM offers a near-native extracellular matrix, which is an ideal substrate for epithelial cell proliferation and adhesion. This application stands in contrast to traditional strategies, which more commonly use synthetic scaffolds whose biochemical signals may be unsuitable for supporting successful tissue regeneration. Also, the basement membrane of the AM has the additional benefit of anti-inflammatory and anti-scarring properties, which are advantageous in augmenting the therapeutic functions in tissue engineering. With ongoing investigations, the diverse functions and properties associated with the basement membrane will continue to expand its application in biomedical sciences, confirming its pivotal position in epithelial tissue function and regeneration (Figure 4.12).

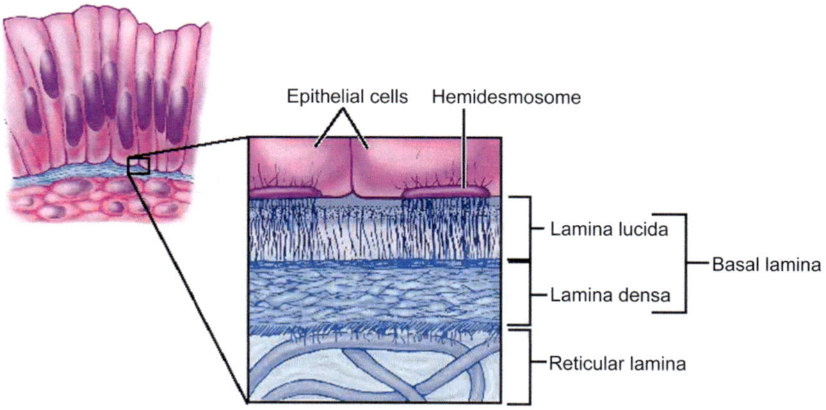

Figure 4.12. Most epithelial cells are separated from the connective tissue by a sheet of extracellular material called the basement membrane. It is formed by the association of two layers: the Basal lamina and the Reticular lamina.

Source: https://rsscience.com/wp-content/uploads/2022/04/basement-membrane-basal-lamina-reticular-lamina.jpeg?ezimgfmt=ng:webp/ngcb1.

Test Your Knowledge

1. What is meant by cell arrangement?
2. What is the polarity of epithelial cells?

4.4. Locations of Epithelial Tissue in the Body

Learning Outcome

1. Describe the skin and outer surfaces;
2. Understand the lining of cavities and organs;
3. Understand the glands.

Epithelial tissue forms a part of various organs and systems within the human body and functions as both a protective barrier and a working interface. Skin, which is made up of stratified squamous epithelium, is arguably the most critical location of epithelial tissue. The multi-layering not only protects from external attack by agents such as pathogens and chemicals but also engages with the senses and with heat regulation. Added to this, epithelial cells of the epidermis are integral to the keratinization process, which enhances the barrier properties of the skin. Epithelial tissue coats the entire gastrointestinal tract, where it facilitates absorption and secretion.

This extensive coverage is a testament to the fact that epithelial tissue is intricately interwoven into the body's functionality as a whole, performing different roles according to where and how it is organized. The respiratory system is the other important location where epithelial tissue is centrally located, i.e., the airway lining. The respiratory tract is lined with ciliated pseudostratified columnar epithelium that acts to trap and remove pathogens and particles. The cilia beat in synchronized fashion to move mucus, secreted by goblet cells within the epithelium, upwards towards the throat, thus clearing the airways. This physiological adaptation enhances the protective function of epithelial tissue in protecting the lungs from infection and irritation. Specialized epithelial cells outside the airways also play essential roles in the olfactory epithelium that gives rise to the sense of smell. The functional extent of the epithelial tissues in these systems highlights their adaptive value during evolution as functional structures. Epithelial tissue placement is also found in the urinary system, where transitional epithelium forms the lining of the bladder and portions of the ureters. Transitional epithelium is specialized epithelium necessary to accommodate urine size changes so that these organs may stretch without bursting. The specialized cell organization of transitional epithelial cells enables them to shift between a relaxed and distended state, reflecting their adaptive reaction to the physiological demand imposed upon them. Moreover, the kidneys are lined with simple cuboidal epithelium, which plays a vital role in filtration and absorption of essential substances. Consequently, the locations of epithelial tissue in the body demonstrate an incredibly varied display, allowing the tissues to fulfill diverse and essential functions relevant to their specific environment and role (Chintapalli et al., 2012Sinclair et al., 2019) (Figure 4.13).

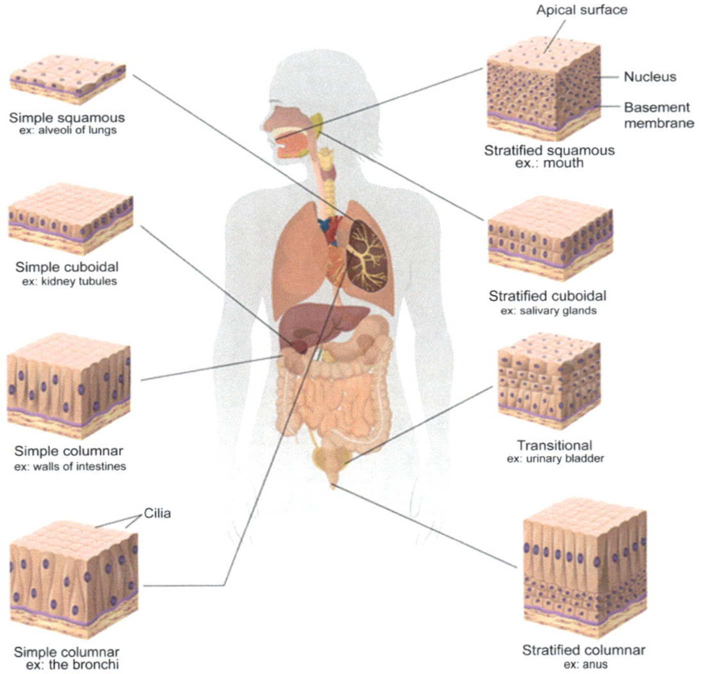

Figure 4.13. Each class of epithelial tissue has a unique shape and number of layers, depending on its location and role in the body.

Source: https://encrypted-tbn0.gstatic.com/images?q=tbn:ANd9GcRELs6wzObsvfsXdPCTsPYloG9qoFCFVHzHrQ&s.

4.4.1. Skin and Outer Surfaces

The skin, the largest organ of the body, is a vital barrier and interface between the internal physiological environment and the external milieu. It is constituted primarily of epithelial tissue and is structured into several layers: epidermis, dermis, and subcutaneous tissue. The epidermis itself, a stratified squamous epithelium, is primarily devoted to protection, regulation, and sensation. Within this most superficial layer, keratinocytes are pivotal in providing strength and mechanical stress and resistance to pathogen invasion. In addition, the interaction between various cell types of the epidermis with the underlying dermis is significant in the maintenance of skin integrity and the healing process after injury. Complexity of skin architecture highlights the importance of ongoing research into its cellular and molecular dynamics, particularly with regard to understanding skin maturation and differentiation; critical topics in research on epithelial tissues in human individuals (Cokus et al., 2019). The uniqueness of the skin's exterior surfaces extends beyond mere structural composition to include functionality and environmental interaction. Many factors, such as UV light, bacteria, and chemical agents, constantly challenge skin integrity with adaptive and protective responses by epithelial tissues. In addition, certain visible features, such as Marxs line on the eyes mucosal surfaces, emphasize the skin role in responding to environmental stressors. This phenomenon has a specific reference to imply that even small epithelial adaptations are going to greatly contribute to tissue health and homeostasis. The dynamic relationship between epithelial integrity and environmental stimulus not only orchestrates local immune response but also controls systemic well-being, revealing the essential need for research into the response of epithelial tissue to varied stimuli in humans (Bron et al., 2011). With research uncovering mechanisms behind the skin and outer skin surfaces, emerging evidence finds that understanding the process is indispensable for the development of effective therapeutic strategies. For instance, knowing the specific roles of different types of epithelial cells in skin can provide insight into the complexities of wound repair and tissue renewal. Also, understanding mechanisms related to epithelial maturation can provide avenues for new therapies of skin disorders and enhanced healing following injury. Discovery of specific molecular markers, underlined by recent studies, could be the foundation for targeted therapies taking advantage of skin epithelial cells' regenerative capacity. Thus, thorough investigation of the skin's epithelial layers will not only increase our understanding of its biological functions but also unveil possibilities for clinical application in dermatology and regenerative medicine (Cokus et al., 2019) (Figure 4.14).

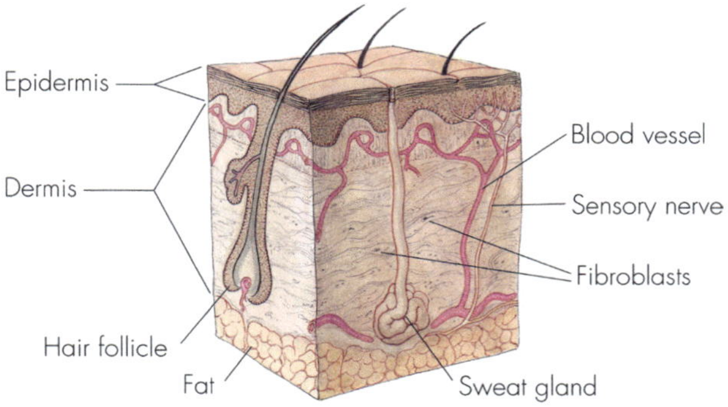

Figure 4.14. Layers of the skin.

Source: https://wtamu.edu/~cbaird/sq/images/300skin1.jpg.

4.4.2. Lining of Cavities and Organs

Epithelial tissue is a key component when lining cavities and organs in the human body, performing crucial functions in protection, secretion, and absorption. This type of tissue is specialized to serve as a barrier between external and internal environments, protecting substances required by the body and barring harmful agents from entering. Epithelial tissue organization varies at different locations; for example, the lining of alveoli in the lungs by simple squamous epithelium facilitates the exchange of gases and the covering of the skin surface by stratified squamous epithelium. In addition, the typical plan of epithelial cells allows them to attain specific functional needs, for example, the cuboidal cells found in glandular tissues that facilitate secretion. The tissue heterogeneity of the epithelium is a reflection of its fundamental function to maintain homeostasis in heterogeneous physiological systems. Aside from protective barrier function, epithelial tissues are important for lining organs and cavities because they can support various physiological processes, such as absorption and secretion. As an example, the columnar epithelium of the intestines is designed for maximal nutrient absorption with microvilli that maximize the surface area. Similarly, the glandular epithelium produces enzymes and hormones needed for digestion and metabolism. The lining of the peritoneal cavity demonstrates the sophisticated interplay between drug delivery systems and epithelial tissue; intraperitoneal (IP) chemotherapy exploits the unique pharmacokinetic properties of the peritoneal-plasma barrier to treat peritoneal metastases. By gaining insights into these dynamic interactions, researchers can venture into novel therapeutic approaches, including the utilization of innovative advancements like IP aerosol therapy and controlled drug delivery systems to boost treatment effectiveness for various types of cancers, as emphasized in recent research (Ceelen et al., 2020). As much as the importance of epithelial linings in organ systems is well established, some epithelial structures need to be explored further to reveal their multifunctional roles. Such an organ is an example of the coagulating gland (CG) in rodents, which, despite its benign disregard in recent reproductive literature, has been discovered to be engaged in local homeostasis and fertility by its renin-angiotensin system. Such glands play roles beyond mere secretion and have a significant impact on male reproductive health, prompting one to think that a similar mechanism may also be present in the human body (Sengupta, 2017). This provokes a re-evaluation of our current understanding of epithelial tissue and highlights the importance of rigorous investigation. Investigating more poorly understood epithelial structures allows us to most comprehensively appreciate the intricate functions that epithelial tissues both play in health and disease and provide opportunities for novel medical interventions and advancing our overall understanding of human biology (Figure 4.15).

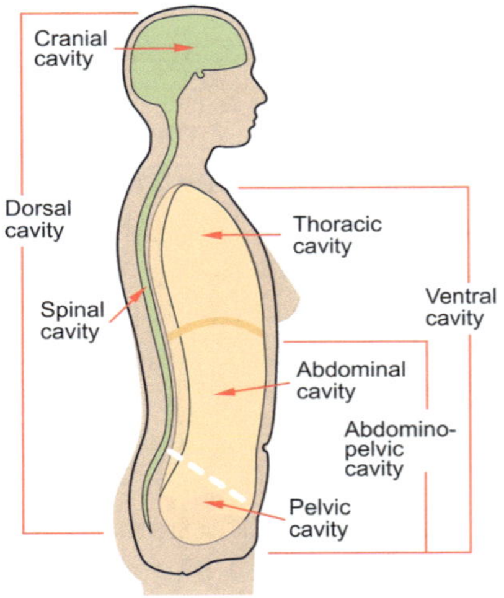

Figure 4.15. Cross-section showing cavities in the human body, the dorsal and ventral body cavities labelled.

Source: https://upload.wikimedia.org/wikipedia/commons/e/ee/Scheme_body_cavities-en.svg.

4.4.3. Glands

Glands are an important component of epithelial tissue in human beings, demonstrating the interdependence of function and structure. Specialized epithelial cells, glands are responsible for synthesizing and secreting chemicals such as hormones, enzymes, and mucus, which play vital roles in regulating physiological functions.

Glands are categorized under two general classes: exocrine and endocrine. Exocrine glands, such as sweat and salivary glands, secrete their product onto epithelial surfaces through ducts, while endocrine glands, like the thyroid and adrenal glands, secrete hormones into the bloodstream. This classification reflects the range of functional roles performed by glands in the body, from metabolism to growth and development, and thus contributes a useful role to homeostasis. The development and function of glands largely rely on epithelial support that maintains glandular tissue. For instance, the control of tight junctions between epithelial layers is important in the control of paracellular transport of substances. Claudins, being a family of proteins required for the formation of tight junctions, play important roles in the permeability and integrity of epithelial cells in various glandular tissues, as seen in studies of mammary glands at various developmental stages (Baumgartner et al., 2017). The dynamic expression and cellular localization of claudins like claudin-3 and claudin-4 during processes like pregnancy and lactation underscore their significance in regulating glandular function by governing solute permeability and cellular interaction. Besides, the interaction of epithelial cells with the environment is also necessary for glandular health and function. Derangement of the signaling pathways that govern glandular function can lead to pathological processes. For example, pathogens from bacteria such as *Clostridium difficile* pose a danger to epithelial integrity by disrupting intercellular junctions and the actin cytoskeleton, as seen in experimental models (Bier et al., 2020). Not only do these disruptions prevent normal secretory functions, but they can also cause inflammatory reactions, which once again points toward the importance of intact epithelial barriers in glandular well-being. Knowledge of the mechanisms underlying gland function and regulation in epithelial tissues is important in developing therapeutic interventions to manage gland-related diseases (Figure 4.16).

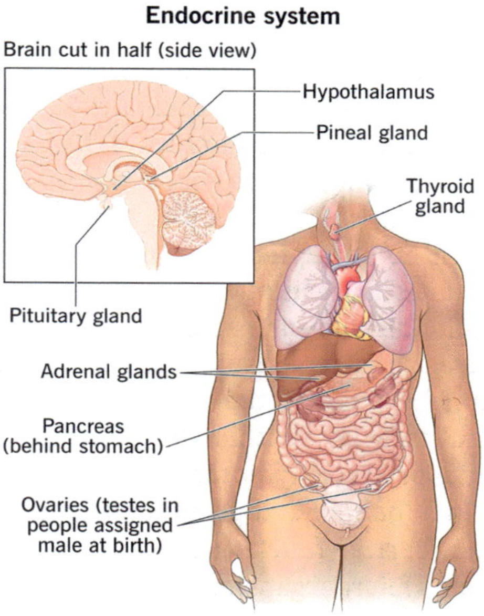

Figure 4.16. Endocrine system consists of the tissues (mainly glands) that create and release hormones.

Source: https://my.clevelandclinic.org/-/scassets/images/org/health/articles/21201-endocrine-system.

Test Your Knowledge

1. What is the skin?
2. What is the lining of the organs and body cavities?

4.5. Epithelial Tissue and Disease

Learning Outcome

1. Understand hotel maintenance management and its impact
2. Perform preventive maintenance
3. Discuss about breakdown maintenance

Epithelial tissue is a crucial barrier and interface of the human body, and its health is a prerequisite for general well-being. Epithelial tissue covers the organs, cavities, and surfaces of the body and permits functions such as absorption, secretion, and protection. However, the integrity of epithelial tissue can be disrupted by numerous diseases and conditions, leading to significant clinical effects. Conditions such as Crohn's disease and ulcerative colitis demonstrate how inflammatory mechanisms possess the potential to disrupt epithelial integrity within the gastrointestinal tract and produce symptoms of diarrhea and abdominal pain. Furthermore, disruption of epithelial barrier function can grant access for pathogenic microorganisms to enter into tissue, thus assisting in the development of disease.

These implications do underscore the close relationship between epithelial tissue health and disease states, and also emphasize the relevance of knowledge regarding epithelial pathophysiology as part of an overall appreciation of health issues. Systemic illnesses as well as chronic infection may detract from epithelial tissues. Immunocompromised individuals, such as those with HIV, display a range of oral epithelial disorders relative to their reduced ability to fight infections. Studies highlight that the majority of individuals infected with HIVexperience impairing oral infections that correlate with disease progression. Testimony to the complex interaction between immune response and epithelial integrity is provided by experiments with SIV infection leading to chronic inflammation activation within the mucosa. This dysregulation may cause decreased epithelial formation and facilitate colonization by bacterial pathogens, indicating that faulty epithelial tissue can be both a marker and a permissive factor for disease advancement (Ocon et al., 2013). In addition, fibrosis is a significant characteristic of epithelial tissue-associated illnesses, linking chronic inflammation and injury with escalating tissue dysfunction. Renal tubulointerstitial fibrosis in the kidney is a global pathological effect of chronic kidney disease (CKD), with large-scale deposition of extracellular matrix disrupting normal epithelial function.

It is a convergent pathway for the majority of kidney diseases and is strongly associated with worsening renal function. The pathologic mechanisms behind renal fibrosis need to be known to create good treatment plans for CKD. When considering epithelial health from the clinic, the relationship among chronic inflammation, tissue remodeling, and organ function should be extensively examined with special focus, since ongoing scientific research continues to uncover novel targets of therapy for countering disease impact on epithelial tissues (Elliott et al., 2015) (Figure 4.17).

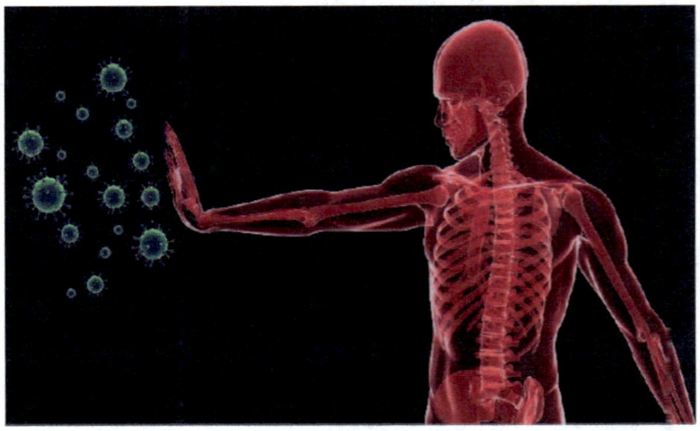

Figure 4.17. Human epithelial cells.

Source: https://www.lifelinecelltech.com/wp-content/uploads/2016/02/Immune-System-v5.jpg.

4.5.1. Cancer and Tumors

The relationship between epithelial tissue and cancer is key to understanding tumor development in the human organism. Epithelial cells happen to be on the receiving end of the outside environment's interface with the body's internal systems and hence become the target of preference for the majority of carcinogens, both chemical agents and ultraviolet radiation. If exposed to such deleterious agents, epithelial cells might acquire genetic mutations that disrupt normal cell division control mechanisms. The derangement of the processes leads to uncontrolled cell proliferation, characteristic of tumors. In addition, the immune response initiated by epithelial cells, as delineated by the inflammation cascade in response to stress, can contribute both for and against tumorigenesis. Although immune surveillance presumably protects against malignancies, the activation of specific pathways may inadvertently establish a tumor-permissive environment, thereby promoting cancer development (Dalessandri & Strid, 2014). The mammary gland constitutes a significant example of the relationship between epithelial biology and oncogenesis. The gland consists mainly of epithelial cells that also experience gigantic regeneration cycles during lactation, which are coordinated by mammary stem cells (MaSC). The stem cells are key to the maintenance of tissue architecture and response to physiological needs. However, the mechanisms regulating MaSC activity can become altered, leading to abnormal proliferation and differentiation and providing a conducive environment for the development of breast cancer. Breast cancer complexity stems from the different signal pathways regulating epithelial differentiation as well as the mammary gland microenvironment. It is crucial to comprehend the processes: not just does it uncover the mammary tumor pathophysiology, but it also gives a glimpse into therapeutic interventions that could potentially employ stem cell dynamics in reversing malignancies (Borena et al., 2013). Moreover, the implication of epithelial tissue in immune response against carcinogenic stress makes the process of cancer development even more intricate. Where epithelial integrity is compromised, such as in chronic inflammation or infection, the type 2 immune response can be redirected. Although the intent of this type of immune response is protective, it can inadvertently facilitate tumor growth by enhancing chronic inflammation that is known to support the survival and growth of cancer cells. Paradoxical is thus the nature of epithelial-driven immunity with significant implications for treatment and prevention of cancer. A profound understanding of how immune mechanisms interact with epithelial stress responses could lead to new therapeutic approaches that target the tumors directly but also manipulate the local microenvironment to efficiently combat cancer formation (Dalessandri & Strid, 2014) (Figure 4.18).

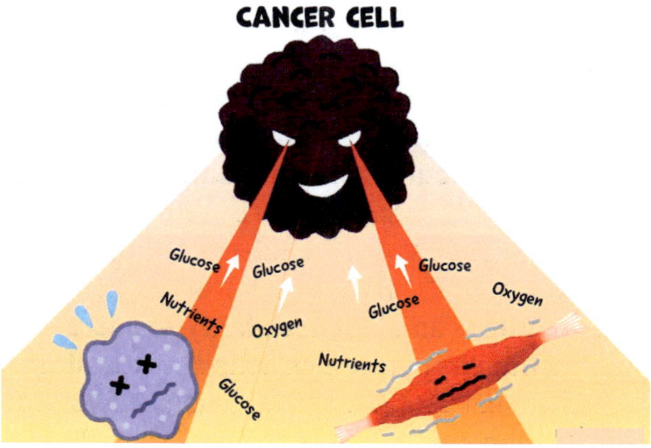

Figure 4.18. Cancer cells plunder the nutrients from surrounding cells and tissues to sustain the rapid growth of tumors.

Source: https://rsscience.com/wp-content/uploads/2022/03/cancer-cells-take-nutrient-from-other-cells.jpg?ezimgfmt=ng:webp/ngcb1.

4.5.2. Inflammatory Conditions

Epithelial tissue is at the heart of inflammatory disorders, since epithelial tissue is the first line of defense against pathogens and environmental insults. Epithelia are more than passive barriers and are actively involved in innate immune responses through the secretion of antimicrobial peptides and cytokines. The inflammatory reaction, a coordinated response to injury or infection, often triggers a cascade of cellular and molecular changes within the epithelial layer. For instance, when inflammatory signals are detected, the epithelial cells may undergo changes that alter their permeability such that immune cells can migrate into the zone to target perceived threats. It is interaction between the epithelial cells and the extracellular matrix that is of critical significance, as their dysregulation leads to chronic inflammation and is involved in inflammatory bowel disease, asthma, or, as has been observed in *Helicobacter pylori* infections, various gastric diseases, which are very closely associated with epithelial damage and repair mechanisms (Hu et al., 2018). The capacity of epithelial tissues to promote inflammation is more than that of a passive defense system since these cells are also pivotal in the modulation of the inflammatory process. In chronic inflammation, i.e., that due to chronic infections or autoimmune diseases, epithelial cells acclimatize by entering into a process called epithelial-to-mesenchymal transition (EMT). EMT equips epithelial cells with migratory and invasive ability, encouraging the recruitment of immune cells and sustaining the inflammation further. But it is pathological and can lead to fibrosis and tissue remodeling, which is common in chronic inflammatory diseases. These diseases cause disruption of normal epithelial architecture, which may promote more serious conditions, like tumorigenesis. Research on organoid models of such conditions finds them to be effective in uncovering major insights into epithelial tissue responses to chronic inflammatory stimulus, hence highlighting pathways that could be targeted for therapeutic intervention (Hu et al., 2018). Understanding mechanisms of inflammation in epithelial tissues could have bearing on the development of targeted therapies that would counter inflammatory disorders. Given the complex nature of host-pathogen interactions, particularly in infections like *Helicobacter pylori*-induced infections, it is certain that inflammation is regulated by both the host's immune system as well as microbial virulence factors. *H. pylori* can induce a low-grade chronic inflammation without being cleared by immunity; it is a prime example of the subtle balance maintained by epithelial cells. This multifaceted relationship is used to demonstrate the importance of comprehending epithelial responses to inflammatory stimuli, both in health and disease. Through the use of advances in organoid technologies and tissue engineering, researchers are well-positioned to model such conditions and ultimately inform our understanding of epithelial pathobiology throughout the spectrum of inflammatory disorders (White et al., 2015).

4.5.3. Genetic Disorders

The intricate interaction between the integrity of human epithelial tissue and genetic disorders has a significant role to play in understanding the pathologic diseases. Epithelial tissues, which perform the function of protection as well as execute a multitude of biological functions, can be greatly influenced by genetic mutations. The disorders may be because of a single-gene mutation or polygenic interactions and can lead to alterations in cellular arrangement and function. These disturbances can be described in terms of diseases of the gastrointestinal tract, respiratory tract, and other epithelial-lined organs. When genetic mutations disrupt the homeostasis of epithelial cells, it may result in conditions such as enhanced permeability, healing defects, and abnormal cell proliferation. These processes must be understood not only for diagnosis but also to develop targeted therapeutic interventions for restoring epithelial health and function. Research has indicated that certain genetic mutations are directly disrupting signal pathways important to the integrity of epithelial tissue. For example, the GUCY2C pathway is an important pathway in the intestinal epithelium that controls many physiological processes that are essential to epithelial homeostasis. Dysregulation of the pathway has been involved in the pathogenesis of several gastrointestinal conditions, including inflammatory bowel disease and colorectal cancer. Genetic mutations that disable the function of GUCY2C can potentially lead to disruption of the secretion of fluid, microbiome homeostasis, and regeneration of epithelial cells. The connection of these genetics with epithelial disease highlights the urgency for further study into how the manipulation of such mechanisms promises new therapeutic interventions. The potential for employing genetic data to enhance the robustness of epithelial cells is a critical focus of research in biomedical science. New stem cell technology holds encouraging potential for the therapy of epithelial tissue genetic disease, particularly where conventional therapies have proved wanting. New advances in culturing adult human intestinal stem cells (ISCs) hold the prospect of new therapies for monogenic and polygenic intestinal failure, in which organoids could be grown that reproduce the structure and function of the epithelium. These advances, combined with genome-editing technologies like CRISPR/Cas9, make it possible to correct the genetic mutations in the stem cells and establish a means towards personalized regenerative medicine approaches. The ability to generate functional epithelial tissue from cells derived from the patient not only gives insight into the pathophysiology of genetic disease but also offers an arena upon which new interventions might be examined in a controlled environment. With ongoing research, the usability of treating genetic diseases that affect epithelial tissues will keep expanding, with improved patient outcomes and better understanding of epithelial tissue biology (Dunn et al., 2016; Rappaport & Waldman, 2018).

Test Your Knowledge

1. What is the role of epithelial tissue in inflammatory conditions?
2. What are genetic disorders?

SUMMARY

Briefly, epithelial tissue plays a critical role in human physiology as a protective barrier and facilitates many of the body's required functions, such as absorption, secretion, and sensation. This tissue is not only critical for maintaining regulation of homeostasis in the body but also in the interface between internal biological mechanisms and external environments. The variability of epithelial tissues, ranging from their diverse structures and functions of simple glandular cuboidal cells to stratified squamous cells of the skin, bestows upon them an overwhelming capacity to adapt to many physiological demands. The in-depth investigation of epithelial tissue still unravels the complexity of depicting how the loss of epithelial integrity leads to many conditions of disease, as seen in chronic infection and inflammation. Moreover, epithelial tissue changes are of great importance to disease onset and to health outcomes. As the evidence that SIV infection is capable of inducing oral microbiome dysbiosis indicates, there is a clear interaction between microbial homeostasis in the body and epithelial health (Ocon et al., 2013). This dysbiosis not only shows the impact of viral infection on epithelial cells but also indicates the significance of maintaining epithelial integrity to prevent opportunistic infections. Findings obtained through such studies underscore the significance of epithelial tissue not just in local but in systemic health and point out that an insight into the biology of such cells plays a pivotal role in developing therapeutic measures to counteract diseases associated with epithelial dysfunction. Briefly, the significance of epithelial tissue cannot be overstated because it transcends mere structural roles to assume crucial functions in immune defense and microbial interactions. Ongoing research on epithelial tissue promises to shed even greater light on the mechanisms of many pathological conditions, such as those occasioned by bacterial infections, attested to by ongoing research on pathogens such as Salmonella (Bernard et al., 2000). As researchers delve deeper into the complex dynamics between epithelial cells, their microbiome, and general health, it becomes increasingly clear that a complete comprehension of the tissue is essential to advancing the field of medical science and improving patient care. In this manner, an interdisciplinary approach incorporating microbiology, immunology, and cell biology is essential in comprehending the totality of epithelial tissue functions and how they contribute to human disease.

Epithelial tissue is one of the critical parts of human physiology because it supplies a protective covering and enables functions in the body. Epithelial tissue exists in different types and encompasses simple and stratified epithelia, each of which is customized to achieve certain purposes depending on location and function. Simple squamous epithelium, for example, is located in places where there is a need for quick diffusion, i.e., the alveoli of the lungs, and stratified epithelium offers protection in places that are exposed to abrasion, e.g., the skin. Epithelial tissue also possesses special features, e.g., polarity, where opposite surfaces have different functions, enabling functions like absorption and secretion. Having this good understanding of these fundamental properties is crucial for ongoing research into how epithelial tissues contribute to overall health and disease processes. Furthermore, epithelial tissue's function is not just passive physical defense; it is also part of complex physiological processes. For example, epithelial cells communicate with the microbiome by regulating the flow of nutrients and immune function. New evidence suggests a role for short-chain fatty acids (SCFA), produced by fermentation of dietary fiber in the gut, that enhance metabolic control and potentially reduce cardiovascular disease risk. In this case, epithelial cells contribute to gut barrier function and immune regulation, and their central role in promoting metabolic well-being and disease prevention is underscored. Study of these interactions has opened up new avenues of therapeutic treatments against gut health, demonstrating the ubiquitous role of epithelial tissue in disease and health. Furthermore, improvements in tools of research, such as the development of three-dimensional co-culture models, have significantly improved the understanding of the role of epithelium in interaction with pathogens. Recent studies employing these models demonstrate significant *in vivo*-like behavior of epithelial tissue in response to infections, including those caused by Salmonella. The capacity of these models to incorporate macrophages allows for a greater comprehension of host-pathogen interactions, including complex dynamics that occur upon infection. Such research demonstrates how tissue architecture and cellular structure of epithelial tissue can be employed to regulate microbial colonization and the immune response. This emerging knowledge brings to the forefront the importance of epithelial tissue not just in its ancient roles but also in its complex relationships with both health-enhancing and disease-producing organisms in the human body.

KEY TERMS FROM THIS CHAPTER

Absorption
Autoimmune disorders
Cancer research
Chemical exposure
Epithelial cells
Epithelial tissue
Exocrine glands
Immune system
Pathogens
Protection
Regenerative medicine
Secretion
Sensation
Simple epithelium

CRITICAL THINKING QUESTIONS

1. **Epithelial tissue primarily functions in:**
   a. Support and structure
   b. Movement
   c. Covering and lining surfaces
   d. Transmission of impulses
2. **Epithelial tissue lacks:**
   a. Blood vessels
   b. Nerve supply
   c. Cells
   d. A basement membrane
3. **The epithelial tissue composed of a single layer of flat cells is called:**
   a. Simple squamous epithelium
   b. Simple cuboidal epithelium
   c. Simple columnar epithelium
   d. Stratified squamous epithelium
4. **Which type of epithelial tissue is found lining the kidney tubules?**
   a. Simple squamous epithelium
   b. Simple cuboidal epithelium
   c. Simple columnar epithelium
   d. Transitional epithelium
5. **Pseudostratified columnar epithelium is characterized by:**
   a. Multiple layers of columnar cells
   b. Cells of different heights giving a stratified appearance
   c. Flattened cells with no nuclei
   d. Only one cell layer with uniform cell height

Short Answer Questions

1. Define the epithelial tissue.
2. Why is epithelial tissue important in the human body?
3. List the types of epithelial tissue.
4. What are the functions of the epithelial tissue?
5. What is the structure of the epithelial tissue?

Answers to Critical Thinking Questions

1. (c); 2. (a) ; 3. (a); 4. (b); 5. (b)

REFERENCES

1. Abbott, N., Covert, J., Dubielzig, R., Isseroff, et al. (2014). *PDGF-BB does not accelerate healing in diabetic mice with splinted skin wounds.* https://core.ac.uk/download/323070343.pdf (accessed on 7th August 2025).
2. Dalessandri, T., & Strid, J. (2014). Beneficial autoimmunity at body surfaces - immune surveillance and rapid type 2 immunity regulate tissue homeostasis and cancer. *Frontiers in immunology, 5,* 347. https://doi.org/10.3389/fimmu.2014.00347(accessed on 7th August 2025).
3. Ahmadiani, A., Ghanavi, J., Jorjani, M., Niknejad, et al. (2008). *Properties of the amniotic membrane for potential use in tissue engineering.* https://core.ac.uk/download/1684261.pdf (accessed on 7th August 2025).
4. Chintapalli VR, Terhzaz S, Wang J, Al Bratty M, Watson DG, Herzyk P, et al. (2012) Functional Correlates of Positional and Gender-Specific Renal Asymmetry in *Drosophila*. PLoS ONE 7(4): e32577. https://doi.org/10.1371/journal.pone.0032577(accessed on 7th August 2025).
5. Alberca Zaballos, M., Calonge Cano, M., Fernández Martínez, I., Galindo de la Rosa, et al. (2019). *A proof-of-concept clinical trial using mesenchymal stem cells for the treatment of corneal epithelial stem cell deficiency.* https://core.ac.uk/download/288886968.pdf (accessed on 7th August 2025).
6. Alvaro, D., Cardinale, V., Carpino, G., Franchitto, et al. (2018). *Contribution of resident stem cells to liver and biliary tree regeneration in human diseases.* https://core.ac.uk/download/188824417.pdf (accessed on 7th August 2025).
7. Andrews-Polymenis, H. L., Bäumler, A. J., Fierer, J., Godinez, et al. (2010). *A rapid change in virulence gene expression during the transition from the intestinal lumen into tissue promotes systemic dissemination of Salmonella.* https://core.ac.uk/download/12175814.pdf (accessed on 7th August 2025).
8. Hu, J. L., Todhunter, M. E., LaBarge, M. A., & Gartner, Z. J. (2018). Opportunities for organoids as new models of aging. *The Journal of cell biology, 217*(1), 39–50. https://doi.org/10.1083/jcb.201709054https://core.ac.uk/download/323074761.pdf (accessed on 7th August 2025).
9. Barrila, J., Brenneman, K., Clemett, S. J., Crabbé, et al. (2017). *Three-dimensional organotypic co-culture model of intestinal epithelial cells and macrophages to study Salmonella enterica colonization patterns.* https://core.ac.uk/download/84045916.pdf (accessed on 7th August 2025).
10. Bartlett, J. D., DenBesten, P., Diekwisch, T. G. H., Duverger, et al. (2017). *Meeting report: A hard look at the state of enamel research.* https://core.ac.uk/download/323074729.pdf (accessed on 7th August 2025).
11. Basil, M. C., Chapman, H. A., Engler, A. E., Guo, et al. (2020). *The cellular and physiological basis for lung repair and regeneration: Past, present, and future.* https://core.ac.uk/download/305124289.pdf (accessed on 7th August 2025).
12. Cunha, G. R., Sinclair, A., Ricke, W. A., Robboy, S. J., Cao, M., & Baskin, L. S. (2019). Reproductive tract biology: Of mice and men. *Differentiation; research in biological diversity, 110,* 49–63. https://doi.org/10.1016/j.diff.2019.07.004(accessed on 7th August 2025).

13. Liaw, A., Cunha, G. R., Shen, J., Cao, M., Liu, G., Sinclair, A., & Baskin, L. (2018). Development of the human bladder and ureterovesical junction. *Differentiation; research in biological diversity, 103*, 66–73. https://doi.org/10.1016/j.diff.2018.08.004(accessed on 7th August 2025).

14. Sinclair, A. W., Cao, M., Pask, A., Baskin, L., & Cunha, G. R. (2017). Flutamide-induced hypospadias in rats: A critical assessment. *Differentiation; research in biological diversity, 94*, 37–57. https://doi.org/10.1016/j.diff.2016.12.001 (accessed on 7th August 2025).

15. Baumgartner, H. K., Bitler, B. G., Burns, V., Kobayashi, et al. (2017). *Developmental Expression of Claudins in the Mammary Gland.* https://core.ac.uk/download/82893751.pdf (accessed on 7th August 2025).

16. Beebe, D., Dana, B., Huang, A., Huang, et al. (2016). *Expression profiling of ascorbic acid-related transporters in human and mouse eyes.* https://core.ac.uk/download/212866507.pdf (accessed on 7th August 2025).

17. Welsh, I. C., Hart, J., Brown, J. M., Hansen, K., Rocha Marques, M., Aho, R. J., Grishina, I., Hurtado, R., Herzlinger, D., Ferretti, E., Garcia-Garcia, M. J., & Selleri, L. (2018). Pbx loss in cranial neural crest, unlike in epithelium, results in cleft palate only and a broader midface. *Journal of anatomy, 233*(2), 222–242. https://doi.org/10.1111/joa.12821(accessed on 7th August 2025).

18. Berloco, B. P., Boitani, C., de Rooij, D. G., Di Persio, et al. (2017). *Spermatogonial Kinetics in Humans.* https://core.ac.uk/download/158327988.pdf (accessed on 7th August 2025).

19. Bernard, S., Brown, D. J., Casadesús, J., Leori, et al. (2000). *Host Adapted Serotypes of Salmonella Enterica.* https://core.ac.uk/download/11686965.pdf (accessed on 7th August 2025).

20. O'Boyle N, Sutherland E, Berry CC, Davies RL (2018) Optimisation of growth conditions for ovine airway epithelial cell differentiation at an air-liquid interface. PLoS ONE 13(3): e0193998. https://doi.org/10.1371/journal.pone.0193998(accessed on 7th August 2025).

21. Bier, E., Franc, N. C., Guichard, A., Roy, et al. (2020). *A Drosophila model for Clostridium difficile toxin CDT reveals interactions with multiple effector pathways.* https://core.ac.uk/download/323065186.pdf (accessed on 7th August 2025).

22. Bonaccorsi di Patti, M. C., Cutone, A., Ianiro, G., Lepanto, et al. (2020). *Lactoferrin's anti-cancer properties. Safety, selectivity, and wide range of action.* https://core.ac.uk/download/296244729.pdf (accessed on 7th August 2025).

23. Borena, B. M., Burvenich, C., Bussche, L., Duchateau, et al. (2013). *Mammary Stem Cell Research in Veterinary Science: An Update.* https://core.ac.uk/download/55798803.pdf (accessed on 7th August 2025).

24. Ceelen, W., Braet, H., van Ramshorst, G., Willaert, W., & Remaut, K. (2020). Intraperitoneal chemotherapy for peritoneal metastases: an expert opinion. *Expert opinion on drug delivery, 17*(4), 511–522. https://doi.org/10.1080/17425247.2020.1736551Bron, A. J., Gaffney, E. A., Tiffany, J. M., Yokoi, et al. (2011). *A solute gradient in the tear meniscus I: A hypothesis to explain Marx's line.* https://core.ac.uk/download/pdf/1634057.pdf (accessed on 7th August 2025).

25. Burgener, A., Carroll, T., Corey, L., Farr Zuend, et al. (2019). *Acute infection and subsequent subclinical reactivation of herpes simplex virus 2 after vaginal inoculation of rhesus macaques.* https://core.ac.uk/download/323068087.pdf (accessed on 7th August 2025).

26. Spaas, J. H., Chiers, K., Bussche, L., Burvenich, C., & Van de Walle, G. R. (2012). Stem/progenitor cells in non-lactating versus lactating equine mammary gland. *Stem cells and development, 21*(16), 3055–3067. https://doi.org/10.1089/scd.2012.0042(accessed on 7th August 2025).

27. Carrasco, E., Mittelbrunn, M., & Soto-Heredero, G. (2019). *The role of extracellular vesicles in cutaneous remodeling and hair follicle dynamics.* https://core.ac.uk/download/343444084.pdf (accessed on 7th August 2025).

28. Chambers, E. S., Frost, G., Morrison, D. J., Preston, et al. (2018). *Role of gut microbiota-generated short chain fatty acids in metabolic and cardiovascular health.* https://core.ac.uk/download/161513799.pdf (accessed on 7th August 2025).

29. Cirio, M. C., Davidson, A. J., de Caestecker, M. P., de Groh, et al. (2013). *Kidney Regeneration: Common Themes from the Embryo to the Adult.* https://core.ac.uk/download/159296304.pdf (accessed on 7th August 2025).

30. Cokus, S. J., De La Torre, M., Medina, E. F., Ramirez-Gutierrez, et al. (2019). *Tissue-specific transcriptomes reveal gene expression trajectories in two maturing skin epithelial layers in zebrafish embryos.* https://core.ac.uk/download/323076243.pdf (accessed on 7th August 2025).

31. Parvy, J. P., Hodgson, J. A., & Cordero, J. B. (2018). *Drosophila* as a Model System to Study Nonautonomous Mechanisms Affecting Tumour Growth and Cell Death. *BioMed research international, 2018,* 7152962. https://doi.org/10.1155/2018/7152962 (accessed on 7th August 2025).

32. Das, S., Foretz, M., Ghosh, P., Ibeawuchi, et al. (2020). *The stress polarity signaling (SPS) pathway serves as a marker and a target in the leaky gut barrier: Implications in aging and cancer.* https://core.ac.uk/download/323065864.pdf (accessed on 7th August 2025).

33. Raj, P. A., & Dentino, A. R. (2002). Current status of defensins and their role in innate and adaptive immunity. *FEMS microbiology letters, 206*(1), 9–18. https://doi.org/10.1111/j.1574-6968.2002.tb10979.x (accessed on 7th August 2025).

34. Donaldson, G. P., Lee, S. M., & Mazmanian, S. K. (2016). *Gut Biogeography of the Bacterial Microbiota.* https://core.ac.uk/download/33123998.pdf (accessed on 7th August 2025).

35. Dunn, J. C. Y., Hong, S. N., Martín, M. G., Stelzner, et al. (2016). *Concise review: The potential use of intestinal stem cells to treat patients with intestinal failure.* https://core.ac.uk/download/323078733.pdf (accessed on 7th August 2025).

36. Elliott, J., Jepson, R. E., Lawson, J. S., Syme, et al. (2015). *Renal fibrosis in feline chronic kidney disease: Known mediators and mechanisms of injury.* https://core.ac.uk/download/36777966.pdf (accessed on 7th August 2025).

37. Galluzzi, L., Vitale, I., Aaronson, S. A., Abrams, J., Adam, D., Agostinis, P., Alnemri, E. S., et al. (2018). Molecular mechanisms of cell death: Recommendations of the Nomenclature Committee on Cell Death 2018. *Cell Death and Differentiation, 25,* 486–541. https://doi.org/10.1038/s41418-017-0012-4 (accessed on 7th August 2025).

38. Robert B. Tallitsch and Ronald Guastaferri (2022). "Histology: An Identification Manual" (2022). *Open Textbooks.* https://digitalcommons.augustana.edu/open_textbooks/1

39. (accessed on 7th August 2025).

40. Hoffmann, K., Berger, H., Kulbe, H., Thillainadarasan, S., Mollenkopf, H. J., Żemojtel, T., Taube, E. T., et al. (2020). Stable expansion of high-grade serous ovarian cancer organoids requires a low-Wnt environment. *The EMBO Journal, 39*. https://doi.org/10.15252/embj.2019104013 (accessed on 7th August 2025).

41. Mueller, G. (2010). *Oral protein therapy for the future – Transport of glycolipid-modified proteins: Vision or fiction?* https://core.ac.uk/download/16432284.pdf (accessed on 7th August 2025).

42. Rappaport, J. A., & Waldman, S. A. (2018). *The guanylate cyclase C-cGMP signaling axis opposes intestinal epithelial injury and neoplasia*. https://core.ac.uk/download/213441819.pdf (accessed on 7th August 2025).

43. White, J. R., Winter, J. A., & Robinson, K. (2015). Differential inflammatory response to Helicobacter pylori infection: etiology and clinical outcomes. *Journal of inflammation research, 8*, 137–147. https://doi.org/10.2147/JIR.S64888(accessed on 7th August 2025).

44. Sengupta, P. (2017). *An update on coagulating gland renin-angiotensin-prostaglandin system: A new hypothesis on its renin function*. https://core.ac.uk/download/477852823.pdf (accessed on 7th August 2025).

45. Ocon, S., Murphy, C., Dang, A. T., Sankaran-Walters, S., Li, C. S., Tarara, R., Borujerdpur, M., Dandekar, S., Paster, B. J., & George, M. D. (2013). Transcription profiling reveals potential mechanisms of dysbiosis in the oral microbiome of rhesus macaques with chronic untreated SIV infection. *PloS one*, *8*(11), e80863. https://doi.org/10.1371/journal.pone.0080863(accessed on 7th August 2025).

CONNECTIVE TISSUE

5

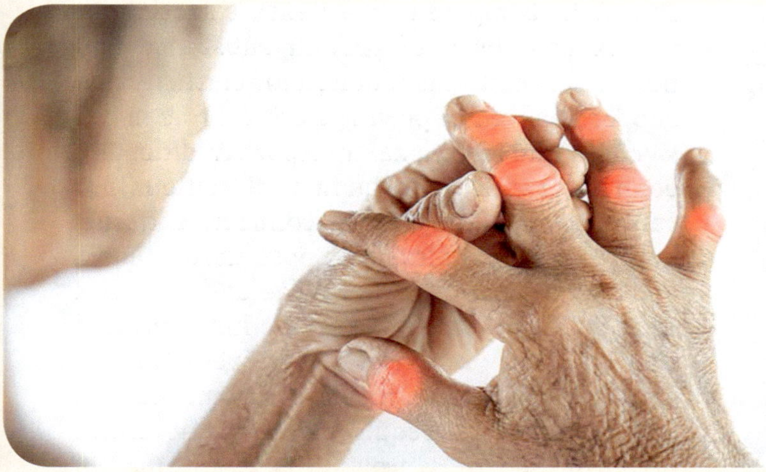

LEARNING OBJECTIVES

After studying this chapter, you will be able to:

1. Explain the types of connective tissue;
2. Describe the functions of connective tissue;
3. Explain the components of connective tissue;
4. Understand the connective tissue disorders.

Introduction

Connecting various components of the human body, connective tissue plays a pivotal role in maintaining the structure intact and supporting physiological activities. One of the four types of major tissues, along with epithelial, muscle, and nervous tissues, connective tissue is a diverse collection of subtypes with specific functions. Bone, adipose (fat) tissue, blood, cartilage, and the specialized connective tissues supporting organs and nerves fall within this category of tissue. Its matrix composition, vastly different from one subtype to another, sets the properties and functions of each connective tissue. That level of variation allows adaptation of structural and functional properties to the challenges posed by environmental or physiological changes and thus is an essential blueprint for body function. The plasticity of connective tissue is also observed through its response to various stimuli. For instance, the musculoskeletal connective tissues, like tendons, ligaments, and cartilage, possess a high capacity to remodel when subjected to mechanical stressors. A good illustration is long-term weightlessness that is experienced by astronauts, where the musculoskeletal system undergoes extreme alterations due to the lack of gravitational forces. Knowing these adaptive mechanisms is crucial to create countermeasures that protect against potential impairment due to extended periods of disuse, as suggested in NASA's "MUSCULOSKELETAL DISCIPLINE SCIENCE PLAN" (1991). The plasticity of connective tissues allows the body to regain homeostasis and can have a profound impact on overall health and function, highlighting its significance in both usual and extraordinary circumstances. Furthermore, connective tissue is also researched in its physiological and pathological context rather than anatomically.

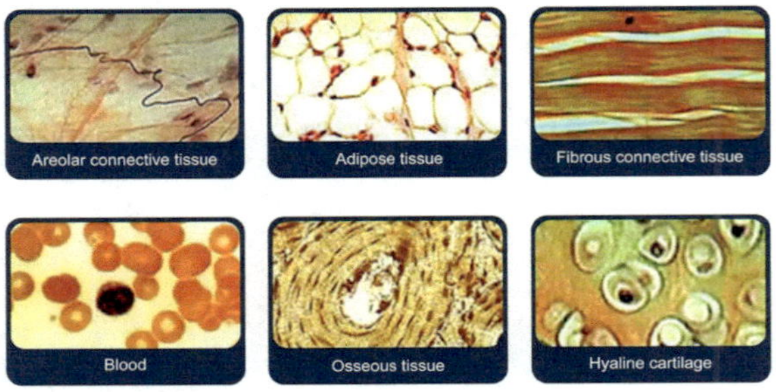

Figure 5.1. Diagram of connective tissue.

Source: https://media.geeksforgeeks.org/wp-content/uploads/20240404111132/Diagram-of-Connective-Tissue.webp.

The interactions among different types of connective tissue have a significant impact on the general body function, for instance, wound healing and inflammatory response. As Merker (2004) highlights, the interactions between neural processes and cognitive functions are also influenced by the composition and structure of connective tissue.

Therefore, the investigation of connective tissue in the overall context of human disease and health is vital to furthering our knowledge of a wide range of medical conditions. By highlighting its role in being multifaceted, this chapter will explore the intricacies of connective tissue, making parallels with its relevance to normal physiological function as well as the obstacles created by pathology or disuse (Figure 5.1).

Definition of Connective Tissue

Connective tissue is a crucial component of the human body, with the same serving multifaceted roles that are tasked with providing structural support in numerous organs and systems. It is characterized by its relatively loose cell structure, compared to a dense extracellular matrix composed of ground substance and fibers. This matrix is required for elasticity and support, as well as playing a critical role in cell signaling and nutritional transport. Additionally, connective tissue is further classified into subtypes, including loose connective tissue, dense connective tissue, adipose tissue, blood, and specialized forms like bone and cartilage. Each subtype possesses specific functions and characteristics, representing the versatility of connective tissue in meeting the mechanical and physiological requirements of the entire organism and thus proving its importance in health and disease. With an extensive array of cell types, connective tissue includes fibroblasts, adipocytes, macrophages, and mast cells, to mention a few, which are all accountable for its multifaceted functions. Fibroblasts, for instance, are important in the formation of the extracellular matrix, while adipocytes are responsible for energy storage in fat form. The presence of immune cells, for instance, macrophages in connective tissue, underscores its role in the immunological defense within the body against causative agents of disease. The interaction between these components of the cell and the extracellular matrix highlights the dynamic function of connective tissue since, while it offers structural support, it is also involved in the constant processes of repair and regeneration. By being involved in these processes, connective tissue maintains homeostasis and responsiveness to the external environment, thus reiterating its importance within the larger context of human biology. The structural support of connective tissue is more than such fundamental groundwork; it also plays a vital role in the body's metabolic processes and overall physiological homeostasis. Blood, for instance, one of the specialized tissues of connective tissue, is necessary for the transport of nutrients and waste products, thereby facilitating cellular communication and metabolic exchange. In addition, the adipose tissue, which is a type of connective tissue, is a system associated with the storage of energy and is involved in thermoregulation and hormonal function. Evidently, the connective tissue scaffold is responsible for creating networks to support organs such that the body's various systems are effectively functioning and coordinated. Hence, due to its intricate nature and extensive array of functions, connective tissue stands forth as an important contributor to the body's overall health, thus underscoring the crucial need for ongoing research on its characteristics and role in clinical studies and therapy interventions.

Importance of Connective Tissue in the Human Body

Connective tissue is an elementary component of the human body that serves as a supporting structure, keeping organs and systems together. It is a heterogeneous population with several subtypes , such as loose connective tissue, dense connective tissue, adipose tissue, blood, and bone, which all contribute in varying ways to the functions of the body. One of the key roles played by connective tissue is to provide stability and support so that organs are maintained in an intact state. For instance, muscles are attached to bones and bones are attached to other bones by tendons and ligaments, which are dense connective tissues, thus ensuring proper functioning of the musculoskeletal system. Without proper connective tissue integrity, structural weakness could lead to injury or chronic disease, demonstrating the significance of these tissues to health and wellness. In addition to its role in structural support, connective tissue plays a vital function in metabolic activity within the body. For example, fat tissue is not only a reservoir of energy but also an endocrine organ that releases hormones , such as leptin and adiponectin, which regulate appetite and glucose metabolism. It takes on a particular importance with regard to chronic diseases; studies have shown that dysfunction in the connective tissue can lead to diseases , such as obesity and diabetes mellitus. The intricate interactions between the connective tissue and the metabolism regulation illustrate its worth beyond structural support. In cases of declining connective tissue health, such as in diabetes mellitus, the impacts can lead to severe complications, such as increased risk of renal disease, illustrating the importance of ongoing research into the protective roles of the connective tissue in metabolic disease (Fernando & Zhou, 2015). Moreover, the pathophysiologic characteristics of connective tissue highlight its role in disease progression. Overproduction of collagen and fibrotic changes within connective tissue, for example, characterize systemic sclerosis, a disorder that results in frank functional impairment of multiple organ systems. A range of growth factors initiates the fibrotic process of systemic sclerosis, further exacerbating tissue remodeling and propagating the severity of disease. Recent studies have shown that this dysregulation of connective tissue is not only pathogenic but also can identify targets of therapy, as modulation of the fibrotic response can provide some relief from systemic sclerosis symptoms (Castro et al., 2010). An understanding of the pathophysiology of connective tissue disease can also provide further insights into treatment, showing the importance of connective tissues in bearing physiological loads and participation in sophisticated biochemical pathways that underlie health.

5.1. Types of Connective Tissue

Learning Outcome

1. Understand the loose connective tissue;
2. Understand the dense connective tissue;
3. Describe the role of specialized connective tissue in the human body.

The classification of the diverse types of connective tissue in humans into different types is based on its multifunctional roles within the body, and these are grouped into many types , such as the loose connective tissue, dense connective tissue, adipose tissue, cartilage, bone, and blood. Loosely connective tissue, which typically forms under epithelial layers, functions to provide support and padding to tissues and organs and facilitates the flow of waste and nutrients. Dense connective tissue, such as ligaments and tendons, consists of tightly packed collagen fibers that provide strength and elasticity. Such tissue is essential in attaching muscles to bones and in joint fixation, thus reacting to mechanical stresses when there is exercise. This singular structural make-up of connective tissues emphasizes their functional significance in maintaining the body's wholeness and integrity, the expression of a system finely tuned to multiform biological requirements. Cartilage, the second most significant type of connective tissue, is an elastic and resilient supportive matrix for the skeletal system. It is categorized as hyaline, elastic, and fibrocartilage—each with specialized functional requirements in various locations throughout the body. Hyaline cartilage, for example, occurs frequently in embryonic skeletons and articular surfaces of joints, and it provides a smooth surface to avoid friction and as a shock material when the body makes movements. Elastic cartilage, in the ear and epiglottis structures, contributes to strength and elasticity so that these areas are able to maintain their shapes. Conversely, fibrocartilage is the strongest type, which occurs in intervertebral discs and knee menisci, where it resists maximum compressive loads. The diversity in properties of the types of cartilage demonstrates the sophisticated nature of connective tissues and their irreplaceable roles in enabling efficient biomechanical function in human physiology. Bone and blood are also specialized types of connective tissue with characteristic compositions and functions. Bone tissue is categorized into compact and spongy types, which serve structural support, mineral storage, and housing for the bone marrow where hematopoiesis occurs.

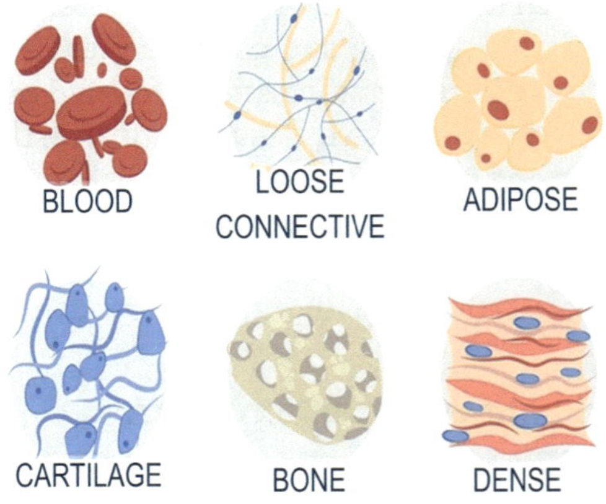

Figure 5.2. Types of connective tissue.

Source: https://www.shutterstock.com/image-vector/types-connective-tissue-medical-vector-600nw-2180225021.jpg.

Bone stiffness is owed to the mineralized matrix that is packed with calcium phosphate, giving it strength and resistance to mechanical stress. On the other hand, blood, at times considered to be liquid connective tissue, is composed of suspended cells in plasma and plays a role in transport and immune protection. Blood facilitates the delivery of oxygen and nutrients to tissues and the removal of waste products. Significantly, the relationship between these various categories of connective tissues shows their synergistic function in general health and functionality of the human body, reinforcing the significance of understanding connective tissues as a whole for future medical research and treatment processes (NASA's MUSCULOSKELETAL DISCIPLINE SCIENCE PLAN, 1991; Riley, 2004) (Figure 5.2).

5.1.1. Loose Connective Tissue

Loose connective tissue, typically comprised of a fibrous matrix with abundant ground substance, serves several functions in the human body. Comprising elastin and collagen fibers predominantly, loose connective tissue provides the body with its structure while allowing it to move and bend. The various cells found in loose connective tissue, such as fibroblasts, macrophages, and mast cells, are the reason behind its dynamism to repair and respond upon being injured. This adaptability is particularly important in areas subjected to stress or in motion, since loose connective tissue serves as a cushion or cover. Thus, its unique structure not only maintains the continuity of neighboring tissues but also plays a key role in immune responses and overall body homeostasis of the environment. Loose connective tissue functions as an important reservoir of nutrients and cellular signaling stimuli. The semi-fluid ground substance serves as a medium for oxygen and nutrient diffusion to the cells and waste elimination. The extracellular matrix also includes various molecules, such as glycoproteins and proteoglycans that facilitate communication between cells and tissue compartments. This interstitial space plays a significant role in sustaining tissue function and health. For instance, the process of healing of loose connective tissue is central to wound healing, where recruitment of cells , such as fibroblasts, is required for collagen deposition and formation of new tissue structure. Therefore, understanding the delicate interactions between elements in loose connective tissue can be of practical value in understanding a variety of disease states, e.g., chronic inflammation. Moreover, loose connective tissue is directly associated with the functions that have been assigned to some organ systems, particularly in the peripheral nervous system (PNS). Loose connective tissue in this case plays the structural support of the nerves while embracing the quick response essential for repairing and regenerating nerves. Glial cells, including Schwann cells, reside within the loose connective matrix, which facilitates the processes of healing following nerve injury. Such a regenerative capability highlighted in PNS illustrates the significant role loose connective tissue has in maintaining neurological health and repairing damage. The relative functioning of glial cells in the PNS to glial cells in the CNS is used to show the flexibility of loose connective tissue and its very nature for preserving tissue function and repair following trauma (Barton et al., 2017). Generally, the diverse roles of loose connective tissue emphasize its critical importance within the broader group of connective tissue in human beings (Figure 5.3).

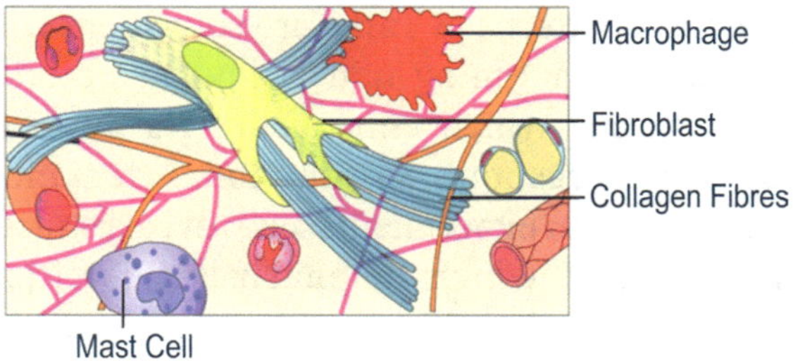

Figure 5.3. Loose connective tissues.

Source: https://media.geeksforgeeks.org/wp-content/uploads/20220531174843/tissue2.png.

5.1.2. Dense Connective Tissue

Dense connective tissue possesses a central role in providing structural support and stability throughout the human body. In a high concentration of collagen fibers, this type of connective tissue is critical to the formation of tendons and ligaments that connect muscles to bones and bones to bones, respectively. The collagen fiber alignment of dense connective tissue can be regular or irregular and influences its mechanical characteristics. Ordinary dense connective tissue, such as in tendons, exhibits aligned fibers in a parallel pattern, thereby giving tensile strength in one direction. However, irregular dense connective tissue, like in the dermis, exhibits a disorganized pattern, and therefore, it can offer resistance to extension in any direction. Such structures have the key function of maintaining the integrity and function of various physiological systems, providing support to movement and stability to joints. The biological role of dense connective tissue extends beyond that of mechanical strength; it also serves as a form of cell-to-cell communication and tissue repair. For example, recent studies have shown that tenomodulin (Tnmd), a type II transmembrane glycoprotein, is critical in dense connective tissues, particularly in healing. Tnmd is involved in enhancing the cell adhesion in tendons and ligaments, which is important in sustaining and maturing the tissues. The expression patterns of Tnmd are coincident with tooth eruption timing and following occlusal force loading, which emphasizes its dynamic property to respond to functional demands. Tnmd-knockout experiments also reveal reduced cell adhesion, which emphasizes its critical role in connective tissue homeostasis (Chung et al., 2013). By regulating cell adhesion and tissue integrity, Tnmd emphasizes the complex relationship between cellular elements and the extracellular matrix in dense connective tissue. The application of ontological knowledge can further augment our understanding of dense connective tissue and its subtle interplay with other biological systems. Ontologies provide an orderly method for the fusion of disparate information related to dense connective tissue so that it becomes simpler to discover and share knowledge in a large variety of research areas. The application of standard terms and definitions helps to improve scientists' communication in order to enable a more uniform understanding of dense connective tissues' properties and functions. Hence, a clearly defined ontology not only aids in unifying disparate research results but also serves as a premise for creating new ideas in connective tissue biology (Seppälä et al., 2017). By promoting consistency in the representation of dense connective tissue-related information, ontologies can become important tools for elucidating the intricate mechanisms underlying connective tissue function and disease (Figure 5.4).

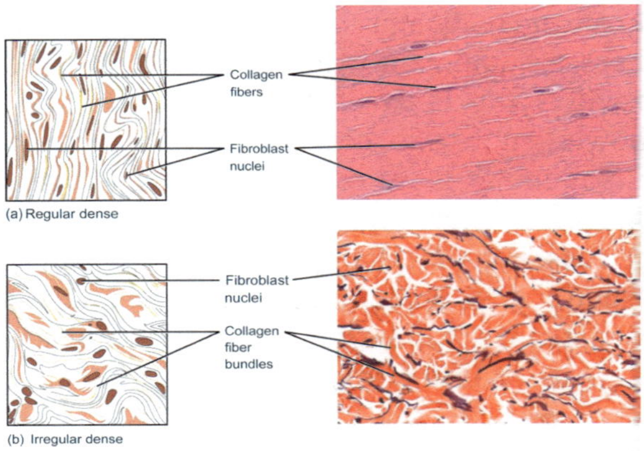

Figure 5.4. Dense Connective Tissue. (a) Dense regular connective tissue consists of collagenous fibers packed into parallel bundles. (b) Dense irregular connective tissue consists of collagenous fibers interwoven into a mesh-like network.

Source: https://s3-us-west-2.amazonaws.com/courses-images-archive-read-only/wp-content/uploads/sites/18/2014/07/19181052/411_Reg_Dense-Irregular_Dense.jpg.

5.1.3. Specialized Connective Tissue

Specialized connective tissues play central roles within the human body and do more than support and connect. Such tissues include cartilage, bone, adipose tissue, blood, and the various specialized types of connective tissue. All are crucial to the proper functioning of organs and systems. Each possesses structural specializations and functions that are directed towards the fulfillment of special physiological needs. For instance, cartilage provides joints with flexible support, and bone provides hard structure and protection for internal organs. This specialization that arises from differences in the composition and organization of the extracellular matrix, which is tailored to meet each tissue's specific mechanical and biological requirements, shows the versatility of the connective tissues towards the organism's needs. In specialized connective tissues, the function of cell types and their relationship with the extracellular matrix cannot be overstressed. In dense connective tissues , such as tendons and ligaments, the expression of certain proteins has been linked with mechanical function and functional integrity. Tnmd, for instance, plays a crucial role in the structural integrity and maturation of the periodontal ligament (PDL). Its expression is consistent with mechanical stress during tooth eruption, highlighting the dynamic relationship between tissue and functional load. It has been established through research that Tnmd controls cell adhesion in a positive manner, which is critical for dense connective tissue integrity, further justifying the assumption that specialized connective tissue is not a passive structure but an active contributor to biological processes conducive to durability and flexibility of the tissue (Chung et al., 2013). In addition, specialized connective tissues are also multifaceted in their functions of storage and metabolic activities. Adipose tissue is a case in point with its energy storage function and its involvement in thermoregulation and hormone secretion. The storage role expounds on the metabolic activity of adipose tissue in regulating energy homeostasis and how even the seemingly simple connective tissues have multifaceted roles in related systemic processes. Apart from their metabolic and mechanical roles, specialized connective tissues are also important in the repair and regeneration of body structures in case of damage. For example, their cellular and fiber arrangement enables them to sustain healing reactions as well as reactions to physiological changes. Therefore, specialized connective tissues are fundamental aspects of maintenance and resistance in the human body, an indication of their inherent significance to general function and well-being (Merker, 2004) (Figure 5.5).

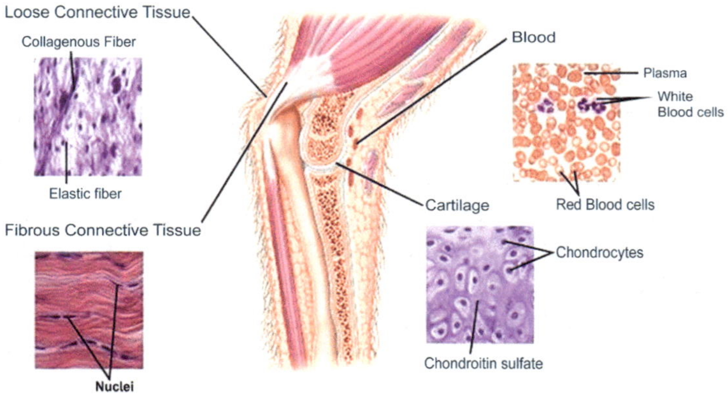

Figure 5.5. Specialized connective tissue.

Source: https://media.geeksforgeeks.org/wp-content/uploads/20220531174828/tissue.png.

Test Your Knowledge

1. List the various types of cell found in loose connective tissue.
2. What is dense connective tissue?

5.2. Functions of Connective Tissue

Learning Outcome

1. Describe the role of connective tissue in providing support and structure within the human body;
2. Understand the transportation of substances within the human body;
3. Understand the storage of energy and nutrients in connective tissue.

Connective tissue plays a role in maintaining the structural integrity of the human body by providing support and coherence to various organs and systems. Composed of a heterogeneous population of cell types and extracellular matrix components, connective tissue not only supports organs but also enables them to communicate with one another. Connective tissue is categorized into different subtypes, including loose connective tissue, dense connective tissue, cartilage, bone, blood, and fat tissue, each playing a specialized function. For example, loose connective tissue is a flexible framework supporting tissues and cushioning them, whereas dense connective tissue forms strong fibrous structures , such as tendons and ligaments, which are essential for movement and stability in the musculoskeletal system. The multitrack nature of the function of connective tissue demonstrates its essential contributions to global physiological homeostasis. Connective tissue is involved in nutritional and metabolic supply, too. Certain connective tissues, such as adipose tissue, also serve as reservoirs of energy by accumulating lipids and helping in the regulation of metabolism. Connective tissue also helps in transporting nutrients, hormones, and waste products within the body via its vascular elements. The blood itself is a specialized form of connective tissue and is transported throughout the body, delivering substances essential for cells and picking up the waste products of metabolism. Moreover, connective tissue also supports immune reactions; for example, reticular connective tissue forms the structural basis for lymphoid organs, providing a site where immune cells can congregate and respond to pathogens. Consequently, the integrative roles of connective tissue in immunity and nutrition also illustrate its indispensable functions in the human body. Additionally, the protective roles of connective tissue play a vital part in preventing organs from physical damage and potential pathogens. The heterogeneous matrix proteins of the connective tissue, such as collagen and elastin, impart tensile strength and elasticity to structures ranging from skin to large vessels, thus aiding in protection against trauma generated by exterior forces.

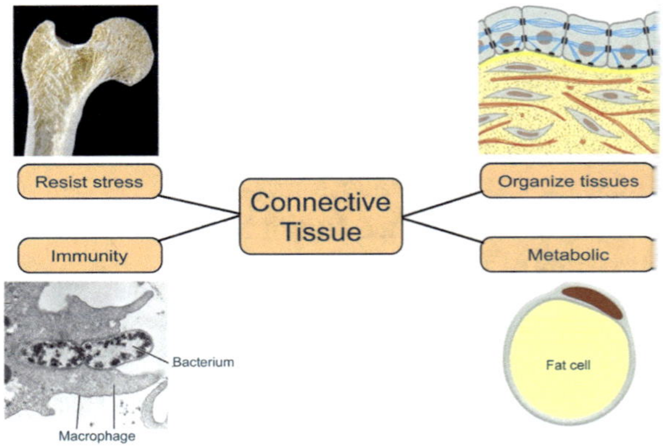

Figure 5.6. Connective tissue serves a variety of functions throughout the body.

Source: https://yalehistology.s3.us-east-2.amazonaws.com/connective_tissue/connective_tissue_types.jpg.

Cartilage is employed as a shock-absorbing cushion above joints, making movement silky smooth, and bone provides rigid protection to structures , such as the brain and heart. In addition, certain connective tissues, such as the dermis of skin, aid in barrier functions that keep pathogens and chemicals out. Dynamic response to the needs of the body, in terms of transforming to injury and inflammation through methods that may involve remodeling and repair, is facilitated by the intricate structure of connective tissue.

This versatility is emphasized by recent disease state research, including tendinopathy, where understanding the molecular pathobiology of connective tissues can give a clue to treatment (Riley, 2004). Overall, the multifunctional nature of connective tissue in protection, support, and flexibility highlights its important role in human health (Figure 5.6).

5.2.1. Support and Structure

The role of connective tissue to provide support and structure to the human body is multifaceted and is critical to general function. The tissue is used as a framework and as a binding tissue, providing support to organs for retention in place while also facilitating movement and pliability. Composed of various subtypes—including loose connective tissue, dense connective tissue, and specialized forms like cartilage and bone—each subtype has its own unique functions. Loose connective tissue, for example, provides cushion and support to organs, while dense connective tissue, composed of a high amount of collagen fibers, offers more tensile strength, which is critical for structures , such as tendons and ligaments. The presence of collagen, the principal structural protein of connective tissue, is vital to provide the stability of various body structures, illustrating how structure and support are interdependent through organization and composition. Moreover, connective tissue also participates in physiological processes, like growth, repair, and the regulation of the movement of joints. As a person grows old, the reduction in the synthesis of collagen causes apparent changes in most tissues, which weaken their ability to support the musculoskeletal load. The skin is a clear-cut example of such a change; it suffers from progressively increasing atrophy of elastin and collagen fibers, leading to its fragility and reduced elasticity. This loss can result in increased susceptibility to injury and reduced healing potential, particularly in the aged, where hormonal changes further exacerbate the issue. Evidence attests that estrogen replacement therapy following menopause can stimulate collagen production and firm up skin, thereby suggesting potential recovery processes for impaired connective tissue support (Calleja-Agius et al., 2007). The interplay of aging and the nature of connective tissue emphasizes the importance of structure in providing resilience and vitality to human physiology. While it functions as a mechanical support system, connective tissue also plays a critical role as a communicator of the body in linking various systems and as part of the immune system. For instance, the extracellular matrix, one of the essential components of connective tissue, allows for the exchange of nutrients and signals between cells, thereby maintaining homeostasis. Research suggests a relationship between oxidative stress and chronic diseases, such as periodontitis, where food antioxidants may prevent damage to connective tissue (Bullon, 2015). This directs our attention to how the structural integrity of connective tissues is not only a passive scaffolding matter but also plays an active role in physiological regulation and defense. Combined, these activities demonstrate how connective tissue support and structure are essential to proper function by way of maintaining body frameworks or facilitating complex biological processes.

5.2.2. Transportation of Substances

Transportation of chemicals within the human body is one of the fundamental roles of the connective tissues, particularly in relation to the blood and lymph functions. Blood, which is a specialized type of connective tissue, plays a crucial role in the transport of nutrients, oxygen and carbon dioxide, hormones, and waste materials throughout the body. The circulatory system, consisting of the heart, blood vessels, and blood, facilitates this transport process so that required substances , such as oxygen, are delivered to tissues and carbon dioxide is removed for exhalation. Plasma, the liquid component of blood, also contains proteins and other solutes that contribute to osmotic balance and pH values, which are crucial for homeostasis. This intricate matrix shows not just the efficiency of substance transport but also the overall significance of connective tissue in ensuring the survival and proper functioning of human physiology. A further very crucial role of substance transport is the role of connective tissues in the lymph system. The lymphatic system, made up of lymph, lymph nodes, and lymph vessels, transports lymph, a fluid comprising immune cells, proteins, and waste products. The lymphatic system plays a vital role in immune function by assisting in filtering out infectious agents and facilitating the transport of immune cells to a site of infection or damage. In addition, the lymphatic system is involved in the digestion of fats in the diet through special lymph vessels called lacteals that exist in the intestinal lining. The two functions undertaken by the lymphatic system prove the role of connective tissues not just in transport but also in immune surveillance and nutrient absorption, further contributing to the coordination and functioning of the body's. Furthermore, connective tissues also interact dynamically with other organ systems to ensure the maximization of the delivery of substances, particularly in the occurrence of diseases , such as diabetes mellitus. According to recent studies, zinc has been referred to as a vital trace element that plays a significant role in regulating carbohydrate metabolism and influencing the manner in which glucose is transported and metabolized within the body. Studies indicated that zinc supplementation could reverse some renal pathological alterations relevant to diabetes, i.e., by lowering oxidative stress and glomerular injury, thereby emphasizing the interaction between connective tissues, transport of nutrients, and overall health (Fernando & Zhou, 2015). There is a need to keep researching the long-term effects of zinc on controlling diseases , such as diabetes in order to know its therapeutic potential better (Miadzelets & Bobr, 2005). This intricacy highlights the central function of connective tissues to facilitate substance transport within the human body and maintain general health (Figure 5.7).

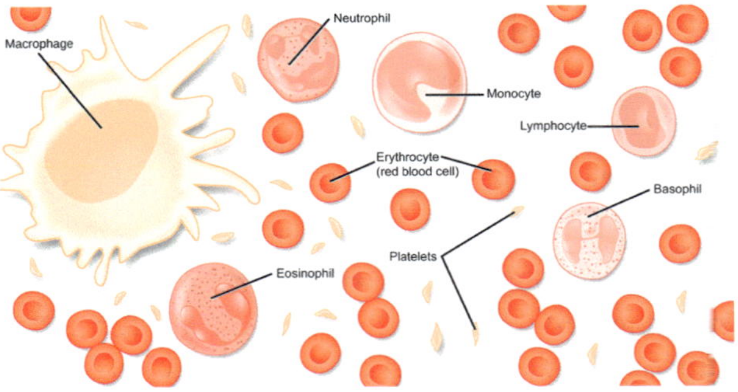

Figure 5.7. Blood is a connective tissue that has a fluid matrix, called plasma, and no fibers. Erythrocytes (red blood cells), the predominant cell type, are involved in the transport of oxygen and carbon dioxide. Also present are various leukocytes (white blood cells) involved in immune response.

Source: https://s3-us-west-2.amazonaws.com/courses-images/wp-content/uploads/sites/3206/2018/05/03191918/Figure_33_02_11.jpg.

5.2.3. Storage of Energy and Nutrients

Storage of energy and nutrients in connective tissue is a necessary process for total health and functioning. Adipose tissue, a specialized form of connective tissue, is primarily used for lipid storage, which serves as an efficient reservoir of energy. It is not just needed for energy reserve but also provides insulation and cushioning for internal organs. The ability of adipocytes to expand and reduce in accordance with energy needs accentuates the dynamic nature of connective tissue in responding to metabolic changes. Under conditions of energy deficit, the stored fatty acids in adipose tissue can be mobilized to support body functions, indicating a crucial relationship of connective tissue with energy metabolism. Connective tissue also has an important role in storing nutrients other than lipids. Glycogen, the polysaccharide found predominantly in liver and muscle tissue, is a reservoir for readily available glucose to generate energy. Glycogen is not stored in connective tissue directly, but the mobilization and control of glycogen are influenced by the structure and function of the connective tissue. The ECM of connective tissue helps in the transport of nutrients, along with the removal of metabolic waste products. Ideal ECM composition sustains tissues in their structural integrity and optimizes nutrient and energy transport, providing a platform for ideal metabolic function throughout the body. The connective tissues also help in the homeostasis of essential nutrients, such as vitamins and minerals, beyond energy storage. The role of antioxidants in the health of connective tissue is notable, and dietary components , such as vitamins E and C are involved in the protective function against oxidative stress. Efficient use of the nutrients can ensure the structural integrity of the connective tissues to promote resilience through various mechanisms. However, research indicates that a deficiency in some antioxidants can compromise the strength of connective tissues, with potential implications for diseases , such as periodontitis, and affect general health (Bullon et al., 2015). Therefore, the connection between dietary nutrients and connective tissue confirms the importance of a balanced diet to maintain the metabolic processes and structural demands of the body (Bosch et al., 2012).

Test Your Knowledge

1. What is the transportation of substances in the body?
2. What is the storage of energy and nutrients in connective tissue?

5.3. Components of Connective Tissue

Learning Outcome

1. Understand the extracellular matrix;
2. Describe the cells involved in connective tissue;
3. Describe the fibers present in connective tissue.

Connective tissue is a key component of the structural organization of the human body, which is further characterized by a diverse array of components with necessary roles. By its very nature, connective tissue contains three principal elements: fibers, cells, and ground substance. The cells are usually classified as resident cells, such as fibroblasts and macrophages, and transient cells, such as lymphocytes and mast cells, which enter the tissue after getting signals from the immune system. Fibers , such as collagen, elastin, and reticular fibers provide the tensile strength and elasticity to the tissue so that it can withstand mechanical stress without compromising its integrity. The ground substance, which has a gel-like matrix, suspends the fibers and cells and facilitates exchange of nutrients and cellular communication. Together, these provide the properties that allow connective tissue to perform its many functions, from structural support to participating in metabolic functions. Of especial interest is the role of connective tissue in disease, as exemplified by its role in fibrotic diseases. Fibrosis, with the abnormal excess of extracellular matrix components, severely compromises normal tissue structure and function. Myofibroblasts, fibroblast-derived cells that mediate wound healing, are the central effectors of these diseases through coordinating the deposition of collagen and other extracellular matrix proteins. Dysregulation underlies the chronicity of the fibrotic diseases, which involve multiple organs and systems and represent a gigantic public health issue globally. An in-depth knowledge of the molecular mechanisms of fibrosis, with intricate interactions between cytokines and growth factors, is essential to the development of successful therapies. It becomes clear that interfering with these pathways has the promise of lowering the disability imposed by fibrotic diseases on human health (Rosenbloom et al., 2013).

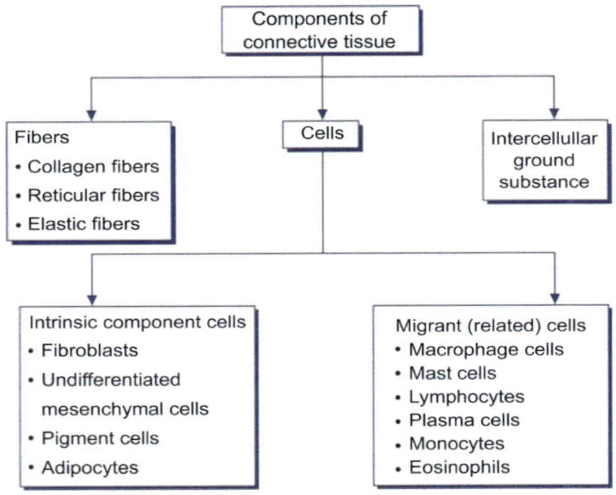

Figure 5.8. Components of connective tissue.

Source: https://d45jl3w9libvn.cloudfront.net/jaypee/static/books/9789385999321/Chapters/images/41-2.jpg.

In addition, research into the structure of connective tissue has a concurrent development in the field of tendinopathy, where pathogenesis underpins clinical practice. Tendinopathy with pain and dysfunction in tendons is extensively attributed to degeneration in the tendon matrix and not solely to inflammatory reactions. Research points to the importance of biochemical and molecular approaches in demystifying the composition of tendons, highlighting the role of the types of collagen and proteoglycans in facilitating healthy tendons. Despite limitations of human tendinopathy biopsies, comparisons with animal models provide leads towards the path of therapy. The integration of new information about the molecular pathology can potentially provide new therapies aimed at preventing pain and promoting healing among the affected population, leading to a better quality of life among patients with tendon disorders (Riley, 2004) (Figure 5.8).

5.3.1. Extracellular Matrix (ECM)

The ECM is pivotal in the structure and function of human connective tissues. Composed of an advanced array of proteins and polysaccharides, the ECM not only provides mechanical strength but also biochemical signals that regulate cellular action. Various components , such as collagen and elastin provide tensile strength and elasticity to tissues so that they can withstand various physiological stresses. Cell-to-cell communication is facilitated by the ECM through biochemical signals, triggering processes , such as cell proliferation, differentiation, and migration.

As such, the correct composition and structure of the ECM are fundamental to maintaining tissue function and integrity and thus its significance in the broader context of connective tissue biology. Furthermore, the dynamics of the ECM profoundly influence injury response, particularly of the tendon, where its degradation is a defining feature of tendinopathy. Tendon pathologies are defined by a complex interaction between the ECM and cellular activity that leads to degeneration and healing processes. Rupture or tendon pain of a chronic nature is normally caused by alterations in the structure of the ECMs due to an imbalance between the synthesis and degradation of the components of the matrix. Most tendon pathology is marked by an active cell-mediated process of degeneration with increased turnover and remodeling of the extracellular matrix, in which metalloproteinases play a central role in the degradation of matrix proteins, mediating cellular reactions, and facilitating tissue repair (Riley, 2005).

These studies have extended our understanding of cellular processes in tendinopathy, which offers promise for future therapeutic avenues. Uncovering the etiology and pathogenesis of conditions of the tendon has developed into the primary field of research, as traditional treatment strategies have often been poorly based on science. Notably, the usage of biochemical and molecular techniques in animal and human studies has drawn the curtain aside for the pathogenesis of these conditions, emphasizing the central position played by the tendon matrix in their generation. This molecular pathology is not only important for grasping the injury processes but also for developing focused approaches that may optimize treatment outcomes in chronic tendon diseases (Riley, 2004) (Figure 5.9).

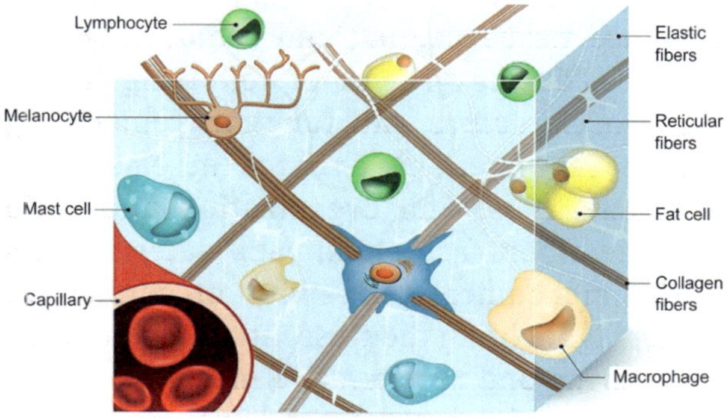

Figure 5.9. The extracellular matrix (ECM) and common cells.

Source: https://biologydictionary.net/wp-content/uploads/2020/10/fibersmatrixcell.jpg.

5.3.2. Cells Involved in Connective Tissue

Connective tissues play the primary role of providing structural and functional integrity to various organs and systems of the human body. The very core of the tissues consists of specialized cells that have distinct functions. The predominant cell types are fibroblasts, which play the role of manufacturing the extracellular matrix and collagen and thereby providing strength and flexibility to connective tissues. In addition, adipocytes are fat-storage cells, and macrophages are immune cells through the phagocytosis of pathogens and detritus. Both cell types create an interactive system in which cell-to-cell signaling is crucial to tissue integrity, repair, and overall homeostasis. The interaction and equilibrium between these numerous diverse cell types are critical to the maintenance of the integrity of connective tissues and, by extension, of the entire organism's health. Another significant category of cells involved in connective tissue is the mesenchymal stem cells, which possess multipotency and can differentiate into numerous types of cells under suitable conditions. The stem cells can differentiate into chondrocytes (cartilage cells), osteocytes (bone cells), and adipocytes and hence play a significant role in repair and regeneration activities in the body. These cells in the connective tissue allow for injury repair as well as a response to disease states. Of specific interest, the dental neural crest-derived progenitor cells (dNC-PCs) represent an interesting example of mesenchymal stem cells within the third molar pad with multipotentiality for differentiation into neural, chondral, and osteogenic lineages (Degistirici et al., 2008). This multipotency is highlighted as a critical aspect in developmental biology and regenerative medicine. Moreover, communication within the microenvironment of the connective tissue involves a vast array of signaling molecules, hormones, and cytokines that regulate the functions of these heterogeneous cell types.

For instance, mechanotransduction is a crucial process that determines how environmental mechanical stresses regulate cell function and behavior. This process is especially significant in musculoskeletal connective tissues, where adaptation to forces of a physical nature is crucial for maintaining structural integrity (N/A). Disruptions in such signaling processes can lead to pathological states, thus it is important to understand the cellular elements of connective tissues. In summary, the intricate interactions among various cells in connective tissues not only maintain homeostasis but also facilitate responses to environmental changes and stresses throughout an individual's life (Figure 5.10).

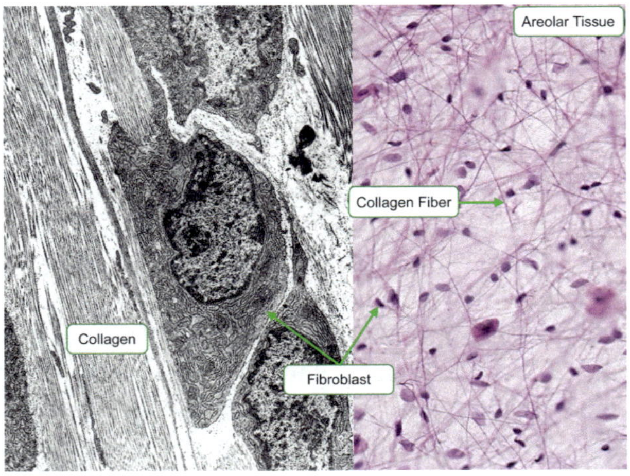

Figure 5.10. Fibroblasts are prominent in connective tissue and synthesize most of the protein components.

Source: https://s3.us-east-2.amazonaws.com/yalehistology/connective_tissue/fibroblasts.jpg.

5.3.3. Fibers Present in Connective Tissue

Connective tissue, a vital component of the human organism, is a multifarious matrix by virtue of its various fiber types. The most significant fibers in connective tissue are collagen, elastin, and reticular fibers, each of which adds distinct functional characteristics. Collagen fibers, which are abundant and firm, withstand tensile stress and enable tissues to withstand stretching and deformation. Elastin fibers, however, give elasticity so tissues can be stretched and then recoil back to their original state. This interaction between collagen and elastin is crucial for structures that need both strength and elasticity, like skin and blood vessels. In addition, reticular fibers create a supporting mesh network that gives framework stability to soft tissues and organs, with the help of which structural integrity is improved. Working together, these fibers enable connective tissues to perform a variety of diverse functions, from providing support structures to enveloping essential components of the circulatory and lymphatic systems that are crucial for general human health. An understanding of fiber composition in detail is necessary to know how connective tissues work under various physiological conditions. For example, collagen fibers in tendons and ligaments are closely packed, and thus these tissues can withstand stress and still offer stability and support to skeletal movement. Alternatively, some connective tissues, like the walls of arteries, contain higher elastin levels that support the pulsatile nature of the blood circulation at the expense of vascular integrity. These variations in fiber composition can also influence tissue healing and remodeling. For instance, during growth or following injury, tissue architecture and function remodeling can be regulated by changes in elastin-to-collagen ratios. The organization and ratio of these fibers are significant determinants of the mechanical properties of connective tissue, highlighting their essential role in tissue engineering and regenerative medicine, where replication of natural mechanical properties in engineered tissue is paramount. Fiber composition implications also extend beyond the structural support boundaries; they extend to affect functional organ and system potential. More particularly, in the muscular and nervous systems, the nature and quality of the connective tissue play a part in the transmission of forces and performance in general. Muscle connective tissues containing strict collagenous structures, for instance, affect muscle force generation and endurance and thereby overall motor function. Research has confirmed that variations in connective tissue fiber types have significant effects on locomotor functions and strength, as in experiments using animal models like piglets, where muscle function is comparable to the fiber composition (Aerts et al., 2019). Additionally, new bioinspired solutions, such as tensegrity-based structures in robotics, show the versatility of connective tissue and the functionality of its fibers. These bio-inspired geometries utilize compliance and flexibility like human joints, illustrating that connectivity to connective tissue fibers can be applied to enhance both biological and synthetic systems (Agogino et al., 2016). As a whole, studies on connective tissue fibers enhance our knowledge of human physiology and inform applied uses in medicine and engineering (Figure 5.11).

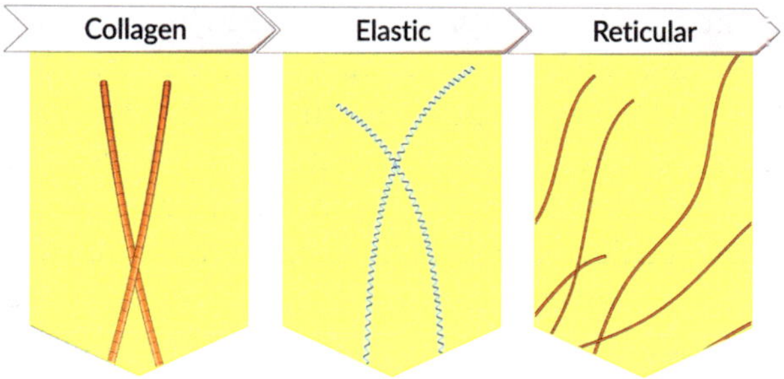

Figure 5.11. Connective tissue fibers.

Source: https://cloudfront.jove.com/files/media/science-education/science-education-thumbs/13981.jpg.

Test Your Knowledge

1. What type of cells are found in connective tissue?
2. Which fibers are present in connective tissue?

5.4. Connective Tissue Disorders

Learning Outcome

1. Understand the common connective tissue disorder;
2. Describe the genetic disorders affecting connective tissue;
3. Describe the impact of lifestyle on connective tissue health.

Connective tissue disorders are a broad range of genetic and acquired disorders that have a marked impact on the structural integrity and functioning of the connective tissues in the human body. These syndromes are caused by deficiencies in such structures as collagen, elastin, and glycosaminoglycans, leading to a range of symptoms and complications. Marfan syndrome, for instance, is caused by vascular complications and skeletal deformity, while Ehlers-Danlos syndrome leads to hypermobility, fragile skin, and bruising tendency. The identification of these disorders not only entails an awareness of genetic predisposition but also addresses factors like the environment and lifestyle decisions that could exacerbate symptoms. Early intervention and detection can stem the development of these disorders and draw attention to clinical awareness as well as a need for ongoing research on their pathophysiology and treatment. The new approach to the treatment of certain connective tissue diseases indicates the persistent advance of medical science. PXE and GACI, for instance, are caused by some inactivating mutations that lead to ectopic calcification in tissues. Research has demonstrated that oral administration of inorganic pyrophosphate (PPi) markedly reduces calcification in such conditions. This represents a paradigm shift in treatment, from symptomatic treatment to targeted therapeutic modalities based on the correction of the underlying biochemical abnormalities. These advances highlight the central place of targeted therapy and molecular diagnosis in the treatment of genetic connective tissue diseases, holding promise of improved patient outcomes and quality of life. The United States Food and Drug Administration's clearance of PPi as a safe and effective intervention means it promises to be a cost-effective therapy for many recalcitrant disorders because of connective tissue calcification (Arányi et al., 2017).

Tendinopathy, a very common and often misconstrued disorder of connective tissues, is especially difficult both in diagnosis and treatment. Despite a voluminous body of literature that has dealt with the etiology and clinical presentation of tendinopathy, there exists a tremendous lack of robust scientific evidence supporting most treatment protocols. The complexity of tendinopathy's pathogenesis, combined with the relative rarity of tendon biopsies before injury, complicates the interpretation of the condition. The principles gleaned from the animal model, though educational, frequently turn out to be inapplicable to human conditions due to differences in healing responses. However, advances in the biochemical and molecular techniques are shedding considerable light on the molecular pathophysiology of tendons and presenting a tighter understanding of such debilitating diseases. This growing cache of information is invaluable in developing evidence-based treatment modalities capable of successfully addressing the problems of tendinopathy and improving clinical outcomes for the affected patients (Riley, 2004) (Figure 5.12).

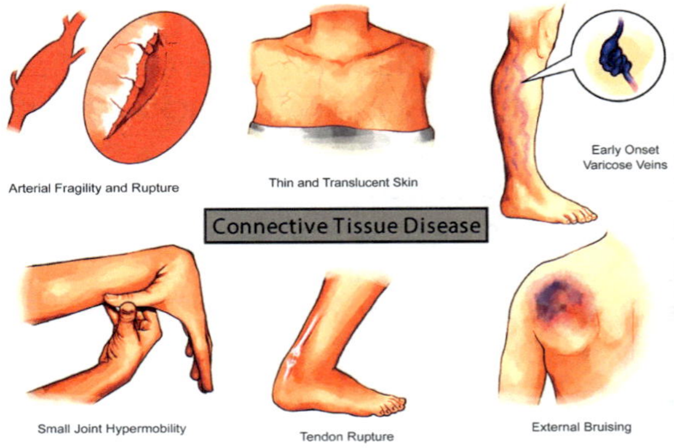

Figure 5.12. Connective tissue disease.

Source: https://www.umassmed.edu/globalassets/dermatology/blog/connective-tissue-disease.jpg.

5.4.1. Common Disorders (e.g., Arthritis and Lupus)

It is important to understand common disorders , such as arthritis and lupus in studying connective tissue, since they impact quality of life and health. Arthritis, in its various forms , such as osteoarthritis and rheumatoid arthritis, is most frequently found in the synovial joints, leading to cartilage and the overlying tissues' inflammation and destruction. This degeneration causes pain, stiffness, and decreased mobility and significantly worsens daily function.

The pathophysiology involves immune processes that can attack joint tissue, yet again emphasizing the interaction between connective tissue and the immune system. Research into these diseases not only provides information regarding inflammation and tissue repair mechanisms but also emphasizes the need for directed therapy to minimize symptoms and modulate disease progression. Lupus, systemic lupus erythematosus (SLE), is a significant disorder that emphasizes the pathology in connective tissues. Lupus is an autoimmune illness that can be expressed in different organ systems, including the skin, joints, and kidneys, demonstrating the immense implications of derangement in connective tissue. Research shows that inflammatory mediators, such as interleukin-2 (IL-2), are significant determinants of lupus disease activity.

A study revealed a strong correlation of elevated serum levels of IL-2 with the SLE disease activity index, suggesting potential avenues for monitoring and treatment in affected patients (Sedighi et al., 2014). Lupus being seen in a vast array of presentations , such as fatigue, arthralgia, and rashes, understanding the involved mechanisms in connective tissues becomes essential in creating effective management protocols unique to each patient's condition.

The link between systemic autoimmune diseases and sensory symptoms also illustrates the intricacy of connective tissue disease. Research indicates that immune-mediated inner ear disease may occur in systemic autoimmune disease patients and result in sensorineural hearing loss, tinnitus, and vestibular impairment. These audiovestibular symptoms may be indistinguishable from primary inner ear disease, and diagnosis, as well as treatment, becomes complicated (Ralli et al., 2018). Interestingly, early identification and effective corticosteroid therapy can significantly improve hearing results, underscoring the importance of understanding the interconnectedness between systemic signs and connective tissue health. These results also corroborate the need for a multidisciplinary treatment approach in these conditions, emphasizing the connections between immune regulation, connective tissue integrity, and patient health (Figure 5.13).

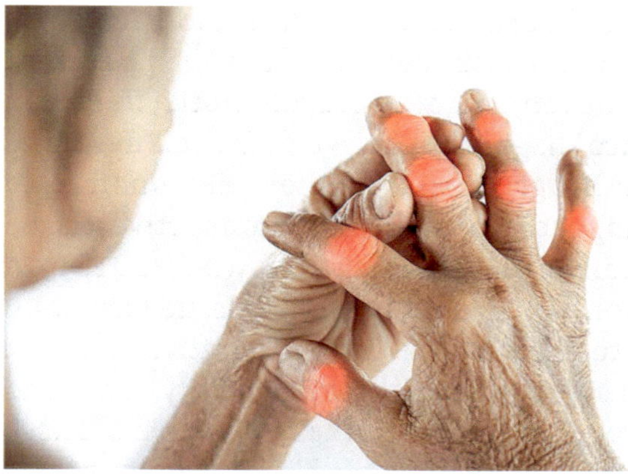

Figure 5.13. Arthritis.

Source: https://nextcare.com/wp-content/uploads/2022/09/Joint-Img-Web.jpg.

5.4.2. Genetic Disorders Affecting Connective Tissue

Connective tissue genetic disorders represent a diverse group of diseases that lead to impairment in the structural integrity and function of connective tissues within the human body. Such disorders often occur because of mutations in genes coding for various proteins, such as collagen or elastin, required for tissue strength and elasticity. For instance, Marfan syndrome is a type of genetic disorder of connective tissue caused by fibrillin-1 coding mutations in the FBN1 gene and leading to tall stature, long limbs, and susceptibility to cardiovascular-related complications. Other syndromes, such as Ehlers-Danlos syndrome, are characterized by hypermobility and elastic, brittle skin, which indicates a direct relationship between genetic defects and the mechanical characteristics of connective tissue. It highlights the significant impact of genetics on the physical condition of human beings and bodily function. The impacts of genetic disorders of connective tissue extend beyond manifestations and reach other functions and systems in the body. For example, connective tissue is crucial in the development and functioning of bones, an aspect that can be greatly impacted in people with genetic disorders. The fetus's biomechanical environment is relevant since inefficient fetal movement or fixed amniotic fluid can produce diagnoses of developmental dysplasia or arthrogryposis, further demonstrating the importance of healthy connective tissue function in development (Nowlan, 2015). In addition, abnormal connective tissue formation leads to chronic pain or degenerative arthritis, which significantly decreases quality of life and generates greater healthcare burdens. These illnesses thus illustrate the highly complex nature of interactions between genetic impact and overall physiological outcome. Breakthroughs in medical and genetic research offer promising directions for more effective management of connective tissue disorders. New advances in gene therapy, for instance, hold the promise of curing or mitigating the genetic abnormalities underlying these illnesses. New therapies target not just symptom reduction but also the genetic cause of conditions like osteogenesis imperfecta or loose type Ehlers-Danlos syndrome. Moreover, complete comprehension of the interaction between hormonal influence and environmental determinants with hereditary predispositions can enhance treatment modalities, particularly for those diseases that vary in men and women (Creel, 2008). Recent research emphasizes the need for comprehensive interventions that involve the integration of genetics with lifestyle modification and treatment protocols and holds promise for the better management of genetic disorders of connective tissue.

5.4.3. Impact of Lifestyle on Connective Tissue Health

The wellness of connective tissues , such as cartilage, tendons, and ligaments, is also significantly influenced by lifestyle , such as diet, exercise, and health care. Exercise is an integral part of ensuring the strength and resilience of such tissues. Engaging in regular exercise can reverse the deterioration of connective tissue integrity that occurs naturally with age. Older adults participating in competitive sports have been discovered to have their connective tissue in good health without excessive susceptibility to injuries normally related to age. This trend demonstrates that a lifestyle with consistent exercise not only increases functional ability but also potentially reduces the onset of degenerative disease in connective tissue, as reflected in studies of master's athletes (Baker, 2015). Therefore, an active lifestyle can become a protective factor, establishing healthy connective tissue over the lifespan. Nutrition also plays a vital role in the integrity of connective tissue, with the emphasis on a proper diet with appropriate necessary nutrients. Necessary vitamins and minerals , such as vitamin C, vitamin D, and zinc, are particularly important for collagen synthesis, a basic part of the structure and function of connective tissue. Lack of these nutrients can lead to impaired connective tissue, with ramifications , such as osteoarthritis or chronic pain syndromes. Moreover, the addition of anti-inflammatory food sources—, such as omega-3 fatty acids found in fish—to a diet helps decrease inflammation and speed up healing of connective tissues. Studies have also identified that sufficient micronutrient levels are associated with positive outcomes in tissue repair and regeneration. This, as such, implies that a prudent nutrition plan can go a long way in controlling one's connective tissue health and overall well-being, complementing the relationship between lifestyle habits and bodily well-being. In addition, lifestyle factors affecting connective tissue health extend beyond body exercise and nutrition to include overall management of health habits, including stress management and staying hydrated. Inflammatory responses can eventually make connective tissues deteriorate if there is chronic stress. Stress management activities , such as mindfulness, yoga, or regular sleep patterns, will ensure connective tissue health by maintaining overall inflammation levels low and allowing for healing of tissue. Adequate hydration is also imperative, as lubrication and nutrient supply to connective tissues demand adequate fluid levels. In addition, awareness of the interplay of conditions like diabetes with connective tissue health underscores the significance of integrative health care strategies. Diabetes, for instance, is associated with susceptibility to connective tissue disorders and thus requires preventive action by lifestyle modification (Fernando & Zhou, 2015). Recognition of the interconnected relationship between lifestyle and the health of connective tissue can lead to informed choice with optimal quality of life and functional capacity (Figure 5.14).

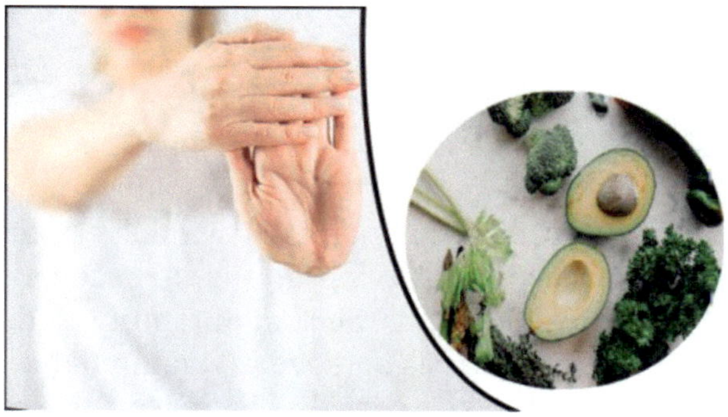

Figure 5.14. Diet for a connective tissue patient.

Source: https://www.stemcellcareindia.com/wp-content/uploads/2023/07/Diet-tips-for-Connective-tissue.jpg.

Test Your Knowledge

1. What is the most common connective tissue disorder?
2. What genetic disorder affects connective tissue?

SUMMARY

In interwoven the intricate functions of connective tissue in the biology of humans, one finds that this tissue is a key element in the structural role and functional processes of most organs. Connective tissue is critical as scaffolding, not only for support but also for cellular communication and tissue repair functions. As we delve into the complexities of connective tissues, particularly their composition and variations, it becomes possible to grasp how they adapt and respond to physiological demands. Such adaptability, with the capacity to be adjusted, allows connective tissue to create homeostasis and overall maintenance of health. Beyond this, understanding the complexity of connective tissue can also increase the knowledge of pathological conditions that result from the dysregulation of connective tissue, emphasizing the importance of continued research (Rosse & Mejino, 2008). The response of connective tissue to various disease states, as outlined in the above sections, emphasizes the tissue's role in influencing local and systemic health. Conditions , such as fibrosis, where there is abnormal connective tissue deposition, illustrate how disease changes can lead to chronic pain and reduced mobility (Reis, 2011). The underlying biological processes of such changes need to be investigated in terms of biochemical and mechanical properties of connective tissue, as such properties are the determinants of the disease course and response to therapy. The art of understanding the nuances of connective tissue function and the participation of connective tissue in disease allows researchers and clinicians to create targeted therapies that reverse the ill effects of connective tissue diseases. Finally, the continuous innovation of diagnostic and therapeutic measures relied on our understanding of connective tissue to enhance patient care and outcomes. New technologies in fields , such as molecular biology and biochemistry enable us to unravel the complexity of connective tissue interaction with other biological systems. This information is not only critical to the design of effective therapies but also to preventive regimens that will prevent connective tissue pathology throughout the entire human life cycle. As we reach the end of this journey of discovery through the study of connective tissue in humans, it is critical to emphasize the importance of interdisciplinary investigation and cooperation in seeking new therapeutic regimens that are capable of changing the approach to patient management and improving quality of life (Rosse & Mejino, 2008).

Understanding the nature of connective tissue is required for the appreciation of its varied roles in the human body, including structural support, protection, and facilitation of nutrient transport. Various forms of connective tissues exist, which include loose connective tissue, dense connective tissue, cartilage, bone, and blood. All these tissues have a unique and fundamental function to perform. For instance, loose connective tissue is a yielding supporting structure, and dense connective tissue is characterized by tensile strength and is found in tendons and ligaments. Cartilage is a padding at joint surfaces, and bone is a firm, supportive structure that holds the body together. Such complex classification accounts for the variety of connective tissues and their function in supporting overall bodily integrity and function. One of the more intriguing aspects of connective tissues is their association with injury, or more particularly, tendons and associated pathologies. Tendons, composed predominantly of type I collagen, are necessary to attach muscles to bones to facilitate movement and the conveyance of force. However, tendinopathy, a chronic condition involving the tendon, is one that is particularly refractory to treatment. The pathology often arises due to alterations in the tendon matrix and is defined by the expression of collagen and matrix remodeling. Of particular interest is the role of metalloproteinase enzymes, specifically ADAM-12 and MMP-23, which play a role in both normal tendon integrity and degeneration visible in tendinopathy. Knowledge of these molecular movements is vital to the development of treatment modalities and suggests the complexity of connective tissue responses to injury and stress (Riley, 2008). Further, the relevance of connective tissue also extends beyond the field of musculoskeletal health, founded on its applications to a variety of clinical disorders, such as spastic cerebral palsy. These children characteristically exhibit enhanced muscle spasticity due to changes in muscle and tendon length and consequently impacts their range of motion. Recent studies have indicated that effective stretching can elicit significant increases in muscle and tendon length, recording plasticity of the connective tissue. These findings highlight the need for condition-specific rehabilitation that fully appreciates the complexity of connective tissue adaptation to mechanical challenge. By combining an understanding of the behaviors of connective tissue, healthcare providers can create more effective treatment protocols that consider the individual needs of patients with various conditions, ultimately resulting in increased mobility and quality of life (Theis et al., 2013).

KEY TERMS FROM THIS CHAPTER

- Central nervous system
- Connective tissue
- Elastin fibers
- Glycoproteins
- Organs
- Peripheral nervous system
- Specialized connective tissues
- Collagen
- Dense connective tissue
- Extracellular matrix
- Loose connective tissue
- Periodontal ligament
- Proteoglycans
- Systemic sclerosis

CRITICAL THINKING QUESTIONS

1. **The primary function of connective tissue is:**
    a. Absorption and secretion
    b. Support and protection
    c. Transmission of impulses
    d. Contraction and movement
2. **Which of the following is classified as loose connective tissue?**
    a. Bone
    b. Adipose tissue
    c. Hyaline cartilage
    d. Blood
3. **Which type of connective tissue provides strength and flexibility and is found in tendons?**
    a. Areolar tissue
    b. Dense regular connective tissue
    c. Reticular connective tissue
    d. Cartilage
4. **Blood is considered a connective tissue because it:**
    a. Contains a liquid extracellular matrix
    b. Provides structural support
    c. Is involved in contraction and movement
    d. Has no cells
5. **The extracellular matrix of connective tissue is composed of:**
    a. Cells and organelles
    b. Ground substance and fibers
    c. Lipids and carbohydrates
    d. Actin and myosin

Short Answer Questions

1. What is connective tissue?
2. Why is connective tissue important in the human body?
3. Name the 3 types of connective tissue.
4. What are the functions of connective tissue?
5. List the components of connective tissue.

Answers to Critical Thinking Questions

1. (b); 2. (b) ; 3. (b); 4. (a); 5. (b)

REFERENCES

1. Abuja, A., Akdemir, M., Anthony, S., et al. (2018). *The physiological mechanisms of effect of vitamins and amino acids on tendon and muscle healing: A systematic review.* https://core.ac.uk/download/287581405.pdf (accessed on 7th August 2025).
2. Abzhanov, A., Baggiolini, A., Baroffio, A., Beverdam, A., Chevallier, A., et al. (2019). *Molecular and cellular mechanisms underlying the evolution of form and function in the amniote jaw.* https://core.ac.uk/download/323079229.pdf (accessed on 7th August 2025).
3. Ralli, M., D'Aguanno, V., Di Stadio, A., De Virgilio, A., Croce, A., Longo, L., Greco, A., & de Vincentiis, M. (2018). Audiovestibular Symptoms in Systemic Autoimmune Diseases. *Journal of immunology research, 2018*, 5798103. https://doi.org/10.1155/2018/5798103(accessed on 7th August 2025).
4. Aerts, P., Ayuso, M., Prims, S., Van Cruchten, et al. (2019). *Does intrauterine crowding affect the force generating capacity and muscle composition of the piglet front limb?* https://core.ac.uk/download/287940318.pdf (accessed on 7th August 2025).
5. Agogino, A., Asper, W., Baltaxe-Admony, L. B., Castro, et al. (2016). *A bio-inspired tensegrity manipulator with multi-DOF, structurally compliant joints.* http://arxiv.org/abs/1604.08667 (accessed on 7th August 2025).
6. Ahmadi, R., Anjomshoa, M., Fard, M., Hejazi, et al. (2015). *Application of allogeneic fibroblast cells in cellular therapy of recessive dystrophic epidermolysis bullosa.* https://core.ac.uk/download/227982916.pdf (accessed on 7th August 2025).
7. Albandar, J. M., Baldi, D., Berlucchi, M., Boltchi, F. E., Borghetti, P., Bouchard, P., Bruno, J. F., et al. (2018). *The effect of partially exposed connective tissue graft on root-coverage outcomes: A systematic review and meta-analysis.* https://core.ac.uk/download/213085713.pdf (accessed on 7th August 2025).
8. Theis, N., Korff, T., Kairon, H., & Mohagheghi, A. A. (2013). Does acute passive stretching increase muscle length in children with cerebral palsy?. *Clinical biomechanics (Bristol, Avon), 28*(9-10), 1061–1067. https://doi.org/10.1016/j.clinbiomech.2013.10.001(accessed on 7th August 2025).
9. Anderson, R. A., Baron, C., Beysens, D., Block, M. I., Boyce, T. M., Boyde, A., Britz, M., et al. (2011). *Investigation of bone resorption within a cortical basic multicellular unit using a lattice-based computational model.* http://arxiv.org/abs/1105.5093 (accessed on 7th August 2025).
10. Arányi, T., Dedinszki, D., Kozák, E., Pomozi, et al. (2017). *Oral administration of pyrophosphate inhibits connective tissue calcification.* https://core.ac.uk/download/95349730.pdf (accessed on 7th August 2025).
11. Bachl, N., Collins, M., Cook, J., Derman, et al. (2008). *International Olympic Committee consensus statement: Molecular basis of connective tissue and muscle injuries in sport.* https://core.ac.uk/download/2776587.pdf (accessed on 7th August 2025).
12. Baker, J. R. (2015). *The prevalence and risks of injury for masters athletes: Current findings.* https://core.ac.uk/download/211331646.pdf (accessed on 7th August 2025).
13. Barton MJ, John JS, Clarke M, Wright A, Ekberg J. The Glia Response after Peripheral Nerve Injury: A Comparison between Schwann Cells and Olfactory Ensheathing Cells and Their Uses for Neural Regenerative Therapies. *International Journal of Molecular Sciences.* 2017; 18(2):287. https://doi.org/10.3390/ijms18020287 (accessed on 7th August 2025).

14. A. D. Miadzelets, A. A. Bobr (2005). *Selected Themes of Histology, Cytology and Embryology Core*; Vitebsk State Medical University. - Vitebsk : VSMU, 2005. - 180 p. https://core.ac.uk/download/80150430.pdf (accessed on 7th August 2025).

15. Bosch, G., Depauw, S., Hendriks, W. H., Hesta, et al. (2012). *Fermentation of animal components in strict carnivores: A comparative study with cheetah fecal inoculum.* https://core.ac.uk/download/30640688.pdf (accessed on 7th August 2025).

16. Calleja-Agius, J., Muscat-Baron, Y., & Brincat, M. P. (2007). Skin ageing. *Menopause international, 13*(2), 60–64. https://doi.org/10.1258/175404507780796325(accessed on 7th August 2025).

17. Bullon, P. (2015). *Antioxidantes dietéticos para la prevención de la periodontitis crónica y su tratamiento: Una revisión de las evidencias actuales procedentes de estudios en animales y humanos.* https://core.ac.uk/download/286563546.pdf (accessed on 7th August 2025).

18. Castro, S. V., Jimenez, S. A., & Piera-Velazquez, S. (2010). *Role of growth factors in the pathogenesis of tissue fibrosis in systemic sclerosis.* https://core.ac.uk/download/83050041.pdf (accessed on 7th August 2025).

19. Chung, U. I., Docheva, D., Hiraki, Y., Hojo, et al. (2013). *Tenomodulin expression in the periodontal ligament enhances cellular adhesion.* https://core.ac.uk/download/12175517.pdf (accessed on 7th August 2025).

20. Creel, M. E. (2008). *Gender differences in survival in idiopathic pulmonary fibrosis and following lung transplant.* https://core.ac.uk/download/12209464.pdf (accessed on 7th August 2025).

21. Degistirici, O., Götz, W., Jaquiery, C., Martin, et al. (2008). *Defining properties of neural crest-derived progenitor cells from the apex of human developing tooth.* https://core.ac.uk/download/18240097.pdf (accessed on 7th August 2025).

22. Fernando, J., & Zhou, S. (2015). *The role of zinc in renal pathological changes in diabetic status.* J Nutr Disorders Ther 2015, 5:3 https://core.ac.uk/download/130975189.pdf (accessed on 7th August 2025).

23. Grange, S. (2011). *Current issues and regulations in tendon regeneration and musculoskeletal repair with mesenchymal stem cells.*

24. Hetherington, C. S. (2019). *Myofascial Release.* https://core.ac.uk/download/289198166.pdf (accessed on 7th August 2025).

25. Heufelder, A. E., Scriba, P. C., & Wenzel, B. E. (1996). *Antigen receptor variable region repertoires expressed by T cells infiltrating thyroid, retroorbital, and pretibial tissue in Graves' disease.* https://core.ac.uk/download/12175984.pdf (accessed on 7th August 2025).

26. Rosenbloom, J., Mendoza, F. A., & Jimenez, S. A. (2013). Strategies for anti-fibrotic therapies. *Biochimica et biophysica acta, 1832*(7), 1088–1103. https://doi.org/10.1016/j.bbadis.2012.12.007(accessed on 7th August 2025).

27. Khatri, P., Roedder, S., Sarwal, M. M., Vitalone, et al. (2011). *Biomarkers in solid organ transplantation: Establishing personalized transplantation medicine.* https://core.ac.uk/download/323074810.pdf (accessed on 7th August 2025).

28. Riley G. (2008). Tendinopathy--from basic science to treatment. *Nature clinical practice. Rheumatology, 4*(2), 82–89. https://doi.org/10.1038/ncprheum0700(accessed on 7th August 2025).

29. Rosse, C., Mejino, J.L.V. (2008). The Foundational Model of Anatomy Ontology. In: Burger, A., Davidson, D., Baldock, R. (eds) Anatomy Ontologies for Bioinformatics. Computational Biology, vol 6. Springer, London. https://doi.org/10.1007/978-1-84628-885-2_4(accessed on 7th August 2025).

30. Merker, B. (2004). *Cortex, countercurrent context, and dimensional integration of lifetime memory*. https://core.ac.uk/download/pdf/87204.pdf (accessed on 7th August 2025).

31. MUSCULOSKELETAL DISCIPLINE SCIENCE PLAN (1991) SPACE NATIONAL PHYSIOLOGY AND COUNTERMEASURES PROGRAM LIFE SCIENCES DIVISION AERONAUTICS AND SPACE ADMINISTRATION WASHINGTON, D.C.ASA-TM-108039 https://core.ac.uk/download/pdf/42808673.pdf (accessed on 7th August 2025).

32. Nowlan, N. C. (2015). *Biomechanics of Foetal Movement*. https://core.ac.uk/download/76995826.pdf (accessed on 7th August 2025).

33. Quantock, A., Hopkinson, A., Connon, C. J., Worthington, C. R., Hukins, D. W. L., Stuart, E. L., et al. (2007). *The Biomechanics of Amnion Rupture: An X-Ray Diffraction Study*. https://core.ac.uk/download/354141.pdf (accessed on 7th August 2025).

34. Reis, C. P. (2011). *P2 purinoceptors signaling in fibroblasts of rat subcutaneous tissue*. https://core.ac.uk/download/15568458.pdf (accessed on 7th August 2025).

35. Richman, E. (2022). *Interdisciplinary Perspectives in Lifetime Wellness*. https://core.ac.uk/download/519914321.pdf (accessed on 7th August 2025).

36. Riley, G. P. (2004). *The Pathogenesis of Tendinopathy: A Molecular Perspective*. https://core.ac.uk/download/2776643.pdf (accessed on 7th August 2025).

37. Riley, G. P. (2005). *Chronic Tendon Pathology: Molecular basis and Therapeutic Implications*. https://core.ac.uk/download/2776642.pdf (accessed on 7th August 2025).

38. Seppälä, S., Ruttenberg, A., & Smith, B. (2017). *Guidelines for Writing Definitions in Ontologies*. https://core.ac.uk/download/144579347.pdf (accessed on 7th August 2025).

39. Sedighi, S., Aghaei, M., Musavi, S., Nomali, et al. (2014). *Relationship between serum level of interleukin-2 in patients with systemic lupus erythematosus and disease activity in comparison with control group*. https://core.ac.uk/download/52204560.pdf (accessed on 7th August 2025).

ADIPOSE TISSUE

6

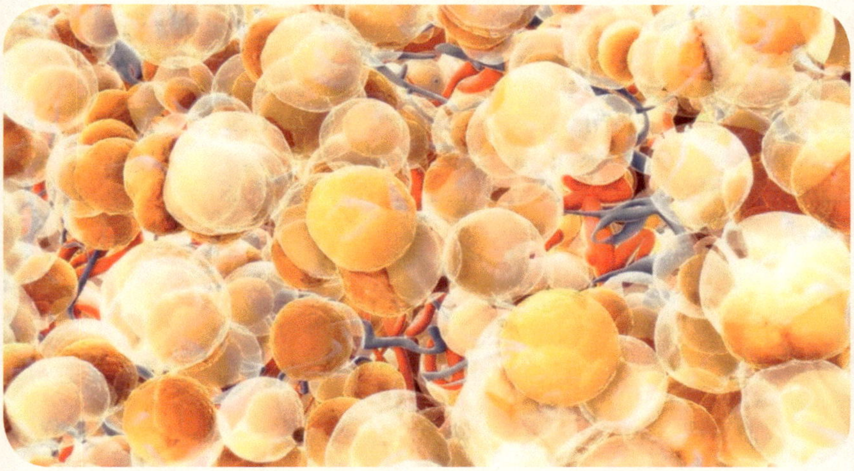

LEARNING OBJECTIVES

After studying this chapter, you will be able to:

1. Describe the types of adipose tissue;
2. Explain the functions of adipose tissue;
3. Understand the development of adipose tissue;
4. Describe the adipose tissue in aging.

Introduction

Studies on adipose tissue in human beings have gained extensive interest in the last few years, primarily due to its fundamental roles in the regulation of metabolism and energy homeostasis. Adipose tissue is not just a reservoir for lipids but is an active endocrine organ that produces a multitude of bioactive molecules. These secreted factors have a pivotal role in modulating metabolism, immune responses, and overall energy balance. With the rising prevalence of obesity globally, research into the forms of adipose tissues, i.e., white, brown, and beige adipose tissues, has become essential in understanding the subtleties of human health and disease. This complex tissue holds more than just an insight into energy storage and expenditure processes, but also of the possible therapeutic targets that might reverse metabolic diseases of obesity. Brown adipose tissue (BAT) is especially noteworthy due to its thermogenic role, which differentiates it from the more prevalent white adipose tissue (WAT). Research to date has highlighted the potential of BAT as a therapeutic strategy in combating obesity and the associated metabolic diseases. While enormous numbers of studies in rodent models have illuminated BAT's molecular and functional characteristics, human investigations have been compromised due to the challenges of safely biopsying. However, with technologies like positron emission tomography and computed tomography-guided Bergström needle biopsy technique, it became possible to collect human BAT samples from areas like the supraclavicular space. The proper application of this method, evidenced by recent studies, enhances the scientific community's ability to explore the human BAT biology and its relationship with metabolic health, providing a foundation for future therapeutic developments (Annamalai et al., 2015). Furthermore, exploration of beige adipocytes with characteristics from both white and brown fat has opened new avenues for potential therapeutic measures. Recent findings reveal newly discovered mechanisms in support of the thermogenic program of beige adipocytes and agents activating their differentiation from white adipose tissue. Discovery of these mechanisms is important since they give hints about new strategies in preventing obesity and obesity-related metabolic diseases. The identification of endogenous secreted factors that induce beige adipocyte activation is particularly intriguing, suggesting a way to use the physiological processes characteristic of these cells. Such knowledge of beige adipogenesis and thermogenesis might lead to new therapeutic targets, amplifying the potential of engineered solutions to address the obesity epidemic and its implications for human health (McQueen et al., 2018) (Figure 6.1).

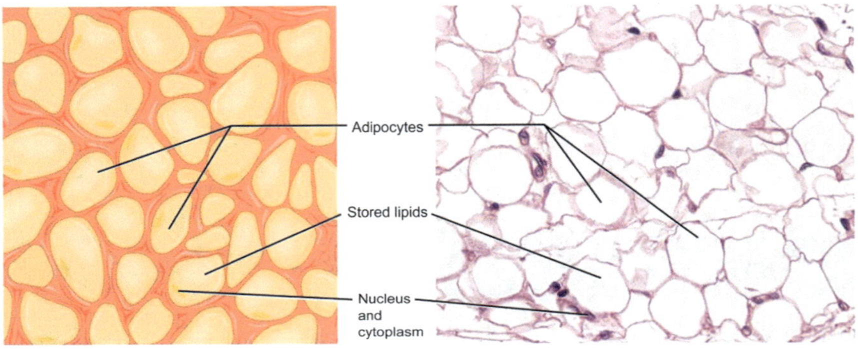

Figure 6.1. Adipose tissueis a loose connective tissue that consists of fat cells with little extracellular matrix. It stores fat for energy and provides insulation.

Source: https://s3-us-west-2.amazonaws.com/courses-images-archive-read-only/wp-content/uploads/sites/18/2014/07/19181049/409_Adipose_Tissue.jpg.

Definition of Adipose Tissue

Body fat or adipose tissue, as it is popularly called, is a specialized connective tissue in human physiology with a multi-functional role. It plays a primary role as an energy depot, storing calories in excess form as triglycerides, which are mobilized during times of energy deficiency. Such a role not only achieves metabolic homeostasis but also overall energy balance. In addition to its role in energy metabolism, adipose tissue is also an endocrine organ, secreting several adipokines—hormones that possess the potential to modulate appetite, affect insulin sensitivity, and inflammatory reactions. This dynamic interplay between storage and hormone roles indicates the critical importance of adipose tissue in the maintenance of metabolic health, necessitating further exploration of its role in conditions like obesity and diabetes, as hypothesized in more recent work

(Bianco et al., 2018). There are two major types of adipose tissue: white adipose tissue (WAT) and brown adipose tissue (BAT), which serve distinct physiological functions. WAT is the most prevalent type in adults and is primarily responsible for energy storage and secretion of various hormones regulating appetite and metabolism. It gives cushioning and insulation, serving to maintain body temperature and shield organs from mechanical injury. In contrast, BAT is more compact in infants and plays a role in thermogenesis, the generation of heat from the combustion of calories. The presence of mitochondria in BAT highlights its energetic functional significance. With increasing studies, the unique characteristics and the therapeutic potential of these different types of adipose tissue become clearer, and their role in the specific treatment of metabolic diseases comes into focus (Argano et al., 2019). In addition, the evolving understanding of adipose tissue involves its link to systemic inflammation and metabolic disorders. The existing evidence indicates that dysfunction in adipose tissue can initiate a pro-inflammatory condition and exacerbate disease states , such as obesity, cardiovascular illness, and type 2 diabetes. The subsequent release of pro-inflammatory cytokines by hypertrophied adipocytes is capable of inhibiting insulin signaling and causing insulin resistance, and it is an example of the multifaceted nature of adipose tissues' contribution to disease and health. Using the integration of multi-omic approaches, researchers are now beginning to define potential biomarkers of adipose tissue dysfunction and thus moving toward personalized treatment strategies for cardiometabolic diseases. As the relationship of adipose tissue with general well-being comes to the forefront, adding gender medicine has the ability to further refine knowledge and treatment, highlighting sophisticated interactions that regulate human health (Argano et al., 2019; Bianco et al., 2018) (Figure 6.2).

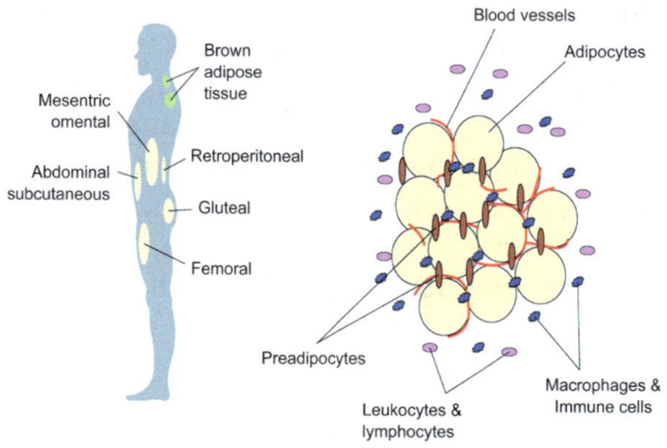

Figure 6.2. Diagram of adipose tissue.

Source: https://media.geeksforgeeks.org/wp-content/uploads/20240516145518/Adipose-Tissue.png.

Importance of Adipose Tissue in the Human Body

Adipose tissue plays a far-reaching role in human physiology, not merely as an energy depot but also as an important endocrine organ. It is mainly composed of adipocytes that store triglycerides and release fatty acids when there is an energy deficit. Besides its function in energy storage, adipose tissue also secretes hormones and signaling molecules known as adipokines that influence metabolic functions throughout the body. For instance, adiponectin sensitizes cells to insulin, and leptin regulates appetite and energy expenditure. Disruption in the synthesis or function of these adipokines can lead to metabolic disorders , such as obesity and type 2 diabetes. It is thus important that one is aware of the hormonal characteristics of adipose tissue so that one may comprehend its impact on health as a whole and metabolism. Secondly, the function of adipose tissue extends into metabolic health even further by means of redox homeostasis and oxidative stress. The presence of peroxisomes in adipocytes has fundamental functions in fatty acid metabolism and control of ROS (Klein et al., 2019). They are involved in maintaining the homeostasis between oxidative and reductive reactions, which is required in preventing damage to the cells and normal adipocyte functioning. Dysregulation of these activities has been associated with increased oxidative stress, increased inflammation and insulin resistance, typical of obesity and metabolic syndrome.

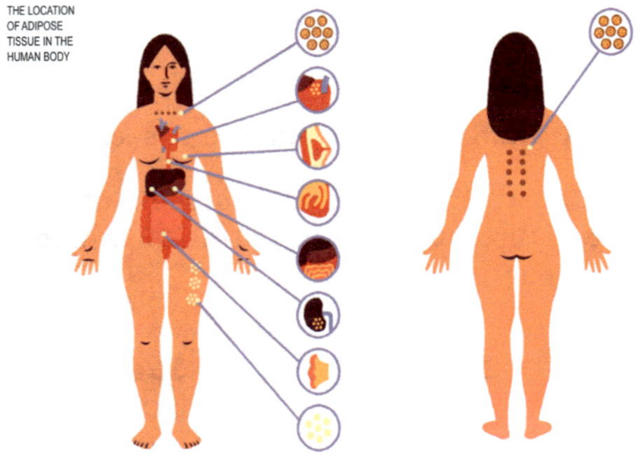

Figure 6.3. The location of adipose tissue in the human body.

Source: https://www.researchgate.net/publication/365193936/figure/fig1/AS:11431281095809130@1668028200307/The-location-of-adipose-tissue-in-the-human-body-In-the-human-body-there-are-three-major.ppm.

Thus, the intricate interaction between adipose tissue metabolism, redox regulation, and metabolic health mirrors the complexity of the adipose tissue as well as the significance of its existence in the human organism. Besides, the role of adipose tissue in thermogenesis and energy balance has gained greater emphasis during the last few decades. BAT, distinct from WAT), is differentiated by the capacity to generate heat through uncoupling mitochondrial respiration, hence being a key mediator in energy dissipation and thermoregulation. Stimulation of BAT has been linked with increased lipoprotein lipase activity, which enhances fat storage and metabolism (McMinn, 1984). Elucidation of the mechanisms of BAT activation has fascinating therapeutic potential for the development of therapeutic interventions for obesity. As researchers continue to disentangle the intricacies of adipose tissue physiology, it is increasingly becoming clear that this tissue is not merely a passive energy depot, but an active component in the body's metabolic network, with roles in energy homeostasis and health (Figure 6.3).

6.1. Types of Adipose Tissue

Learning Outcome

1. Understand the white adipose tissue (WAT);
2. Understand the brown adipose tissue (BAT);
3. Describe the beige adipose tissue.

WAT is primarily the energy reservoir of the body, serving as an insulator and protector of vital organs. It stores surplus energy in the form of triglycerides and serves as a fatty acid source when energy supply is required. WAT is also known to be involved in endocrine function, with the secretion of a number of hormones , such as leptin and adiponectin, which have important roles to play in regulating metabolism and appetite. Also, in obesity, a significant change has been found in WAT lipid metabolism and inflammation, revealing the tissue's importance in health and metabolic disease (Gonzalez-Periz et al., 2014). In contrast to WAT, BAT is essential in thermogenesis during cold exposure. BAT generates heat through a process termed non-shivering thermogenesis, which is predominantly mediated by the presence of uncoupling protein 1 (UCP1) in its mitochondria. This unique characteristic allows BAT to waste energy and generate heat, thereby being involved in energy homeostasis. Earlier research has commented on the possibility of BAT as a drug target for the treatment of obesity and metabolic disease since it can burn calories rather than store them. However, it has been challenging to gain knowledge on the molecular and functional properties of human BAT due to the challenges in obtaining human samples. New biopsy techniques, such as the recently developed for the sampling of human BAT in the supraclavicular region, are now viable means of expanding our knowledge base about this essential adipose tissue (Annamalai et al., 2015).

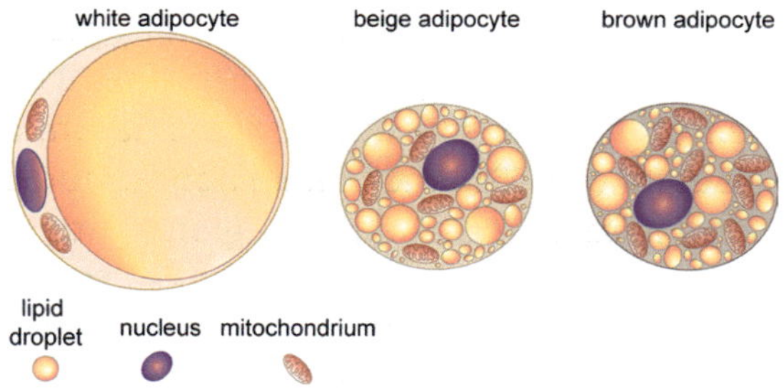

Figure 6.4. Types of adipose tissue.

Source: https://www.researchgate.net/publication/324476714/figure/fig2/AS:614524717633538@1523525518478/Three-types-of-adipocytes-The-morphological-differences-between-the-three-types-of.png.

Both adipose tissues are important to the regulation of metabolic balance, yet they possess different cellular characteristics and functions that contribute to overall health. The interaction between WAT and BAT can significantly regulate a person's susceptibility to metabolic illnesses, including obesity and type 2 diabetes. Add-on treatments aimed at enhancing BAT activity or transdifferentiating WAT towards a more active, metabolically brown-like adipose tissue are being studied. Moreover, the role of inflammatory pathways and signaling molecules derived from adipose tissue , such as prostaglandins, complicates our understanding of the dialogue between these tissues and various physiological processes. From an understanding of these mechanisms, researchers seek new ways to combat obesity and improve metabolic health through targeted management of adipose tissue (Gonzalez-Periz et al., 2014) (Figure 6.4).

6.1.1. White Adipose Tissue (WAT)

White adipose tissue (WAT) is a key component of the human body's energy balance. Consisting primarily of adipocytes characterized by a single large lipid droplet, WAT is present in two primary depots, subcutaneous and visceral. Subcutaneous WAT, located beneath the skin, serves as an insulating barrier and mechanical cushioning, while visceral WAT surrounds large organs, playing a role in visceral fat deposition. This unusual pattern of WAT is interesting because it has implications for metabolic well-being; excess accumulation of visceral fat is typically linked to increased risks of metabolic disease in the form of type 2 diabetes and cardiovascular disease. WAT adipocytes are very plastic and can be changed in size and quantity according to individual metabolic conditions, thus contributing to energy balance and global metabolic homeostasis (Jenkins III, 2022). WAT, aside from its established function in energy storage, is increasingly being recognized as a necessary endocrine organ. Adipocytes release a number of signaling molecules known as adipokines that have significant impacts on systemic metabolism and are also involved in inflammation. Among these, leptin, identified in the first half of the 1990s, plays a significant role in regulating energy balance, affecting appetite and energy expenditure. Leptin and other adipokines exhibit pro-inflammatory or anti-inflammatory activity, thereby linking adipose tissue with the immune system and metabolic pathways. This endocrine function of WAT highlights its dual nature of both maintaining energy homeostasis and contributing to obesity pathologies, thereby bringing its further comprehension and significance for human health to the fore (Cuevas-Ramos et al., 2019). The regulatory processes of WAT functionality are complex and multifactorial and are regulated by many biological pathways. Specifically, WAT and FGF21 interaction has emerged in the spotlight because it can regulate adipocyte differentiation and thermogenesis. FGF21 boosts the expression of uncoupling protein 1 (UCP1), much like the mechanisms of action in BAT, linking WAT to energy expenditure under some conditions, like cold or exercise. These findings tell us that WAT is not only a passive energy reservoir but an active participant in energy metabolism and heat regulation. The study of how to regulate WAT to optimize metabolic well-being remains an area of investigation, which represents a shift in perspective regarding adipose tissue as part of disease and health (Jenkins III, 2022) (Figure 6.5).

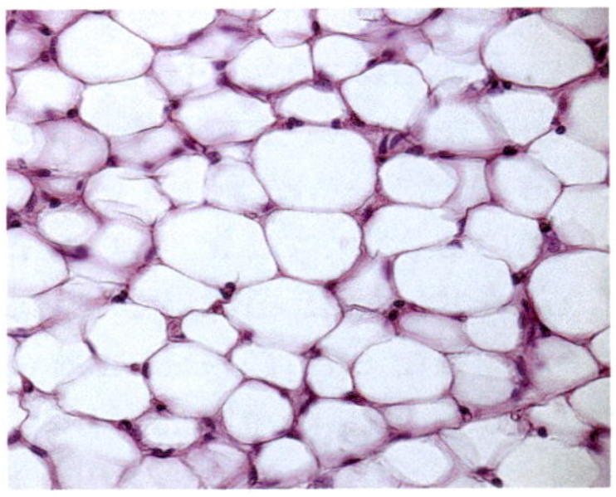

Figure 6.5. White adipose tissue (WAT).

Source: https://www.shutterstock.com/image-photo/light-micrograph-white-adipose-tissue-600nw-185476955.jpg.

6.1.2. Brown Adipose Tissue (BAT)

The pertinence of BAT in human physiology extends much beyond its initial categorization as merely a heat-generating tissue. Brown fat consists of a special form of adipocyte characterized by their ability for non-shivering thermogenesis, a metabolic response essential for the maintenance of body temperature during cold exposure. The presence of (UCP1) within the mitochondria of such cells plays a central role in this process, allowing for energy loss in the form of heat rather than retaining it as chemical energy. This unique mechanism highlights BATs potential role in regulating energy balance and metabolism, quite different from (WAT), which is primarily an energy storage reservoir in the long term. As studies continue, understanding the special function and control of BAT is increasingly important, especially against the background of rising rates of obesity and metabolic disease affecting modern populations (Jenkins III, 2022). Recent evidence has indicated that adult human beings possess significant deposits of BAT, dispelling the current paradigm that it is predominantly present in infants. Experiments have indicated that the activity of BAT can be modified by environmental temperature, suggesting that its function is dynamic and adaptive to the environment. Moreover, the anatomical distribution of BAT in the human body is notably localized in certain anatomical regions, with rich blood supply and innervation, further supporting BAT's role in physiological thermogenesis. Such versatility highlights the potential of BAT as a drug target for therapeutic strategies against obesity. Exploiting the thermogenic potential of BAT, researchers are seeking ways of causing weight loss and enhancing metabolic health, and in so doing, are highlighting the necessity to respect underlying mechanisms that govern BAT function (Jenkins III, 2022). New research confirms the presence of beige adipose tissue, a unique phenotype that shares characteristics of both BAT and WAT, further enriching the knowledge on the adipogenic reactions in human beings. Beige adipocytes can emerge from white fat through a process referred to as browning, with increased mitochondrial load and thermogenic capacity comparable to BAT. This is controlled by a variety of endogenous regulators and extrinsic stimuli, which could initiate the differentiation process. There are newly identified mechanisms causing the thermogenesis of beige adipocytes independent of classical pathways associated with UCP1. This advance provides a very promising potential for the therapeutic targeting of beige adipose tissue for obesity and metabolic disease, underpinning the importance of both mechanisms of browning and the regulatory components controlling beige adipocyte biology (Figure 6.6).

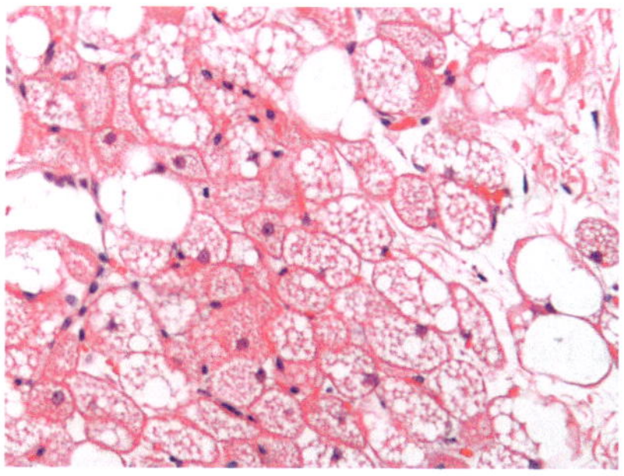

Figure 6.6. Brown adipose tissue (BAT).

Source: https://medcell.org/histology/connective_tissue_lab/images/brown_adipocytes.jpg.

6.1.3. Beige Adipose Tissue

Classification of adipose tissue has become more sophisticated after the discovery of beige adipose tissue, which is a unique type intermediate between white and brown adipose tissues. Unlike white adipocytes, which are primarily set aside for energy storage, beige adipocytes are critical for thermogenesis, releasing energy to generate heat. This thermogenic potential is very much facilitated by theUCP1, which diverts energy to heat and not to stored fat. In humans, beige adipose tissue is found predominantly in subcutaneous fat depots, and these assume increasing relevance in the context of obesity and metabolic derangements. Understanding the physiological and biochemical mechanisms of beige adipocyte development and activity promises the development of therapeutic interventions for the treatment of obesity-related disease, outlining a potential path to enhanced metabolic health by manipulation of body composition and fat distribution. There has been evidence of environmental control influencing beige adipose tissue behavior markedly. For example, cold exposure has been demonstrated to stimulate the differentiation of white adipose tissue into beige adipocytes, while excessive nutrients and higher temperatures may reduce their abundance. This development tests the responsiveness of beige fat to external cues, bringing to the fore the complex physiological mechanisms underlying its control. Remarkably, studies indicate that the maintenance of beige adipocyte features, such as thermogenic gene expression, is reversible, and the term beige adipocyte renaissance has been used to describe this process. This reversibility suggests that environmental manipulation may be a tactical method for enhancing the thermogenic potential of beige adipose tissue, and this provides opportunities for the effective control of obesity and metabolic modulation in human populations (Wang et al., 2017). Besides, recent advances uncover the basic molecular pathways underlying beige adipocyte physiology, highlighting secreted factors that drive thermogenesis. Specific pathways and factors have been identified to stimulate beige adipogenesis and promote the maintenance of activation of thermogenic programs in these cells. The role of liver kinase B1 and histone deacetylase 4 has also been indicated in these mechanisms, indicating a system of intricate regulation that aids in the maintenance of the features of beige adipocytes at different life stages. This evidence supports the therapeutic potential of targeting these mechanisms towards the enhancement of beige adipose function in obesity-prone patients. By accessing the advances in understanding beige adipose tissue biology, researchers can produce novel strategies to treat obesity, highlighting the therapeutic significance of inducing metabolic well-being by modulating the composition of adipose tissue (McQueen et al., 2018).

Test Your Knowledge

1. What's the difference between white and brown adipose tissue?
2. What is beige adipose tissue?

6.2. Functions of Adipose Tissue

Learning Outcome

1. Describe the energy storage and metabolism in adipose tissue;
2. Understand the insulation and temperature regulation;
3. Describe the hormonal regulation and signaling.

The functions of adipose tissue go beyond energy storage as they play vital roles in energy metabolism, heat generation, and endocrine regulation. There are primarily two forms of adipose tissue: (WAT) and (BAT), where the former is utilized as an energy depot and the latter for heat production via non-shivering thermogenesis. WAT contains mainly triglycerides, releasing fatty acids during fasting or energy demand, thereby ensuring energy homeostasis. In contrast, BAT, being highly mitochondrial and (UCP1) rich, ensures the dissipation of stored energy as heat, especially important in newborns and hibernating mammals. The intricate interaction between these two types of adipose tissue is an expression of their complementary function, crucial for thermoregulation and countering varying metabolic demands in human individuals. Moreover, research has revealed the complex signaling role of adipose tissue that regulates systemic metabolic activities. Specifically, WAT is an active endocrine organ releasing multiple adipokines , such as leptin, adiponectin, and resistin. These signaling molecules are involved in appetite, insulin sensitivity, and inflammation. Leptin, for instance, signals satiety to the hypothalamus and therefore regulates energy expenditure and intake. Adiponectin, however, enhances insulin sensitivity and fatty acid oxidation which are important in glucose metabolism. The secretion of these hormones encapsulates not just the metabolic state of adipose tissue but also its significant connotations within the context of obesity pathology, including type 2 diabetes and cardiovascular disease. This multi-valent functionality encapsulates the meaning behind realizing adipose tissue dynamics within broader metabolic health contexts.

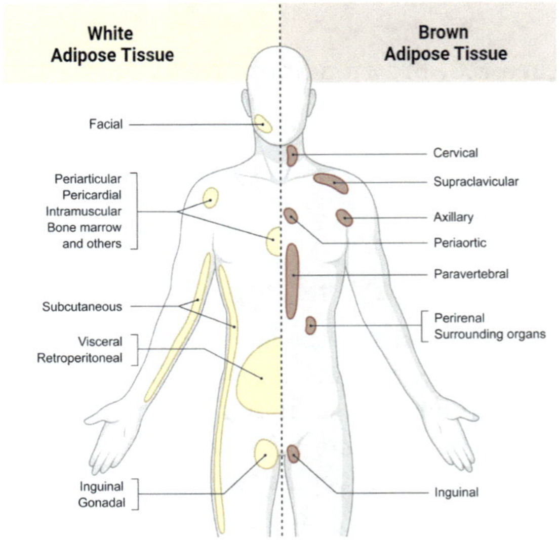

Figure 6.7. Endocrine function of adipose tissue.

Source: https://endoconsult.b-cdn.net/wp-content/uploads/adipose-tissue.png.

Additionally, bone marrow adipose tissue (BMAT) is another crucial but less-prominent subtype of adipose tissue that has a unique function in metabolic regulation. BMAT appears to possess distinctive mechanisms from traditional WAT and BAT, and mounting evidence suggests that it plays a role in glucose metabolism and insulin sensitivity. Transcriptome profile analyses demonstrate that BMAT exhibits disrupted glucose regulation and decreased insulin sensitivity, which may affect global systemic glucose homeostasis. Recent research employing advanced imaging techniques, for instance, PET/CT has established that while BMAT is insulin-resistant towards glucose uptake, it still maintains a greater basal glucose uptake than other tissues , such as skeletal muscle. This distinctive role emphasizes BMAT's possible effect on metabolic wellness and warrants further investigation to define its specific roles in human physiology, particularly in obesity and metabolic disease (Czech et al., 2017; Suchacki et al., 2020) (Figure 6.7).

6.2.1. Energy Storage and Metabolism

Energy storage and metabolism of the adipose tissue are critical components of human physiology with important implications for many aspects of disease and health. Adipose tissues constitute the major reservoir of energy in the body, wherein excess calories are deposited as triglycerides. Such a storage unit is critical to maintain the body in energy equilibrium, particularly in the condition of caloric deficit, wherein fat may be metabolized for use. The metabolic functions of adipose tissue extend beyond storage; they involve the regulation of lipid metabolism through intricate biochemical processes that include lipoprotein lipase and other enzymes. In this context, how adipose tissue responds to various hormonal stimuli, including testosterone, is essential to appreciating its role in body fat distribution and metabolism, especially in states like obesity and hypogonadism (Santosa & Jensen , 2012). The differential storage of fatty acids in adipose tissue also helps explain the complexity of energy metabolism. It was established by research that chronic hypogonadism results in abnormal patterns of storage for fatty acids, and for such individuals, a greater proportion of consumed fatty acids is stored in subcutaneous fat. This is linked to the activity of specific enzymes , such as acyl-CoA synthetase, whose function is pivotal in the activation of fatty acids and their subsequent integration into triglycerides. Stimulation of these pathways illustrates how hormonal state can have a significant influence on energy storage capabilities and metabolic health. In addition, differences in the role of adipose tissue emphasize the need for targeted interventions in obesity treatment, particularly those targeting the hormonal regulators of energy metabolism (Santosa & Jensen , 2012). In addition, the broader context of explaining energy storage and metabolism involves the participation of systemic regulators of metabolic rates. The individuality in energy expenditure arises due to both behavioral patterns as well as intrinsic physiological mechanisms, increasing the complexity of the energy-balance equation. Plausible mechanisms, such as the differential activities of lipoprotein lipase and the role of brown adipose tissue in thermogenesis, are worthy of study in human obesity. Available literature provides insights into the multifaceted interaction of metabolic rates, hormonal control, and capacity for fat storage. By establishing our understanding of these determinants, researchers are better able to conceptualize obesity and potential interventions that can decrease its prevalence, leaving open the promise of treatments that are aimed at the metabolic intricacies of adipose tissue (Figure 6.8).

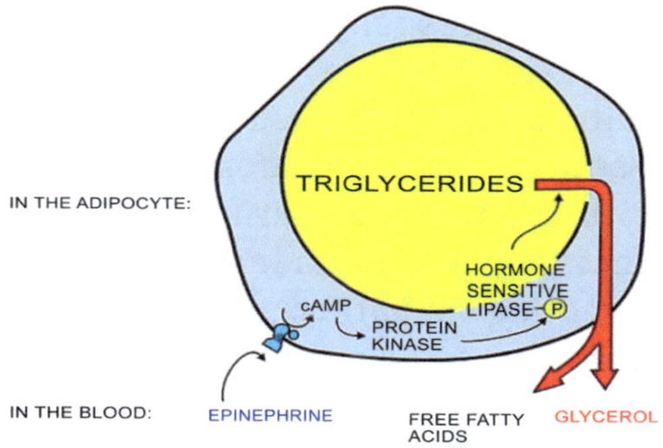

Figure 6.8. Lipolysis – a source of energy from stored fats.

Source: https://biologydictionary.net/wp-content/uploads/2021/06/lipolysis.jpg.

6.2.2. Insulation and Temperature Regulation

Adipose tissue plays a significant role in human body insulation and thermal regulation and general thermal homeostasis as well. The tissue was also storing energy in the form of fat and working as a necessary insulating layer that reduces cold-induced loss of heat. The insulating role of adipose tissues is most evident in subcutaneous fat, which serves as a cover against cold environments by preventing conduction of heat away from the body. Interestingly, the relationship between adipose tissue and the circulatory system also supports thermoregulatory activities, providing a regulated distribution of heat between regions of the body. These mechanisms are required for the maintenance of core body temperature, especially during thermal stress, such that optimal physiological function is preserved under extreme conditions (Kaciuba-Uscilko & Greenleaf, 1989). Thermogenesis in adipose tissue is also important to control the temperature, especially upon cold stress. Cold exposure initiates a series of physiological mechanisms, including the stimulation of specific pathways that induce heat production in brown adipose tissue, which is a type of fat tissue rich in mitochondria. Not only does this adaptive response increase metabolic rate, but it also involves considerable energy expenditure, as evidenced by experiments demonstrating the stimulation of β-adrenergic receptors in adipocytes during cold exposure. The thermogenic mechanism is essential in preventing hypothermia by generating heat through non-shivering thermogenesis. Understanding processes that regulate adipose tissue thermogenesis is thus crucial in formulating effective strategies in maintaining body temperature as well as boosting energy metabolism (Tajima et al., 2020). Advances in recognizing adipose tissue mechanisms have also enabled the development of new technologies in optimizing temperature control mechanisms. The optogenetic approach to inducing thermogenesis in adipose tissue is only one such example. Employing selective stimulation of calcium signaling pathways in adipocytes, researchers have demonstrated the potential to initiate fat thermogenesis outside of external cold exposure. This advancement not only provides us with more understanding of adipose function but also promises therapeutics for preventing obesity. Given that the regulation of temperature is growing in significance in the context of issues from climate change and metabolic disease, ongoing research into adipose tissue function is important. Its complicated status as a balancer of energy and insulator makes it an attractive subject for future study with a perspective towards its health improvement in various populations (Tajima et al., 2020).

6.2.3. Hormonal Regulation and Signaling

The intricate interaction between hormone signaling and regulation plays a key role in unraveling the dynamics of adipose tissue in the physiology of humans. Insulin, leptin, and adiponectin are a few of the important hormones in the regulation of adipose tissue metabolism with both lipid storage and mobilization effects. Insulin, for instance, not only activates the uptake of glucose by adipocytes but also inhibits lipolysis, thus facilitating lipid storage. Conversely, leptin, which is secreted by adipocytes, provides the central nervous system with feedback regarding energy reservoirs and assists in appetite regulation and energy expenditure. The delicate equilibrium of these hormonal messages is a reflection of how vital the hormonal regulation is to maintaining homeostasis in the adipose tissue and how advanced energy balance mechanisms are in humans. In recent years, research has been carried out to study the molecular processes of hormonal signaling pathways in adipose tissue. Circadian rhythms have been found to be crucial in influencing the rhythm of hormonal secretion, thus affecting metabolic functions. Coordination of hormonal function with the circadian clock is essential, as disruption of this timing will lead to metabolic diseases , such as obesity and type 2 diabetes. By establishing a more precise concept for these relationships, researchers can identify novel targets for therapy aimed at the modulation of thermogenic signaling within fat tissue, which can offer new therapeutic avenues to the regulation of metabolic disease. Moreover, this growing literature highlights the interconnectedness of endocrine function and circadian rhythm, revealing possible means of preventing metabolic dysregulation (Gnocchi & Bruscalupi, 2017). The impact of such hormonal signaling mechanisms extends past mere metabolic control; they also have important implications for overall health. Adipose tissue, long thought to be a passive depot, is also an active participant in endocrine function, releasing cytokines and adipokines that modulate a wide range of physiological responses. In disease, such as obesity, the deregulation of these hormonal signals within changed secretion can lead to chronic inflammation and insulin resistance, exacerbating metabolic disease. Understanding of the mechanisms controlling such hormonal interactions is key to effective intervention design. As a study shown enhanced understanding of hormonal control may pay dividends in the form of new therapeutic approaches to endocrine and metabolic disease, ultimately enhancing health outcomes in populations worldwide (Chen et al., 2015) (Figure 6.9).

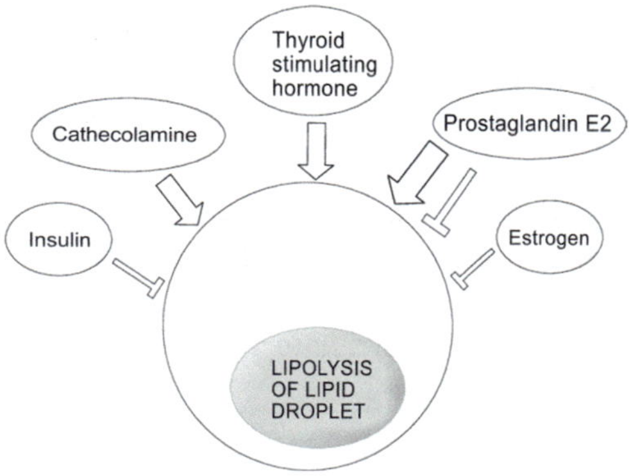

Figure 6.9. Regulation of adipose tissue lipolysis.

Source: https://www.researchgate.net/profile/Harry-Luglio/publication/271592707/figure/fig1/AS:392159028105224@1470509406993/Regulation-of-adipose-tissue-lipolysis.png.

Test Your Knowledge

1. How is energy stored in adipose tissue?
2. What is relationship between hormonal regulation and signaling?

6.3. Development of Adipose Tissue

Learning Outcome

1. Understand the process of adipogenesis for the development and differentiation of adipocytes;
2. Describe the factors influencing adipose tissue development;
3. Understand the role of genetics in adipose tissue distribution.

Human adipose tissue formation is a multi-stage process that initiates early in fetal life and extends into the adult years. The adipogenesis, or the formation of fat cells, is also regulated by genetic, environmental, and hormonal influences. In the growth of the body, preadipocyte differentiation to mature adipocytes is an essential mechanism regulating the overall amount of adipose tissue. This process is not a passive energy reservoir, but actually an active participant in the control of metabolism and energy homeostasis. Clarifying the mechanisms of adipose tissue deposition may yield critical information regarding conditions of health, particularly obesity that has now spread like an epidemic in the majority of the world. By analyzing intrinsic and extrinsic factors on adipogenesis, researchers aim to disclose potential therapeutic candidates for metabolic disease with obesity associated adipose tissue. Considerable attention has been focused on the possible role of various pathogens in adipose tissue formation. For instance, studies indicate that certain viral infections, e.g., human adenovirus 36 (Adv 36), are capable of promoting adipogenesis. The presence of Adv 36 was discovered in biopsies of adipose tissue in patients with severe obesity, which suggests that such infective entities are critically involved in the determination of fat storage and distribution in the body. This finding is of utmost concern in terms of how infection influences metabolic pathways and results in overaccumulation of adipose tissue. Therefore, it is crucial to expand studies into the relationship between infections and adipose tissue development. It points to the need for a more integrated model of causes of obesity beyond traditional diet and lifestyle, placing infectious causes in a broader context of metabolic health. In addition, the impact of obesity status on the physiology of adipose tissue has been described in evidence from varied omics studies, providing an integrated summary of how body weight affects tissue function.

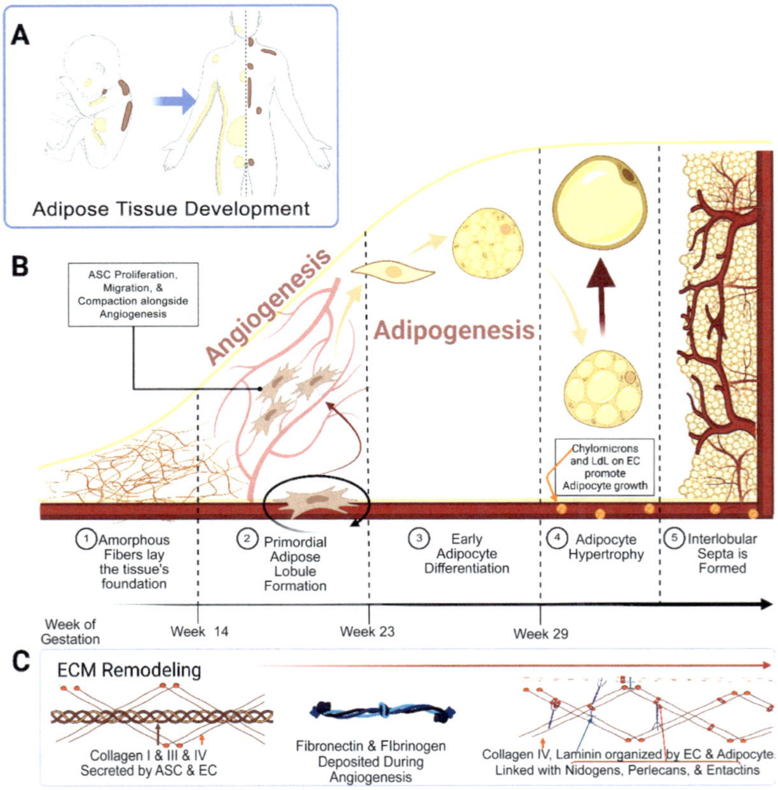

Figure 6.10. Caption first, then explanation of the figure.Schematic representations of (A) the localization of white adipose tissue (yellow) and brown adipose tissue (brown) in a developing neonate and adult human; (B) the breakdown of adipose tissue development into the 5 specified stages; (C) the prominent Extracellular Matrix (ECM) components over the course of adipose tissue development.

Source: https://encyclopedia.pub/media/item_content/202210/6357395beacd5biomedicines-10-02227-g001.png.

In one study, comparing monozygotic twin pairs of differing body mass indices, in the heavier twins, both augmented transcriptional changes were observed in the adipose tissue. These changes included upregulation of inflammatory pathways and downregulation of mitochondrial functions and represent metabolic profile changes that are characteristic of over-adiposity. Additionally, pro-inflammatory lipids were observed at elevated levels in the adipose tissue of these twins. These findings exemplify the dynamic interaction between adipose tissue and obesity, highlighting that adipose tissue plays a pioneering role in metabolic dysfunctions , such as dyslipidemia and insulin resistance. Elucidation of these pathogenic processes forms the backbone of the development of effective measures against obesity complications and preservation of metabolic well-being among various groups (Salehian et al., 2010; van der Kolk et al., 2021) (Figure 6.10).

6.3.1. Adipogenesis and Differentiation of Adipocytes

Adipogenesis is the process of differentiation and development of adipocytes, which are the units of adipose tissue. Adipogenesis is a multistep process that begins with the activation of preadipocytes, which finally mature to become lipid-storing adipocytes. At the heart of the process is regulation by a number of transcription factors, most prominently peroxisome proliferator-activated receptor gamma (PPARγ), which triggers the expression of genes controlling lipid metabolism and accumulation. Bone morphogenetic proteins (BMPs) have also been found to be powerful regulators of adipogenesis, through complex pathways that influence not just the rate of differentiation but also the characteristics of the adipocytes produced. Interestingly, studies have shown that BMP antagonists, such as Noggin, are crucial here by modulating adipogenesis and, in this way, impacting metabolic conditions like obesity (Blázquez-Medela et al., 2019). Incorporating gender differences into the study of adipogenesis means translating into nuanced distinctions in how adipocytes respond to hormonal and environmental stress. Research identifies that Noggin deficiency exacerbates obesity in old age to a significant extent, particularly in female mice, with an overwhelming decrease in brown adipose marker and thermogenic gene expression, such as PGC1alpha and UCP1. This indicates gender-specific susceptibility towards obesity development because females exhibited serious lipid metabolism and thermogenesis impairments compared to males. Conversely, males had some early signs of metabolic change but still possessed relatively preserved adipogenic activity at early stages of Noggin deletion.

The findings indicate the complexity of adiposity, regulated by intrinsic endocrine and genetic determinants that control differential patterns of metabolism in adipocytes (Blázquez-Medela et al., 2019). The modulation of oxidative stress and adipogenesis also accounts for the molecular machinery of adipocyte differentiation. Peroxisomes, which are the organelles that play a crucial role in lipid metabolism, play a critical role in redox homeostasis mediation in adipocytes. The organelles carry out such critical processes as fatty acid oxidation and detoxification of ROS and thus influence the cellular redox status. A balance of redox is necessary to provide optimal adipocyte function and differentiation. Disruption of peroxisomal functions can have the possibility of leading to a dysregulated adipogenic process with inflammation, which can exacerbate obesity and metabolic disease. Understanding the peroxisomal function-adipocyte differentiation relationship provides an opening for the development of targeted therapeutic approaches to reverse obesity and obesity-linked metabolic disorders and is an exciting future research direction (Figure 6.11).

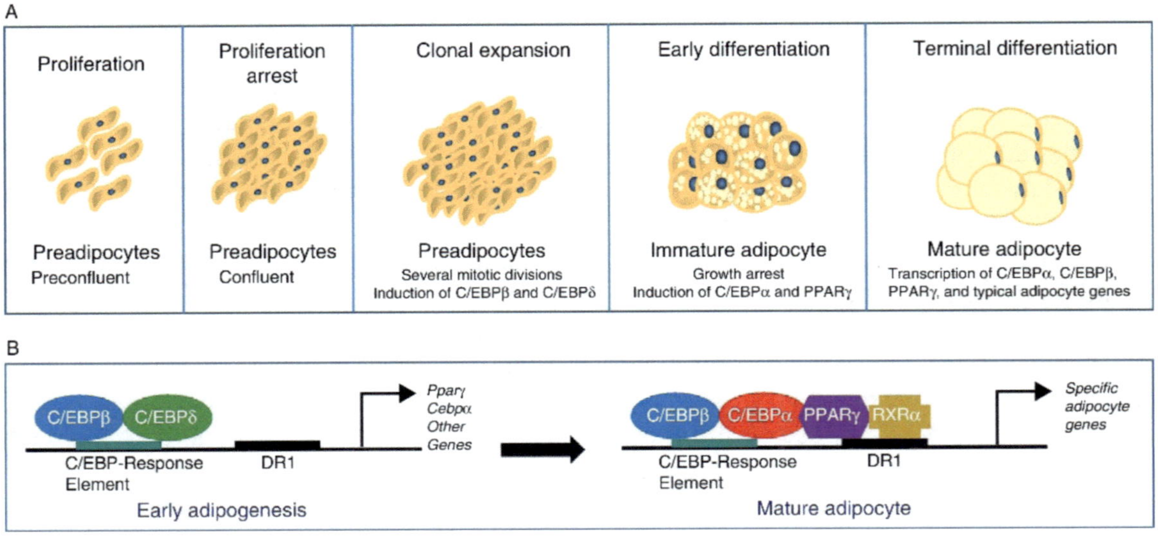

Figure 6.11. Differentiation of preadipocytes into adipocytes. (A) Scheme of the transition process from preadipocyte to mature adipocyte, including the different stages. (B) Sequential model of transcriptional control during adipogenesis.

Source: https://static.elsevier.es/multimedia/21735093/0000006100000002/v1_201403140305/S2173509314000336/v1_201403140305/en/main.assets/gr6.jp eg?xkr=ue/ImdikoIMrsJce rZ+w997EogCnBdOOD93cPFbanNf23BIP/DWE pPOpuWlfofny59eNEDq11r0z12hWOP+26sL WrrtA9M3g3Ke4eNG3dLuiRtxG2ChobSscP5t4ezl6 spwXZw5jsta+VP5li3dYGgRveIk9NjIPJqG DRXKwX66tnMt6ig97TaUfwfeb0juIY8SGcCQ7FcoEno34wcSaYNQiOsh4H/LbIfPAEb+F1/ByfVzpqM pGb9J2mgrYz3NacTu0XM09PyHUGuilzQ5+J6goaDK8I4n+EDkwWE5dGD0=.

6.3.2. Factors Influencing Adipose Tissue Development

Adipose tissue development is a multifaceted process influenced by an interwoven system of physiological, genetic, and environmental factors. Central to this mechanism is the interaction between energy expenditure and intake, which dictates the amount of fat the body can deposit. When regular caloric intake surpasses energy expenditure, the result is a positive energy balance, supporting the growth of adipose tissue. The composition of dietary intake has extremely important impacts on energy balance; there are nutrients that can influence metabolism and endocrine reactions and hence fat deposition. For instance, intake of whey protein has been reported to reduce intake of energy intake, boost expenditure of energy expenditure, and enhance insulin sensitivity, all of which lead to negative energy balance that may avert or minimize excessive gain of adipose tissue (McAllan et al., 2012). Understanding such food influences on the accrual of adipose tissue provides insight into potential therapies for obesity and related metabolic ailments. Besides the dietary factors, the influence of environmental toxins on adipose tissue formation cannot be overemphasized. Persistent organic pollutants (POPs) are generally distinguished by their persistence and bioaccumulation in biological organisms. They can interfere with normal metabolic processes in adipose tissue. There is evidence that such contaminants can change energy balance and metabolic properties in different species and with potential human health implications. For instance, studies on grey seal pups have shown that intense exposure to POPs has been demonstrated to change adipose tissue function, affecting glucose metabolism and rates of lipolysis based on feeding status. The alterations are significant, particularly at life stages where there is considerable fat deposition and mobilization (Bennett et al., 2018). Accordingly, the role of exposure to POPs in the environment must therefore be accounted for in the assessment of the factors that contribute to developing adipose tissue and consequently to its final metabolic impact. The genetic predispositions also control one's susceptibility to developing adipose tissue. Gene variations controlling metabolic functions and fat storage influence adipocyte differentiation and proliferation, dictating the heterogeneity in adipose tissue distribution as well as function. Specific genetic polymorphisms have correlated with susceptibility to obesity, indicating a hereditary component in the regulation of adipose tissue. Furthermore, epigenetic alterations , such as DNA methylation and histone modification are subject to lifestyle factors like diet and exercise and therefore may be altering gene expression associated with adipogenesis. This new field of science brings to the fore the complex process of adipose tissue formation, where genetic and epigenetic factors intersect with environmental and nutritional influences to create an individual's metabolic landscape. Addressing these various causative factors is critical to building efficacious interventions for the prevention of obesity and the concomitant health risk.

6.3.3. Role of Genetics in Adipose Tissue Distribution

Clarification of the genetic factors for adipose tissue distribution is critical to illuminating the inherent causes of obesity and its accompanying metabolic disturbances. Genetic predisposition has been found to influence fat accumulation sites within the body, with persons sharing differences in the fat distribution patterns, e.g., subcutaneous versus visceral fat. Variability is significant because it represents individualized threats to health, e.g., cardiovascular disease and type 2 diabetes. For instance, visceral fat is most directly associated with metabolic disturbances due to its proximity to key organs, while subcutaneous fat, despite being considered less harmful, remains a threat to the collective obesity threat. Genetic research pinpointed some polymorphisms affecting the adipocyte function and fat distribution patterns, with the hope that uncovering these genetic determinants would reveal personalized intervention in managing obesity. Another essential region of adipose tissue genetics is connected with epigenetic regulation, which can modify gene expression without altering the main DNA structure. Recent studies show that DNA methylation is a significant component in adipose tissue biology and controls not just the development of adipocytes but also overall metabolic processes of fat pads. The study reveals that such epigenetic modifications can even be passed down through generations and thus potentially perpetuate obesity and concomitant metabolic diseases within families. Furthermore, disease-specific adipose tissue, characterized by abnormal patterns of DNA methylation, has been linked to obesity and type 2 diabetes and thus emphasizes the importance of further research with a view to epigenetic mechanisms. Understanding these processes is also necessary for the recognition of new therapeutic targets in treating the epigenetic control of adiposity disorders and enhancing metabolic well-being in individuals at risk for obesity disease (Ma & Kang, 2019). The cross-talk between genetics and body fat distribution is also a contributor to health heterogeneity in obesity. Not everybody with the same body mass index (BMI) is at equal risk for metabolic disease, as what happens in those who are classified as metabolically healthy obese would demonstrate. Differences in genes can explain this variation by altering the functional properties of different depots of adipose tissue, such as their hormonal regulation and sensitivity to inflammation. For example, perivascular adipose tissue (PVAT) is critical to the vessels' health and is determined by the distribution of fat in the area, having implications for cardiovascular risk. Identification of the genetic determinants of fat deposition in adipose tissue can clarify why some individuals are more safeguarded from the pathologic impacts of obesity, and hence highly individualized measures for handling obesity must be adopted, giving consideration to both environmental and genetic determinants in shaping the metabolic profiles of individuals (Costa et al., 2018) (Figure 6.12).

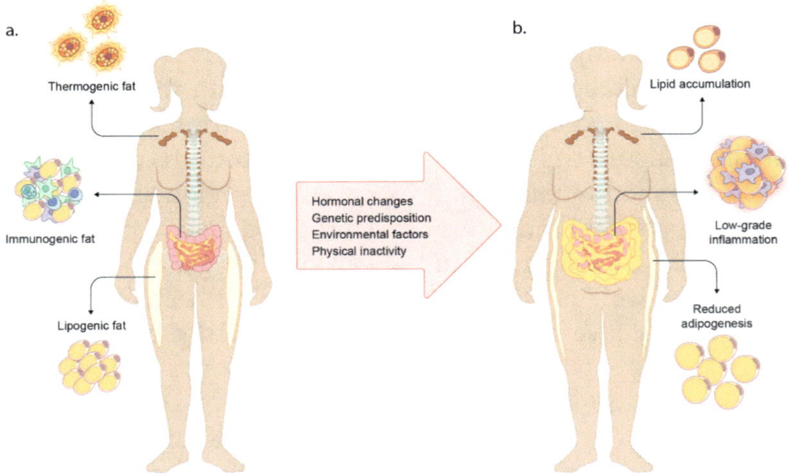

Figure 6.12. Loss of functions of adipose tissues in relation to metabolic dysfunction. In a healthy state (a), thermogenic fat (brown adipose tissue) is sympathetically activated in response to cold, producing heat and taking up glucose and fatty acids from the circulation. Several factors including hormonal changes, genetic predisposition, environmental factors and physical inactivity, contributes to metabolic dysfunction (b). Thermogenic depots lose their capacity of substrate uptake and thermogenesis.

Source: https://media.springernature.com/full/springer-static/image/art%3A10.1038%2Fs44324-024-00036-z/MediaObjects/44324_2024_36_Fig1_HTML.png?as=webp.

Test Your Knowledge

1. What is the process of adipogenesis?
2. What is the role of genetics in adipose tissue distribution?

6.4. Adipose Tissue in Aging

Learning Outcome

1. Understand the changes in adipose tissue distribution with age;
2. Describe the effects of aging on adipocyte function;
3. Understand the implications of adipose tissue for health and longevity.

The dynamic process of aging has a marked effect on the dynamics of adipose tissue, leading to dramatic body composition alterations. With aging, there is a tendency for the loss of lean muscle mass, a state that is called sarcopenia, which is usually followed by elevated adiposity. Fat gained with advancing age is not only a volume issue, i.e., accumulation of adipose tissue, but also an issue related to redistribution of the fat, with very important consequences for therapy. Specifically, the balance between declining muscle mass and rising stores of fat is responsible for reduced physical performance and heightened risks of disability, hospitalization, and death in older people.

Here, the understanding of the intricate interaction between adipose tissue and muscle dynamics is essential to surmount the health problem of the elderly, since changes in body composition in these compartments are linked with undesirable outcomes that emphasize the significance of adipose tissue in the aging process (Carter et al., 2019). Moreover, the changes in adipose tissue physiology during aging are not only confined to mass changes. The adipose tissue secretory phenotypes and cellularity are significantly impaired with increased inflammation and metabolic dysregulation. Adipocyte capacity to respond to maximum metabolic stress declines progressively as age increases, leading to lipotoxicity, where there is excessive spilling of lipids to non-adipose tissues, including skeletal muscle. This inter-organ communication is particularly cause for concern since it can adversely affect muscle quality, further exacerbating the sarcopenic process. The cross-talk between fat accumulation beyond metabolic requirements and metabolic dysfunction is a central axis for describing aging-related changes in physical function and health. Hence, the correction of the biochemical and physiological changes in adipose tissue can offer therapeutic intervention strategies to improve the quality of life in older individuals (Carter et al., 2019). Finally, the regenerative potential of stem cells in the context of age-related changes in adipose tissue presents a fascinating prospect for investigations and therapeutic targeting.

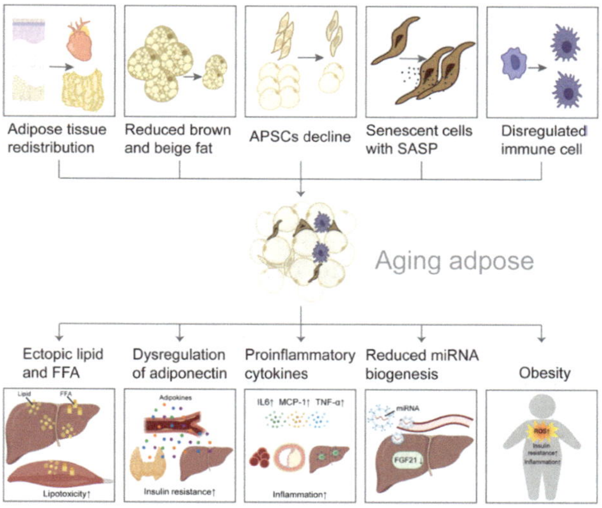

Figure 6.13. The role of adipose tissue in the aging process.

Source: https://media.springernature.com/full/springer-static/image/art%3A10.1038%2Fs41419-022-04752-6/MediaObjects/41419_2022_4752_Fig4_HTML.png?as=webp.

As the efficacy of regenerative processes with advancing age decreases, particularly in the presence of metabolic syndromes, the therapeutic potential of stem cells in reversing or mitigating the influence of aging becomes increasingly more prominent. Techniques , such as growth factor pre-treatment of the stem cells or synthetic scaffolding can improve them for treating adipose tissue dysfunction in the elderly. Discovering how the stem cells communicate with adipose tissue in late life could reveal new ways to rejuvenate metabolic homeostasis and healthy tissue. Therefore, the integration of regenerative medicine knowledge with research on aging adipose tissue could contribute to feasible pathways for building resistance to metabolic age-related diseases (Figure 6.13).

6.4.1. Changes in Adipose Tissue Distribution with Age

Aging in man is accompanied by the occurrence of dramatic alterations in adipose tissue distribution, which have considerable impacts on the health and metabolic function of the organism. Among the earliest alterations is the shift in subcutaneous fat deposition to visceral fat accumulation. The encasing of organs by this visceral fat is associated with enhanced risk of metabolic disease and cardiovascular disease. Research indicates that this redistribution results from the effects of hormonal changes and reduced physical activity with age, both of which alter the site and quantity of fat deposition within the body.

The ramifications of this are considerable, particularly given the realization that visceral fat accumulation has been shown to be correlated with increased insulin resistance and other metabolic syndromes prevalent in the elderly, thereby expanding health risks of aging. In addition to the altered fat distribution, senescence brings alterations in the physiologic characteristics of adipose tissue itself. Adipose tissue changes cellularity and inflammation patterns, revealing a more dynamic nature of fat tissue function. As explained in some reports, including those that examine the level of adipokines like vaspin, the interaction between body mass index (BMI) and metabolic health also becomes more complex in advanced ages. Excess fat mass in older persons may exceed the oxidative capacity of adipose tissue, and ectopic fat deposition in non-adipose tissue, such as skeletal muscle, will follow. This will not only increase the risk for metabolic derangements but also contribute to the reduced muscle strength and quality observed, compounding the mysteries of the aging process and physical functioning of older adults (Carter et al., 2019).

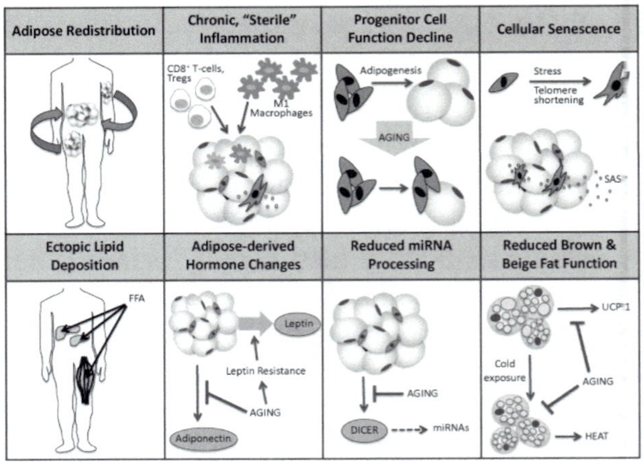

Figure 6.14. Adipose tissue changes with aging.

Source: https://www.researchgate.net/profile/Allyson-Palmer/publication/296479019/figure/fig4/AS:341301401800712@1458384003456/Adipose-tissue-changes-with-aging.png.

Moreover, the aging-related fat distribution changes coincide with the state of sarcopenia, which is characterized by the decline of muscle mass and strength of the skeletal system. The enhancement of fat tissue, particularly in visceral compartments, combined with the reduction of muscle mass, represents a twofold danger to old age health. Particularly, the presence of surplus fat can have a more inflammatory tissue composition around muscles, which will impair muscle contractility and functionality. It emphasizes the importance of considering fat distribution when evaluating the body performance impacts of sarcopenia. Clarifying these interactions is significant because they offer insight into the broader implications of adipose tissue changes, ultimately paving the way for focused interventions addressing not just weight regulation but activity as well to optimize muscle retention throughout the trajectory of aging (Carter et al., 2019) (Figure 6.14).

6.4.2. Effects of Aging on Adipocyte Function

Aging impacts adipocyte function in important and multifactorial ways that result in changes in body composition with profound health implications. With advancing age, there is an appreciable increase in adiposity accompanied by a decrease in lean muscle mass, a condition termed sarcopenia. This change in body composition is clinically relevant since the increase in fat mass, particularly when redistributed into the ectopic spaces of skeletal muscle, can interfere with the optimal physiological function. Dynamics of adipose tissue aging involve changes in cellularity, secretory profile, and inflammatory signals, all of which produce an adverse environment for muscle function. Consequently, the coincidence of aging and adipocyte dysfunction would thus affect mobility and bodily function, lending credence to the assumption that the aging process remodels adipose tissue as well as its role in metabolic well-being and holds tremendous implications for older adults (Carter et al., 2019). In addition to structural remodeling, adipocyte function is significantly controlled by hormonal regulation, namely glucocorticoids, with rising frequency as age progresses. These steroid hormones play an essential role in metabolic adaptation but elicit adverse effects on chronic exposure, including insulin resistance and dyslipidemia. It is observed that increased glucocorticoid levels may exacerbate the aging-related diseases by promoting the dysregulation of adipocytes, which compromises metabolic homeostasis. Especially, glucocorticoid signaling by the intracellular glucocorticoid receptor may lead to aberrant lipid storage dynamics in adipose tissues. In older adults, the endocrine disruption may lead to diminished thermogenic stimulation of brown fat and promote the white adipose phenotype, which also contributes to metabolic decline. It is thus crucial to understand the interaction between glucocorticoid signaling and aging in order to appreciate the complexity of adipocyte function during older age (Harris et al., 2018). Furthermore, age-related accumulated adipose tissue is not an inert organ; it is also an actively engaged tissue that engages in a dynamic crosstalk with other tissues, culminating in a condition of chronic low-grade inflammation. An elevated level of pro-inflammatory cytokines secreted by defective adipocytes can cause systemic inflammation, destabilizing metabolic homeostasis and promoting age-related disease. This biased secretory profile is particularly harmful because it initiates a vicious cycle of muscle loss and increased fat deposition. Research has established that the lipotoxicity caused by adipose tissue excess negatively affects muscle quality, meaning the deleterious effect on contractility and muscle architecture. The alteration in adipocyte function with aging therefore takes precedence to warrant particular interventions that address the metabolic as well as the inflammatory aspects of adipose tissue to avert the detrimental effects of aging on overall health and physical capability (Carter et al., 2019) (Figure 6.15).

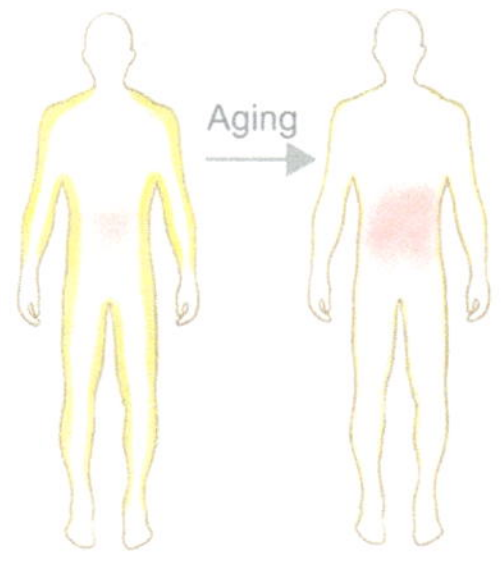

Figure 6.15. The age-related redistribution of adipose tissue.

Source: https://media.springernature.com/full/springer-static/image/art%3A10.1038%2Fs41419-022-04752-6/MediaObjects/41419_2022_4752_Fig1_HTML.png?as=webp.

6.4.3. Implications for Health and Longevity

Adipose tissue is of a multifunctional nature in the human body, exerting a major influence on health and longevity. Energy storage is its primary function; however, it is also an endocrine organ, releasing a number of hormones and cytokines that regulate metabolism, inflammation, and energy balance. Dysregulation of fat tissue also leads to metabolic diseases, such as obesity, with concomitant risks of diabetes, cardiovascular disease, and certain cancers. This pathological adipose tissue is not a local effect but has systemic consequences that can compromise overall health, reflecting the tissue's central function in maintaining metabolic health. An adequate understanding of these dynamics is required, considering the trend of modern lifestyles towards excess adiposity, hence worsening these risks and causing longevity issues by further linking longevity with chronic inflammation caused by dysfunctional adipose tissue. The connection between adipose tissue and aging is strongly exemplified through sirtuin functions, a family of proteins involved in cellular regulation and longevity. Sirtuins, whose activity is defined by the availability of nicotinamide adenine dinucleotide (NAD+), have been proven to control pivotal metabolic reactions, linking cell energy budgets to aging mechanisms. Research shows that NAD+ levels decline with older age and consequently sirtuin action follows (Imai & Guarente, 2016). This decline not only jeopardizes the communication between the mitochondria and the nucleus of cells but also disrupts the signaling between the hypothalamus and the fat tissue. These disruptions are pertinent in the sense that they unleash a chain reaction of age-related functional decline, further stressing the importance of impaired fat tissue regulation to longevity and overall health outcomes. In considering the health implications of adipose tissue, it becomes clear that enhancing NAD+ levels and sirtuin activity offers promising avenues for treatments that promote longevity and reduce age-related disease. Supplementation with NAD+ has been researched recently with interest as a means to restore sirtuin function, thus optimizing metabolic health that comes with progressive aging. Not only does this new field of research corroborate the relationship between aging and adipose tissue function but also offer practical ways to reverse metabolic dysfunctions related to aging. Furthermore, the healthful maintenance of adipose tissue through modification of such lifestyle factors as right nutrition and proper exercise may boost the availability of NAD+ and activate sirtuins. These forward-looking measures would lead to better pathways of aging, hence improving quality of life and longevity in the population (Chen et al., 2015).

Test Your Knowledge

1. What are the effects of aging on adipocyte function?
2. What are the implications of adipose tissue for health and longevity?

SUMMARY

The physiology of man's adipose tissue reveals its function diversified beyond simple oil storage and as an integral part of metabolic regulation and general homeostasis. Adipose tissue influences many physiological processes, including energy balance, endocrine function, and immune defense. Based on the evidence derived from research studies, variability in adipose tissue function and disposition has a significant bearing upon an individual's susceptibility to obesity and related metabolic diseases. For instance, bone morphogenetic protein (BMP) and of its antagonists, for example, Noggin, has been found to have a significant role to play in adipogenesis and obesity during aging. The BMP signaling might thus prove to be a new intervention for the control of health problems brought about by obesity (Blázquez-Medela et al., 2019). Furthermore, microRNA function, including miR-34a, in the control of inflammation and lipid metabolism in adipose tissue has also been highlighted by recent research. High expression of miR-34a has been identified as linked with increased inflammation, a feature of obesity and type 2 diabetes. By comparing wild-type and miR-34a−/− mouse models, scientists established that the lack of this microRNA led to increased weight gain and altered features of adipocytes when fed on a high-fat diet. These findings underpin the significance of miR-34a's role in both the inflammatory processes and metabolic pathways involved in adipose tissue functionality, ultimately revealing its therapeutic potential as a target for obesity management (Baker et al., 2016). In this way, research into adipose tissue mechanisms has far-reaching implications for how obesity and its consequences can be understood and treated. The intricate dance between several molecular actors like BMPs and microRNAs demonstrates that an integrated strategy to research adipose tissue is the need of the hour. Such a strategy could lead to new therapeutic strategies that leverage the biological complexity of adipose tissue to modulate metabolism optimally and mitigate the adverse effects of obesity. Through continued deconstruction of mechanisms governing adipose tissue biology, clinicians and scientists can better enable more efficient treatments and preventive medicine against obesity and related disorders, ultimately contributing to better public health.

Adipose tissue, a component of human physiology, plays a part in the regulation of metabolism and the maintenance of energy homeostasis. As highlighted in recent research, adipose tissue dysregulation is significantly associated with rising epidemics of type 2 diabetes and obesity, with consequent serious health, social, and economic issues. Understanding the intricate biology of adipose tissue is pivotal to the creation of suitable therapeutic options. Key findings indicate epigenetic regulations, particularly DNA methylation, as vital in regulating adipose tissue development and expression of metabolic genes. This makes it essential to study the epigenetic profile of adipocytes in an attempt to identify new drug targets for the management of obesity and T2D, since dysregulation within this region can result in dysfunctional adipose tissue leading to elevated metabolic disorders (Ma & Kang, 2019). The second vital function of adipose tissue is that it interacts with environmental factors, particularly exposure to persistent organic pollutants (POPs). Experiments have established that these toxic chemicals can be sequestered in the adipose tissue and disrupt metabolic processes, thereby influencing energy balance. For instance, it has been discovered through studies on marine mammals, including grey seal pups, that endogenous loads of POPs can influence metabolic characteristics , such as utilization of glucose and rates of lipolysis. These findings suggest that already at the early stages of life, adipose tissue is significantly affected by environmental toxicants, potentially disturbing energy regulation and fitness. Such findings emphasized on the importance of considering both ecological and biological contexts while addressing the issues resulting from dysregulated adipose tissue (Bennett et al., 2018). In summary, the understanding of adipose tissue is more than the traditional notion of a basic energy reservoir; it is indelibly tied to metabolic well-being and disease susceptibility. The dual-pronged strategy of epigenetic factors and environmental factors provides a timely overview of how adipose tissue intersects with the greater scheme of human health. By determining the interactions between extrinsic pollutant exposure, genetic control, and metabolic dynamics, researchers can discern possible therapeutic pathways. In the end, an integrated approach combining both intrinsic and extrinsic factors is required for the management of adipose tissue dysregulation and its implications in the prevention of obesity and T2D (Bennett et al., 2018; Ma & Kang, 2019).

KEY TERMS FROM THIS CHAPTER

- Adiponectin
- Adipose tissue
- Beige adipose tissue
- Bone marrow adipose tissue
- Brown adipose tissue
- Cardiovascular diseases
- Computed tomography
- Hypothalamus
- Leptin
- Metabolic disorders
- Mitochondria
- Oxidative stress
- Positron emission tomography
- Redox homeostasis

CRITICAL THINKING QUESTIONS

1. The primary function of adipose tissue is:

a. Protein synthesis

b. Energy storage and insulation

c. Bone support

d. Immune response

2. Adipose tissue is classified as:

a. Epithelial tissue

b. Connective tissue

c. Nervous tissue

d. Muscular tissue

3. The main cell type in adipose tissue is:

a. Fibroblast

b. Chondrocyte

c. Adipocyte

d. Osteocyte

4. The two main types of adipose tissue are:

a. Dense and loose adipose tissue

b. Elastic and reticular adipose tissue

c. White and brown adipose tissue

d. Fibrous and areolar adipose tissue

5. Which hormone is secreted by adipose tissue to regulate appetite and energy balance?

a. Insulin

b. Leptin

c. Ghrelin

d. Glucagon

Short Answer Questions

1. What is adipose tissue?
2. Why is adipose tissue important in the human body?
3. List the types of adipose tissue.
4. What are the main functions of adipose tissue?
5. How does adipose tissue develop?

Answers to Critical Thinking Questions

1. (b); 2. (b) ; 3. (c); 4. (c); 5. (b)

REFERENCES

1. Cuevas-Ramos, D., Mehta, R., & Aguilar-Salinas, C. A. (2019). Fibroblast Growth Factor 21 and Browning of White Adipose Tissue. Frontiers in physiology, 10, 37. https://doi.org/10.3389/fphys.2019.00037 (accessed on 7th August 2025).
2. van der Kolk, B. W., Saari, S., Lovric, A., Arif, M., Alvarez, M., Ko, A., Miao, Z., Sahebekhtiari, N., Muniandy, M., Heinonen, S., Oghabian, A., Jokinen, R., Jukarainen, S., Hakkarainen, A., Lundbom, J., Kuula, J., Groop, P. H., Tukiainen, T., Lundbom, N., Rissanen, A., ... Pietiläinen, K. H. (2021). Molecular pathways behind acquired obesity: Adipose tissue and skeletal muscle multiomics in monozygotic twin pairs discordant for BMI. Cell reports. Medicine, 2(4), 100226. https://doi.org/10.1016/j.xcrm.2021.100226(accessed on 7th August 2025).
3. Annamalai, P., Cesani, F., Chao, T., Chondronikola, et al. (2015). A percutaneous needle biopsy technique for sampling the supraclavicular brown adipose tissue depot of humans. https://core.ac.uk/download/323070870.pdf (accessed on 7th August 2025).
4. Arafat, A. M., Isken, F., Loeffelholz, C. von, et al. (2010). Circulating vaspin is unrelated to insulin sensitivity in a cohort of nondiabetic humans. https://core.ac.uk/download/46325.pdf (accessed on 7th August 2025).
5. Arble, D. M., Bass, J., Behn, C. D., Butler, et al. (2015). Impact of sleep and circadian disruption on energy balance and diabetes: A summary of workshop discussions. https://core.ac.uk/download/213087763.pdf (accessed on 7th August 2025).
6. Argano, V., Balistreri, C. R., Giarratana, R. M., Lio, et al. (2019). On the road to accurate biomarkers for cardiometabolic diseases by integrating precision and gender medicine approaches. https://core.ac.uk/download/268910274.pdf (accessed on 7th August 2025).
7. Salehian, B., Forman, S. J., Kandeel, F. R., Bruner, D. E., He, J., & Atkinson, R. L. (2010). Adenovirus 36 DNA in adipose tissue of patient with unusual visceral obesity. Emerging infectious diseases, 16(5), 850–852. https://doi.org/10.3201/eid1605.091271(accessed on 7th August 2025).
8. Avitabile, D., De Falco, E., Gambini, E., Spaltro, et al. (2016). Physiological conditions influencing regenerative potential of stem cells. https://core.ac.uk/download/54531370.pdf (accessed on 7th August 2025).
9. Baker, A. H., Caslake, M., Collier, A., Donnelly, et al. (2016). miR-34a-/- mice are susceptible to diet-induced obesity. https://core.ac.uk/download/42371340.pdf (accessed on 7th August 2025).
10. Suchacki, K. J., Tavares, A. A. S., Mattiucci, D., Scheller, E. L., Papanastasiou, G., Gray, C., Sinton, M. C., Ramage, L. E., McDougald, W. A., Lovdel, A., Sulston, R. J., Thomas, B. J., Nicholson, B. M., Drake, A. J., Alcaide-Corral, C. J., Said, D., Poloni, A., Cinti, S., Macpherson, G. J., Dweck, M. R., ... Cawthorn, W. P. (2020). Bone marrow adipose tissue is a unique adipose subtype with distinct roles in glucose homeostasis. Nature communications, 11(1), 3097. https://doi.org/10.1038/s41467-020-16878-2(accessed on 7th August 2025).
11. Bennett, K. A., Debier, C., Eppe, G., Hall, et al. (2018). Persistent organic pollutant burden, experimental POP exposure and tissue properties affect metabolic profiles of blubber from grey seal pups. https://core.ac.uk/download/237029622.pdf (accessed on 7th August 2025).
12. Bianco, A., Castaldo, C., D'Alicandro, G., Di Meglio, et al. (2018). Effects of physical exercise on

adiponectin, leptin, and inflammatory markers in childhood obesity: Systematic review and meta-analysis. https://core.ac.uk/download/188826572.pdf (accessed on 7th August 2025).

13. Blázquez-Medela, A. M., Boström, K. I., Fogelman, A. M., Guo, et al. (2019). Noggin Depletion in Adipocytes Promotes Obesity in Mice. https://core.ac.uk/download/323080402.pdf (accessed on 7th August 2025).

14. Gnocchi, D., & Bruscalupi, G. (2017). Circadian Rhythms and Hormonal Homeostasis: Pathophysiological Implications. Biology, 6(1), 10. https://doi.org/10.3390/biology6010010(accessed on 7th August 2025).

15. Carter, C. S., Justice, J. N., & Thompson, L. (2019). Lipotoxicity, Aging, and Muscle Contractility: Does Fiber Type Matter? https://open.bu.edu/bitstream/2144/40625/7/carter_justice_thompson_Lipotoxicity_paper_04302019.pdf (accessed on 7th August 2025).

16. Wang, Y., Paulo, E., Wu, D., Wu, Y., Huang, W., Chawla, A., & Wang, B. (2017). Adipocyte Liver Kinase b1 Suppresses Beige Adipocyte Renaissance Through Class IIa Histone Deacetylase 4. Diabetes, 66(12), 2952–2963. https://doi.org/10.2337/db17-0296(accessed on 7th August 2025).

17. Chen, L., Delville, C., Derous, D., Douglas, et al. (2015). The effects of graded levels of calorie restriction: II. Impact of short term calorie and protein restriction on circulating hormone levels, glucose homeostasis and oxidative stress in male C57BL/6 mice. https://core.ac.uk/download/30435896.pdf (accessed on 7th August 2025).

18. Costa, R. M., Lobato, N. S., Neves, K. B., Tostes, et al. (2018). Perivascular adipose tissue as a relevant fat depot for cardiovascular risk in obesity. https://core.ac.uk/download/153572426.pdf (accessed on 7th August 2025).

19. McAllan L, Cotter PD, Roche HM, Korpela R, Nilaweera KN (2012) Bioactivity in Whey Proteins Influencing Energy Balance. J Metabolic Synd 1:107. doi:10.4172/2167-0943.1000107 (accessed on 7th August 2025).

20. Czech, M. P., Danai, L. V., Guilherme, A., Henchey, et al. (2017). Adipocyte lipid synthesis coupled to neuronal control of thermogenic programming. https://core.ac.uk/download/84911330.pdf (accessed on 7th August 2025).

21. Tajima, K., Ikeda, K., Tanabe, Y. et al. Wireless optogenetics protects against obesity via stimulation of non-canonical fat thermogenesis. Nat Commun 11, 1730 (2020). https://doi.org/10.1038/s41467-020-15589-y(accessed on 7th August 2025).

22. Gonzalez-Periz, A., Neuhofer, A., Pirraco, A., Vidal-Puig, A., Dobrian, A. D., Oliveira, A. G., Hevener, A. L., et al. (2014). Prostaglandin profiling reveals a role for hematopoietic prostaglandin D synthase in adipose tissue macrophage polarization in mice and humans. https://core.ac.uk/download/77407781.pdf (accessed on 7th August 2025).

23. Hanna Kaciuba-Uscilko and John E. Greenleaf(1989). Acclimatization to Cold in Humans. NASA Technical Memorandum 101 01 2 https://core.ac.uk/download/pdf/42828156.pdf (accessed on 7th August 2025).

24. Imai, Si., Guarente, L. It takes two to tango: NAD^+ and sirtuins in aging/longevity control. npj Aging Mech Dis 2, 16017 (2016). https://doi.org/10.1038/npjamd.2016.17 (accessed on 7th August 2025).

25. Santosa S, Jensen MD (2012) Effects of Male Hypogonadism on Regional Adipose Tissue Fatty Acid Storage and Lipogenic Proteins. PLoS ONE 7(2): e31473. https://doi.org/10.1371/journal.pone.0031473 (accessed on 7th August 2025).
26. Harris, C. A., Lee, R. A., & Wang, J. C. (2018). Glucocorticoid Receptor and Adipocyte Biology. https://core.ac.uk/download/323081126.pdf (accessed on 7th August 2025).
27. Jenkins, S. W. III. (2022). The role of perivascular adipose tissue and infiltrating macrophages in vascular dysfunction with inflammatory bowel disease. https://mospace.umsystem.edu/xmlui/handle/10355/95153 (accessed on 7th August 2025).
28. Ma, X., & Kang, S. (2019). Functional Implications of DNA Methylation in Adipose Biology. Diabetes, 68(5), 871–878. https://doi.org/10.2337/dbi18-0057(accessed on 7th August 2025).
29. Klein, S., Liu, J., Lu, W., Shi, et al. (2019). Peroxisomal Regulation of Redox Homeostasis and Adipocyte Metabolism. https://core.ac.uk/download/231816688.pdf (accessed on 7th August 2025).
30. McQueen, A. E., Koliwad, S. K., & Wang, J. C. (2018). Fighting obesity by targeting factors regulating beige adipocytes. Current opinion in clinical nutrition and metabolic care, 21(6), 437–443. https://doi.org/10.1097/MCO.0000000000000509(accessed on 7th August 2025).
31. Kyrou, I., Randeva, H. S., Tsigos, C., Kaltsas, G., & Weickert, M. O. (2018). Clinical Problems Caused by Obesity. In K. R. Feingold (Eds.) et. al., Endotext. MDText.com, Inc.(accessed on 7th August 2025).
32. Lawson, H. A., & Miranda, M. A. (2018). Ironing out the details: Untangling dietary iron and genetic background in diabetes. https://core.ac.uk/download/212866727.pdf (accessed on 7th August 2025).
33. McMinn, M. R. (1984). Mechanisms of Energy Balance in Obesity. https://digitalcommons.georgefox.edu/cgi/viewcontent.cgi?article=1276&context=gscp_fac (accessed on 7th August 2025).

CARTILAGE

7

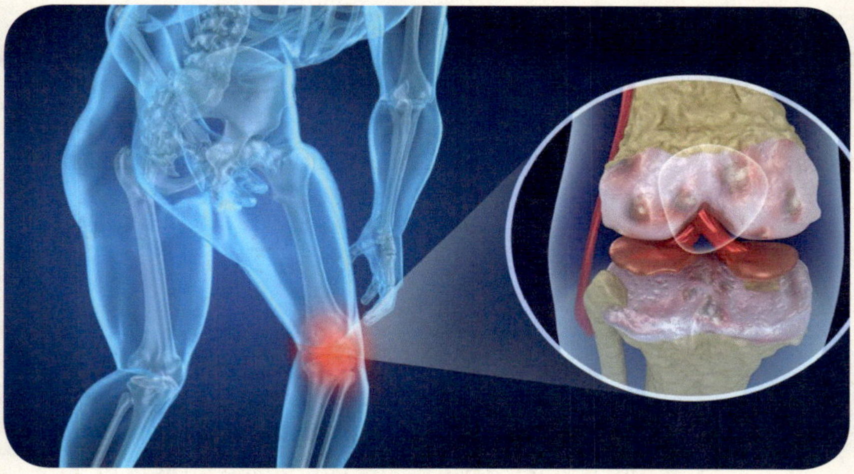

LEARNING OBJECTIVES

After studying this chapter, you will be able to:

1. Describe the types of cartilage;
2. Describe the structure and functions of cartilage;
3. Learn about cartilage in health;
4. Explain the cartilage disorders.

Introduction

The significance of cartilage in human physiology and anatomy cannot be overstated, as it is a fundamental connective tissue necessary for joint function, structural support, and growth. Cartilage is primarily composed of a dense extracellular matrix, which contains various types of collagen and proteoglycans, thus making the tissue elastic and resistant. This unique architecture allows cartilage to support compressive stress, particularly in weight-bearing joints like the knees and hips. Interestingly, articulation of bones is also a function of cartilage, thereby providing smooth motion and reducing friction in locomotion. Understanding of the intricacy of cartilage structure and function is vital in its handling of the many pathologies of its degeneration, e.g., osteoarthritis and other degenerative arthropathies, that significantly impact the quality of life for individuals around the world. Aside from its biomechanical functions, cartilage plays a vital role in development processes encountered within the human body. It is a vital element in the embryogenesis of various structures, particularly endochondral bone development, in which cartilage serves as a precursor to the bone tissue. Cartilage interaction and coordination with the surrounding tissues are mediated by molecular signaling cascades as well as mechanical forces, which guide cell behaviors throughout development. For instance, the cranial neural crest mesenchyme plays a critical role in the development of the jaw complex, and its importance is underscored on how malformations in the process of cartilage formation lead to congenital defects and other pathologies. The utility of cartilage goes beyond the mere structural elements since it participates in a wide array of biological functions critical in normal growth and functional adjustment, thus underscoring the necessity for further study.

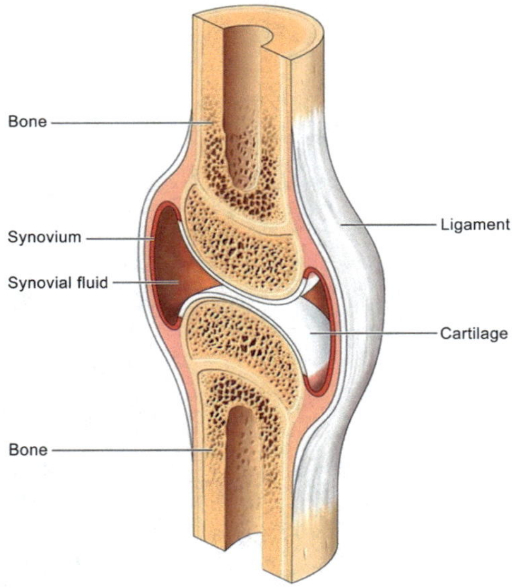

Figure 7.1. Cross-section through a typical synovial joint, showing the bone, synovial membrane, synovial fluid, cartilage and ligament.

Source: https://d2jx2rerrg6sh3.cloudfront.net/image-handler/ts/20170720020555/ri/673/picture/2017/7/shutterstock_280030736.jpg.

The clinical relevance of cartilage science is profound, particularly in terms of the therapeutic alternatives for cartilage pathology. Advances in tissue engineering and regenerative medicine are laying the groundwork for revolutionary treatments that will replace or repair injured cartilage. For instance, early intervention processes, such as condylectomy in unilateral condylar hyperplasia, focus on the application of biological principles in the effective management of disorders with great results in patient's aesthetic and functional parameters (Almeida et al., 2018). Besides, continuous exploration of cellular and molecular mechanisms regulating cartilage biology will enable the development of targeted therapies to rectify present shortcomings and promote tissue repair mechanisms. As the disease and injury of cartilage involve a high percentage of the population, an in-depth understanding of cartilage biology is required to increase therapeutic potential and patient care in musculoskeletal health (Figure 7.1).

Definition of Cartilage

Cartilage is a specialized connective tissue that plays a vital role in the human body. Cartilage is a tough and elastic tissue composed largely of a dense extracellular matrix containing collagen fibers and proteoglycans. Its unique composition allows cartilage to withstand compressive forces, hence providing support and structure to the various parts of the body. The three primary types of cartilage — hyaline, elastic, and fibrocartilage — all function differently; for example, hyaline cartilage forms the joint ends of bones and the tracheal framework, while fibrocartilage, in intervertebral discs, withstands tension and absorbs shock.

The presence of cartilage is essential not only for the adult skeleton but also for enabling movement and friction reduction of joints during life. Growth and maintenance of cartilage are regulated by many biological occurrences and extrinsic factors. An awareness of the histological makeup of cartilage reveals its low vascularization, which influences the diffusion of nutrients and the self-healing capacity of the tissues. Compared to bone, cartilage's healing process is more sluggish due to the absence of a direct blood supply, and this may lead to degenerative ailments and vulnerability to injury. Recent studies have highlighted the intricacy of this connective tissue, showing variation among species and age groups, with the advances in molecular biology further establishing the cellular processes of growth and degeneration of cartilage. For example, research into the composition of the extracellular matrix reveals that aberrations in regulatory proteins can cause cartilage-related disease and strengthens the case for ongoing research into this subject. Clinical relevance of cartilage health extends to other fields, more so in the context of joint disease , such as osteoarthritis.

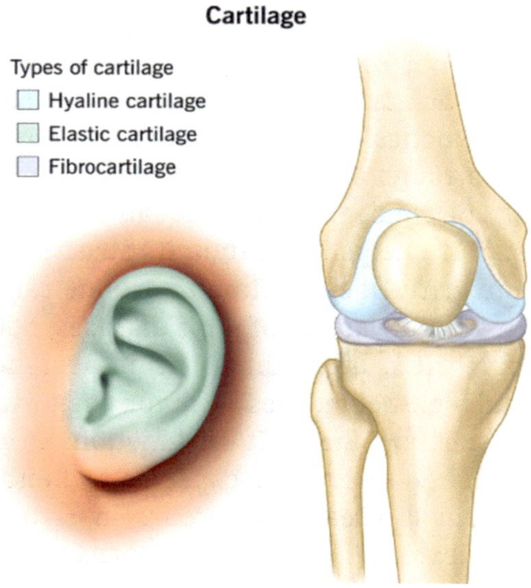

Figure 7.2. The three types of cartilage in your body are hyaline cartilage, elastic cartilage and fibrocartilage.

https://my.clevelandclinic.org/-/scassets/Images/org/health/articles/23173-cartilage-final

As cartilage degenerates through wear and tear with time, it loses its ability to withstand compressive loads, leading to pain and loss of mobility. This degeneration is typically further perpetuated by factors , such as aging, ob(‑‑'y, and repetitive strain. Research into cartilage pathology has advanced the knowledge of mechanisms for conditions like tendinopathy, where the extracellular matrix is disrupted by increased turnover and remodeling. The intricate interaction of cellular and molecular factors responsible for tendon and cartilage health supports an urgent requirement for the development of targeted therapies directed at preventing degeneration and facilitating regeneration. New technology in regenerative medicine can potentially harness the knowledge gained from pathology in cartilage and tendon to create new treatments which would reestablish function and enhance quality of life for those affected (Riley, 2005; Sánchez-Villagra & Forasiepi, 2017) (Figure 7.2).

Importance of Cartilage in the Human Body

Cartilage has multiple significant roles within the human body, which encompass mobility and general skeletal health. Composed of specialized connective tissue, cartilage forms a smooth, resilient surface for the articulation of joints, allowing bones to glide over one another easily with minimal friction when in motion. This dampening effect, necessary in weight-bearing joints , such as the hips and knees, shields against degeneration and potential joint disease, including osteoarthritis.

0In addition, cartilage supports the structure of areas of the body more distal to joints, including the nose, ears, and rib cage, proving useful beyond joints. Cartilage's composition, primarily collagen and proteoglycans, provides it with resistance to compression and support for bearing load without compromising its structure, proving useful in maintaining physiological stability as well as mobility. Further, cartilage's regenerative capacity is the focus of research on substantial bulk. In contrast to the rest of the body tissues, cartilage has limited self-healing ability as it is avascular and metabolically inactive. Such an absence of a mechanism makes it a dismal task to heal cartilage injuries, particularly in athletes who are repeatedly subjected to such damage. The present studies to find ways of healing cartilage have led to innovative approaches, such as designing hybrid biomaterials that mimic the extracellular matrix and facilitate cell growth and repair. By integrating artificial and biological components, researchers aim to produce scaffolds capable of maintaining tissue regeneration with an adaptive response to the unique properties of cartilage (Abalymov et al., 2020).

The quest for useful treatments underscores the essential importance of cartilage not only in joint health but in regenerative medicine in general. Furthermore, knowledge of the molecular mechanisms involved in cartilage degeneration is also crucial to the establishment of preventive strategies and useful therapies. Modern research is starting to bring about the understanding of pathogenesis of diseases , such as tendinopathy, where the healthy function of connective tissues like cartilage is impaired.

Tendon lesions have also been observed to mirror the pathologies present in cartilage disease, which speaks to the interdependency of these tissues and to the overall implications of musculoskeletal health (Riley, 2004). Through such exploration of these interactions and the physiology of cartilage integrity, medical professionals can more effectively treat degenerative diseases and create comprehensive treatment protocols. Finally, realizing the multi-functionality importance of cartilage, the need for continued research and development in this area is unquestionable, towards further therapeutic treatments and better results in patients.

7.1. Types of Cartilage

Learning Outcome

1. Describe the hyaline cartilage;
2. Understand the elastic cartilage;
3. Know about fibrocartilage.

Types of cartilage are crucial in the human body and primarily fall under three heads: hyaline, elastic, and fibrocartilage, differing in structure and function. Hyaline cartilage, the most prevalent type, is characterized by its glassy, polished appearance and is of vital importance to the development of fetal skeletons. It can be found in areas , such as the articular surfaces of joints, costal cartilages uniting ribs to the sternum, and in the trachea and bronchi (Mironova et al., 1996). This cartilage not only acts as a cushion to joints but also facilitates the free movement between adjacent bones. The presence of chondrocytes within a tough extracellular matrix comprised mainly of collagen and proteoglycans that do not rupture helps it to retain its structural role and integrity. Degeneration of hyaline cartilage may lead to a variety of joint diseases, such as osteoarthritis, highlighting its importance in skeletal well-being. Less common than hyaline, elastic cartilage has critical functions in areas of the body where the capacity to bend and hold form is greater. It occurs in structures like the external ear and epiglottis, where it must withstand bending or flexing without deformation. Composed of a dense matrix of elastic fibers loosely scattered with collagen, elastic cartilage yields the elasticity needed by these regions (Nakayama et al., 2016). Because of its unique structure, it can recover from deformation to its original form, and thus it is needed for the functioning of elastic tissues. Its ability to sustain a form in place, even though it involves dynamic motions, emphasizes the importance of elastic cartilage anatomically and physiologically. Furthermore, understanding the organization and function of elastic cartilage contributes to general knowledge of cartilage function in human growth and health. Fibrocartilage, whose collagen fibers are highly concentrated, occupies a vital space in the human body where resistance to tension and support are essential. It is found in intervertebral discs, the pubic symphysis, and knee menisci as a cushion for shock absorption and load distribution between joints (Nakayama et al., 2016). Due to the structural properties of fibrocartilage, it can sustain high levels of stress and strain, and therefore, it is essential in maintaining joint stability and musculoskeletal health. As opposed to elastic and hyaline cartilage, fibrocartilage lacks a perichondrium and therefore has limited regenerative capacity once injured. Consequently, fibrocartilage injury can significantly compromise mobility and chronic pain if left untreated. An understanding of these types of cartilage and their specific functions will enhance our management approach to cartilage injury and disease, allowing improved patient outcomes (Figure 7.3).

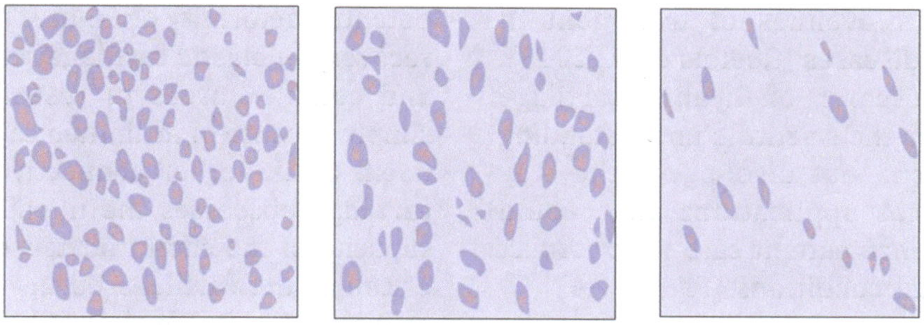

Figure 7.3. Three different types of cartilage: elastic (A), hyaline (B), and fibrous (C).

Source: https://biologynotesonline.com/wp-content/uploads/2023/06/Cartilage_types.jpg.

7.1.1. Hyaline Cartilage

Hyaline cartilage is an important structure in human anatomy and physiology and serves as a body structural component. It is a type of specialized connective tissue that has a glassy color and consists of Type II collagen fibers, which provide it with strength and elasticity. It is found in most places, like the joint articular surfaces of joints, the costal cartilages of ribs, and the nose. Hyaline cartilage is a smooth gliding surface for skeletal movement and development. Its highly extracellular matrix consisting of proteoglycans and hyaluronic acid enables it to ably absorb compressive loads. Hyaline cartilage is essential to joint function and structure, so essential to effective locomotion in man. Regenerative medicine seeks to repair the loss and degeneration of hyaline cartilage, notably osteoarthritis and trauma. Failure of internal healing processes in avascular cartilage tissue necessitates an intervention in many cases to initiate repair. Recent development in orthobiologics, including the use of platelet-rich plasma (PRP) and bone marrow aspirate concentrate (BMAC), has been reported to possess promise for enhancing the regenerative capacity of hyaline cartilage. These medications can be combined with biomaterials like organic scaffolds or synthetic polymers to create hybrid systems supporting cartilage repair processes. Experiments have indicated that such combinatorial strategies were able to induce cellular function and enhance outcome in preclinical as well as clinical contexts, thereby emphasizing the potential for innovation in the treatment of cartilage injury (Yamaguchi et al., 2019). Investigation into hyaline cartilage is not only focused on examining regenerative strategies but also examines the inherent biological processes that control its function and longevity. Research has identified the critical role played by some of the signaling pathways and the influence of mechanical loading on cartilage homeostasis. Comprehension of these pathways is significant since they underpin therapeutic measures with the ability to reduce the severity of cartilage degradation. Also, widespread support of this field has been complemented by organizations , such as Arthritis Research UK that fund, on a fundamental level, research aimed at the discovery of new avenues of treatment in cartilage-related diseases (Roelofs et al., 2013). Thus, ongoing research on hyaline cartilage not only enhances the scientific understanding of this vital tissue but also paves the way for future clinical applications that could significantly enhance patient care with respect to musculoskeletal conditions (Figure 7.4).

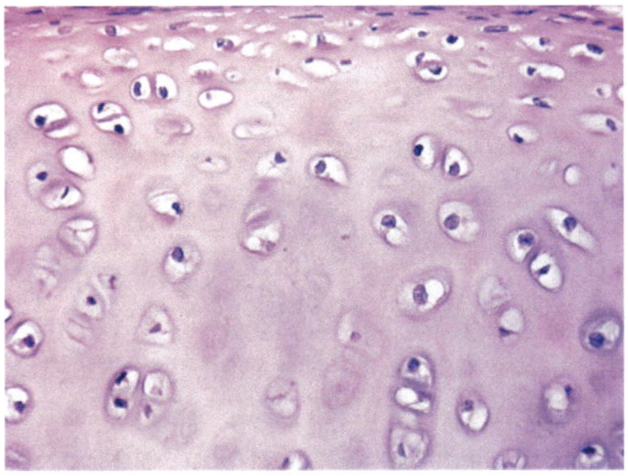

Figure 7.4. Hyaline cartilage.

Source: https://medcell.org/histology/connective_tissue_lab/images/hyaline_cartilage.jpg.

7.1.2. Elastic Cartilage

Elastic cartilage, due to its elasticity and flexibility, is a significant characteristic of many anatomical locations in the human body. This cartilage is specialized mainly for areas that require strength along with flexibility, such as the outer ear (auricle), the epiglottis, and parts of the larynx. The structure of elastic cartilage, which is different from others, has a high content of elastic fibers arranged in a loose network held by collagen fibers, allowing them to be bent repeatedly without changes in form. That elasticity is crucial to the functions these structures perform, emphasizing the function of elastic cartilage within the overall functioning of the human musculoskeletal system. Its elasticity serves not only to provide structural support but also to safeguard underlying tissues, emphasizing the importance of healthy cartilage to prevent potential deformity or failure. The regrowth and recovery of elastic cartilage remain challenging and complex areas of research in medicine simply because of its limited capacity for healing itself. Unlike other connective tissues, elastic cartilage possesses the impaired regenerative capacity of the chondrocytes, the primary type of cell of the cartilage tissue, owing to its low cellularity and limited ability to proliferate. Recent cartilage pathology also highlights the molecular mechanism of degeneration, which is generally most frequently associated with increased turnover of the extracellular matrix, even in elastic cartilage. Studies indicate that degradation of the cartilage matrix can lead to conditions like osteoarthritis, which has a direct impact on mobility as well as the quality of life. With a better understanding of these degenerative processes, therapeutic agents attacking the retardation of cartilage disease are feasible. Emerging technologies are being devised to reverse the defect of repair of elastic cartilage, with the integration of bioengineering approaches. Advances through 3D-printing technologies have proved successful in recent studies to reconstruct elastic cartilage morphology, particularly in areas like the auricle where considerations of both form and function are critical. With the aid of a porous, empty mold and autologous diced cartilage and platelet-rich plasma, researchers have developed scaffolds with chondrocyte survival support and stimulation of synthesis of essential extracellular matrix components. The study shows immense potential in cartilage reconstruction, with an apparent path to promoting surgical results in patients requiring elastic cartilage reconstruction. As the topic continues to progress, knowledge of how mechanical properties relate to biological integration will be critical to maximizing the efficacy of such regenerative strategies and ensuring enhanced patient outcomes for cartilage-specific pathologies (Riley, 2005; Chen et al., 2019) (Figure 7.5).

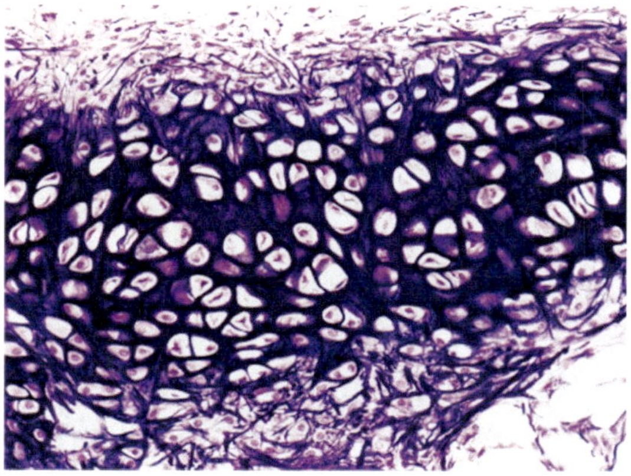

Figure 7.5. Elastic cartilage.

Source: https://medcell.org/histology/connective_tissue_lab/images/elastic_cartilage.jpg.

7.1.3. Fibrocartilage

Fibrocartilage is an essential element in the function and structure of various joints of the human body, performing as a key feature that enables enhanced load-bearing ability of cartilage. Fibrocartilage is distinct from hyaline cartilage in having a dense matrix in the form of packed collagen fibers, which provides it with increased tensile strength and shear resistance. This particular type of cartilage is found mainly in areas that are subjected to great mechanical stress, such as the intervertebral disks, knee menisci, and the pubic symphysis. Fibrocartilage composition lends it tolerance of compressive and tensile stress, and it plays a critical role in joint stability and overall musculoskeletal well-being. Knowledge of the biomechanical properties of fibrocartilage is critical in the resolution of several orthopedic problems and cartilage diseases, hence the significance of the tissue in human anatomy and physiology. Fibrocartilage's ability to regenerate is a significant area to study, particularly concerning injury and degenerative conditions. Fibrocartilage possesses poor inherent healing capacity relative to other types of cartilage, hence challenging the recovery of its function if it is injured. The latest studies examine the use of orthobiologic therapies, such as platelet-rich plasma (PRP) and bone marrow aspirate concentrate (BMAC), to enhance the healing mechanisms of fibrocartilage. Biomaterials serve as delivery mediums for such therapies, promoting the release of regenerative factors to the target areas and the restoration of the musculoskeletal system.

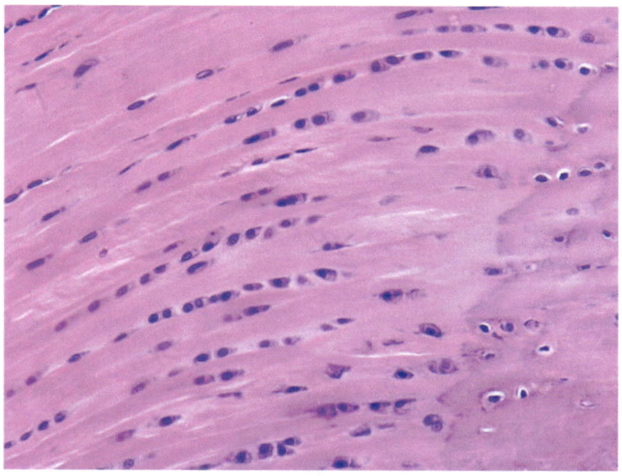

Figure 7.6. Fibrocartilage.

Source: https://medcell.org/histology/connective_tissue_lab/images/fibrocartilage.jpg.

The integration of these innovative therapeutic strategies is becoming a turning point in clinical research aimed at assisting in the rehabilitation of fibrocartilage, ultimately hoping to alleviate the symptoms of cartilage degeneration and the function of joints. With ongoing exploration, the potential for new therapies for fibrocartilage damage only expands, a future in regenerative medicine looking bright (Yamaguchi et al., 2019). Fibrocartilage is also found to have a significant relationship with hormonal signaling and fibrocartilage, and implications for health and disease. For instance, alterations in estrogen levels have been implicated in the disease pathology of temporomandibular joint disease (TMD), depicting the impact of hormonal alterations on cartilage integrity during different stages of life. Women, especially, have a higher occurrence of oral diseases like periodontal diseases associated with TMD, which may be reflected by the fluctuating levels of estrogen throughout their lives. An understanding of the estrogen signaling pathway may yield clues to mechanisms that control fibrocartilage homeostasis and reactions to exogenous stressors like pregnancy and menopause. These discoveries can pave the way to the development of novel drug therapies that act to preserve the integrity of fibrocartilage, demonstrating the intersection of hormonal regulation and cartilage integrity in the grand tapestry of human biology (Chen et al., 2020) (Figure 7.6).

Test Your Knowledge

1. What is hyaline cartilage?
2. What is elastic cartilage?

7.2. Structure of Cartilage

Learning Outcome

1. Describe the composition of cartilage;
2. Describe the types of cells in cartilage;
3. Learn about the extracellular matrix and its components.

The structure of cartilage plays an important role in its functioning in the human body, and therefore, a detailed research of its various constituents is important. Cartilage is made up of a strong mesh of collagen fibers and gel matrix, and it provides flexibility along with hardness. The matrix includes predominantly proteoglycans, enormous molecules that trap water, creating a strong cushioning system. This particular structure allows cartilage to withstand compressive stresses and facilitate smooth joint movement. Cartilage is avascular, i.e., it lacks blood vessels, and thus relies on diffusion for nutrient delivery and waste removal. This characteristic contributes to its low regenerative capability, and thus, its appreciation is very important in regenerative medicine and cartilage injury repair. Different types of cartilage—hyaline, elastic, and fibrocartilage—share specialized structural features suited to their specific functions. Hyaline cartilage, the most widespread type in human joints and ribcage, has a smooth, glassy appearance, minimizing friction against movement. Its matrix is high in type II collagen concentrations, which facilitates tensile strength while allowing it to possess an appropriate amount of elasticity. Conversely, elastic cartilage, found in such structures as the ear, has a higher density of elastic fibers and is therefore better suited to holding its shape and reverting to its original shape when deformed. Fibrocartilage, which is found in intervertebral discs and menisci of joints, contains a dense matrix of collagen fibers that contributes additional strength and resistance to shear forces. Such heterogeneity of cartilage structure is a testament to its evolution with the varied mechanical requirements in different anatomical locations. The synergy between cartilage structure and function is also a testament to the fact that pathological conditions resulting from its breakdown are evidence of the same. Osteochondromas, for instance, are benign bone tumors that are formed on cartilage, which remind us of the rudimentary requirement of cartilage in developing and repairing the skeleton (Flohr et al., 2017). Research also reveals the impact of pharmacologic treatments on cartilage health, particularly osteoarthritis. Experiments have suggested that drugs , such as alendronate may play protective functions in cartilage by mitigating subchondral bone changes and degeneration in response to joint injury, but long-term efficacy remains unclear (Khorasani et al., 2015). This interaction of structure and health also emphasizes the importance of ongoing research into cartilages complex biology, particularly as it may influence therapeutic approaches to joint disease and move us closer to an understanding of cartilage's role in human health (Figure 7.7).

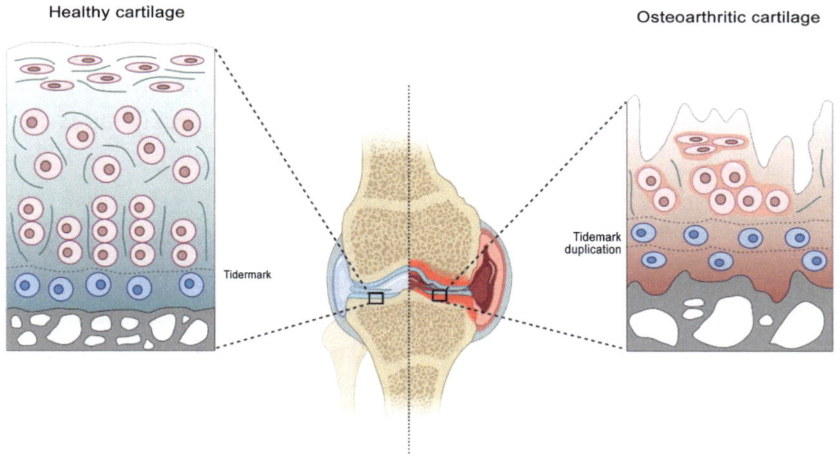

Figure 7.7. Cartilage structure in normal (left) and OA (right) tissues.

Source: https://www.mdpi.com/processes/processes-11-01014/article_deploy/html/images/processes-11-01014-g002.png.

7.2.1. Composition of Cartilage

The cartilage structure is a significant parameter that lends support to its mechanical and biological functions in the organism. Cartilage is primarily composed of a dense extracellular matrix, which comprises water, proteoglycans, and collagen fibers in large proportions. Collagen, particularly type II collagen, lends tensile strength and structural rigidity, and cartilage withstands compression as well as shear stresses. The proteoglycans, such as aggrecan, play a vital role in retaining water within the matrix, which is key in providing cushioning and resilience. The interactive dynamics between these molecules create a unique composite material that allows cartilage to support its function in joints and elsewhere. With respect to depth in cartilage, the arrangement and proportion of these components can be extremely variable, depending on the complexity of architecture to fulfill its multi-directional mechanical demands. Composition of cartilage in depth exhibits a high degree of variability, which has important implications for its functional properties. In the superficial zone, collagen fibrils align parallel to the surface and provide the initial resistance to extrinsic loads, while proteoglycan densities are maximal to react to compressive loads. Moving towards the cartilage interior, collagen orientation becomes increasingly randomized, which increases the compressional tolerance of the tissue. In particular, studies using advanced imaging techniques have measured such variations and reported variations of activation energy for relaxation processes in cartilage with depth, having decreased activation energies in shallower depths, indicating a varying molecular environment (Binks et al., 2017). This depth gradient affects not just the mechanical properties but also affects cartilage's response to damage or degeneration with increasing time. Furthermore, research shows how the composition of cartilage can differ significantly under pathological conditions , such as osteoarthritis (OA).

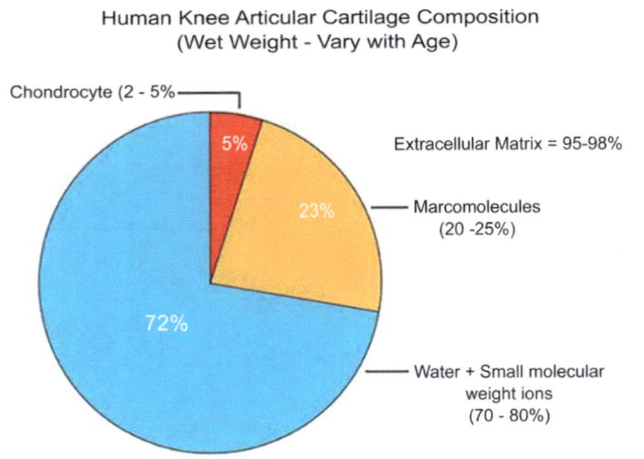

Figure 7.8. The composition of wet weight in the knee joint cartilage of the human adult reveals that chondrocytes constitute a mere 2%–5% of the total weight, while the bulk of 95%–98% is composed of the extracellular matrix. This matrix is largely comprised of tissue fluid and low molecular weight ions. It is worth noting that the wet weight of the macromolecules in knee articular cartilage differs based on both age and the specific anatomical location.

Source: https://cdnintech.com/media/chapter/1165716/1730917164-367556923/media/F2.png.

During the initial stages of OA, the collagen fiber orientation and the distribution of proteoglycans within cartilage's superficial zone are greatly disrupted, disturbing its normal structural pattern (Saarakkala et al., 2010). As degeneration progresses, loss of collagen content becomes more severe, particularly in later stages, compromising the mechanical strength and raising the risk for tissue failure when loaded. These findings underscore the importance of understanding what constitutes cartilage, both with regard to developing therapeutic interventions to reverse degenerative diseases as well as in furthering regenerative approaches. By knowing the biochemical and structural differences that exist in cartilage, scientists are in a better position to predict how the changes will influence tissue function and integrity at different ages in life (Figure 7.8).

7.2.2. Types of Cells in Cartilage

In the intricate structure of cartilage, there are a number of cell types that are responsible for its function and maintenance of integrity. The primary cells involved in cartilage synthesis and maintenance are chondrocytes, which reside in the extracellular matrix (ECM). Chondrocytes are derived from precursor mesenchymal stem cells and possess the special ability to produce collagen and proteoglycans required in cartilage composition. The action of chondrocytes is not only central to initial cartilage development but also in the ongoing repair and maintenance processes.

Also, information concerning the life cycle and functional properties of the chondrocytes is mandatory as it determines treatment modalities for degenerative joint diseases, e.g., osteoarthritis, in which these cell functions become dysfunctional and can lead to significant morbidity in such affected individuals. Besides chondrocytes, cartilage also possesses other special cells, i.e., chondroblasts and chondroclasts, each playing a specific function in cartilage homeostasis. Immature chondrocytes, called chondroblasts, are the ones that synthesize the components of the

ECM before undergoing full differentiation into mature chondrocytes. Chondroblasts are most active during early development and growth of cartilage. Chondroclasts, however, have a role in the resorption of cartilage tissue, controlling turnover of the ECM, thus contributing to the dynamic balance between cartilage breakdown and synthesis.

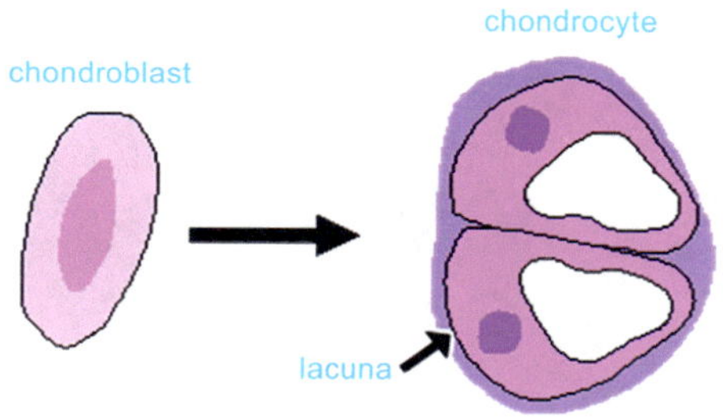

Figure 7.9. Types of cells in cartilage.

Source: https://www.histology.leeds.ac.uk/bone/assets/chondrocyte.gif.

This balance is critical in maintaining healthy joint function, as alterations can lead to such conditions as osteoarthritis, wherein increased degradation with a dearth of repair further enhances cartilage loss. Knowing cellular makeup within the cartilage also has interests in applied fields of tissue engineering and regenerative medicine. Recent advances in biomaterials have used knowledge from cartilage cell biology to develop hybrid constructs that mimic native tissue behavior. Single-phase polymer-based biomaterials tend to target soft tissues, but including inorganic content allows for the replication of the mechanical strength or biochemical properties of harder tissues and hence greater integration and function in tissue reconstruction. These innovations hold a promising future in repairing cartilage injury and degenerative states through the utilization of engineered constructs with specific cell types in consideration, ultimately aiming to restore the natural health and function of cartilage within human joints (Riley, 2004; Abalymov et al., 2020) (Figure 7.9).

7.2.3. Extracellular Matrix (ECM) and Its Components

The ECM is a crucial component of cartilage, providing mechanical strength and biochemical support that the tissue needs for function. Comprised primarily of proteoglycans, collagen fibers, and non-collagenous proteins, the ECM regulates many cellular events, including cell proliferation, differentiation, and migration. Glycosaminoglycans (GAGs), extremely hydrophilic proteoglycan components, provide cartilage viscoelasticity that enables resistance to compressive stresses. Type II collagen, the most prevalent subtype of collagen present in cartilage, is the key to maintaining the tensile character and structural scaffold of the ECM. Cartilage homeostasis needs a dynamic balance between ECM synthesis and degradation, and derangements in this equilibrium may result in pathologies , such as osteoarthritis, in which loss of ECM components is a defining characteristic (Cucchiarini et al., 2007). The role of ECM elements in OA highlights their importance in cartilage health. Osteoarthritis is defined by extensive loss of synthesis of major ECM elements, like type II collagen and proteoglycans, resulting in cartilage failure and dysfunction. Experiments demonstrate that gene therapy approaches, such as rAAV-mediated SOX9 overexpression, can replenish the synthesis of these important elements, allowing cartilage repair and regeneration. These therapies target the ECM directly to strengthen its structure and function, demonstrating the therapeutic potential of adjusting ECM composition in degenerative joint diseases. Widespread use of these methods will revolutionize current treatment modalities for osteoarthritis, highlighting the need for further research into the mechanisms of ECM integrity maintenance and repair (Cucchiarini et al., 2007). Current advances in regenerative medicine have also emphasized the role of ECM components in attempting to rebuild cartilage. For example, the use of three-dimensional (3D) printing technology enables the creation of hollow, porous structures that can be implanted with cartilage grafts to regenerate tissue. In such strategies, autologous diced cartilage with platelet-rich plasma creates a conducive environment for chondrocyte proliferation and survival in a 3D matrix with the highest retrieval of cartilage-specific ECM components like collagen II and GAGs. This innovative method not only enhances the biomechanical integrity of the newly formed tissue but also underscores the important role played by the ECM in the support of cellular activities essential for successful cartilage engineering. As research goes on to advances, understanding of ECM dynamics will inform the development of increasingly efficacious treatments for cartilage regeneration and repair (Figure 7.10).

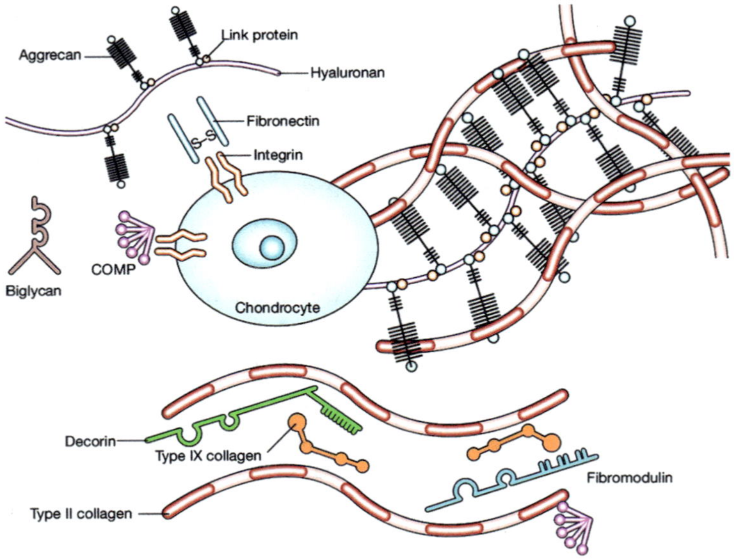

Figure 7.10. Extracellular matrix of cartilage. Three classes of proteins exist in articular cartilage: collagens (mostly type II collagen); proteoglycans (primarily aggrecan); and other noncollagenous proteins (including link protein, fibronectin, cartilage oligomeric matrix protein) and the smaller proteoglycans (biglycan, decorin and fibromodulin). The interaction between highly negatively charged cartilage proteoglycans and type II collagen fibrils is responsible for the compressive and tensile strength of the tissue, which resists load *in vivo*.

Source: https://www.researchgate.net/profile/Rocky-Tuan-2/publication/6855196/figure/fig1/AS:667198494359558@1536083925181/Extracellular-matrix-of-cartilage-Three-classes-of-proteins-exist-in-articular.png.

Test Your Knowledge

1. List the types of cells in cartilage.
2. What is extracellular matrix and its components?

7.3. Functions of Cartilage

Learning Outcome

1. Describe the support and flexibility;
2. Understand the shock absorption;
3. Describe the role of cartilage in joint movement.

Cartilage fulfills several crucial functions in the human body, most importantly, structural support and accommodating flexible movement. Cartilage is a specialized form of connective tissue produced by chondrocytes in an extracellular matrix that provides it with specific mechanical properties, making it capable of carrying out functions. Such functions are essential in regions , such as joints, where articular cartilage minimizes friction between bones when under motion, cushions impacts and creates a smooth articulation. Moreover, in the respiratory pathway, cartilage maintains open airways to permit free passage of air. Cartilage is of a kind that can be modified under varied conditions of stress and loading, providing stability along with resilience, both significant for locomotion in general and physical function. Apart from its mechanical functions, cartilage also plays a crucial role in bone development and growth through endochondral ossification. This is particularly evident in the long bone growth plates, where cartilage serves as a template for bone formation. Cartilage is transformed into bone as part of a dynamic process regulated by an orderly progression of biochemical signals, one that is vital to skeletal development. TGFβRI-signaling pathways, as seen from studies using mice, have an immense impact on cartilage function and development. Significantly, the removal of specific receptors in cartilage has been found to induce severe developmental abnormalities that prove how critical cartilage is to normal bone development and skeletal function (Wang et al., 2019). Evidently, cartilage is not only an inactive structural component but also actively contributes to skeletal health and development. Moreover, cartilage is key to regulating a variety of biological processes, including inflammation and tissue repair. While often considered in structural function, cartilage is also involved in the biomechanical response to stress, which may influence cellular activity and contribute to damage repair. Studies in cartilage have shown it to interact with other signaling factors; for instance, TGFβRI has been found to control signaling pathways that, interestingly, show it suppresses BMP signaling, again proving the intricacy of cartilage in physiology (Wang et al., 2019). These interactions underscore their importance as well as serving as support structures; they are essential to the maintenance of homeostasis in joint environments and the integration of stressor reactions. Ultimately, the varied functions of cartilages emphasize their irreplaceable status in human health, influencing not only physical function but also the intricacy of growth and repair mechanisms (Figure 7.11).

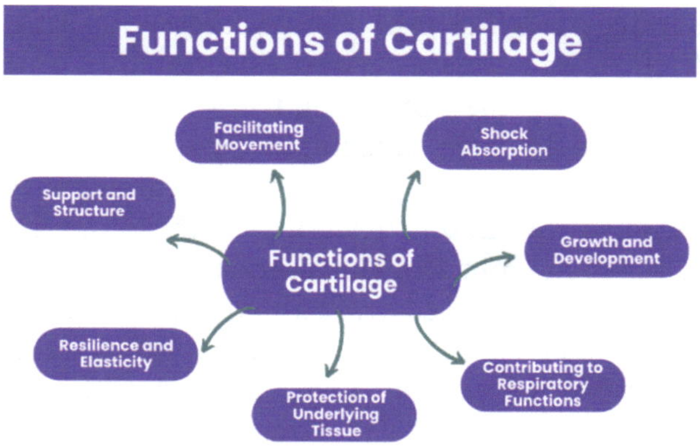

Figure 7.11. Functions of Cartilage.

Source: https://images.examples.com/wp-content/uploads/2024/05/Functions-of-Cartilage-1.png

7.3.1. Support and Flexibility

The unique nature of cartilage, particularly the combination of support and flexibility, is involved in most physiological functions within the human body. Cartilage is a form of connective tissue that provides structural support to various components of the skeletal system, such as joints, ribcage, and the nasal and auricular structures. This structural support arises due to the unique nature of cartilage, comprising collagen fibers and proteoglycans. The architecture of these components gives cartilage resistance to compressive forces but is still flexible enough for smooth movement and absorption of shock when there is exercise. This duality is crucial not just for mobility but also for cushioning the underlying bones from excessive stresses and strains, illustrating how the biochemical architecture of cartilage accommodates its mechanical requirements in load-carrying conditions. In addition to its mechanical support, the flexibility of the cartilage plays a large role in many parts of the body. As an illustration, the most abundant form of hyaline cartilage is the most abundant form, a dense padding in the joints that permits smooth motion while it supports it. Its minimal deformation upon loading enables the articular surfaces to glide over one another with little friction and thus enhances the function and lifespan of the joint. Similarly, the elastic cartilage in such structures as the ear and epiglottis enables not only structural support but also the inbuilt flexibility of these organs to function optimally. This particular adaptation demonstrates the evolutionary advantages of various types of cartilage to specialized functions in various anatomical regions in the human body. The complementarity of support and elasticity of cartilage comes next to the tissue engineering advance that could improve its regenerative ability. Researchers are examining synthetic and hybrid biomaterials that mimic cartilage's inherent characteristics for repairing or replacing damaged tissue efficiently. As highlighted in recent studies, inorganic element-containing polymers can create scaffolds that are well-suited for cartilage tissue growth. These have been targeted as remedies for curing pathological disease, such as osteoarthritis, where cartilage loss causes pain and loss of mobility. By sustaining cell proliferation and extracellular matrix formation in such engineered tissues, scientists are not only targeting repair of cartilage structure but also its mechanical function, hence having the prospect of a cartilage damage-management and healing future where support and flexibility in engineered as well as natural tissues are prioritized (Bronner & LeDouarin, 2012; Abalymov et al., 2020).

7.3.2. Shock Absorption

The ability of cartilage to absorb shock is a critical component that is the foundation of its role in human joints. This ability is largely attributed to the outstanding structure and composition of articular cartilage with an anatomical organization for enduring recurring mechanical stresses associated with body movements. Cartilage contains a gel matrix with collagen fibers, proteoglycans, and water that creates an environment that is effective in disseminating forces across the joint surface. On impact, cartilage's porous structure allows for deformation of its matrix and thus enables energy absorption and minimization of stress passed to underlying bone structures. Not only is this useful in the maintenance of joint integrity, but also in general mobility and performance while moving, which indicates the significance of cartilage in maintaining musculoskeletal health as individuals engage in day-to-day activities and sports. The shock-absorbing mechanism of cartilage is also enhanced by the synovial fluid, which plays a crucial role in lubricating the joint surfaces while providing additional cushioning. The fluid is secreted from the synovial membrane and fills the matrix of the cartilage, creating a hydrodynamic system that facilitates smooth movement, hence reducing friction and wear. Advances in research have begun exploring the synovial fluid motion dynamics within cartilage and examining its influence on load distribution upon joint operation. According to current studies, such as research on the analytical models of joint mechanics, quantitative analysis of interaction between synovial fluid and cartilage can be conducted to assess its performance in shock absorption across various loads (Ruggiero et al., 2011). These results highlight the complex interplay between the cartilage's structural characteristics and the biomechanical factors of joint lubrication in providing maximal shock-absorbing functions. In addition, cartilage degeneration, as observed in diseases like osteoarthritis, can significantly compromise its shock-absorbing function, resulting in worsened joint pain and dysfunction. When cartilage deteriorates, it is unable to maintain maximum hydration and structural integrity, resulting in compromised energy absorption during load-carrying movements. Physical stressors tend to exacerbate this deterioration, thereby demonstrating the double role of biological as well as physical mechanisms towards cartilage function. Therefore, it is not just important to understand shock absorption mechanisms to value the normal functioning of cartilage but also for efficient design of therapeutic intervention that aims to preserve cartilage integrity. Current controversies in veterinary medicine regarding physiotherapeutic techniques for enhancing joint well-being reflect the relevance of such research to human and veterinary medicine, indicating rising interest in developing strategies to offset cartilage degeneration and improve shock absorption capabilities (Samoy et al., 2016).

7.3.3. Role in Joint Movement

The role of cartilage in the movement of a joint is intrinsically linked to the unique structural aspects that it exhibits and is involved in shock absorption as well as friction reduction. Articular cartilage that coats the ends of the bones in synovial joints has a smooth surface that enables gliding effortlessly during activities , such as walking, running, and other physical exercises. This avascular connective tissue relies on synovial fluid for waste and nutrition to maintain its augmented biomechanical function. In particular, the composition of cartilage, consisting of collagen fibers and proteoglycans, allows it to withstand compressive loading and distribute loads during joint motion. Hence, healthy cartilage is needed to provide stable joints and prevent suffering or degeneration, which can build up from repeated motion or trauma, making its role invaluable to efficient and pain-free movement within the musculoskeletal system. Cartilage does not have the sole responsibility of moving joints; it's a question of intricate coordination of tendons and muscles functioning around the joints for mobility.

As illustrated in studies of evolution within Archosauria, limb anatomical changes from quadrupedal to bipedal modes of locomotion have long-reaching consequences on mobility at the joints. For example, evolutionary trends in forelimb functionality and anatomy between various groups highlight how changes in joint mechanics, as governed by muscular attachment patterns and movement, affect mobility strategies. Biomechanical model studies between different species illustrate that the articulation-based range of motion within joints can increase or inhibit movement capability, thus being in accordance with evolutionary adjustments to different environments. Such dependence of cartilage function on muscle structure underscores the need for both factors to engage in harmony in order to achieve effective joint movement.

Further, the cartilage-synovial membrane relationship plays a vital role in joint movement, particularly through the mediation of inflammatory and repair responses. Healthy synovial tissue promotes cartilage well-being through proper lubrication and delivery of nutrients via synovial fluid. In pathological states like rheumatoid arthritis, leucocyte infiltration leads to inflammation, compromising cartilage integrity, demonstrating how disturbance in the synovial membrane can shorten joint function. Tissue-resident macrophages' role in cartilage homeostasis highlights the dynamic relationship between immune responses and cartilage health. Their presence within healthy synovial tissue suggests a state of readiness at all times to defend against future trauma and, therefore, successful joint movement depends not only on cartilage's physical properties but also on the underlying biological processes that regulate tissue homeostasis and repair, once more emphasizing the multi-dynamic nature of joint movement in human function (Figure 7.12).

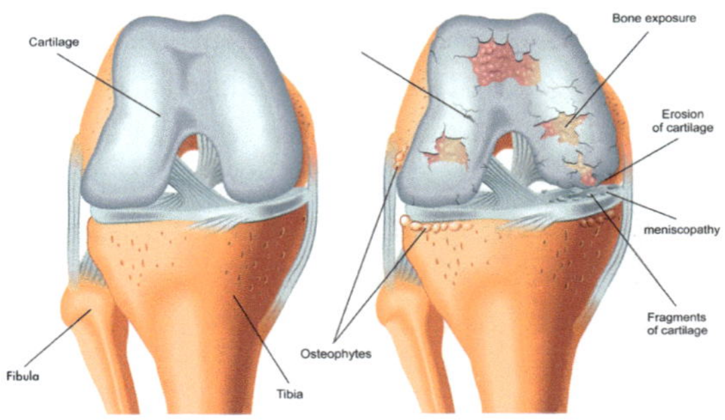

Figure 7.12. Cartilage's role in joint pathologies.

Source: https://cdn.prod.website-files.com/639d6ae0c420837577c9b371/6656204527a5dda4fac5ed64_2-cartilage-role-in-joint-pathologies%20(1).png.

Test Your Knowledge

1. What is meant by shock absorption?
2. What is the role of cartilage in joint movement?

7.4. Cartilage in Health

Learning Outcome

1. Describe the role of cartilage in maintaining joint health;
2. Learn about nutritional factors affecting cartilage;
3. Understand the exercise and its impact on cartilage health.

Cartilage health is significant to provide joint function and total mobility in the human body. Cartilage is a connective tissue with specialized properties, and it serves as a cushion between bones, providing support and elasticity in numerous joints , such as the knees, hips, and elbows. Cartilage is critical for shock absorption in weight-bearing and aids gliding movement, thereby preventing unnecessary wear and tear on the underlying bone. Cartilage structure, made up of water, collagen fibers, and proteoglycans, allows for sustaining heavy mechanical loading with integrity preservation. Proper hydration and nutrition are essential to cartilage maintenance, allowing metabolic activity of chondrocytes, which are responsible for cartilage upkeep. Therefore, an imbalance between these elements leads to cartilage degradation, and thus, requires measures to ensure cartilage integrity throughout the lifespan of humans. Recent findings have put the spotlight on the interaction between vitamin D and cartilage, with emphasis on its protective effect against osteoarthritis (OA). Particularly, 24R,25(OH)2D3 is found to be a bioactive vitamin D analogue suppressing apoptosis of chondrocytes and maintaining cartilage integrity (Boyan et al., 2016). Data suggest that this metabolite of vitamin D could suppress degenerative processes of inflammatory disorders, e.g., IL-1β-induced disorders, by triggering pathways like TGF-β1. With the application of *in vivo* models on animals, it has been established that 24R,25(OH)2D3 treatment significantly reduced cartilage injury of the articular and levels of inflammatory mediators under conditions mimicking OA. Therefore, the role of vitamin D in cartilage is a promising potential towards devising preventive and treatment approaches to promote joint well-being and reduce the incidence of degenerative diseases in advanced age. In exploring pharmacological therapy, bisphosphonates , such as alendronate (ALN) have been recorded to possess chondroprotective properties. Studies on how they function reveal that the use of high doses of ALN can effectively preserve articular cartilage and suppress early trabecular bone loss following knee trauma, demonstrating the beneficial impact during the initial stage of degeneration (Khorasani et al., 2015). However, the long-term success of such measures appears to be constrained by their inability to forestall joint degeneration and osteophyte formation in advanced life. This juxtaposition of short-term benefit with long-term disadvantage serves to underscore the difficulty of controlling cartilage well-being and the need to ensure that treatment plans effectively meet both ephemeral and enduring needs. Continued research into these treatment options is critical to expanding our understanding of cartilage well-being and designing effective methods of combating cartilage diseases in humans.

7.4.1. Role in Maintaining Joint Health

Cartilage's role in the maintenance of joint health cannot be overstated since it is the primary protective covering that protects joints against motion. The elastic, frictionless tissue permits bones to slide against one another, thus making a wide range of motions possible without causing friction or pain. Moreover, cartilage plays a vital role in distributing and absorbing mechanical stresses while walking, running, and lifting. Its function in stress resistance is required to prevent joint damage that can result in diseases , such as osteoarthritis. Cartilage avoids bone contact, thereby preventing the possibility of injury, eventually keeping the overall joint function and lifespan intact. The health of cartilage, therefore, is directly related to maintenance of joint health, a factor that explains why it is crucial to examine factors influencing cartilage integrity, an explanation that shall be elaborated upon in the following sections. In addition to its mechanical functions, cartilage plays an essential role in biochemical signaling in the joint microenvironment. It produces a variety of molecules with responsibility for regulating synovial fluid viscosity and lubrication functions and thereby optimal joint functioning. Besides, cartilage participates in synovial tissue homeostasis, a role that plays a central function in the inflammatory process following joint diseases or injuries. Understanding macrophage function, especially in the synovial tissue, demonstrates how immune cells ensure joint health. According to research, constitutive tissue macrophage presence supports the function of tissue macrophages in synovial homeostasis, and a properly regulated number of macrophages is presumably needed for joint health even during inflammation or injury (Alivernini et al., 2017). So, the intricate relationship between cartilage biomechanics and immunity is important for preserving joint integrity. Furthermore, emerging evidence indicates that therapeutic interventions aimed at protecting cartilage will also enhance joint health. For instance, the application of bisphosphonates , such as alendronate has been discovered to prevent degeneration of joints following injury by sustaining subchondral bone and protecting cartilage from degradation (Khorasani et al., 2015). These findings suggest that pharmacologic interventions have a special function to fulfill in preserving joint health through the repair of the resulting changes in cartilage biochemistry and structure as it ages. Thus, effective joint health preservation regimens will have to consider the biologic characteristics of cartilage as well as the therapeutic potential of medical interventions in making it more durable. In summary, the multifaceted role of cartilage in joint health calls for learning both the physical nature and biological mechanisms involved in its maintenance to counteract degenerative joint disorders.

7.4.2. Nutritional Factors Affecting Cartilage

Nutritional factors play a prominent role in the integrity of cartilage, and they are vital in the maintenance of its function and structure. Vitamins and minerals are essential nutrients that sustain cartilage health by synthesizing collagen and proteoglycans, the building blocks of cartilage. For instance, vitamin C is essential for synthesizing collagen and acts as protection against oxidative stress, which kills cartilage cells. In addition, food intake of omega-3 fatty acids has been shown to inhibit inflammation, a crucial element in the destruction of cartilage typical of conditions , such as osteoarthritis. Consumption of these nutrients in a healthy diet maintains tissue homeostasis and delays the onset of degenerative joint diseases, emphasizing the significant contribution of diet to cartilage health. Further, consumption of certain dietary fats is said to influence cartilage health, although findings from recent studies have yielded controversial data. A study using data from the Osteoarthritis Initiative shows that overall fat intake was not strongly related to hand osteoarthritis prevalence after adjusting for various demographic and lifestyle factors. Instead, the research points out that variables , such as age, gender, and way of life, such as alcohol consumption, appeared more powerful in influencing cartilage quality than dietary fat composition. This implies that while some fats may be beneficial, others may also have the potential to exacerbate cartilage degeneration, thus demonstrating the complexity of dietary influence on articular cartilage and necessitating further studies to fully clarify , such associations (Lacy, 2017). In addition to specific nutrients, the overall dietary pattern is crucial in relation to cartilage health. The high fruit, vegetable, whole grain, and healthy fat intake Mediterranean diet has been associated with decreased joint issues. The eating pattern emphasizes that not only the quality but also the amount of intake contributes to cartilage well-being. The diet-derived nutrients have been shown to exert positive influences on mesenchymal stem cells involved in repairing and regenerating cartilage. The food factor interaction with mesenchymal cell behavior means that nutrition approached in an overall manner can ensure cartilage health and prevent degeneration (Ammendola et al., 2018). As our understanding of such nutritional factors increases, so does the potential for developing specific diet approaches in disease management and prevention of cartilage diseases.

7.4.3. Exercise and Its Impact on Cartilage Health

Adequate physical exercise has a considerable impact on the upkeep and health of cartilage in the human body, an essential component that provides joints with their freedom of movement and general musculoskeletal wellness. Exercise aids in the dissemination of synovial fluid—which feeds and lubricates cartilage—thus enabling nutrient transfer necessary for cellular function and renewal. Since mechanical stress is put on the cartilage when an individual undertakes physical exercise, it stimulates chondrocytes, the primary cells of cartilage, to synthesize significant components of the ECM, including collagen and proteoglycans. Not only does it maintain the integrity of cartilage, but it also renders it resistant to degenerative conditions like osteoarthritis. Consequently, a properly planned exercise regimen may be a preventive force against cartilage degeneration, highlighting the importance of lifelong physical activity among individuals of any age. The type and intensity of exercise dictate its beneficial effect on cartilage status. Both weight-bearing and non-weight-bearing exercises are reported to be helpful, but high-impact exercise has been known to induce elevated tensile forces related to cartilage stiffening. However, the risk of damage from excessive high-impact activity has the potential to result in harm, and a measured response is thus required. Moreover, individual variability in response to exercise due to genetic determinants, health status, and lifestyle habits makes the relationship between physical activity and cartilage health more complex. Factors like dietary intake, levels of stress, and sleep quality also alter the musculoskeletal adaptation to exercise, and therefore, an approach to fitness that is holistic in nature, with exercise supplemented by adequate nourishment and mental health, is crucial. The multi-faceted model is essential for maximizing cartilage health and minimizing joint disorders. As research evolves, understanding personal variability in cartilage responses is essential. For instance, during spaceflight difficulties, considerable differences have been noticed in astronauts' musculoskeletal responses, most probably due to several variables , such as exercise intensity and overall mission conditions. These observations highlight the need for individualized exercise protocols that take into account individual differences in responding to physical activity. Characterizing such individual variation is necessary to advance interventions that can be employed to ensure cartilage health, particularly for at-risk individuals who are most likely to develop joint degeneration. Furthermore, completely eliminating these variances can enhance exercise prescription methods so they can adequately address the needs of variable individuals and ensure long-term cartilage health—a crucial focus in contemporary medicine and athletic training. Thus, with our increasing knowledge, the development of personalized exercise plans will become imperative in promoting maximum cartilage health and joint function.

Test Your Knowledge

1. What is the role of cartilage in maintaining joint health?
2. How does exercise affect cartilage?

7.5. Cartilage Disorders

Learning Outcome

1. Describe the osteoarthritis and its effects on cartilage;
2. Describe the cartilage injuries and their treatment;
3. Learn about genetic disorders affecting cartilage.

Among the numerous conditions of cartilage affecting human health, temporomandibular joint disorders (TMDs) are particularly urgent since they affect the complex anatomical formations surrounding the jaw. According to research, TMD symptoms occur in approximately 60%–70% of adults, commenting on the prevalence of this disorder and its link to pain and dysfunction in routine activities. The pathophysiology of TMDs is typically an inflammatory insult to the integrity of articular tissues, including the articular disc, condylar cartilage, and overlying muscle tissue. Given the multifactorial etiology of TMDs, traditional treatments often are unable to provide significant relief. This deficiency has prompted the development of interest in new therapeutic approaches, particularly those that leverage advances in material science, i.e., hydrogels. Such materials hold potential for repair of articular disc and cartilage regeneration, opening the doors to better future clinical management of TMDs (Wang et al., 2024). Disease of cartilage can be associated with other genetic diseases as well, such as Marfan syndrome (MFS), which is characterized by the profound impact on the body's connective tissue. In MFS, approximately 90% of the conditions are due to mutations in the fibrillin-1 (fbn1) gene, which is the classical basis that can lead to significant cartilage malformations. The effects of such mutations are not merely confined to structural impairments; they can result in extreme, systemic involvement, with cardiovascular as well as skeletal impairment. Recent studies have utilized innovative genomic techniques like whole-exome sequencing to identify new variants in the fbn1 gene for MFS. The acquired information regarding genetic abnormalities not only enhances the characterization of the disorder but also suggests potential therapeutic interventions, linking the study of cartilage disorders to precision medicine in general (Huang et al., 2024).

The interplay between genetic susceptibility and environmental exposure underlies the spectrum of cartilage disorders that afflict individuals. Further study of the pathophysiologic pathways of such diseases is crucial for the development of therapeutic modalities. Emerging technologies, such as CRISPR/Cas9, hold the promise to delineate the functional impact of discrete mutations in cartilage genes. Specifically, the ability to study such mutations in model organisms, i.e., zebrafish, allows investigators to gain insights into morphological and functional pathology in cartilage disease. As science advances, the future of personalized medicine approaches ever nearer, paving the way for specifically targeted treatments to counteract the shortcomings of cartilage disease. The combining of gene study and fresh ways of treatment is a multidisciplinary approach to addressing the complex problems of cartilage health in humans.

7.5.1. Osteoarthritis (OA) and Its Effects on Cartilage

OA is an arthropathy in which the cartilage of a joint progressively degenerates, leading to severe discomfort and disability for affected people. Cartilage, which allows for the smooth functioning of a joint, gradually loses its structural homogeneity because of a multitude of reasons, including mechanical stress and biochemical changes. The chondrocytes, which maintain the cartilage healthy, undergo apoptosis—programmed cell death—aggravating the condition further. It happens with growing alarm as loss of chondrocytes diminishes the repair mechanisms in cartilage and leads to irreversible damage. Studies have also shown that decreased circulating concentrations of vitamin D have been linked to the formation of OA, which is indicative of the complex relationship between nutrition and cartilage (Boyan et al., 2016). The action of OA on cartilage is more than a matter of a straightforward reduction in tissue volume; it encompasses alterations in the biochemical composition of the cartilage matrix. In OA, degradation of the proteoglycans—crucial components that confer compressive strength to cartilage—leads to compromised resilience in response to mechanical loading. Evidence based on animal models suggests that therapeutic strategies aimed at modulating the inflammatory environment have tremendous promise in sustaining cartilage health. For instance, compounds like 24R,25(OH)2D3 have been demonstrated to shorten inflammatory responses in chondrocytes, thereby sustaining their viability and function (Boyan et al., 2016). These findings, therefore, demonstrate the necessity for definite therapeutic interventions against both the symptoms and mechanisms accountable for cartilage degradation within osteoarthritis. Furthermore, an understanding of the interface between subchondral bone changes and cartilage degradation is imperative in the development of comprehensive OA management strategies. Subchondral bone carries the overlying cartilage, and changes in it can dramatically affect cartilage integrity. Recent research involving bisphosphonates like alendronate has shown significant effects on preserving the health of subchondral bone and preventing cartilage deterioration in the immediate aftermath of joint trauma. Treatment with high-dose alendronate has been shown to be useful in maintaining articular cartilage and preventing initial trabecular bone loss after trauma, though its effectiveness in long-term joint degeneration is still limited. This data suggests that effective OA management may demand a multifaceted strategy addressing cartilage and bone maintenance for optimal joint salvage (Figure 7.13).

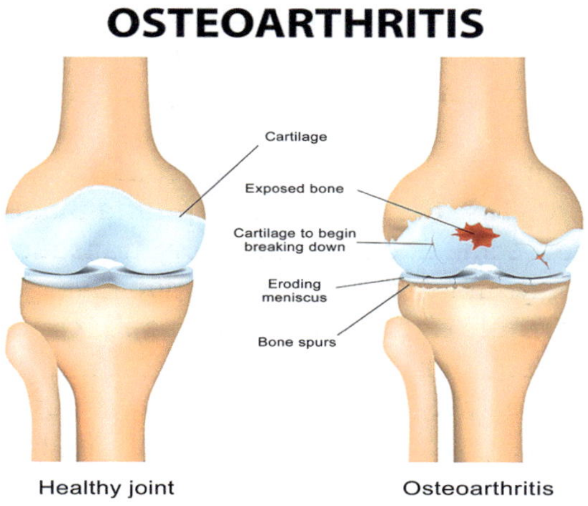

Figure 7.13. Osteoarthritis.

Source: https://www.kovilpattivenkateswarahospitals.com/wp-content/uploads/2022/10/cartilage-defect.jpg.

7.5.2. Cartilage Injuries and Their Treatment

Cartilage's function in human joints cannot be overstressed, particularly with regard to its vulnerability to injury caused by trauma, overuse, or degenerative disease. Injury to the cartilage will usually lead to intense pain, swelling, and loss of range of motion, significantly affecting one's quality of life. Athletes are particularly vulnerable since the force of their sports can lead to acute cartilage damage. In addition, degeneration with age can exacerbate these injuries in the geriatric age group. Current methods of treatment aim to minimize symptoms and influence repair, but are many times incomplete, leaving partial pain and disability. Understanding the subtleties of cartilage structure and function is essential to developing effective treatment protocols that can effectively treat cartilage trauma with minimal long-term joint integrity consequences. Emerging developments in regenerative medicine have ushered in promising therapy for cartilage injury. Included in these are the uses of orthobiologic therapies , such as platelet-rich plasma (PRP) and bone marrow aspirate concentrate (BMAC) as novel interventions compared to traditional ones. These interventions tend to supplement the body's intrinsic healing processes, with the potential capability in stimulate the regeneration of cartilage and reduce symptoms. Notably, some biomaterials have been explored as carriers of PRP and BMAC to increase the regenerative capacity of these treatments. A proper combination of these biologic therapies with an appropriate biomaterial can yield useful results in cartilage injury treatment. Clinical trials continue to explore the efficacy of such synergistic therapies, pushing the boundaries of traditional treatment for cartilage conditions and holding promise for relief to those suffering from chronic injury (Yamaguchi et al., 2019). Although promising, the future of regenerative medicine holds, treatment for injuries to the cartilage continues to be filled with challenges.

The lack of replicability of outcomes raises the question of whether existing treatment is effective. While technical advances like arthroscopic surgery and grafting have shown promise, they never go so far as to fully restore cartilage function. Additionally, the threat of abuse of growth factors or cell-based therapies for sporting enhancement has led to regulation by governing bodies, and clinical use of these emerging therapies is complicated (Ljungqvist et al., 2008). As the science progresses, continued research and close adherence to ethical principles will be essential to unlocking the promise of these treatments so that they benefit victims of cartilage damage without compromising the integrity of sport and athletic competition.

7.5.3. Genetic Disorders Affecting Cartilage

The cartilage disorders demonstrate a complex interaction between heredity and the structural integrity of this important tissue. Various genetic mutations have the potential to lead to disorders , such as osteogenesis imperfecta and achondroplasia, both of which have severe impacts on cartilage growth and function. These conditions are a result of mutations in one or more of the key genes important for cartilage matrix synthesis and maintenance, leading to joint function derangements and musculoskeletal health. This genetic origin necessitates a better understanding of how these mutations result in the phenotypic presentation seen in affected individuals.

Thus, ongoing research is key to the identification of the specific genetic pathways that influence cartilage formation and degradation and illuminate potential avenues of therapy for the management of related disorders. Furthermore, the role of environmental factors in addition to genetic determinants cannot be overstated. Nutritional factors, particularly dietary, have been found to play a role along with cartilage-related genetic susceptibility. A diet of fruit and vegetables has been observed in one study to offer protective factors for preventing the development of osteoarthritis, something worthy of consideration in light of an increase in the prevalence of the disease associated with cartilage degeneration.

The presence of alliums containing compounds like diallyl disulfide demonstrates a potential mechanism that may be able to reduce matrix-degrading enzyme expression in chondrocytes, suggesting that nutritional therapy may enhance genetic predispositions toward better cartilage health. Thus, an understanding of the interplay of genetic factors with lifestyle factors may be important in the management of cartilage disorders. Regarding pain perception and the hereditary aspect of cartilage disease, research has established that heritability plays a role in pain disorders resulting from cartilage degeneration, e.g., low back pain resulting from intervertebral disc dysfunction. The genes involved in cartilage structural integrity, as well as those regulating inflammatory response and nociceptive sensory transduction pathways, must be considered. Individual genes responsible for inflammation and collagen synthesis, for instance, directly influence cartilage integrity and predispose patients to develop chronic pain following injury or degeneration. By determining genetic risk profiles for osteoarthritis and chronic pain syndromes, clinicians can formulate targeted interventions considering both psychosocial factors and genetic factors. This multifaceted strategy is compatible with the nascent field of personalized medicine, which seeks to optimize patient outcomes by implementing customized treatment protocols that incorporate genetic data about cartilage well-being.

Test Your Knowledge

1. What is osteoarthritis and its effects on cartilage?
2. Describe the genetic disorders affecting cartilage.

SUMMARY

In forming a conclusive point on the role and purpose of cartilage within the human body, it is worth noting its major role in joint health and overall mobility. Cartilage, as a strong connective tissue, is what is required in cushioning bones against each other to avoid friction and wear when an organism is in motion. This is perfectly observed on such joints as knees and hips, where cartilage softens the shocks and enables free movement. The clinical relevance of cartilage degeneration, as observed in osteoarthritis, underscores the need to understand cartilage biology and susceptibility to parameters like age, trauma, and load. Knowledge gained from recent studies can be used to inform therapeutic intervention, potentially enhancing cartilage homeostasis and joint function. Moreover, recent studies suggest that it is necessary to investigate pharmacological agents that could potentially prevent cartilage degeneration, such as bisphosphonates. A study of the effects of alendronate therapy revealed that earlier treatment with this anti-resorptive drug is utilized to avoid loss of trabecular bone as well as cartilage degradation after injury, though it cannot cure established long-term joint conditions (Khorasani et al., 2015). This finding produces additional exploration of the time and classes of therapy for individuals at risk of cartilage loss. Apparently, treatment of the complexities of cartilage health requires a multidisciplinary approach consisting of lifestyle modification, therapeutic progress, and drug therapy to achieve improved joint disorder control. Finally, cartilage's evolutionary and functional significance requires increased research focus, particularly as it pertains to its adaptation according to biomechanical demand in different species. Research into the evolutionary significance of cartilage, specifically in terms of locomotor behavior, provides a fascinating addition to this debate. Describing the role of the centrale in hominoid wrists, for instance, places cartilage within an evolutionary context and relates physical changes to functional pressures (Püschel et al., 2020). This association not only illustrates the biological importance of cartilage in human beings but also its intricate relationship with our evolutionary heritage. Effectively, the future of cartilage research is where clinical use and evolutionary biology meet to shed more holistic perspectives into dealing with and understanding cartilage well-being in various populations.

The study of cartilage in human beings gives vital details concerning its structure, function, and importance in health. Cartilage, which is a hard connective tissue, is the main facilitator of smooth joint movement, a shock absorber, and a structural framework for various body parts. The hypothesis of cartilage pathology relies on an understanding of its composition, which includes a dense matrix of collagen fibers and proteoglycans that provide tensile strength and elasticity. Significantly, the determinants of cartilage integrity have been noted by researchers to be age, mechanical loading, and metabolic activity. The interdependency of the mentioned factors reflects the need for cartilage health in order to provide overall joint function and has accordingly remained a focus in research relevant to such disorders as osteoarthritis. Contemporary research has investigated the role of pharmacological intervention in the health of cartilage, particularly for degenerative joint disease. For example, bisphosphonates , such as alendronate have been a focus of attention since they can affect bone remodeling. Investigations have established that the administration of high doses of alendronate is effective in inhibiting early bone loss in the trabecula and degeneration of cartilage after injury, as evident through impressive findings of micro-computed tomography analysis (Khorasani et al., 2015). The long-term efficacy of such treatments is in question, particularly considering that they may not effectively counteract ongoing degeneration in joints. This complex interaction highlights the delicate interplay between bone and cartilage health and emphasizes the importance of ongoing research in the field of targeted therapies for the preservation of cartilage in varying states of physiology and pathology. Furthermore, the evolutionary history of musculoskeletal adaptations and cartilage presents a fascinating track to explore in delineating its development and role. The carpal fusion, for instance, of the centrale with the scaphoid in primates, shows functional locomotor adaptations, that is, knuckle-walking (Püschel et al., 2020). Finite element inferences show that such morphologies are biomechanically advantageous and suggest structural adaptations to meet certain definite functional demands. Such evolutionary insight not only sheds light on the origin of human joint mechanics but also emphasizes the strength and plasticity of cartilage confronted with an array of evolutionary stresses. Through investigation of these evolutionary relationships, researchers can better comprehend cartilage's function in health and disease, advancing the discovery and prevention of therapy for joint disease.

KEY TERMS FROM THIS CHAPTER

- Cartilage
- Condylectomy
- Fibrocartilage
- Hybrid biomaterials
- Osteoarthritis
- Proteoglycans
- Temporomandibular joint disease
- Collagen fibers
- Elastic cartilage
- Hyaline cartilage
- Orthobiologics
- Platelet-rich plasma
- Regenerative medicine
- Tendinopathy

CRITICAL THINKING QUESTIONS

1. **Cartilage is classified as:**
   a. Nervous tissue
   b. Epithelial tissue
   c. Connective tissue
   d. Muscular tissue
2. **The main cell type found in cartilage is:**
   a. Osteocyte
   b. Chondrocyte
   c. Fibroblast
   d. Adipocyte
3. **The most abundant type of cartilage in the body is:**
   a. Elastic cartilage
   b. Fibrocartilage
   c. Hyaline cartilage
   d. Articular cartilage
4. **Elastic cartilage is found in:**
   a. The intervertebral discs
   b. The external ear (pinna)
   c. The trachea
   d. The epiphyseal plates
5. **Fibrocartilage is characterized by:**
   a. A high content of elastic fibers
   b. A dense arrangement of collagen fibers
   c. Its role in rapid growth
   d. The absence of the extracellular matrix

Short Answer Questions

1. What is cartilage?
2. Why is cartilage important in the human body?
3. Name the three types of cartilage.
4. What are the functions of the cartilage?
5. Describe the various cartilage disorders affecting human health.

Answers to Critical Thinking Questions

1. (c); 2. (b) ; 3. (c); 4. (b); 5. (b)

REFERENCES

1. Abalymov, A., Parakhonskiy, B., & Skirtach, A. (2020). *Polymer- and hybrid-based biomaterials for interstitial, connective, vascular, nerve, visceral and musculoskeletal tissue engineering.* https://core.ac.uk/download/299792280.pdf (accessed on 7th August 2025).
2. Aberle, H., Agarwal, S., Agrawal, A., Aladin, J., Anderson, P., Andersson, L., Annunen, et al. (2009). *Current evidence for a modulation of low back pain by human genetic variants.* https://core.ac.uk/download/14527638.pdf (accessed on 7th August 2025).
3. Acheson, T., Adler, P., Allen, B., Anderson, C., Arie, J., Atsumi, et al. (2016). *Skeletal immaturity, rostral sparing, and disparate hip morphologies as biomechanical causes for Legg-Calvé-Perthes' disease.* https://core.ac.uk/download/151159396.pdf (accessed on 7th August 2025).
4. Alivernini, S., & Kurowska-Stolarska, M. (2017). *Synovial Tissue Macrophages: Friend or Foe?* https://core.ac.uk/download/143476600.pdf (accessed on 7th August 2025).
5. Allen, V., Hutchinson, J. R., Otero, A., Pol, D., et al. (2017). *Forelimb muscle and joint actions in Archosauria: Insights from Crocodylus johnstoni (Pseudosuchia) and Mussaurus patagonicus (Sauropodomorpha).* https://core.ac.uk/download/141887609.pdf (accessed on 7th August 2025).
6. Almeida, L. E., Botero, J. R., & López, D. F. (2018). *Early Condylectomy: Biological Considerations.* https://core.ac.uk/download/213089642.pdf (accessed on 7th August 2025).
7. Almeida, L. E., Castrogiovanni, P., Chiarenza, G. P. S., Imbesi, G., et al. (2016). *ADAM10 localization in temporomandibular joint disk with internal derangement: An ex vivo immunohistochemical study.* https://core.ac.uk/download/213079027.pdf (accessed on 7th August 2025).
8. Ammendola, S., Cocchiola, R., Lopreiato, M., Scotto D'Abusco, A., et al. (2018). *Effects of nutrients, mainly from Mediterranean dietary foods, on mesenchymal stem derived cells: Growth or differentiation.* https://core.ac.uk/download/188823135.pdf (accessed on 7th August 2025).
9. Khorasani, M. S., Diko, S., Hsia, A. W., Anderson, M. J., Genetos, D. C., Haudenschild, D. R., & Christiansen, B. A. (2015). Effect of alendronate on post-traumatic osteoarthritis induced by anterior cruciate ligament rupture in mice. *Arthritis research & therapy*, *17*(1), 30. https://doi.org/10.1186/s13075-015-0546-0(accessed on 7th August 2025).
10. Hu, J. L., Todhunter, M. E., LaBarge, M. A., & Gartner, Z. J. (2018). Opportunities for organoids as new models of aging. *The Journal of cell biology*, *217*(1), 39–50. https://doi.org/10.1083/jcb.201709054Augello, A., & De Bari, C. (2010). *The Regulation of Differentiation in Mesenchymal Stem Cells.* https://core.ac.uk/download/177373.pdf (accessed on 7th August 2025).
11. Babic, M., van der Giet, M., Herrmann, J., Schuchardt, M., et al. (2020). *Research models for studying vascular calcification.* https://core.ac.uk/download/323258131.pdf (accessed on 7th August 2025).
12. Ljungqvist, A., Schwellnus, M. P., Bachl, N., Collins, M., Cook, J., Khan, K. M., Maffulli, N., Pitsiladis, Y., Riley, G., Golspink, G., Venter, D., Derman, E. W., Engebretsen, L., & Volpi, P. (2008). International Olympic Committee consensus statement: molecular basis of connective tissue and muscle injuries in sport. *Clinics in sports medicine*, *27*(1), 231–xi. https://doi.org/10.1016/j.csm.2007.10.007(accessed on 7th August 2025).
13. Wang, W., Chun, H., Baek, J., Sadik, J. E., Shirazyan, A., Razavi, P., Lopez, N., & Lyons, K. M. (2019). The TGFβ type I receptor TGFβRI functions as an inhibitor of BMP signaling

in cartilage. *Proceedings of the National Academy of Sciences of the United States of America, 116*(31), 15570–15579. https://doi.org/10.1073/pnas.1902927116(accessed on 7th August 2025).

14. Bemben, D., Bloomfield, S., Hunter, S. K., Ploutz-Snyder, L., et al. (2014). *Effects of Sex and Gender on Adaptation to Space: Musculoskeletal Health*. https://core.ac.uk/download/213078847.pdf (accessed on 7th August 2025).
15. Binks, D. A., Damion, R. A., Foster, R. J., McGonagle, D., et al. (2017). *Imaging of nuclear magnetic resonance spin–lattice relaxation activation energy in cartilage*. https://core.ac.uk/download/161514353.pdf (accessed on 7th August 2025).
16. Boyan, B. D., Coutts, R. D., Healey, R., Hyzy, S. L., et al. (2016). *24R,25-dihydroxyvitamin D3 protects against articular cartilage damage following anterior cruciate ligament transection in male rats*. https://core.ac.uk/download/79819409.pdf (accessed on 7th August 2025).
17. Bricca, A., Juhl, C. B., Roos, E. M., Steultjens, M., et al. (2018). *Impact of exercise on articular cartilage in people at risk of, or with established, knee osteoarthritis: A systematic review of randomized controlled trials*. https://core.ac.uk/download/293885617.pdf (accessed on 7th August 2025).
18. Bronner, M. E., & LeDouarin, N. M. (2012). *Development and Evolution of the Neural Crest: An Overview*. https://core.ac.uk/download/6103405.pdf (accessed on 7th August 2025).
19. Püschel, T. A., Marcé-Nogué, J., Chamberlain, A. T., Yoxall, A., & Sellers, W. I. (2020). The biomechanical importance of the scaphoid-centrale fusion during simulated knuckle-walking and its implications for human locomotor evolution. *Scientific reports, 10*(1), 3526. https://doi.org/10.1038/s41598-020-60590-6(accessed on 7th August 2025).
20. Chang, L. W., McAlinden, A., Varghese, N., Wirthlin, L., et al. (2013). *Differentially expressed microRNAs in chondrocytes from distinct regions of developing human cartilage*. https://core.ac.uk/download/70382017.pdf (accessed on 7th August 2025).
21. Chen, J., Chen, Y., He, B., Li, D., et al. (2019). *Auricle Shaping Using 3D Printing and Autologous Diced Cartilage*. https://core.ac.uk/download/323068973.pdf (accessed on 7th August 2025).
22. Chen, J., Johnson, P. M., Kister, K., Robinson, R., et al. (2020). *Estrogen signaling impacts temporomandibular joint and periodontal disease pathology*. https://core.ac.uk/download/344443832.pdf (accessed on 7th August 2025).
23. Cucchiarini, M., Kohn, D., Madry, H., Terwilliger, E., et al. (2007). *Restoration of the extracellular matrix in human osteoarthritic articular cartilage by overexpression of the transcription factor SOX9*. https://core.ac.uk/download/pdf/10700253.pdf (accessed on 7th August 2025).
24. Flohr, S., Gomez, S., Kierdorf, H., Kierdorf, U., et al. (2017). *Multiple osteochondromas of the antlers and cranium in a free-ranging white-tailed deer (Odocoileus virginianus)*. https://core.ac.uk/download/148067969.pdf (accessed on 7th August 2025).
25. Sánchez-Villagra, M.R., Forasiepi, A.M. On the development of the chondrocranium and the histological anatomy of the head in perinatal stages of marsupial mammals. *Zoological Lett* **3**, 1 (2017). https://doi.org/10.1186/s40851-017-0062-yf (accessed on 7th August 2025).
26. Huang, S., Lei, L., & Zhang, R. Y. (2024). Exome sequencing identifies a novel FBN1 variant in a Chinese family with Marfan syndrome that includes aberrant right

subclavian artery. *European Heart Journal*. https://www.semanticscholar.org/paper/c36cf6a8b40f6ff83ae6adfcf7384867baf4fe0a (accessed on 7th August 2025).

27. Nakayama, N., Lee, J. Y., Matthias, N., Umeda, K., Yan, Q., & Huard, J. (2016). Cartilage Regeneration Using Pluripotent Stem Cell-Derived Chondroprogenitors: Promise and Challenges. InTech. doi: 10.5772/63052 (accessed on 7th August 2025).

28. Inui, A., Iwakura, T., & Reddi, A. H. (2012). *Human Stem Cells and Articular Cartilage Regeneration*. https://core.ac.uk/download/323071679.pdf (accessed on 7th August 2025).

29. Saarakkala, S., Julkunen, P., Kiviranta, P., Mäkitalo, J., Jurvelin, J. S., & Korhonen, R. K. (2010). Depth-wise progression of osteoarthritis in human articular cartilage: investigation of composition, structure and biomechanics. *Osteoarthritis and cartilage*, *18*(1), 73–81. https://doi.org/10.1016/j.joca.2009.08.003(accessed on 7th August 2025).

30. Lacy, A. (2017). *Dietary fat and the prevalence of hand osteoarthritis: Data from the Osteoarthritis Initiative*. https://core.ac.uk/download/142080935.pdf (accessed on 7th August 2025).

31. Ruggiero, A., Gòmez, E. & D'Amato, R. Approximate Analytical Model for the Squeeze-Film Lubrication of the Human Ankle Joint with Synovial Fluid Filtrated by Articular Cartilage. *Tribol Lett* **41**, 337–343 (2011). https://doi.org/10.1007/s11249-010-9710-5 (accessed on 7th August 2025).

32. Mironova, N., Pilmane, M., & Skidenko, N. (1996). *Spectrophotometrical alterations in the support tissue of large bronchi in humans*. https://core.ac.uk/download/427509176.pdf (accessed on 7th August 2025).

33. Riley, G. P. (2004). *The Pathogenesis of Tendinopathy: A Molecular Perspective*. https://core.ac.uk/download/2776643.pdf (accessed on 7th August 2025).

34. Riley, G. P. (2005). *Chronic Tendon Pathology: Molecular Basis and Therapeutic Implications*. https://core.ac.uk/download/2776642.pdf (accessed on 7th August 2025).

35. Roelofs, A. J., Alegre-Aguaron, E., Augello, A., Barbero, M., Bentley, G., Boneberg, M., et al. (2013). *Cell-based approaches to joint surface repair: A research perspective*. https://core.ac.uk/download/20443940.pdf (accessed on 7th August 2025).

36. Rowan, A. D., Cassidy, A., MacGregor, A. J., Valdes, A. M., Olafsdottir, A. S., Teucher, B., et al. (2010). *Dietary garlic and hip osteoarthritis: Evidence of a protective effect and putative mechanism of action*. https://core.ac.uk/download/2776285.pdf (accessed on 7th August 2025).

37. Samoy, Y., Saunders, J., & Van Ryssen, B. (2016). *Physiotherapy in Small Animal Medicine*. https://core.ac.uk/download/154408470.pdf (accessed on 7th August 2025).

38. Yamaguchi, F. S. M., Shams, S., Silva, E. A., & Stilhano, R. S. (2019). PRP and BMAC for Musculoskeletal Conditions via Biomaterial Carriers. *International journal of molecular sciences*, *20*(21), 5328. https://doi.org/10.3390/ijms20215328(accessed on 7th August 2025).

39. Wang, X., Liu, F., Wang, T., He, Y., & Guo, Y. (2024). Applications of hydrogels in tissue-engineered repairing of temporomandibular joint diseases. *Biomaterials Science*. https://www.semanticscholar.org/paper/029382ebb73f9fde2566e968c7f86a51f49ff3fe (accessed on 7th August 2025).

BONE

8

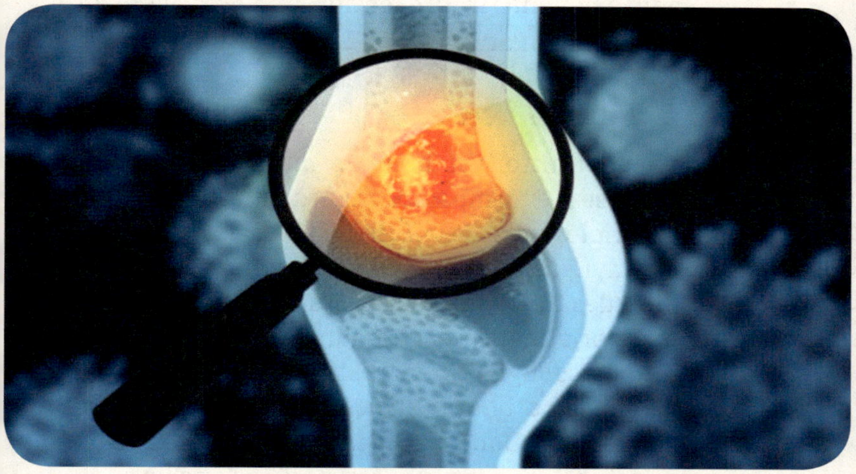

Introduction

Bone is an important contribution of the human body as it is the framework that offers support and protection to various organs, aids in movement, and assists in metabolic processes. Bone, whose science also has the name osteology, is not only interested in the anatomy and physiology of bone but also in development and pathology. This comprehensive branch of study reveals the complexity of bone makeup, which is not merely a static scaffold but a dynamic and active tissue undergoing constant remodeling throughout one's life. Knowing the complexity of the bone biology serves to elucidate variables influencing bone health and can prepare preventive interventions for the disease osteoporosis that so badly afflicts the elderly. It is crucial to comprehend the intricate function of bone to appreciate its importance in the entire physiology of the human body and thus to pave a firm foundation to pursue deeper into this life-giving tissue (Patwardhan, 2008). Besides, the intricate processes in forming and maintaining bone are controlled by cellular mechanisms that couple multiple biological systems.

LEARNING OBJECTIVES

After studying this chapter, you will be able to:

1. Describe the composition and functions of bones;
2. Understand the bone development and growth;
3. Describe the types of bones;
4. Learn about bone health and diseases;
5. Describe the diagnostic techniques for bone health.

Recent developments in molecular biology have clarified the interaction among bone cells, signaling pathways, and the extracellular matrix. For instance, that of cranial neural crest mesenchyme highlights the complex cell orchestration that has been behind the shaping of not only the jaw but also other elements of the skeleton. These interactions between cells are fundamental in determining the size, shape, and overall morphology of bones, thereby making adaptive evolution over the years possible. This information is invaluable, providing a glimpse into the reasons why bone structure can vary from individual to individual and species to species as a function of developmental factors and environmental signals. To interpret the full complexity of bone function, it is important to consider not only its structural aspects but also the sub-processes responsible for its formation and adaptation (Woronowicz et al., 2019).

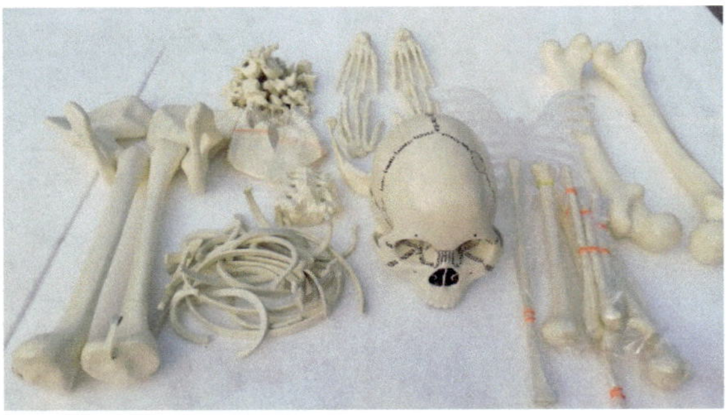

Figure 8.1. Bones.

Source: https://m.media-amazon.com/images/I/61ouqApZ2ML.jpg.

The value of bone is not just in support; it is also crucial in the storage of minerals, blood cell production, and the regulation of many body functions. Bones are mineral reservoirs , such as calcium and phosphorus and play a crucial role in ensuring homeostasis in the body. Bone marrow of certain bones is also engaged in the process of blood cell production, and that again reflects the interdependence of skeletal and hematologic well-being. Pricing these multifunctionality aspects ultimately results in a better integrated appreciation of human physiology. Consequently, studying bone not only educates regarding the knowledge of bone ailments but also enlightens one on general systemic health upkeep. With ongoing progress in science and technology, ongoing investigation into bone biology's complexity is likely to enhance our understanding of human disease and health, paving the way for advancements in prevention and treatment in the future (Patwardhan, 2008) (Figure 8.1).

Definition of Bone

The definition of bone is multi-dimensional because it encompasses its structural, functional, and biological features. Bone in its simplest form is a dynamic and living connective tissue that provides the human skeletal system. Comprising most of a matrix of inorganic mineral salts, as well as collagen fibers, bone serves not only to support the body's structure but also to have metabolism. Bone provides support to the body's structure, allowing movement when anchored to muscles and serving as a protective cage around vital organs. In addition, bones also serve as a reservoir for minerals, such as calcium and phosphorus, which are responsible for various physiological functions. Therefore, knowledge of bone entails an appreciation of its complexity as a living tissue that remains in remodeling under mechanical stress and metabolic needs. Beyond its physiologic structure, bone morphology is crucial in accounting for its multifaceted functions. There are two types of human bone: cortical bone which makes up the dense outer layer and cancellous or trabecular bone with a spongy structure. Cortical bone provides strength and solidity, while trabecular bone provides lightweight support and functions in producing blood cells in the marrow. Microscopic structures of the bones , such as osteons and lamellae, reflect their intricate organization that adapts to stress and strain through physical activity. Of course, one should also consider that bone microarchitecture and density vary with age and health and influence the material properties and fracture risk. The study of these features is crucial to facilitating our understanding of bones' function in human health and disease, especially in disciplines , such as orthopedics and regenerative medicine, where accurate bone parameter assessment is of significance (Andreis et al., 2017). Research has more and more focused on the study and understanding of normal bone parameters, especially in comparative research among species. Other research identifies that animals like pigs are able to make conclusions regarding the human bone anatomy due to comparable morphology and composition. For instance, studies of porcine bone architecture and mineral content yield useful reference values enhancing human bone growth and pathology knowledge (Stegner et al., 2014). This information is vital in enhancing surgical techniques, prosthetic models, and therapeutic plans for bone pathologies. By establishing a clear set of criteria for what is normal bone, scientists can then better interpret clinical findings and build good interventions. The entire definition of bone, then, not only encompasses its biological and structural properties but also underscores the significance of continuing research in enabling us to better comprehend the complexity of this vital tissue in the human body (Figure 8.2).

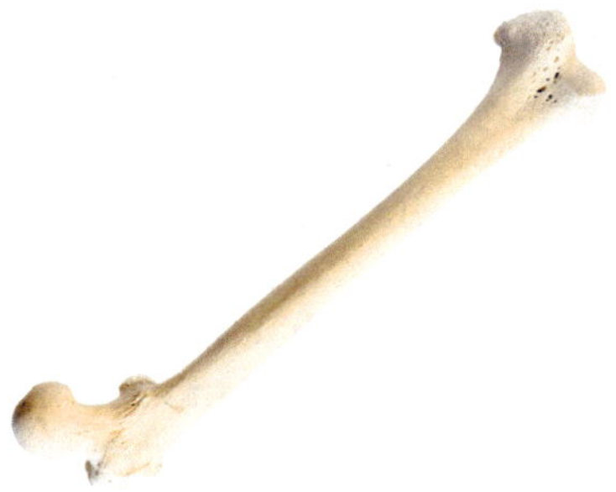

Figure 8.2. The Long Bone.

Source: https://cdn.prod.website-files.com/6022fbd4e8b6ac659f5b49a9/604ea9ffe9f5d3c0f56cd478_long-bones-nav%20copy.png.

Importance of Bones in the Human Body

The skeletal system is a key structural framework of the human body, whose function is to provide support and protect sensitive organs. Bones are not only passive structures; they are dynamic tissue that plays an active role in numerous biological mechanisms. Each bone contributes to general strength in the skeleton, such that a varied range of motion becomes feasible. Furthermore, the various shapes and sizes of bones reflect their unique purposes, ranging from the weight-bearing femur to the minuscule bones of the inner ear for hearing. Such functionality indicates the evolutionary significance of bones since they have developed to address the necessity of movement and overall survival across distinct environments. Furthermore, bones serve as a reservoir for minerals like calcium and phosphorus, which play crucial roles in various functions of the body and thus, apart from serving as structural support alone, exhibit their utility in this function. Bones play a significant role in the production of blood cells through a process known as hematopoiesis, along with structural and protective roles. Bone marrow, which is found in certain bones, is the primary location for the manufacturing of red blood cells, white blood cells, and platelets. Such production is most significant in maintaining a healthy immune system, as white blood cells are crucial in helping to defend the body against infection. Furthermore, regulation and blood cell production in proportion is a very developed mechanism to accommodate the body's requirements, and it illustrates the interactivity of the skeletal system with other physiological processes. The systemic nature of bone functions holds equally for its impact on overall health; disease or imbalance of bones, such as osteoporosis, has far-reaching effects on the production of blood and immune response, demonstrating integration of the skeletal system in overall human physiology (Patwardhan, 2008). Biomechanics further emphasizes the contribution of bones to facilitating movement and providing leverage to the musculoskeletal system. The coordination of bones and muscles enables a range of activities from simple movements , such as walking to complex movements , such as sports performance. Greater examination reveals that evolutionary modification of certain bones, particularly the wrist, is specific evidence of locomotor activity, such as knuckle-walking. Experiments conducted through finite element simulations have revealed that certain bone fusions in the wrist enhance the bearing capacity of the wrist during these activities, which indicates functional adjustment to locomotion modes of our ancestors (Püschel et al., 2020). This biomechanical perspective not only corroborates the function of bones to facilitate movement but also underscores the significance of skeletal adjustments in the context of evolutionary biology. Therefore, bones are not just critical to structural strength but also to functional perfection, highlighting their role in the human body in several ways.

8.1. Composition of Bone

Learning Outcome

1. Describe the types of bone tissue;
2. Understand the mineral content and its significance;
3. Describe the role of collagen in bone structure.

The bone structure is a complicated matter involving organic and inorganic compounds that enter into its unique structural and functional features. Organic matrix, composed predominantly of collagen fibers and non-collagenous proteins, accounts for about 30% of the mass of bones and plays an essential role in the provision of tensile strength and pliability. Collagen is a fibrous protein that creates a scaffold allowing bones to resist deformation when subjected to stress. In comparison, the inorganic portion, which consists of hydroxyapatite crystals comprising calcium and phosphate, accounts for approximately 70% of the mass of bones. The mineral content gives bone its stiffness and bearing capacity, which is why it is required for the overall support of the human skeleton. The combination of organic and inorganic materials results in a bone structure that is both resilient and strong to support the integrity and functionality of the body itself. Moreover, the cellular constituents of the bone tissue form the center of its composition, including osteoblasts, osteocytes, and osteoclasts. The formation of bones is facilitated by osteoblasts, which develop organic bone matrix components and create space for mineralization. They differentiate into osteocytes once embedded within the matrix to be in charge of bone tissue homeostasis and engage with other bone cells to regulate remodeling processes. Osteoclasts, on the contrary, are specialized cells charged with resorbing bone, breaking down the matrix and assisting in maintaining calcium homeostasis within the blood. This dynamic balance between these cellular constituents is critical for bone strength and resistance, allowing bones to adjust to varying physiological stresses , such as mechanical stress or hormonal stimuli. A knowledge of these cellular interactions is thus important to address disorders of the bone as well as to encourage enhanced skeletal health. Besides its physical composition, bone also serves as a reservoir of the two primary minerals, calcium and phosphorus, essential to most physiological processes. The bone matrix not only offers structural support but also plays a critical role in the storage and release of minerals so that the body can retain and stabilize minerals and maintain metabolic activity. The ability of bone to serve as a reservoir for minerals is particularly valuable in bone remodeling, where the alternating resorption and formation supply for continuous adaptation of bone shape to changes in mechanical stress. The composition of bone can also be controlled by a variety of factors, including dietary intake, exercise, and hormone levels, and those that affect rates of bone resorption and bone formation. Thus, understanding the intricate makeup of bone reveals its function and the implications for diseases like osteoporosis and other metabolic bone diseases (Figure 8.3).

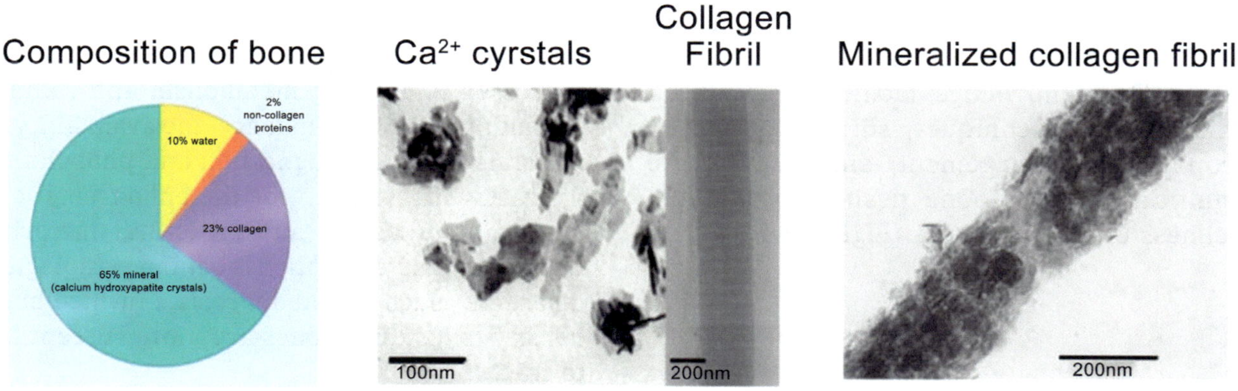

Figure 8.3. The major structural components of bone are calcium-phosphate crystals and type I collagen.

Source: https://yalehistology.s3.us-east-2.amazonaws.com/bone/bone_composition.jpg.

8.1.1. Types of Bone Tissue

Bone tissue in the skeleton is divided into several different types, all of which are crucial to human physiology. These are the two primary types of bones: compact and spongy bone. Compact bone, or cortical bone, is the strong outer covering of bones and is responsible for their structural integrity and strength. Compact bone consists of dense osteons, or Haversian systems, and is what makes it resistant to compressive force. On the other hand, cancellous bone or spongy bone is found mostly at the ends of long bones and within others. Its porous and trabecular nature permits effective stress and weight transmission, as well as hematopoietic tissue formation in the bone marrow, to facilitate the formation of blood cells. Hence, the understanding of the variability of bone tissue is important to the overall comprehension of skeletal function. Furthermore, within the two major categories, bone tissue is further classified as woven and lamellar bone according to its age of development and pattern of structure. Woven bone, by virtue of its random collagen fiber structure, is usually present in bone formation in its earlier stages and during injury. It is less dense and is progressively substituted by lamellar bone in the aging organism and healing process. Lamellar bone, on the other hand, is organized into parallel layers, with greater tensile strength and resilience owing to its ordered matrix. The mechanism of woven to lamellar bone replacement illustrates the dynamic state of the skeletal system, which can adapt to shifting mechanical stress and biological demands. This adaptability is not only necessary for normal growth but also in healing processes following fractures or trauma. The significance of bone tissue types extends beyond mere structural considerations, with implications for various aspects of health and clinical practices. For example, understanding the differences in bone composition will maximize techniques for the treatment of bone diseases. Diseases such as osteoporosis and osteoarthritis are impacted by the ratio of the types of bone present. In osteoporosis, the trabecular bone loss substantially increases the risk of fracture, while osteoarthritis involves cartilage and subchondral bone alterations that compromise joint function. Moreover, advances in biotechnology, such as the development of dental implants, underscore the importance of knowledge in bone tissue biomechanics for establishing flawless integration and function within the human body (Grenoble & Knoell, 1973). This knowledge facilitates enhanced rehabilitation techniques, surgery, and even prophylactic management, emphasizing the significant role of bone tissue types in the wellness of human beings (Figure 8.4).

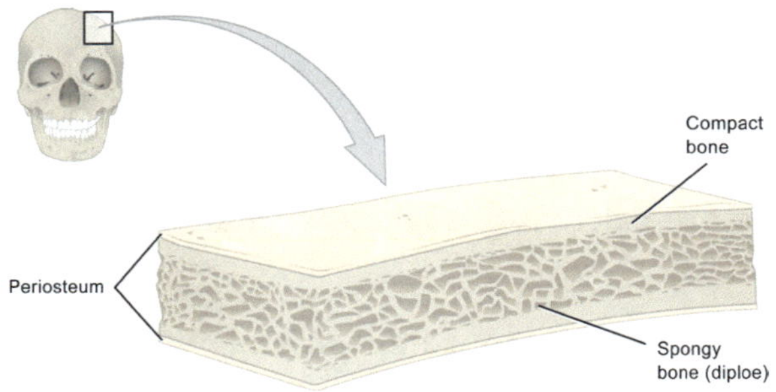

Figure 8.4. Flat bones are typically enveloped by compact bone, with a center of spongy bone.

Source: https://jwu.pressbooks.pub/app/uploads/sites/31/2021/05/Anatomy_of_a_Flat_Bone.jpg.

8.1.2. Mineral Content and Its Significance

Mineral content of bone is a vital ingredient to provide skeletal integrity and function. Made largely of hydroxyapatite, a calcium and phosphate crystalline structure, the mineral matrix provides firmness and rigidity to the skeletal system. Bone remodeling and development are facilitated by calcium, and the regulation of osteoblast and osteoclast function and, therefore, bone density and health of the skeleton. Research reveals, appropriate levels of dietary calcium are essential to the maintenance of alveolar bone and, by extension, oral health in general, underlining the importance of minerals not just for overall health but also for specific physiological functions in bone health (Battino et al., 2016). The interdependence of mineral content and structural properties of the bone demonstrates the importance of nutrition to skeletal health over life. Moreover, minerals also interact in complex manners to affect not only the bone's structure but also the biochemical processes underlying metabolism and cellular communication. For instance, the availability of minerals , such as magnesium and phosphorus interacts with calcium for the enhancement of bone mineralization and structural integrity. These minerals' disruption is behind pathological disorders , such as osteoporosis, in which bone density is lost and bones are more susceptible to fractures.

Current evidence highlights the roles of trace minerals in the regulation of inflammation and oxidative stress, both of which have significant impacts on bone. The fine balance of these compounds underscores their worth in food advice and population health plans that reduce the prevalence of bone disorders and promote lifetime skeletal health (Allen et al., 2019). Lastly, the function of minerals in bone wellness is still acknowledged in chronic disease disorders that affect the integrity of the skeleton. For example, chronic kidney disease can lead to mineral metabolism disturbances and has been known to cause chronic kidney disease-mineral bone disorder (CKD-MBD) to develop. In such cases, the body's ability for mineral homeostasis is compromised, resulting in mineralization and structural abnormalities of bone as well as cortical porosity enhancement. Such a change can significantly impact the overall status of health and quality of life. Therefore, the study of the roles of various minerals not only reveals their overt functions in bone strength but also their broader role in general well-being and disease protection, enhancing the preeminent role minerals play in promoting not only skeletal but also systemic health (Allen et al., 2019) (Figure 8.5).

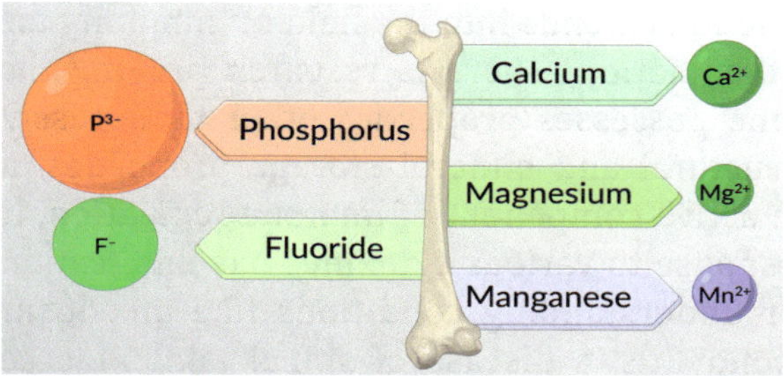

Figure 8.5. Essential minerals for bone health.

Source: https://www.jove.com/files/media/science-education/science-education-thumbs/14021.jpg.

8.1.3. Role of Collagen in Bone Structure

Collagen's role in bone structure is of primary importance as a vital protein, imparting tensile strength and structural integrity to the skeleton. Bone is dominated by collagen type I, which creates a fibrous scaffold that allows for mineral deposition, allowing bones to bear mechanical loads. The specific composition of such a material achieves compatibility between flexibility and rigidity, which is critical for load-bearing under the motion of activities of daily living. Not only is collagen accountable for bone's physical properties, but it also profoundly affects the biological role of bone remodeling and upkeep. Because osteoblasts secrete collagen, they guide the process of mineralization that ultimately builds bone tissue, thus establishing an immediate association between collagen synthesis and bone health. Also important is the intricate arrangement of collagen fibers in bone tissue and its impact on the mechanical performance of the tissue. Collagen molecules are arranged hierarchically, packing into fibrils and aggregating into fibers, eventually forming the structure of bone. Not only does such an arrangement determine the toughness and strength of bones, but also how they respond to growth and repair processes. Collagen synthesis disturbances are associated with various diseases affecting the bones, such as osteogenesis imperfecta and osteoporosis, in which reduced levels of collagen can lead to brittle bones and increase the risk of fractures. This highlights the significance of maintaining healthy levels of collagen via diet and lifestyle, thereby emphasizing the protein's complex role in bone health and human well-being. Aside from its structural functions, the involvement of collagens also includes the signaling pathways of bone metabolism. Collagen has been shown to interact with other signaling molecules and receptors, influencing osteoclast and osteoblast activity. The interaction is crucial in maintaining bone homeostasis since disruption could lead to diseases like osteoporosis, which is characterized by the excessive resorption of bone. Recent research has established that alterations in collagen architecture, e.g., cross-linking differences and variations in the ratio of different collagen types, can affect these control processes. Understanding these control processes is integral to the design of treatment strategies to enhance bone density and strength, particularly in those populations at risk for bone disorders. Thus, collagen is not only a fundamental component in the structural composition of bones but a key player in the intricate web of bone health and remodeling.

Test Your Knowledge

1. List the types of bone tissue.
2. What is the role of collagen in bone structure?

8.2. Functions of Bones

Learning Outcome

1. Describe the support and structure for the body;
2. Learn about the protection of vital organs;
3. Understand the facilitation of movement through joints.

The roles of the bones in the human body are varied and essential to ensure overall well-being and functionality. One of the main functions of bones is to give structural support, constituting a framework that upholds the shape of the body as well as guards essential organs. For example, the backbone protects the spinal cord, and the ribcage guards the lungs and heart from trauma. This strength of structure is required not only for the height of the body, but also for the mobility to move by muscle attachment via tendons, forming a robust mechanism of movement and stability. The function of bones extends beyond stabilization alone; they are also pivotal in the generation of bone marrow, a process which aids the body's ability to produce blood cells, showing how skeletal health is integral to functioning overall. Bone adaptation is governed by various factors, including mechanical stress, which will elicit an effect known as Wolff's Law. This is a law that dictates that bone remodels itself depending on the forces it experiences, thus keeping the skeletal system strong yet light in weight. This adaptive function is very important in athletes and physically active individuals because it can prevent bones from losing density and fractures. In addition, bones serve as reservoirs for essential minerals , such as calcium and phosphorus, which are crucial in the homeostasis process in the body. The mineral reservoir also serves as a buffer system to ensure mineral balance, demonstrating that bones not only provide structural support physically but also have a regulatory function in important biochemical processes within the human body. Additionally, bone tissue function extends into the field of immunity and inflammation. There is research proving that bone possesses properties other than passive structural and mineral storage properties, as an active component of immune regulation. Its response to various cytokines has implications for understanding conditions like ankylosing spondylitis, a disease of spinal joint illnesses that highlights the role of the connective tissue in immunity and inflammation (Owen et al., 2017). In tendinopathy, which also encompasses inflammatory processes involving the tendon-bone interface, understanding bone pathology has provided new therapeutic opportunities, highlighting the significance of a differentiated comprehension of bone functions during health and disease (Riley, 2004). This revised perception of bones reflects their fundamental role in both giving the body its structure and actively engaging in the body's complex system interplay.

8.2.1. Support and Structure for the Body

The adult human skeleton is an essential support framework of the body, with a key role to play in facilitating physical integrity and movement. As a structural support, bones provide the rigidity and stability required for upright posture in bipedal locomotion. Every bone has a unique contribution to the functionality of the entire musculoskeletal apparatus, and the skeletal system is extremely specialized. Bones do not just bear organs but also protect vulnerable structures , such as the brain, within the cranial cavity. The importance of this structural support lies in the complex relationship between different bones and muscle groups that need to work together to provide smooth movement, weight-bearing, and interaction with the outside world. Thus, learning about the supportive role of bone is essential to comprehend human physiology and biomechanics. Besides its structural role, bone is an active tissue that participates in many physiological functions. They are also repositories for the essential minerals calcium and phosphorus, which are indispensable to a myriad of metabolic processes. Furthermore, bone tissue plays a key part in hematopoiesis, the development of blood cells within the bone marrow. This multifaceted function is the reason why bones are not only static structures but also dynamic participants in the body's total physiology. Modern anatomical research underlines the intricacy of the associations, which illustrate how bone support must extend beyond structural characteristics. As an example, the Digital Anatomist Foundational Model of Anatomy illustrates a comprehensive symbolic model consisting of anatomical relations and physical attributes necessary to describe the complexity of organization in the human body, illustrating the way in which bone engages other life systems to support life (Rosse & Mejino, 2004).

Besides, a skeletal anatomy study reveals noticeable differences in complexity and integration among species, even that of human beings. Recent times have seen studies of network analysis highlighting the distinctive adaptation in the fore- and hindlimb anatomical structures of human beings compared to our closest living relations, e.g., chimpanzees. Notably, human hindlimb possesses a level of complexity in competition with that of chimpanzees, although the forelimb is less anatomically complex. These findings contradict traditional concepts of limb function and reveal that human evolution has shaped anatomical networks in specific manners to optimize mobility and dexterity. Interpreting these complex configurations has not only the potential to enlighten evolutionary biology but also to inform clinical practice within orthopedics and rehabilitation. Thus, bone architecture and support analysis will further advance with the help of cutting-edge methodologies that reveal the intricate web of interactions sustaining the human musculoskeletal system (Esteve-Altava et al., 2018) (Figure 8.6).

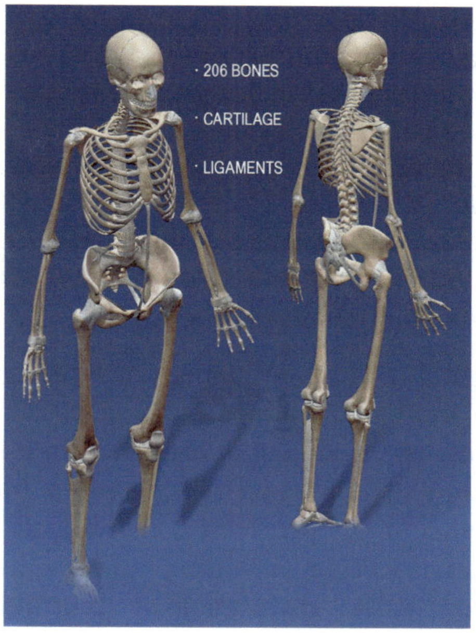

Figure 8.6. Skeletal system.

Source: https://www.visiblebody.com/hs-fs/hub/189659/file-2382117556.jpg.

8.2.2. Protection of Vital Organs

The most critical function of the skeletal system far exceeds structural support; it also participates in protecting vital organs in the human organism. Encasing delicate and important structures, the bones themselves form a sturdy shield that lessens damage. A case is the rib cage encasing the heart and lungs, a sturdy shield against outside pressures. The cranium shields the brain from injury and other environmental hazards by encasing it. Such protection is not random but represents an inherent aspect of bone architecture, supporting the role that skeletal structures play in sustaining life and sustaining homeostasis. As disease involving bones becomes increasingly common, understanding how these systems function in protecting vital organs is more critical as researchers seek to develop treatments and interventions promoting the health of bones and enhancing overall protective mechanisms of the body (Baldin et al., 2021). Furthermore, tissue engineering achievements have also brought into focus the role of bone in organ protection. Researchers are currently more interested in creating scaffolds that would promote bone regeneration, particularly where injury or disease compromises the structural integrity of skeletal structures. In addition to maintaining structural support, such scaffolds must also respond to biological signals to promote healing appropriately.

By developing new biomaterials, researchers aim to promote bone repair and hence reinforce the protective function of the skeleton for vital organs. This phenomenon between healthy bone and organ protection extends to other fields of medicine, including orthopedics and dentistry, where restoration of bone integrity can lead to healthier results. Thus, exploring the intersection of bone regeneration and organ protection continues to be a topic of research, reflecting the double-duty functions that bones play in general health (Baldin et al., 2021). As such, the protection of vital organs is an integral function of the skeleton, further underscoring the central role that bones play in human body anatomy.

The intricate interplay between bone strength and organ protection highlights the need for novel strategies in bone regeneration and repair. With the increasing incidence of skeletal disease, there is a continually increasing need to better understand how bone tissue can be engineered so that its protective roles are optimized. Further, ongoing developments spurred by institutions like the Biotechnology and Biological Sciences Research Council (BBSRC) demonstrate the ambition to develop successful biomaterials in support of this endeavor. With ongoing discoveries into the protective function of the human skeleton, medical research and treatment vision becomes increasingly defined, eventually informing actions to induce health and longevity (Figure 8.7).

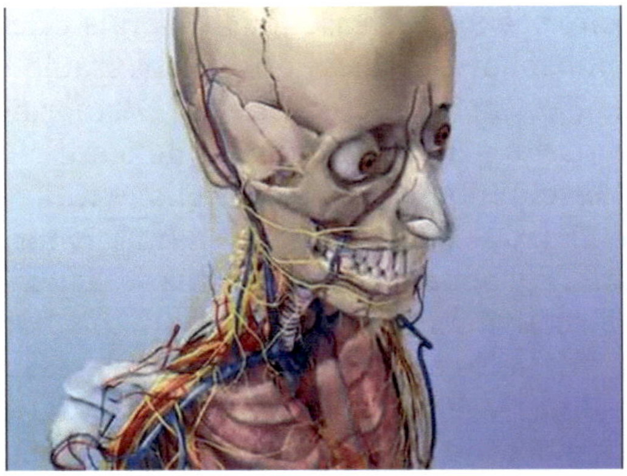

Figure 8.7. Skeleton protects vital organs.

Source: https://i.ytimg.com/vi/F3jJ-AeYQU4/hqdefault.jpg?sqp=-oaymwEmCOADEOgC8quKqQMa8AEB-AHm3IACzgOKAgwIABABGE8gVyhlMA8=&rs=AOn4CLD02idL5muaPgnSS1VDpvGMF6hF-w.

8.2.3. Facilitation of Movement Through Joints

Movement at joints is an advanced process based on the interaction of bones, ligaments, tendons, and the surrounding musculature. Joints act as hinges in the skeletal apparatus to allow extensive varieties of movements required for most physical processes. The type of joint—synovial, fibrous, or cartilaginous—orders the range and kind of movement possible. Synovial joints, for instance, are characterized by the fact that there exists a fluid-filled space within them that lubricates the moving surfaces to reduce friction during movement. Furthermore, the structural arrangement of such joints, e.g., their alignment and stabilization offered through ligaments, enables maximal movement patterns and economy of energy expenditure during walking or running. Such a refined system relies heavily on the mechanical properties of the bones involved as well as on the neuromuscular coordination required to move smoothly and effectively. The joint skeletal frames' anatomy influences the joint movement mechanics to a large extent. Bone positions in joints, coupled with the function of muscles and tendons involved in the movement, are essential to enabling motion. For instance, in walking or running motions, the Achilles tendon's elasticity and fixation to the calcaneus facilitate effective force transmission by the gastrocnemius muscle. As it appears, differences in walking speed could have a significant effect on tendon loading and joint function. Increased walking speed may be used to alter joint forces, as shown in studies that suggest that increased gait speed may result in decreased maximum tendinous forces, with overall work at the ankle increasing (Kharazi et al., 2023).

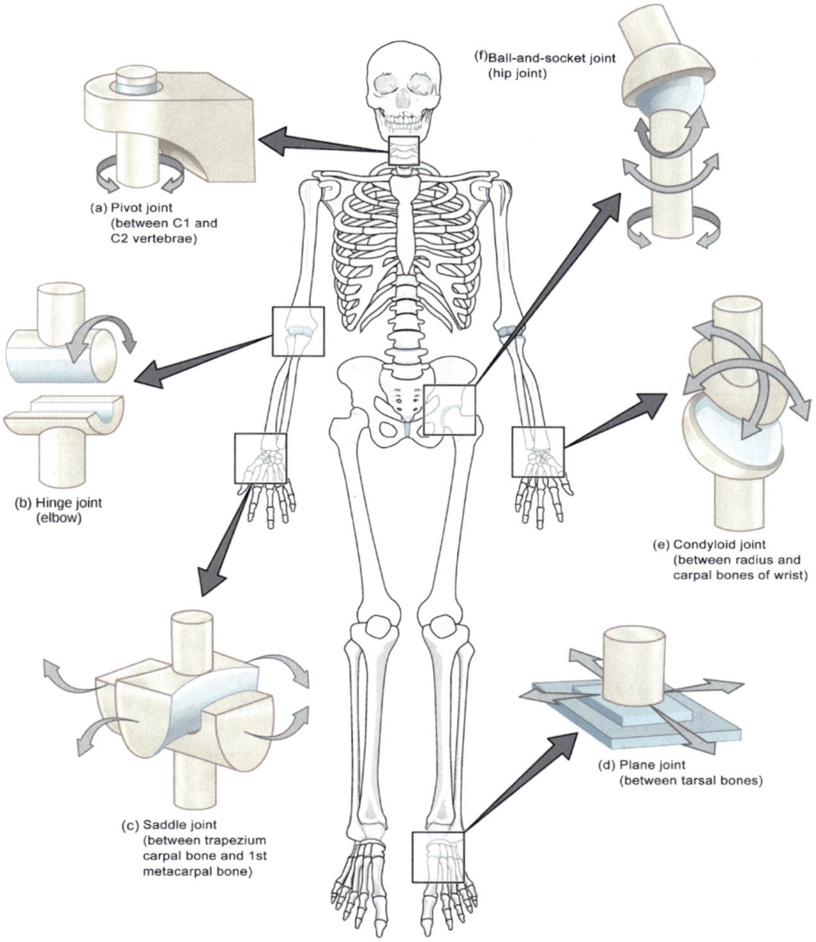

Figure 8.8. Different types of joints allow different types of movement. Planar, hinge, pivot, condyloid, saddle, and ball-and-socket are all types of synovial joints.

Source: https://opentextbc.ca/biology/wp-content/uploads/sites/96/2015/03/Figure_38_03_04.jpg.

Appreciation of such dynamics is not only essential for maximizing athletic performance but also for engineering ways to prevent injury by maximizing joint mechanics. Joint movement facilitation is of broader applicability than mere locomotion, stretching to more general relevance in human health and athletic performance. Improved insight into joint mechanics informs rehabilitation therapy for patients with musculoskeletal injury, as well as prevention strategies for preventing overuse injury. Curiously, it has been demonstrated that regular wear of modern shoes can compromise natural foot and joint function, favoring a higher rate of injury in sportsmen compared to runners who run barefoot or in minimalist footwear (Scarlett, 2018). This biomechanical observation of the effect of shoe wear underscores the importance of personalized interventions to restore natural joint function as well as enhance movement economy. Lastly, through the development of a deep appreciation of how the joints enable joints to move, we are better positioned to appreciate the interconnectedness of the muscular and skeletal systems and their collective effect on physical performance and health (Figure 8.8).

Test Your Knowledge

1. What is the protection of vital organs?
2. What is facilitation of movement?

8.3. Bone Development and Growth

Learning Outcome

1. Understand the process of ossification;
2. Describe the factors influencing bone growth;
3. Understand the changes in bone density with age.

The intricate sequence of bone growth and development in humans involves a series of tightly regulated biological events that progress through easily distinguishable phases, including embryonic development, childhood, and adolescence. Bones first develop through two general mechanisms: intramembranous and endochondral ossification. In intramembranous ossification, mesenchymal stem cells become directly committed to osteoblasts that form flat bones , such as those of the skull. Endochondral ossification, or the sequential replacement of cartilage by bone common in the development of long bones, takes place with conversion being critical to the maintenance of normal bone strength and size. Breaks at any stage can lead to deformities of the skeleton or short stature. Therefore, it is important to be aware of the delicate interplay between these processes if therapies for bone pathologies developing due to developmental abnormalities are to be enhanced. Signaling pathways are essential in bone formation, and various growth factors guide the complex biological process necessary for skeletogenesis. Among these, fibroblast growth factor (FGF) signaling is a vital one that impacts important events , such as limb formation, chondrogenesis, and osteogenesis. In fact, FGF signaling initiates the mesenchymal cell condensation in the limb bud, an important process prior to cartilage and bone formation. Recent studies highlight the contribution of mutations in FGF signaling molecules to skeletal malformation formation, illuminating the significance of the pathway in normal and pathological bone development. Through the study of FGF dynamics and interaction with other pathways, researchers strive to develop novel therapeutic options for genetic diseases that impair bone growth and strength. These discoveries can radically alter the treatment approach for developmental skeletal disease and enhance bone regenerative potential. Moreover, improvements in medical technology are also transforming the area of bone reconstruction and repair, particularly relating to age-related degenerative changes as well as trauma. Bone loss, quite prevalent among older individuals due to aging, periodontal disease, and trauma, presents significant clinical challenges. Orthodox methods most commonly turn to autologous grafting or metallic implant usage; however, these methods are not only expensive but also fall short of restoring the natural form and function of the bone. Emerging technologies like 3D printing have created opportunities for customized prosthetic implants, which can be tailored to fit individual anatomical demands. Combining material engineering and tissue engineering, researchers are developing hybrid implants that facilitate better osseointegration and stimulate bone growth. These advances underscore the power of interdisciplinary research in maximizing bone regeneration and improving patient outcomes for patients with skeletal deficiencies, thus representing a major unmet clinical need (Argárate et al., 2015; Marie et al., 2015) (Figure 8.9).

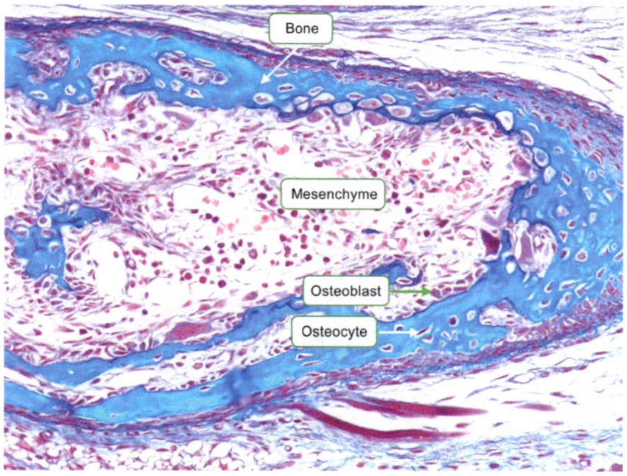

Figure 8.9. Intramembraneous ossification involves bone formation on mesenchymal tissue.

Source: https://s3.us-east-2.amazonaws.com/yalehistology/bone/intramembraneous_ossification.jpg.

8.3.1. Process of Ossification

Ossification is a critical aspect of skeletal development, when the cartilage-based framework is substituted by a bony one. Ossification is a physiological process that constructs the human skeleton prenatally as well as postnatally. Intramembranous and endochondral are the two primary types of ossification. Intramembranous ossification occurs directly in the mesenchymal tissue, primarily for flat bones, the skull being a case in point. In contrast, endochondral ossification involves a model of hyaline cartilage and is primarily responsible for the development of long bones. Regulation of the processes is carefully modulated by several signaling pathways and endocrine control to provide sufficient bone density and structural support as the organism grows. Ossification begins early in fetal life, typically in the sixth week of gestation, as chondrocytes are formed from differentiating mesenchymal cells, establishing a template of cartilage. This cartilage serves as a scaffold for the later bone formation, in which mineralization becomes initiated. Ossification progressed, osteoblasts, or bone cells that form bones, resorb cartilage by bone tissue, while producing new blood vessels simultaneously, especially during endochondral ossification. The interactive dynamics among such cells not only create the beginning of bone growth but also facilitate vascularization necessary for nutrient supply at the site of ossification. Defects in this complicated process can lead to congenital diseases and have an impact on overall bone health, so it is important to know the process of ossification for medical science and orthopedics. Ossification continues to play a vital role in bone maintenance and repair in adult life, most importantly after fractures. Successful healing of the fracture requires a fine-tuned orchestration between osteoblastic and osteoclastic functions to ensure the efficient production of new bone while remodeling existing bone. Evidence suggests that age is one of the factors that has a determining impact on the ability of progenitor cells in ossification to regenerate. For instance, studies indicate that in elderly patients, there is a significant decline in the prevalence and capability of mesenchymal stem cells and endothelial progenitor cells, which are important for bone formation and vascularization, respectively. This reduction results in prolonged recovery times, necessitating new treatment strategies to enhance ossification processes in aging populations, including cellular and pharmacologic approaches aiming to restore optimal skeletal repair function (Clauss et al., 2019) (Figure 8.10).

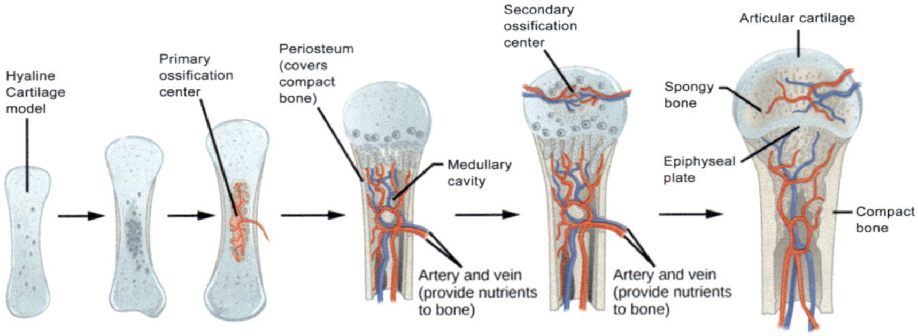

Figure 8.10. Endochondral ossification is the process of bone development from hyaline cartilage. The periosteum is the connective tissue on the outside of bone that acts as the interface between bone, blood vessels, tendons, and ligaments.

Source: https://s3-us-west-2.amazonaws.com/courses-images/wp-content/uploads/sites/1223/2017/02/08000442/Figure_38_02_06-1024x378.jpg.

8.3.2. Factors Influencing Bone Growth

Determinants of bone growth are multifactorial, involving genetic, nutritional, hormonal, and environmental influences. Genetics has a crucial role in determining the formation of an individual's bone structure as well as density, influencing growth patterns throughout development. Genetic heterogeneity for genes expressed in bone development and remodeling can lead to differences in skeletal integrity. Nutritional intake, that is, the consumption of minerals , such as calcium and phosphorus, also plays a major part in the attainment of bone growth. The nutrients act to increase the mineralization process that forms bone matrix. Further, vitamins, especially Vitamin D, increase calcium absorption, hence playing a significant role in the development of bones. Imbalance of these nutrients might result in conditions like osteoporosis or rickets, hence bringing into context the necessity of proper dietary components for proper skeletal growth. Hormones also play a significant role in bone development, with several endocrine factors regulating bone development and bone resorption. Growth hormone and insulin-like growth factors are required to activate bone cell activity during childhood and adolescence and influence bone maturation rate. Sex hormones , such as estrogen and testosterone also significantly affect bone metabolism; they promote bone density and permit the epiphyseal plates to close, which indicates the end of bone elongation. Conversely, diminished secretion of these hormones with age will add to greater bone resorption and decreased bone mass, further enhancing the risk of fracture. This, to this extent, brings to the fore how the changes in hormones might affect bone health, underscoring integrated approaches in the management of bone loss associated with aging, which is critical in maintaining skeletal integrity throughout one's life course. Environmental factors critically contribute to the development of bones, most importantly through exercise and mechanical loading. Exercise putting weight on the body results in the growth of bone mass as mechanical stress forces onto the bone matrix, thus increasing strength and density. Activities stimulate osteoblasts, the bone-building cells. Long-term immobilization or inactivity leads to loss of bone mass and to susceptibility to fractures. Further, exposure to sunlight promotes Vitamin D synthesis, linking lifestyle directly to bone health. Exposure to environmental pollutants from the outdoors is another factor that can have undesirable impacts on bone health, with implications for bone density and strength. Adjustment to these environmental, hormonal, and dietary stimuli is crucial to the formation of healthy bone development and prevention of associated diseases in human populations (Dijcker et al., 2011; Babic et al., 2020).

8.3.3. Changes in Bone Density with Age

With advancing age, there are dramatic changes in bone density primarily resulting from alterations in bone remodeling activities. At adolescence, bone growth comes to predominate the process of resorption, stimulating an increase in bone mass and peak bone density during the second half of adolescence or young adulthood. By the third or fourth decade, however, the equation is inverted. The resorption process, regulated by osteoclasts, comes to dominate as bone density slowly declines. This decline is particularly outstanding in women following menopause due to the decrease in levels of estrogen, crucial in retaining bones. Consequently, older adults are at higher risk of osteoporosis, brittle bones, and higher susceptibility to fractures because the vast loss of bone density with increasing age erodes skeletal strength. The aging process also impacts the bone microarchitecture and results in reduced bone strength that further multiplies the risks associated with low bone density. Evidence suggests that age-dependent changes in bone quality extend beyond mere density measurements; they extend to alterations in the trabecular structure as well as cortical thickness. One such study on cynomolgus monkeys revealed that the lumbar volumetric bone mineral density (vBMD) increases at an accelerated rate until around the age of 10 years, after which it declines drastically, primarily among postmenopausal women. The implication of such findings is dire, as it has been observed that preventive interventions and measures to enhance the quality of bones must be prioritized, especially among predisposed postmenopausal women (Zeng et al., 2023). Knowing the mechanisms behind this leads to the understanding of why interventions regarding age-related loss of bone density are necessary. Lifestyle is also equally influential on age-related bone density changes. Normal weight-bearing exercise, proper intake of calcium and vitamin D in the diet, and refraining from smoking or excessive alcohol use could reduce risks for osteoporosis and resultant fractures. For example, the application of bisphosphonate therapy has revealed encouraging results in promoting bone mineral density in high-risk populations, such as nonambulatory children with reduced bone density (Lee et al., 2024). Not only do these treatments undo the effects of aging on bone structure but also address the overall skeletal health. It should be noted that the fight against the loss of bone density is a complex one, involving a strategy of both medical management and change in lifestyle to promote healthier aging and prevent widespread loss of bones in the aging population (Figure 8.11).

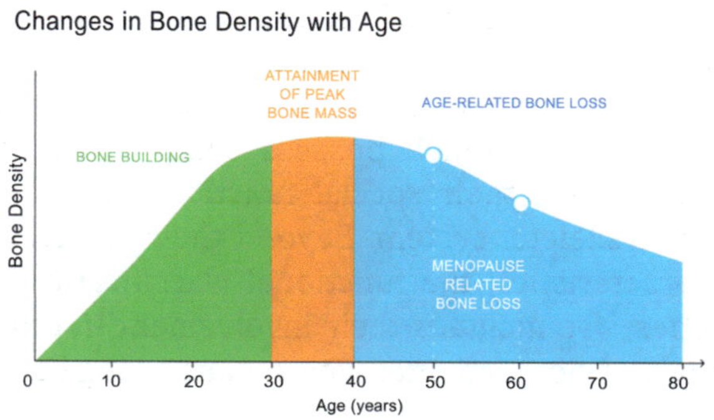

Figure 8.11. Changes in bone density with age.

Source: https://www.austinsimplyfit.com/wp-content/uploads/2021/09/Bone-density-2-e1631577818799-768x471.png.

Test Your Knowledge

1. What is the process of ossification?
2. What are the factors influencing bone growth?

8.4. Types of Bones

Learning Outcome

1. Understand the long bones and their characteristics;
2. Describe the short, flat, and irregular bones;
3. Describe the role of sesamoid bones.

The human skeleton is made up of various classes of bones with varied functions, which are crucial in biomechanics as well as general health. Primarily, bones are classified into four categories: long, short, flat, and irregular bones, which have characteristic structural features and functions. Long bones, such as the femur or humerus, are long bones that allow for motion and bear weight. Short bones, found in the wrists (carpals) and ankles (tarsals), are cuboidal in structure and provide stability and support with little range of motion. Flat bones, such as the skull and ribcage, are primarily for the protection of internal organs and are sites of muscle attachment. Lastly, there are the irregular bones, including vertebrae and facial bones, which possess complex shapes that explain their special functions and roles in the skeletal system. Beyond their structural characteristics, the functional classification of bones also includes their involvement in other physiological activities. For instance, long bones play a significant role in hematopoiesis, a blood cell development process that occurs in the bone marrow held inside them. Meanwhile, flat bones are significant in offering protective coverings for organs, for example, in the thorax, where the ribs offer protection for the lungs and heart. Secondly, irregular shapes of particular bones facilitate articulations that are significant to enhance flexibility and movement. Significantly, unique patterns of anatomical complexity of individual bones have a significant role in human evolution and mobility research. Network analyses show fascinating contrasts, reflecting that while the human forelimb and hindlimb are dissimilar in complexity, they are clearly differentiated for bipedal locomotion and other functional pressures, especially when regarded with our closest relatives, the chimpanzees (Esteve-Altava et al., 2018). The health of these various forms of bones is important in an attempt to preserve a well-functioning skeletal system. Osteoporosis, where bone density is declining, is a disease that can disproportionately affect certain bones, particularly in the elderly, and cause them to be extremely prone to fractures. Solving these issues depends on medical education and technological advancements. For example, the use of multimedia educational packages, such as 3D anatomical models and cadaveric dissections, is a good method for enhancing patient comprehension of the bone condition and the importance of rehabilitation after injury (Buchanan et al., 2014). Through the creation of extensive bone structure and function understanding, patients can more effectively engage in preventative care and comply with treatment instructions, ultimately improving long-term health results related to the skeletal system. Thus, knowledge of the various types of bones and their specific roles favors maintaining the integrity of bones during a lifetime (Figure 8.12).

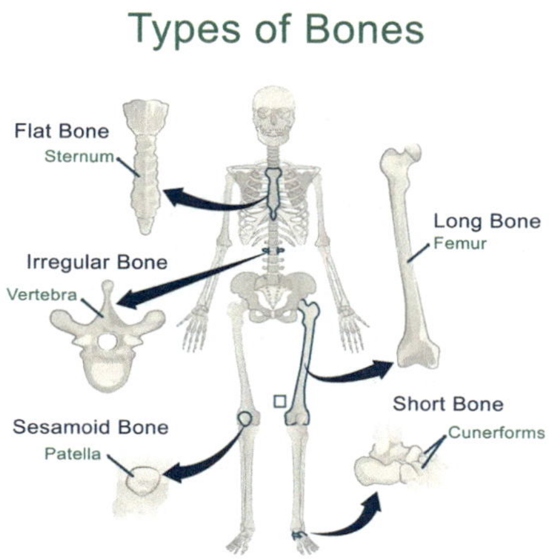

Figure 8.12. Types of bones.

Source: https://media.geeksforgeeks.org/wp-content/uploads/20240326131048/Types-of-Bones.webp.

8.4.1. Long Bones and Their Characteristics

Long bones, which are part of the human skeletal system, exhibit certain characteristics that support their primary functions of movement, support, and protection of important organs. The long bones, including the femur, tibia, and humerus, have their anatomy in common, which includes a diaphysis, epiphyses, and a medullary cavity. The diaphysis, or shaft, is primarily cylindrical and is a structural component contributing to strength, while the epiphyses serve for the joint articulation surfaces. The endosteum-lined medullary cavity holds bone marrow and plays an essential role in hematopoiesis and fat deposition. Such a sophisticated structure allows efficient force transmission during movement, illustrating the evolutionary advancements that have optimized long bones in their various functions in human physiology. The histological organization of long bones reveals crucial information regarding their functioning and strength. Composed primarily of compact bone, which is dense and organized in the shape of structural units known as osteons, long bones are strong enough to withstand severe mechanical loads. The outermost layer, the periosteum, has a dense network of blood vessels and nerves and is involved in the metabolic function and healing processes of the bones. Additionally, the trabecular or spongy bone within the epiphyses internally also enhances the strength-to-weight ratio to allow maximized movement at reduced expense of energy.

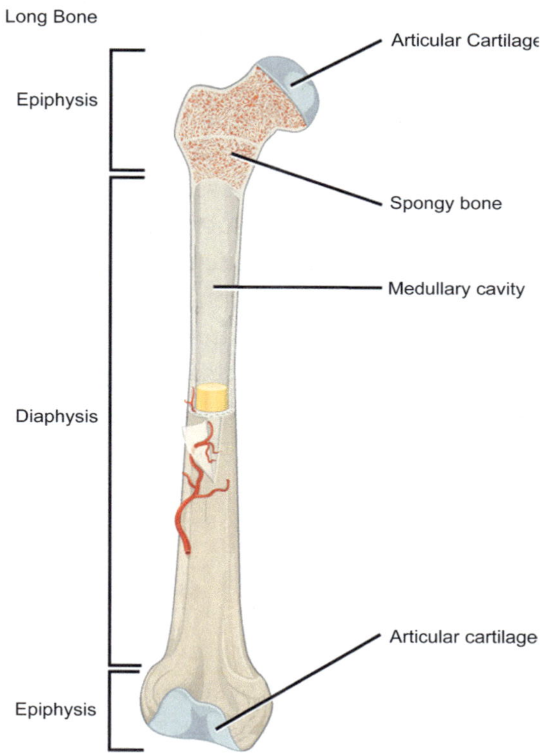

Figure 8.13. The long bone is covered by articular cartilage at either end and contains bone marrow (shown in yellow in this illustration) in the marrow cavity.

Source: https://s3-us-west-2.amazonaws.com/courses-images/wp-content/uploads/sites/1223/2017/02/07235425/Figure_38_02_02.jpg.

Studies have indicated that long bone microarchitecture variations may be associated with physical activity levels and general well-being, and the significance of these characteristics in assessing the skeleton's health and the effect of lifestyle on bone health (Simmons et al., 2016). In addition, the burial and processing of long bones in archaeological sites reveal more about social practice and cultural tradition. By examining the taphonomic processes responsible for bone preservation, conspicuous variation in human remains treatment from other animals has been discerned. For instance, preferential faunal remains modification at certain archaeological sites indicates culturally instituted practices that define the processing of different species, including social positions accorded to them. The analysis of this differentiation has the potential to illuminate broader cultural attitudes towards life and death, which raises questions about human–animal relations in past societies. Knowledge of these practices is crucial, for modern research may uncover the impact of past rituals on existing society norms for handling remains, highlighting the prominence of bone traits in both biological and sociocultural contexts (Madgwick, 2008) (Figure 8.13).

8.4.2. Short, Flat, and Irregular Bones

The human skeletal system contains an assortment of bone types, each with its own special structure and function. Among all of them, short, flat, and irregular bones play very significant roles in offering the integrity and function of the body. Short bones, such as those that exist at the wrists and ankles, are usually cube-shaped and provide stability while allowing the capacity to move slightly. Their design enables them to bear weight and absorb shock, an essential characteristic for the joints they support. In addition, flat bones , such as the skull and ribcage have protective functions, shielding important organs and offering broad surfaces for muscle attachment. Abnormal bones , such as the vertebrae, possess intricate designs allowing them special functions, providing support and flexibility to the spinal cord. These variations in bone type serve to illustrate the marvelous flexibility of the human bony system. Increased investigation of flat bones reveals their essential function in the overall physiology of the body. Flat bones are structurally composed of two parallel compact layers of bone separated by a layer of spongy bone or diploë. This structure provides not only strength and stiffness but also reduces weight, an advantage when considering mobility.

The flat bones in the skull protect the brain and facilitate the attachment of many muscles, crucial in the movement of the head and facial expressions. Furthermore, red bone marrow in flat bones, in their spongy center, is a hematopoietic area where blood cells are generated. This intricate function emphasizes the significance of flat bones in protection and body physiology, emphasizing their need for human health. Irregular bones with asymmetrical shapes also confer some advantages necessary for human function. The vertebrae, one of irregular bones in themselves, not only provide body structure but also protect the spinal cord, part of the nervous system. Each vertebras unique structure permits flexibility and range of motion to provide for bending and twisting activities. In addition, irregular bones typically incorporate various features like spines, wings, or processes that serve as points of attachment for ligaments and muscles. This complexity provides the body's ability to execute a large number of diverse movements and withstand stress. As our knowledge of bone types evolves, work on innovations like regenerative medicine and additive manufacturing is transforming our methods for bone repair and regeneration, promising better results for conditions that impact these fundamental skeletal structures (Tofail et al., 2017; Zakrzewski et al., 2019) (Figure 8.14).

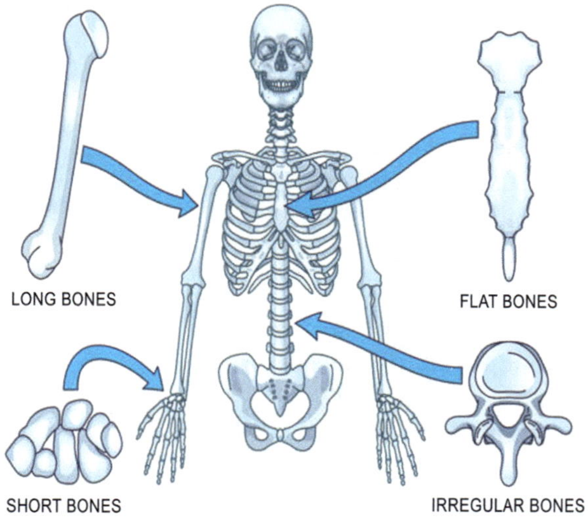

Figure 8.14. Shapes of bones.

Source: https://media.istockphoto.com/id/2082297857/vector/shapes-of-bones-with-anatomical-human-skeleton-shape-division-outline-diagram.jpg?s=612x612&w=0&k=20&c=jdJ_S9xYoRSJgS53vwx3uwPuEAHvw3sJg9P6NYw7YU4=.

8.4.3. The Role of Sesamoid Bones

The human skeleton is highly diverse, consisting of a vast array of bone types, all with specific functions critical to locomotion and support. Among these, sesamoid bones are most crucial, with the sole function of enhancing the mechanical efficiency of joints and tendons. They are tiny oval bones that are key components within tendons, allowing them to deflect forces developed during movement. For instance, the patella, which is the largest of the sesamoid bones, is used to increase the leverage of the quadriceps muscle, thereby increasing the force developed when extending the knee. This indicates the importance of sesamoid bones not only in mechanical advantage but also in lessening tendons' wear and tear, highlighting their importance from both functional and evolutionary viewpoints. The function of sesamoid bones extends beyond mere structural support and demonstrates their presence as an integral part of the dynamics of motion, in effect resulting in effective human movement. In addition to mechanical advantage, sesamoid bones also play a protective function. As a shock absorber between tendons and bone structures around them, sesamoid bones effectively absorb tendons from abrasion and damage caused by friction in stressful movements. The existence of sesamoid bones, therefore, brings a degree of toughness to the musculoskeletal system, particularly to high-impact actions , such as running and jumping. Their dispersed presence in numerous locations, such as the hands and feet, distinguishes their function of having evolved to both bipedal and multi-directional motion. In addition, their unique embryonic development, through differentiation from tendons subjected to mechanical stress, suggests an adaptive advantage in situations requiring vigorous locomotion. Overall, these points highlight the complex functions of sesamoid bones and their complexity within the human skeletal system. Further research also reveals further insight into the potential variability of sesamoid bones among various populations, in the direction of lifestyle and activity adaptation. Awareness of these distinctions can inform us about differences in health and mobility between populations. Furthermore, conditions like sesamoiditis, an inflammation of these bones, suggest the need for further study of their role in both healthy movements and disease. As more recent studies adopting advanced methodologies, such as Anatomical Network Analysis, have now begun to deconstruct intricate musculoskeletal interactions, the role of sesamoid bones also continues to unfold within the greater scheme of human anatomy. The classification of sesamoid bones within this framework not only serves to identify their pertinence to normal physiological function but also the complexity that comes with studying human skeletal adaptations, once more emphasizing their role in the history of bone in humans (Mitchell, 2014; Diogo et al., 2015) (Figure 8.15).

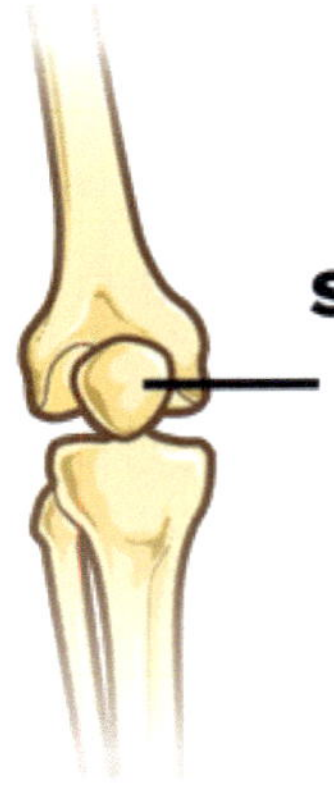

Figure 8.15. The patella is a sesamoid bone found in the knee.

Source: https://images.my.labster.com/v2/LOS/98487eea-860e-499c-bcab-0793dcefaf1d/LOS_SesamoidBones.en.x256.png.

Test Your Knowledge

1. What are the long bones and their characteristics?
2. What is the role of sesamoid bones?

8.5. Bone Health and Diseases

Learning Outcome

1. Describe the common bone diseases;
2. Understand the impact of nutrition on bone health;
3. Understand the importance of physical activity for bone strength.

Bone health and the prevalence of diseases , such as osteoporosis result from the complex interplay of biological, environmental, and lifestyle determinants. Bone density, one of the most important measurements of bone health, is influenced by variable determinants including genes, diet, and physical activity. Of these determinants, nutrition is a modifiable risk factor, particularly in the prevention and management of osteoporotic conditions. Calcium and vitamin D are widely recognized to play roles in bone metabolism, but as evidence mounts, so does the interest in the role of B vitamins. These vitamins have key roles in cellular metabolism, yet evidence has been inconsistent regarding their influence on mineral density and bone turnover. While clinical trials have suggested potential benefits in terms of overall plasma homocysteine concentration, evidence of their effect on fracture risk in the short term remains unclear and further studies are needed to define the mechanisms of these relationships (Ilesanmi-Oyelere & Kruger, 2023). Vitamin D thus stands as one of the key determinants of healthy skeletal structures; lack of vitamin D makes patients prone to greater risks of fragility fracture and chronic diseases. Evidence establishes the necessity of attaining optimal levels of vitamin D not just for bone-related benefits but also for extraskeletal benefits. A position paper by the European Society for Clinical and Economic Aspects of Osteoporosis and Osteoarthritis has accumulated evidence that confirms that certain supplementation in high-risk groups is necessary. Recent guidelines emphasize the need to evaluate the role of vitamin D beyond its function of simple calcium absorption, particularly in light of the promising but inconclusive evidence around its use in treating autoimmune diseases and heart health. Specifically, although certain research supports higher serum concentrations of 25-hydroxy vitamin D, the safety and effectiveness of exceeding threshold guidelines are still to be fully determined, highlighting the need for more thorough studies (Cianferotti et al., 2017). Incorporating a multi-dimensional model of bone health involves understanding both disease prevention strategies and therapeutic care for bone disorders. Modifiable risk factor modification , such as diet and exercise, can also have significant effects on bone health outcomes. Daily weight-bearing physical activity and adequate use of the necessary nutrients , such as calcium and vitamin D, can enhance bone density and lower the risk of osteoporotic conditions. Moreover, public health interventions to inform individuals about the impact of lifestyle choices on bone health are imperative. With an aging population susceptible to bone diseases, targeted education campaigns can help individuals make better choices and enhance their probability of having healthier bones. Lastly, encouraging an integrated understanding of bone health and innovative research will be needed to advance preventative and therapeutic strategies to mitigate the worldwide bone disorder burden (Ilesanmi-Oyelere & Kruger, 2023).

8.5.1. Common Bone Diseases (e.g., Osteoporosis)

Bones' complex organization and fundamental function are often disturbed by prevalent bone diseases, of which osteoporosis, osteoarthritis, and rheumatoid arthritis are significant diseases applicable to the health of elderly populations. Osteoporosis, the loss of bone density and resulting increase in bone fragility, increases the risk of fracture, therefore impairing mobility and overall well-being. This disorder is increasing in prevalence among elderly individuals, particularly among women postmenopause, due to the hormonal changes affecting bone development and resorption. The silent onset of osteoporosis can lead to disastrous skeletal fractures, particularly of the hip, wrist, and spine, making early screening and treatment so vital to manage this disorder. Sophisticated diagnostic methods, such as dual-energy X-ray absorptiometry (DEXA) scans, have made it possible to diagnose early low bone density, making it possible to implement timely therapeutic interventions that are capable of slowing the risk of fractures. In addition to osteoporosis, osteoarthritis is the other common bone disease, characterized primarily by joint cartilage and subchondral bone loss. The pathologic process tends to result in significant pain, stiffness, and functional impairment in the joints, negatively impacting the quality of life of individuals affected. Being a degenerative condition, the incidence of osteoarthritis rises with age, usually compounded by obesity, joint trauma, and genetic susceptibility. The cartilage that enables movement in the joints loses its elasticity and cushion with age, ultimately forming bone spurs and joint lining swelling. Successfully treating osteoarthritis typically involves making lifestyle changes, physical therapy, and pain management methods that can significantly restore mobility while reducing pain. Rheumatoid arthritis, another systemic disorder of the systems of bone and joints, is an autoimmune condition that results in chronic inflammation of the joints, leading to pain and potential joint destruction. Unlike osteoarthritis, which is usually a result of wear and tear, rheumatoid arthritis involves the immune system attacking the synovial membrane inadvertently, resulting in swelling and erosion of bone and cartilage. This long-standing disease may lead to joint deformity and extreme functional impairment as time progresses, particularly if not treated. Rheumatoid arthritis is generally treated with the administration of disease-modifying antirheumatic drugs (DMARDs) and biologics to prevent disease progression and alleviate symptoms. In addition, recent evidence indicates that lifestyle, such as dietary elements like tea, have been implicated in the regulation of inflammation and bone health, and emphasis should be placed on integrated methods for treating prevalent diseases of bone (Xie et al., 2024; Rhee, 2025) (Figure 8.16).

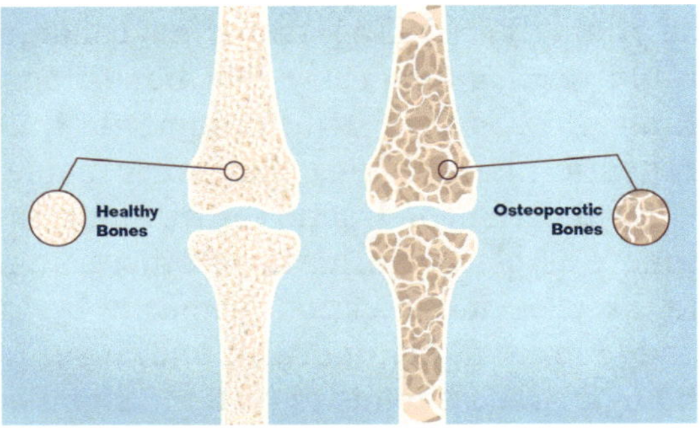

Figure 8.16. Bone diseases.

Source: https://lh7-rt.googleusercontent.com/docsz/AD_4nXdtPKCNy30EAUeYHpzkw6Wkf60W9kWMxxUtsPsqLvx1DDc6Ekzi_VSAerv-q44_n3du99bcEg4EbpqAYIb8UHXqwjBV7SijUPCYLaqYnYK52ewRtHjBHJDXN1pefvpG1shgQH_1NDOio5QH-A5txSrfksYW?key=dISz3DG-Iw54A86ren0bwA.

8.5.2. Impact of Nutrition on Bone Health

Nutrition plays a fundamental role in the maintenance of bone health, as correct intake of nutrients is compulsory for bone density and structural strength. Key nutrients like calcium and vitamin D have been of particular interest because of their roles in bone metabolism. Calcium plays a role in building and maintaining bone tissue, while vitamin D helps in the intake of calcium from the intestines, thereby providing bones with the minerals necessary for maximum strength. The research highlights the need to personalize nutrition strategies to populations, and in particular, women, who may suffer from heightened vulnerability to osteoporosis and its related syndromes in old age. In their appreciation of the interaction between bone health and nutrition, scientists are more likely to provide appropriate dietary interventions that are likely to prevent bone degeneration and associated diseases, hence immensely enhancing health outcomes for at-risk groups, mainly women who tend to be more susceptible to bone health problems throughout their lifespan (Moran, 2022). In addition to calcium and vitamin D, other dietary components , such as protein, magnesium, and vitamin K, play important roles in bone structure. Protein is necessary for the production of collagen, a structural substance of bone tissue, and has been shown to influence bone density positively. Magnesium is also involved in bone construction and is employed to activate vitamin D, once again elevating the uptake of calcium. Vitamin K assists in the formation of proteins needed for the mineralization of bones. All these nutrients taken together in an overall diet can prevent osteoporosis and fractures. Since nutritional science is constantly being updated, there must be more research to determine the best diets that may promote bone health among various groups of people, thereby pointing to the importance of nutrition as part of preventive health measures (Smith, 2000). Lastly, the connection between nutrition and bone health emphasizes the necessity to include dietary assessment in health care management. For instance, those who execute long-duration space travel and experience significant physiological changes, such as bone decalcification, represent a compelling example of the necessity for the evaluation of nutrient metabolism under different conditions. NASA's studies on the nutritional requirements of astronauts highlight the need for individually tailored dietary interventions to offset the specific challenges of microgravity, where traditional nutritional guidance may not be sufficient. These studies focus on essential nutrients, like calcium, which plays a critical role in avoiding bone loss. By fostering a culture that supports continuous research about nutrition's impact on bone health, we can create well-educated diet recommendations that not only benefit astronauts but also extend to the general population, enhancing bone health on a global level (Smith, 2000; Moran, 2022).

8.5.3. Importance of Physical Activity for Bone Strength

Physical activity plays a key role in the preservation of bone strength, particularly through the process of bone remodeling. Through weight-bearing exercise, the mechanical stresses acting on bones will stimulate osteoblasts, the bone-building cells, to reinforce bones and enhance their density. This physical reaction not only maintains skeletal integrity but also reduces the potential for fracture, especially in cohorts like postmenopausal women in whom bone density would otherwise decrease. Exercise can thus actually reverse physiologic bone loss that occurs with age and sedentary lifestyle, establishing the need for active engagement in running, jumping, and resistance-type exercise. When individuals incorporate these activities into their routine, they establish a foundation of bone resilience that provides lifetime musculoskeletal health. Secondly, some high-impact exercises have been found to induce quantifiable changes in bone material properties. A trial of healthy postmenopausal women highlights that a highly designed high-impact exercise program led to a statistically significant 7% improvement in the bone material strength index (BMSi) of the intervention limb within a three-month duration, demonstrating the causative effect between the level of exercise and bone strengthening. These outcomes further confirm the worth of specific physical activities that utilize bone loading, significantly raising both external bone density and the microstructure of the bone itself. This would mean that structured exercise programs should be promoted proactively, particularly in the elderly or at-risk groups, where emphasis is given to interventions enhancing mechanical loading of the skeletal system for improved bone function and quality (Hellgren et al., 2018). Apart from physical disability, nutrition and supplementation also play a critical role in maximizing the effect of physical exercise on bone quality. The interplay of creatine supplementation, for instance, can enhance muscle strength and contribute to improved adaptation to exercise. These adaptations are critical, especially in populations at risk for bone loss or density, as in cancer patients receiving treatments that may lead to diminished muscle mass. With the synergism of nutritional approaches with regular physical activity, people can achieve a superior outcome concerning bone strength and musculoskeletal well-being in general. This multi-component strategy emphasizes that promotion of physical activity, in addition to improvement in nutrition, constitutes a holistic strategy to ensure optimum bone strength, essential in maintaining independence and quality of life in various populations (Fairman et al., 2018) (Figure 8.17).

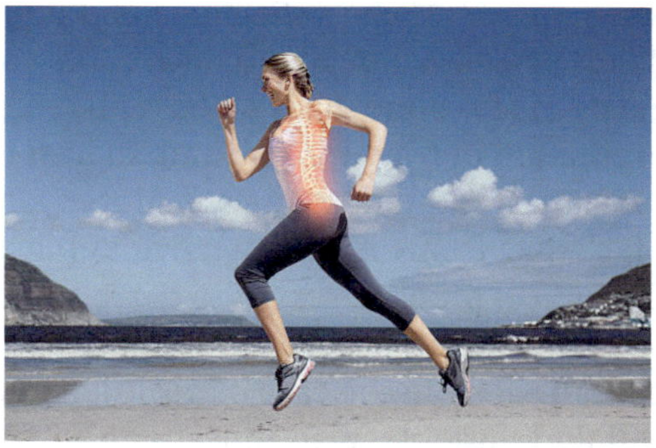

Figure 8.17. Importance of exercise for healthy bones.

Source: https://oaidocs.com/wp-content/uploads/2023/03/istockphoto-479572586-612x612-1.jpg

Test Your Knowledge

1. What is the most common bone disease?
2. What is the importance of physical activity for bone strength?

8.6. Diagnostic Techniques for Bone Health

Learning Outcome

1. Understand the X-rays and their role in bone assessment;
2. Describe the MRI and CT scans for detailed imaging;
3. Understand the bone density tests and their significance.

Bone health assessment is a critical part of human physiology knowledge and the prevention of conditions , such as osteoporosis. Among the numerous diagnostic tests employed, dual-energy X-ray absorptiometry (DEXA) is one of the gold standards to assess the bone mineral density (BMD). This non-invasive imaging technique uses two distinct X-ray beams to compute bone density in regions of greatest risk for osteoporosis, such as the spine and hip. The precision of DEXA not only contributes to the diagnosis of low bone mass diseases but also to the prediction of fracture risk and, therefore, to appropriate treatment guidance. Moreover, the very fact that DEXA is in extensive application within clinical practice serves to corroborate its status as a routine procedure for testing bone health, especially in the case of postmenopausal women and patients aged more than 50 years, wherein cases of osteoporosis are very much prevalent. Other than DEXA, quantitative computed tomography (QCT) is a newer modality with three-dimensional bone density and structure measurement. Unlike DEXA, which is predominantly interested in mineral density, QCT provides valuable information regarding the structure of trabecular and cortical bone, which can identify subtle changes in bone health that cannot be detected with conventional methods. This is especially important in metabolic bone disease, in which bone microstructural change may precede detectable change in BMD. The ability of QCT to quantify volumetric bone density allows for more comprehensive evaluation, a feature that is valuable in the follow-up of the efficacy of therapeutic measures. With the advancement of bone biology, the integration of advanced imaging techniques like QCT into clinical practice could result in earlier diagnosis and improved treatment of bone diseases. Ultrasound technology is also becoming more widely recognized as a non-invasive approach to measuring bone health and holds several advantages over traditional ionizing radiation methods. Specifically, ultrasound can measure the mechanical competency and fracture risk of bones without exposing patients to harmful radiation. It is also very useful in children, where minimizing radiation exposure is of paramount importance. New evidence shows that ultrasound is quite capable of quantifying cortical bone thickness and elasticity, which both have high correlation with conventional bone density measurements. Moreover, the portability and inexpensiveness of ultrasound provide a gratifying option for mass screening programs, particularly in underserved communities. With research continuously developing the application of ultrasound for the diagnosis of bone health, it could augment the current techniques like DEXA and QCT, leading to a more inclusive system of evaluating and maintaining bone health in the population of humans (NASA Publication, 1988) (Figure 8.18).

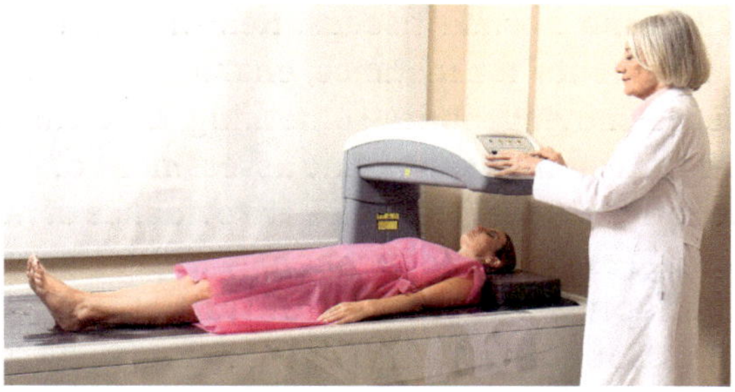

Figure 8.18. Bone density scan (DEXA scan).

Source: https://healthybonesaustralia.org.au/wp-content/uploads/2023/10/dexa-bone-density-scan.jpg.

8.6.1. X-Rays and Their Role in Bone Assessment

The advent of the X-ray technology has brought a new dimension in medical imaging, particularly in assessing bone strength and health. By using high-energy electromagnetic radiation, X-rays can pass through soft tissues but image more dense structures , such as bones. The capability facilitates diagnostic fractures, identifies diseases in bones, and assesses the structural integrity of the skeleton. X-ray imaging not only provides a two-dimensional representation of bone but also allows clinicians to evaluate the alignment and status of numerous disparate skeletal components. Consequently, this non-invasive approach has become a recognized diagnostic modality in both orthopedics and emergency medicine, enabling patient management and treatment planning. Moreover, X-ray imaging is crucial for continuous bone density and skeletal status evaluation, particularly in individuals at risk of osteoporosis development. Bone density is crucial for evaluating bone strength and resistance and to predict fractures and other trauma. Techniques , such as dual-energy X-ray absorptiometry (DEXA) provide precise values of bone mineral density, which gives valuable information regarding an individual's risk factors. Understanding of these factors is essential to preventive medicine, especially among elderly individuals with a high incidence of osteoporosis. X-rays allow for proactive healthcare in this regard through early diagnosis and treatment before clinical fracture, improving patient outcomes greatly through earlier diagnosis and treatment. X-ray technology is constantly evolving, allowing for enhanced imaging and diagnostic quality. Technological innovations , such as digital X-rays give higher picture quality, lower doses of radiation, and quicker data handling, aiding clinicians in their diagnosis. Additionally, growth in 3D imaging techniques aids in more precise evaluations of complex fractures and other abnormalities of bone morphology. All these advancements underscore the pivotal position X-rays play in medical imaging and orthopedic care overall. By being accurate and responsive to technological advancements, X-rays remain a fundamental component of bone assessment, informing treatment and ultimately improving healthcare outcomes for patients with varied skeletal conditions (NASA Publication, 1988; ; Palacio, 2020) (Figure 8.19).

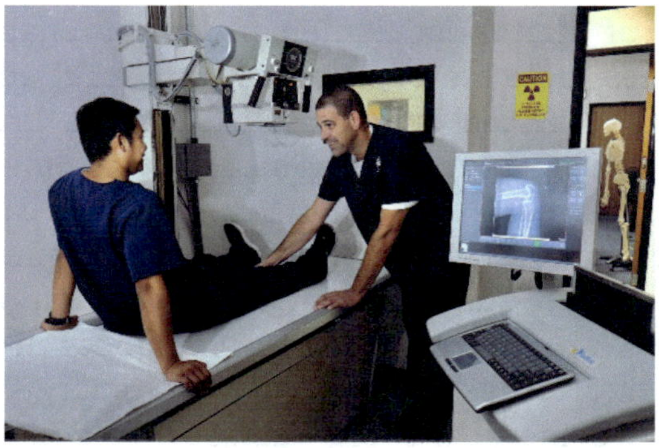

Figure 8.19. X-rays in diagnosing bone fractures.

Source: https://lakezurichopenmri.com/wp-content/uploads/2024/09/X-Rays-in-Diagnosing-Bone-Fractures.jpg.

8.6.2. Magnetic Resonance Imaging (MRI) and Computed Tomography (CT) scans for detailed imaging

The evolution of imaging technologies, particularly MRI and CT, has revolutionized the diagnosis and treatment of bone disorders in humans. Both methods offer precise, subtle details and images of bone anatomy, with the ability to clearly identify fractures, tumors, and other abnormalities. MRI employs strong magnetic fields and radio waves to produce detailed images of soft tissues and bone, thereby enabling an understanding of the intricate anatomical relationships within the musculoskeletal system. CT scans, on the other hand, merge many X-ray images taken from various angles and compile them by means of computer technology in an effort to provide cross-sectional views of bone, which are crucial in determining bone structure and quality. In combination, these imaging techniques provide practitioners with valuable information, enhancing patient care and treatment outcomes in osteology and orthopedics. The incorporation of digital imaging within both MRI and CT has also made them more effective. Recent advances in computer technology have facilitated the processing of data at higher speeds and resulting in sharper and more accurate diagnostic images. Use of digital acquisition processes enables images to be stored, recalled, and acquired in a way that can be accessed without a break on several platforms. These advancements have played a key role in complicated cases where accurate bone information is required, such as pre-surgical planning or post-surgical follow-up. Interestingly, developments in CT imaging techniques, such as dual-energy CT, can provide dual-energy datasets to assist in characterizing bone lesions. Therefore, the ability to create high-quality images at speed literally translates into enhanced clinical decision-making and management of bone health, as both modalities complement each other in providing a comprehensive appreciation of skeletal pathology and anatomy. Both CT scans and MRI also continue to advance with new advancements in contrast agents and imaging equipment. Better contrast agents render bone structures even more visible, as well as improve the ability to differentiate between disease and normal tissues. Real-time imaging advancements, for instance, enable clinicians to observe moving bone, something that can be quite critical in the dynamic assessment of joint function. These technologies are evidence of how ongoing research and technology improvements are shaping the future of radiology. The application of non-invasive angiography via these imaging modalities is further evidence of their usefulness in examining the vascular element associated with bone health. With these continued improvements, CT and MRI scans are today invaluable tools in the modern medical era, ultimately resulting in a better understanding of bone in human anatomy and more effective treatment procedures (N/A, 2004; Vassallo, 2004) (Figure 8.20).

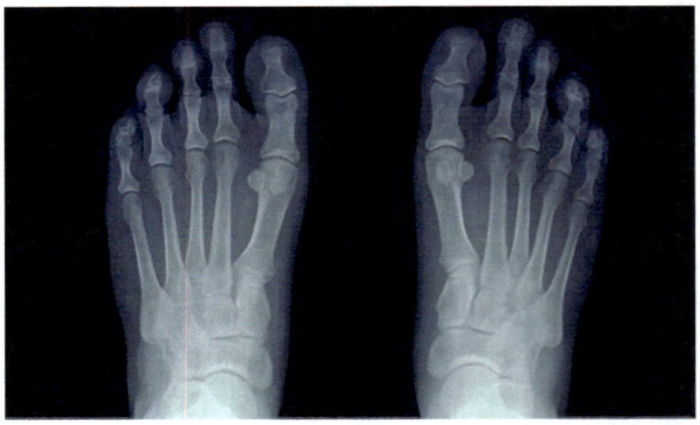

Figure 8.20. Computer tomography (CT) scans for bone imaging.

Source: https://kiranpetct.com/wp-content/uploads/2023/06/CT-scan-bones.jpg.

8.6.3. Bone Density Tests and Their Significance

Bone density tests are significant in assessing skeletal well-being and fracture risk in patients, particularly the old. The most prevalent technique for estimating bone density is dual-energy X-ray absorptiometry (DXA), whereby it measures bone mineral content, which is useful to clinicians with critical information on bone strength. Because there is such a direct relationship between bone mineral density (BMD) and osteoporotic fracture risk, the significance of these tests cannot be overestimated. Better BMD typically means stronger bones, and poorer scores mean increased susceptibility to breakage. With regular screening, especially in vulnerable populations, health care providers can initiate prophylactic therapy aimed at maintaining bone strength and avoiding secondary complicating factors related to fragile bones. New methods have been established in recent studies to complement routine DXA assessment. For instance, near-infrared spectroscopy (NIRS) has emerged with potential as a non-surgical means for assessing intraosseous vasculature and the relationship between vascular health and bone strength. NIRS's ability to measure blood flow through bony structures provides a new methodology for studying the vascular component of bone health because vascular disease has been linked with reduced bone strength. Research has indicated that NIRS-based markers can show correlations with BMD values obtained through DXA and other imaging devices to yield a better understanding of the determinants of bone density (Ball et al., 2021). Such technological advancements not only give us a clearer view of skeletal tissue but also accompany the ever-broadening quest for new types of diagnostic methods in the practice of bone health. Furthermore, the application of bone density measurements extends beyond mere fracture prediction; they detail physiological adaptation and response to exercise. For example, studies involving throwing athletes have shown how mechanical stress can provoke cortical bone parameters to produce increased bone mineral content in areas of strain. The longitudinal adaptations observed between the throwing and non-throwing arm demonstrate the body's adaptive ability, showing how specialized physical activity can optimize bone health (Weatherholt & Warden, 2018). The association reinforces the importance of bone density tests to inform exercise regimens and bone health interventions. Through the convergence of findings from different methodologies, clinicians and researchers can better address the sophistication of bone health and craft personalized strategies that enable improved skeletal development in various populations (Figure 8.21).

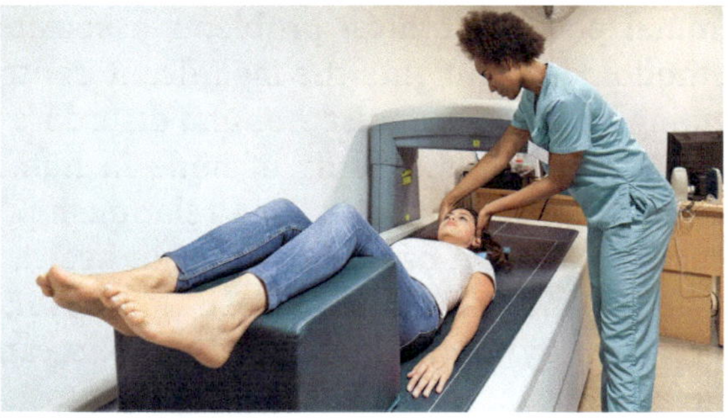

Figure 8.21. Bone density test.

Source: https://media.post.rvohealth.io/wp-content/uploads/2023/10/young-female-bone-density-scan-1296-728-header.jpg.

Test Your Knowledge

1. Why is x-ray used for bones?
2. What is the bone density tests and their significance?

SUMMARY

In the overview of the investigation into bone in man, one needs to take into account the sophisticated functions bone plays in the human body beyond that of structural support. Bones are not dead, static tissues, but are vital and are involved in continuous remodeling throughout life, suggestive of their ability to adapt to altering physiological stress and environmental trauma. The intricate interplay of osteoclasts and osteoblasts illustrates the ongoing processes of bone reabsorption and bone growth, maintaining bone integrity and density. Moreover, the importance of bone health extends to systemic health conditions, most notably osteoporosis and other degenerative conditions that underscore the importance of preventive approaches to preserving bone strength. The full understanding of bone functions directs medical interventions as well as individual health programs, underscoring the importance of additional studies on biological processes regulating such mechanisms. Moreover, with the advancement of imaging technology, our view of bone has expanded as a complex and multifunctional system. Techniques , such as second-harmonic generation microscopy allow researchers to study the microstructural order of collagen fibers within bone tissue, demonstrating how factors, including genetic influences , such as decorin, influence collagen organization and bone strength. Close examination of these structures provides insight into conditions compromising bone integrity, paving the way for targeted therapeutic interventions. As indicated, the ability to study existing data makes possible the combination of bone biology knowledge with minimal possible ethical problems associated with direct human investigation. Such pioneering methodology highlights the significant contribution of imaging specialists and researchers in the ongoing battle against diseases and disorders of bones, marking a milestone in radiographic practice. In total, the understanding of bone in humans is full of biological, medical, and social meaning that goes beyond anatomy. The relationship between bone health and general health has led to it being a focal point of research within health sciences, particularly with increasing health issues to the public, including osteoporosis. Moreover, the role of radiographers in this discipline cannot be overstated; by their expert position, one can access and interpret valuable osteological data that bridges the gaps between imaging diagnosis and clinical practice. As new research emerges, and particularly in collagen remodeling and what it reveals regarding bone pathology, interdisciplinary cooperation needs to be advanced to achieve breakthroughs that are translated into improved clinical outcomes. The integration of technological advances and biological understanding predicts an era in which bone health may be more effectively watched over, sustained, and treated, thereby optimizing the quality of life in individuals at all points of their life cycle.

Understanding the intricacy of bone disease is critical in the design of treatment modalities for the numerous bone diseases. A crucial aspect of bone health is the intricate remodeling processes that involve many cell types, including osteoblasts, osteoclasts, and tenocytes residing in tendons. Cell dynamics are essential to maintain bone integrity, and alterations in their function can result in diseases like osteoarthritis or tendinopathy. For instance, chronic tendon pathology, often characterized by changes in the structure of the extracellular matrix, emphasizes the importance of a balanced remodeling response. Type III collagen and other marker overexpression may indicate repair events but could also indicate an adaptive response to mechanical stressors. Hence, familiarity with these changes deepens our insight into bone pathologies and their treatment (Riley, 2008). Bone remodeling correlates very closely with the biomechanical forces that the skeleton is subjected to, and there exists a direct connection between physical activity and osseous health. Research has shown that mechanical loading stimulates osteogenic activity that increases bone density and the strength of bones. However, insufficient mechanical loading might contribute to atrophy and susceptibility to injury. The efficacy of bisphosphonates and effect on early bone loss, particularly in the context of osteoarthritis, is a classic illustration of this dilemma. Prevention of post-traumatic trabecular bone loss was possible with high-dose alendronate treatment but had no influence on long-term degeneration. This paradox reflects the challenge of successfully treating disease of the bone while leaving intact the adaptive processes of the skeleton. In addition, the bone resorption and formation biochemical markers observed as a response to trauma demonstrate the intricate balance between biological process and mechanical demand (Khorasani et al., 2015). Synthesis knowledge for bone pathologies needs a multi-disciplinary strategy that is concerned with both the biochemical and physiological determinants of bone health. The interrelatedness of tendons and bones, as evidenced by the role of metalloproteinases in tendon matrix degradation, is the interrelated nature of musculoskeletal tissues. Interestingly, chronic disease , such as tendinopathy illustrates how dysregulation of one system can have an impact on others, leading to systemic issues in bone health. In building therapeutic approaches, discovery of specific molecular targets of treatment becomes increasingly vital. Therapy of the causative agents of bone and tendon structural changes has the promise of opening more effective therapies, ultimately enhancing patient outcomes. Continued study of these interactions will not only increase our understanding of bone disease but also refine treatments that will eventually prevent joint and bone degeneration in the long term (Riley, 2008).

KEY TERMS FROM THIS CHAPTER

- Blood cells
- Collagen fibers
- Cortical bone
- Hematopoiesis
- Lamellar bone
- Musculoskeletal system
- Skeletal system
- Cancellous bone
- Compact bone
- Fibrous protein
- Hydroxyapatite
- Morphology
- Osteology
- Spongy bone

CRITICAL THINKING QUESTIONS

1. **The primary function of bones in the human body is:**
   a. Blood filtration
   b. Structural support and protection
   c. Hormonal secretion
   d. Oxygen transportation
2. **Bones are classified as:**
   a. Muscular tissue
   b. Nervous tissue
   c. Connective tissue
   d. Epithelial tissue
3. **The main structural protein in bone is:**
   a. Elastin
   b. Actin
   c. Myosin
   d. Collagen
4. **The femur is an example of a:**
   a. Long bone
   b. Short bone
   c. Flat bone
   d. Irregular bone
5. **Which of the following is an example of a flat bone?**
   a. Tibia
   b. Sternum
   c. Humerus
   d. Carpal

Short Answer Questions

1. What is the simple definition of bone?
2. Why are bones important in the human body?
3. What are the functions of bones?
4. Describe the process of bone development and growth in humans.
5. List the types of bones.

Answers to Critical Thinking Questions

1. (b); 2. (c) ; 3. (d); 4. (a); 5. (b)

REFERENCES

1. Woronowicz, K.C., Schneider, R.A. Molecular and cellular mechanisms underlying the evolution of form and function in the amniote jaw. *EvoDevo* **10**, 17 (2019). https://doi.org/10.1186/s13227-019-0131-8(accessed on 7th August 2025).
2. Aerts, P., Ayuso, M., Prims, S., Van Cruchten, S., et al. (2019). *Does intrauterine crowding affect the force generating capacity and muscle composition of the piglet front limb?* https://core.ac.uk/download/287940318.pdf (accessed on 7th August 2025).
3. Allen, M. R., Chen, N. X., Hill Gallant, K. M., Lachcik, P. J., et al. (2019). *Effect of ovariectomy on the progression of chronic kidney disease-mineral bone disorder (CKD-MBD) in female Cy/+ rats*. https://core.ac.uk/download/227054397.pdf (accessed on 7th August 2025).
4. Khorasani, M. S., Diko, S., Hsia, A. W., Anderson, M. J., Genetos, D. C., Haudenschild, D. R., & Christiansen, B. A. (2015). Effect of alendronate on post-traumatic osteoarthritis induced by anterior cruciate ligament rupture in mice. *Arthritis research & therapy*, *17*(1), 30. https://doi.org/10.1186/s13075-015-0546-0 (accessed on 7th August 2025).
5. Andreis, M. E., Cattaneo, C., Cummaudo, M., Di Giancamillo, A., et al. (2017). *Swine cortical and cancellous bone: Histomorphometric and densitometric characterization*. https://core.ac.uk/download/296280482.pdf (accessed on 7th August 2025).
6. Argárate, N., Arrabal, P. M., Becerra-Ratia, J., Belmonte, J., et al. (2015). *A model of maxilla resection to test new hybrid implants: Macroporous titanium and tissue engineering elements*. https://core.ac.uk/download/62905155.pdf (accessed on 7th August 2025).
7. Aspden, R. M., Bruel, A., Chen, L., Delville, C., et al. (2015). *The effects of graded levels of calorie restriction: I. Impact of short-term calorie and protein restriction on body composition in the C57BL/6 mouse*. https://core.ac.uk/download/30435703.pdf (accessed on 7th August 2025).
8. Babic, M., van der Giet, M., Herrmann, J., Schuchardt, M., et al. (2020). *Research Models for Studying Vascular Calcification*. https://core.ac.uk/download/323258131.pdf (accessed on 7th August 2025).
9. Baldin, E. K., Giròn Bastidas, J., Godoi, T. P. M., Machado, D. C., et al. (2021). *Biomaterials for bone regeneration: An orthopedic and dentistry overview*. https://core.ac.uk/download/479499360.pdf (accessed on 7th August 2025).
10. Ball, S., Casanova, F., Fulford, J., Knapp, K. M., et al. (2021). *In vivo measurement of intraosseous vascular hemodynamic markers in human bone tissue utilizing near infrared spectroscopy*. https://core.ac.uk/download/479013102.pdf (accessed on 7th August 2025).
11. Battino, M., Bullon, P., Giampieri, F., Quiles, J. L., et al. (2016). *A systematic review on the implication of minerals in the onset, severity and treatment of periodontal disease*. https://core.ac.uk/download/161255425.pdf (accessed on 7th August 2025).
12. Benjamin, M., Carciofi, A., Carlson, C. S., Choudhury, D., Craig, L. E., Csuti, B., Dyson, S., et al. (2017). *Skeletal pathology and variable anatomy in elephant feet assessed using computed tomography*. https://core.ac.uk/download/76981012.pdf (accessed on 7th August 2025).
13. Cianferotti, L., Bertoldo, F., Bischoff-Ferrari, H. A., Bruyere, O., Cooper, C., Cutolo, M., Kanis, J. A., Kaufman, J. M., Reginster, J. Y., Rizzoli, R., & Brandi, M. L. (2017). Vitamin D supplementation in the prevention and management of major chronic diseases not related to mineral homeostasis in adults: research for evidence and a scientific statement from the European society for

clinical and economic aspects of osteoporosis and osteoarthritis (ESCEO). *Endocrine, 56*(2), 245–261. https://doi.org/10.1007/s12020-017-1290-9(accessed on 7th August 2025).

14. Buchanan, G., Ma, M., & Rea, P. M. (2014). *A multimedia package for patient understanding and rehabilitation of non-contact anterior cruciate ligament injuries*. https://core.ac.uk/download/16461708.pdf (accessed on 7th August 2025).
15. Bushman, W. A., Campagnola, P. J., Campbell, K. R., Chaudhary, R., et al. (2019). *Second-harmonic generation microscopy analysis reveals proteoglycan decorin is necessary for proper collagen organization in prostate*. https://core.ac.uk/download/220159112.pdf (accessed on 7th August 2025).
16. Püschel, T. A., Marcé-Nogué, J., Chamberlain, A. T., Yoxall, A., & Sellers, W. I. (2020). The biomechanical importance of the scaphoid-centrale fusion during simulated knuckle-walking and its implications for human locomotor evolution. *Scientific reports, 10*(1), 3526. https://doi.org/10.1038/s41598-020-60590-6(accessed on 7th August 2025).
17. Clauss, M., Fennimore, A., Gunderson, Z. J., Kacena, M. A., et al. (2019). *Dysfunctional stem and progenitor cells impair fracture healing with age*. https://core.ac.uk/download/228066279.pdf (accessed on 7th August 2025).
18. Simmons, T., Goodburn, B., & Singhrao, S. K. (2016). Decision tree analysis as a supplementary tool to enhance histomorphological differentiation when distinguishing human from non-human cranial bone in both burnt and unburnt states: A feasibility study. *Medicine, science, and the law, 56*(1), 36–45. https://doi.org/10.1177/0025802415589776(accessed on 7th August 2025).
19. Esteve-Altava, B., Villmoare, B., Rolian, C., et al. (2018). *First anatomical network analysis of fore- and hindlimb musculoskeletal modularity in bonobos, common chimpanzees, and humans*. https://core.ac.uk/download/157769144.pdf (accessed on 7th August 2025).
20. Fairman, C. M., Galvao, D. A., Hart, N. H., Kendall, M., et al. (2018). *The potential therapeutic effects of creatine supplementation on body composition and muscle function in cancer*. https // core.ac.uk/download/213607833.pdf (accessed on 7th August 2025).
21. Flohr, S., Gomez, S., Kierdorf, H., Kierdorf, U., et al. (2017). *Multiple osteochondromas of the antlers and cranium in a free-ranging white-tailed deer (Odocoileus virginianus)*. https://core.ac.uk/download/148067969.pdf (accessed on 7th August 2025).
22. Diogo R, Esteve-Altava B, Smith C, Boughner JC, Rasskin-Gutman D (2015) Anatomical Network Comparison of Human Upper and Lower, Newborn and Adult, and Normal and Abnormal Limbs, with Notes on Development, Pathology and Limb Serial Homology vs. Homoplasy. PLoS ONE 10(10): e0140030. https://doi.org/10.1371/journal.pone.0140030(accessed on 7th August 2025).
23. Grenoble, D. E., & Knoell, A. C. (1973). *Unified Approach to the Biomechanics of Dental Implantology*. https://core.ac.uk/download/pdf/10303373.pdf (accessed on 7th August 2025).
24. Hellgren, M., Kazakia, G. J., Lorentzon, M., Nilsson, A. G., et al. (2018). *High-impact mechanical loading increases bone material strength in postmenopausal women—A 3-month intervention study*. https://core.ac.uk/download/323073929.pdf (accessed on 7th August 2025).
25. Ilesanmi-Oyelere, B. L., & Kruger, M. C. (2023). *B vitamins and homocysteine as determinants of bone health: A literature review of human studies*. https://core.ac.uk/download/642812856.pdf (accessed on 7th August 2025).

26. Kharazi, M. (2023). *Consideration of Monoarticular and Biarticular Mechanisms*. https://core.ac.uk/download/586787679.pdf (accessed on 7th August 2025).

27. Lee, M., Kwon, A., Song, K., Lee, H. I., Choi, H., Suh, J., Chae, H., et al. (2024). Effectiveness and safety of pamidronate treatment in nonambulatory children with low bone mineral density. *Annals of Pediatric Endocrinology & Metabolism, 29*, 46–53. https://www.semanticscholar.org/paper/5e92f52e9c5a5e96856239fd581b77124f1a6483 (accessed on 7th August 2025).

28. Lewis, S. J. (1998). *Some Research Possibilities in Diagnostic Radiography*. https://core.ac.uk/download/364240.pdf (accessed on 7th August 2025).

29. Madgwick, R. (2008). *Patterns in the Modification of Animal and Human Bones in Iron Age Wessex: Revisiting the Excarnation Debate*. https://core.ac.uk/download/4898902.pdf (accessed on 7th August 2025).

30. Marie, P. J., & Ornitz, D. M. (2015). *Fibroblast Growth Factor Signaling in Skeletal Development and Disease*. https://core.ac.uk/download/70381887.pdf (accessed on 7th August 2025).

31. Riley G. (2008). Tendinopathy--from basic science to treatment. *Nature clinical practice. Rheumatology*, *4*(2), 82–89. https://doi.org/10.1038/ncprheum0700(accessed on 7th August 2025).

32. Rosse, C., Mejino, J.L.V. (2008). The Foundational Model of Anatomy Ontology. In: Burger, A., Davidson, D., Baldock, R. (eds) Anatomy Ontologies for Bioinformatics. Computational Biology, vol 6. Springer, London. https://doi.org/10.1007/978-1-84628-885-2_4 (accessed on 7th August 2025).

33. Mitchell, K. (2014). *A Comparative Analysis of Primate First Metatarsals: Implications for Ardipithecus ramidus*. https://core.ac.uk/download/643694581.pdf (accessed on 7th August 2025).

34. Moran J. M. (2022). Nutrition and Women's Bone Health. *Nutrients, 14*(4), 763. https://doi.org/10.3390/nu14040763NASA Publication (1988). *Aerospace medicine and biology: A continuing bibliography with indexes, supplement 190, February 1979*. NASA SP-701j (309) https://core.ac.uk/download/pdf/42870573.pdf (accessed on 7th August 2025).

35. Owen, H. L. (2017). *A Review of Ankylosing Spondylitis*. https://core.ac.uk/download/158970001.pdf (accessed on 7th August 2025).

36. Patwardhan, K. (2008). *Concepts of Human Physiology in Ayurveda*. https://core.ac.uk/download/pdf/87482.pdf (accessed on 7th August 2025).

37. Rhee, S. (2025). Application of deep learning for diagnosis of shoulder diseases in older adults: A narrative review. *The Ewha Medical Journal*. https://www.semanticscholar.org/paper/9e212ce852bbee829aa9de65e92d1eb4ca443f93 (accessed on 7th August 2025).

38. Riley, G. P. (2004). *The Pathogenesis of Tendinopathy. A Molecular Perspective*. https://core.ac.uk/download/2776643.pdf (accessed on 7th August 2025).

39. Scarlett, M. A. (2018). *Can a comprehensive transition plan to barefoot running be the solution to the injury epidemic in American endurance runners?* https://core.ac.uk/download/159384850.pdf (accessed on 7th August 2025).

40. Smith, S. M. (2000). *Nutritional Biochemistry of Space Flight*. https://core.ac.uk/download/pdf/10555799.pdf (accessed on 7th August 2025).

41. Stegner, A., Barnosky, A. D., Holmes, M., Kirchholtes, E., et al. (2014). *Prelude to the Anthropocene: Two new North American Land Mammal Ages (NALMAs)*. https://core.ac.uk/download/322493979.pdf (accessed on 7th August 2025).

42. Tofail, S. A. M., Koumoulos, E. P., Bandyopadhyay, A., Bose, S., O'Donoghue, L., & Charitidis, C. A. (2017). Additive manufacturing: Scientific and technological challenges, market uptake and opportunities. *Materials Today, 21*, 22–37. https://doi.org/10.1016/j.mattod.2017.07.001 (accessed on 7th August 2025).

43. Dijcker, J. C., Plantinga, E. A., van Baal, J., & Hendriks, W. H. (2011). Influence of nutrition on feline calcium oxalate urolithiasis with emphasis on endogenous oxalate synthesis. *Nutrition research reviews, 24*(1), 96–110. https://doi.org/10.1017/S0954422410000351(accessed on 7th August 2025).

44. Vassallo, P. (2004). *Radiology*. https://core.ac.uk/download/46601887.pdf (accessed on 7th August 2025).

45. Velandia Palacio, L. A. (2020). *Development of Third Molar and Third Molar Index: I3M Global Observations*. https://core.ac.uk/download/322780478.pdf (accessed on 7th August 2025).

46. Weatherholt, A. M., & Warden, S. J. (2018). Throwing enhances humeral shaft cortical bone properties in pre-pubertal baseball players: a 12-month longitudinal pilot study. *Journal of musculoskeletal & neuronal interactions, 18*(2), 191–199.(accessed on 7th August 2025).

47. Xie, X., Fu, J., Gou, W., Qin, Y., Wang, D., Huang, Z., Wang, L., et al. (2024). Potential mechanism of tea for treating osteoporosis, osteoarthritis, and rheumatoid arthritis. *Frontiers in Medicine, 11*. https://www.semanticscholar.org/paper/45216832ce15c578983905ce6848e8c51a3f6908 (accessed on 7th August 2025).

48. Zakrzewski, W., Dobrzyński, M., Szymonowicz, M., & Rybak, Z. (2019). Stem cells: Past, present, and future. *Stem Cell Research & Therapy, 10*. https://doi.org/10.1186/s13287-019-1165-5 (accessed on 7th August 2025).

49. Zeng, C., Guo, B., Zhang, S., Zhou, Z., Cai, Q., Hou, L., Tan, Z., et al. (2023). Age-related changes in lumbar bone mineral density measured using quantitative computed tomography in healthy female cynomolgus monkeys. *Quantitative Imaging in Medicine and Surgery, 13*, 2038–2052. https://www.semanticscholar.org/paper/9ab61aa5160d50daba6fc68fdbeca66473e5506e (accessed on 7th August 2025).

BLOOD AND HEMATOPOIESIS

9

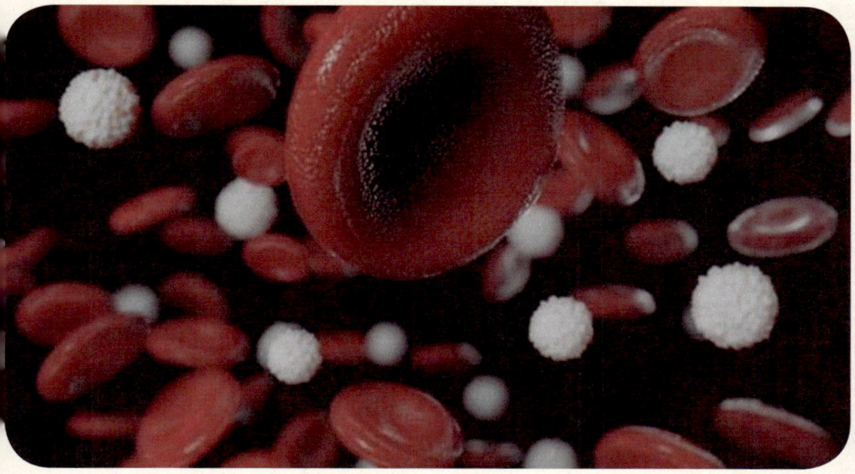

Introduction

Hematopoiesis and the biology of human blood are an intriguing intersection of clinical significance, physiology, and biology. Hematopoiesis, or the generation of blood cells, occurs almost exclusively within the bone marrow and is governed by a complex system of cell-to-cell interactions and signaling cascades. This sophisticated process not only maintains the homeostasis of the body but also allows for a successful defense against infection. It should be noted that hematopoiesis is not only a physiological process but also controlled by various factors including genetic mutations, environmental factors, and availability of nutrients. Relevance of these factors points to the need to address their roles, the relevance of vitamin A and its active metabolite, retinoic acid, whose function to regulate key aspects of hematopoiesis during development and far into maturity has been shown (Cañete et al., 2017). In the last few years, preleukemia has taken on a new connotation with advances in genetic research and diagnostic technologies. Previously applied to describe diseases

LEARNING OBJECTIVES

After studying this chapter, you will be able to:

1. Describe the composition and functions of blood;
2. Understand the process of hematopoiesis;
3. Describe the types of blood cells produced;
4. Understand the regulation of hematopoiesis;
5. Learn about disorders related to blood and hematopoiesis.

, such as myelodysplastic syndromes (MDS) that put patients at risk of acute myeloid leukemia (AML), the preleukemia term is now applied to many other gene mutations and also clonal hematopoiesis. These mutations, with a higher risk of developing leukemia, have not only been identified in patients diagnosed with AML but also in older patients presenting with clonal hematopoiesis that could be a sign of an initial phase of blood malignancies. Comprehending these new categorizations and their implications emphasizes the importance of early diagnosis and intervention practices in hematological disorders (Koeffler & Leong, 2017).

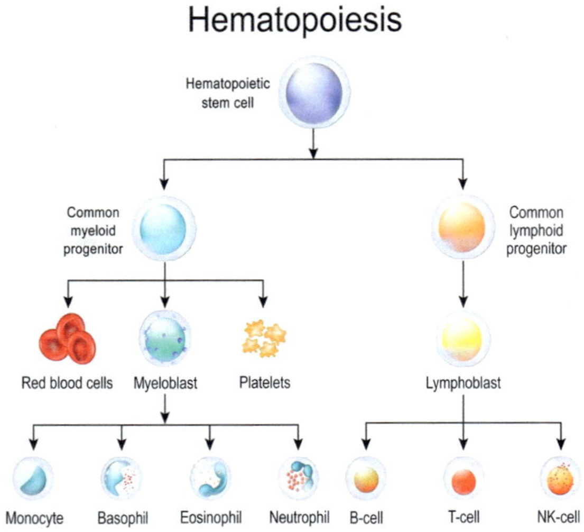

Figure 9.1. Hematopoiesis.

Source: https://media.beckman.com/-/media/stock-images/resource-center/images/hematopoiesis_03_2022.jpg?rev=e17a24c18ea74fa4b4f2f9512b3dfeca.

The dialogue between hematopoiesis and the overall health of the body is a dynamic and multifaceted arena. Several environmental as well as genetic factors can be held accountable for disrupting normal hematopoiesis, leading to anemia and leukemia. Failure to attain critical nutrients , such as vitamin A, will interfere with the differentiation and proliferation of blood cells, as manifested in embryogenesis and adult life (Cañete et al., 2017). Further, the emergence of preleukemic conditions based on genetic predispositions necessitates an in-depth examination of the molecular mechanisms of hematopoiesis. Such a study not only increases understanding of the function of blood but also encourages the development of targeted therapy and prevention in hematologic illnesses, ultimately leading towards improved patient outcomes in illnesses ranging from benign to malignant blood illnesses (Figure 9.1).

Definition of Blood and Its Components

Blood, a vital fluid in the human body, is defined as a specialized connective tissue circulating through the cardiovascular system. The intricate blend comprises many elements, primarily red blood cells (erythrocytes), white blood cells (leukocytes), platelets, and plasma. Each element has its unique role in homeostasis and overall health. Red blood cells carry oxygen from the lungs to tissues and return carbon dioxide for exhalation, while white blood cells are also crucial to the immune response, eliminating infectious agents and foreign invaders. Platelets are also crucial in coagulation, aiding in wound closure through the prevention of unnecessary blood loss by creating clots. The plasma, or the blood fluid matrix, serves not only as a medium for transport of these cell elements but also conveys nutrients, waste products, hormones, and proteins to and from the cells of the body. In the broader sense, the composition of the blood is a reflection of its diversified functions, emphasizing function over mere transport. Plasma occupies about 55% of the blood volume and contains a majority of water, besides dissolved constituents , such as electrolytes, proteins, glucose, lipids, and waste products of metabolism. Of particular interest are the plasma proteins, namely albumin, globulins, and fibrinogen, with the roles of maintaining osmotic equilibrium, immune function, and blood clotting, respectively. Hematopoiesis, or blood cell formation, occurs primarily in the bone marrow, where hematopoietic stem cells mature into a variety of cell types of blood. The process is demonstrated to require factors like oxygen levels since hypoxia and hypoxia-inducible factors (HIFs) regulate stem cell maintenance and differentiation (Aljoufi et al., 2018). An understanding of blood's structure and definition is essential for grasping the complex hematopoiesis processes and the importance of hematopoiesis to human health. Interaction between blood components and their precursors within the bone marrow is closely linked to a range of illnesses of health. For instance, anemia, leukemia, or myelodysplastic syndromes may be caused by dysfunction of hematopoiesis. Furthermore, it is mentioned that determinants of bone marrow, including adiposity and environmental influences, may significantly impact hematopoietic function (Cañete et al., 2017). This intricate relationship leads to the requirement of guarantees that blood components are in a healthy state and underlines the role played by scientific inquiry towards the comprehension of blood and blood disorders and their implication for health in general (Figure 9.2).

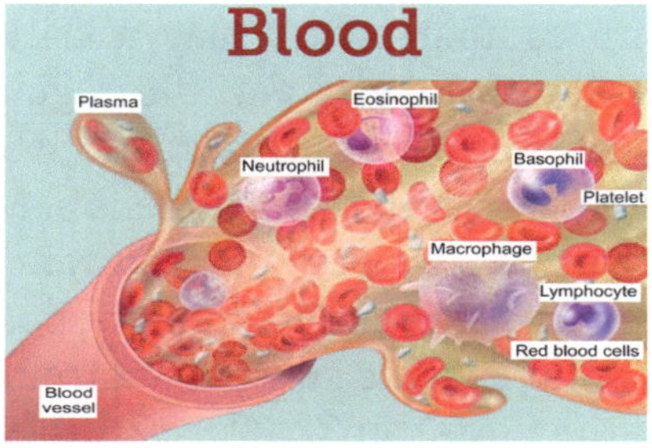

Figure 9.2. Blood.

Source: https://assets.lybrate.com/imgs/tic/enadp/image-of-the-blood.jpg.

Importance of Hematopoiesis in Human Health

Hematopoiesis, or the production of blood cells, is at the forefront of human health due to its critical role in maintaining a balanced, functioning immune system. Hematopoietic stem cells mature into various blood cell types, including red blood cells, white blood cells, and platelets, via hematopoiesis. These functions are performed by each of these constituents: red blood cells transport oxygen, white blood cells defend against disease, and platelets contribute to blood clotting. Disruptions in this function can lead to a host of types of health complications , such as anemia, increased susceptibility to disease, and bleeding disorders. Aside from that, hematopoiesis information is necessary for the identification of treatment for a lot of blood ailments, and so its worldwide significance reaches beyond personal health to public health concerns in general. Hematopoietic discoveries can be easily translated to therapeutic approaches to diseases like leukemia and other blood malignancies. The significance of hematopoiesis to human physiology is also underscored, considering the regulatory role of environmental factors over hematopoiesis. Current studies show that exposure to microbial environments, particularly in early life, is crucial for conditioning the immune system and hematopoietic stem cell behavior. The hygiene hypothesis supposes that reduced microbial exposure may cause the immune system to become biased towards hypersensitivity, and hence hematopoiesis is significant in the modification of immune functions according to environmental conditions (Apostol et al., 2020). Also, the conditions , such as oxygenation in the bone marrow, effectively regulate hematopoiesis; hypoxia-inducible factors (HIFs) are of pivotal importance to maintain hematopoietic stem cell function and differentiate under varied oxygen conditions (Aljoufi et al., 2018). Thus, crosstalk between extrinsic forces and hematopoietic processes is important for maintaining immune fitness. Also, advances in our understanding of hematopoiesis have significant implications for regenerative medicine and treatments aiming to enhance human health. Technologies such as gene therapy and stem cell transplantation utilize discoveries from hematopoietic studies to treat blood diseases and to improve the quality of patient outcomes. , The ability to engineer hematopoietic stem cells for regenerative purposes can treat not just hematological malignancies but also many other disorders. The unrelenting pursuit of hematopoietic stem cell niches, oxygen signaling, and cellular metabolism further broadens the realm of treatable possibilities that can help restore health and resilience among populations. With more probing, the importance of hematopoiesis is not only a pillar of immunological wellness but a foundation of therapeutic innovations in contemporary medicine (Apostol et al., 2020).

9.1. Composition of Blood

Learning Outcome

1. Describe the plasma and its functions;
2. Understand the red blood cells (erythrocytes) and their role;
3. Describe the white blood cells (leukocytes) and their types.

The composition of blood is a complex and broad subject that encompasses its cell and fluid components, responsible for numerous physiological activities. Blood comprises primarily red blood cells (RBCs), white blood cells (WBCs), platelets, and plasma. RBCs, which constitute about 45% of blood volume, are responsible for oxygen delivery, given that they contain hemoglobin. WBCs play a critical role in the immune defense mechanism, safeguarding the body against infection and foreign material. Platelets are responsible for ensuring clotting in the blood, preventing profuse bleeding in case of an injury. Plasma, the fluid component, contains water, electrolytes, nutrients, hormones, and waste products and serves as a transport medium. Understanding this intricate constitution is not only significant in terms of an integrated picture of human physiology but also in the creation of treatments in medicine, as deviations of constituents in the blood may indicate numerous health issues or diseases. The study of hematopoiesis—the development and differentiation of blood cells—is directly intertwined with the constitution of the blood. Hematopoiesis is primarily performed in the bone marrow, where the hematopoietic stem cells give rise to all mature blood cell types. The stem cells undergo many cycles of differentiation, based on intrinsic and extrinsic factors, including the bone marrow microenvironment. Fetal hematopoietic stem cells have been suggested by recent research to be susceptible to environmental factors, particularly microbial exposure during pregnancy, which may play a role in shaping the immune system. Fundamentally, the health and viability of blood cells depend not only on their inherent traits but also on conditions governing their development. Therefore, awareness of such dynamics is essential to comprehend diseases , such as anemia and leukemia when hematopoiesis is compromised. Other than composition and genesis, the constitution of blood is considerably influenced by the microenvironment of hematopoietic cells. Spleen stromal cells that organize the tissue into compartments play a critical role in aiding hematopoiesis and the regulation of immune responses. The interaction between hematopoietic cells and stromal cells plays a vital role in ensuring a proper balanced composition of blood and an effective immune response. The recognition of specific subsets of stromal cells, such as the Sca-1$^+$gp38$^+$Thy1.2$^+$CD29$^+$CD51$^+$ subset, reveals their increased capacity for the support of hematopoiesis, demonstrating the complexity of cell-to-cell contact in the hematopoietic niche. These results underscore the necessity of understanding the cellular microenvironments to have a full picture of how composition of blood can be altered by response to environmental stimuli and conditions of disease, for instance, as suggested by the hygiene hypothesis that reduced microbial exposure may influence immune development and thus impact blood cell function (Lim & O'Neill, 2019; Apostol et al., 2020) (Figure 9.3).

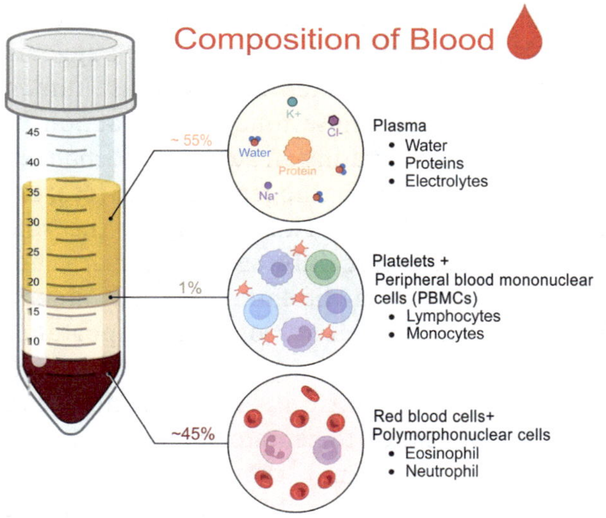

Figure 9.3. Composition of blood.

Source: https://microbenotes.com/wp-content/uploads/2023/04/Composition-of-Blood.jpg.

9.1.1. Plasma and Its Functions

Plasma, the liquid component of blood, plays a key role in homeostasis and the mediation of a number of physiological processes. Comprising approximately 55% of blood volume, plasma is comprised primarily of water, electrolytes, proteins, and dissolved nutrients. Its major functions include the transport of gases, nutrients, hormones, and waste products around and within the body. Plasma proteins , such as albumin, globulins, and fibrinogen, have roles to play in blood osmotic pressure, immunity, and blood coagulation. Also, plasma acts as a carrier for the delivery of essential nutrients and signaling molecules to supply tissues with materials needed for metabolic processes. Plasma composition is dynamic and reflects the body's metabolic status, allowing for prompt changes based on physiological requirements, such as those in hydration status or ingestive events, thereby emphasizing its importance in the overall maintenance of blood and hematopoiesis in humans. The interdependence with other blood cells identifies the central function of plasma in cellular functions and hematopoiesis. Plasma not only provides a medium for cell carriage, like red and white blood cells, but it is also rich in an environment of growth factors and cytokines essential for hematopoietic progenitor cell division and differentiation. For instance, cytokines like erythropoietin are required to stimulate the production of red blood cells in a state of hypoxia. In addition, plasma acts as a reservoir for releasing immune-derived signaling molecules to allow leukocytes to communicate with each other. Plasma composition can be modified by numerous factors, including disease states and environmental toxin exposure, with possible influence on hematopoiesis and immune function as discussed in the context of steroid hormone effects on blood cell development (Burvenich et al., 2004) and benzene's impact on hematologic status (Bechtold et al., 1996). Besides its role in transportation and signaling, plasma is also responsible for the body's response to injury and inflammation. Plasma contains a range of proteins that are involved in the coagulation cascade necessary for hemostasis. Fibrinogen, upon activation, is converted into fibrin, which forms a web trapping the blood cells and is responsible for creating a clot and stopping excessive bleeding. Furthermore, plasma proteins , such as immunoglobulins are very important in the immune system, protecting against infection. Studies of the plasma under situations , such as infection or inflammation prove that the plasma functions in hematopoietic response regulation. Changes in the white blood cell production, initiated by plasma composition change, prove how plasma functions over the delivery function. This connectivity between plasma dynamics and hematopoiesis underscores the significance of maintaining optimal plasma health as the foundation for proper immune function and general welfare (Figure 9.4).

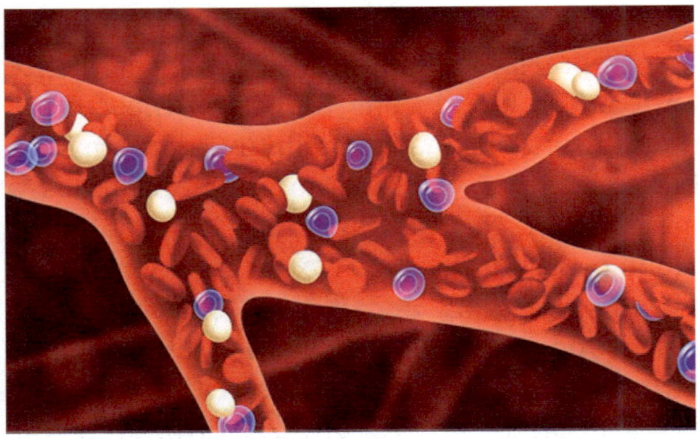

Figure 9.4. Plasma.

Source: https://www.hematology.org/-/media/hematology/images/patients/blood-vessels-with-with-plasma-and-other-blood-cells.png?la=en&h=471&w=765&hash=FAD9B09DEC111953B8C402FCBE7F42EB.

9.1.2. Red Blood Cells (Erythrocytes) and Their Role

Red blood cells (erythrocytes) play a central role in human physiology, primarily through their role in gas exchange. Formed within the bone marrow through a process known as erythropoiesis, erythrocytes transport oxygen from the lungs to body tissues and carbon dioxide from body tissues to the lungs for expulsion. Individual cells are uniquely adapted to perform this role, with their biconcave shape that offers sufficient surface area, as well as allowing for simple gas diffusion. Besides, the presence of hemoglobin, a protein molecule that oxygen attaches to, prepares erythrocytes for carrying sufficient amounts of this essential gas. Erythrocytes are not just passive oxygen carriers, however; they also interact with the immune system in various ways, revealing a richer functional repertoire than simple respiration (Morera & Mackenzie, 2011). Erythrocyte immune interactions also illustrate their multifunctionality in human health. Recent research has indicated that such cells actually participate in the immune response, and they can respond to pathogens and mediate certain immune processes. For example, erythrocytes can interact with viral and bacterial pathogens and not just act as a transport mechanism for the said agents, but also as a place for their possible activation. The evidence suggests that while non-nucleated in mammals, human erythrocytes can show functional reaction to infection, demonstrating an adaptive mechanism for survival under pathogenic attack (Morera & Mackenzie, 2011). This highlights the role of erythrocytes not only as gas carriers, but as active players in the immune environment, which provides evidence of their importance in vertebrate evolutionary roles. Furthermore, erythrocyte formation and function are intrinsically related to hematopoiesis, a complex biological phenomenon that underscores cell differentiation and integrity in the hematopoietic system.

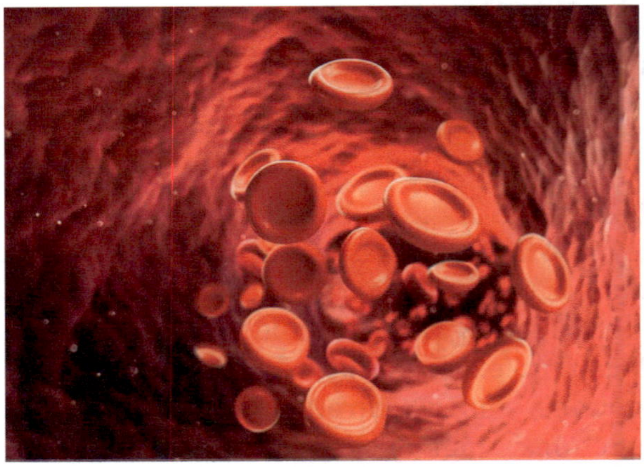

Figure 9.5. Red blood cells.

Source: https://www.hematology.org/-/media/hematology/images/patients/red-blood-cells.png?la=en&h=543&w=759&hash=5146221F14A698D2C8C870E5BF5CDE3C.

Telomerase activity has been found to be significant in hematopoiesis and to exert a modulating influence on erythropoietic differentiation. Zebrafish research demonstrates that knockdown of the telomerase reverse transcriptase led to severe defects in blood cell counts and differentiation, thereby emphasizing telomerase's telomeric-independent roles. This suggests that telomerase activity regulation is crucial for the full development of erythrocytes and even other hematopoietic lineages. The information gained in this research adds to the understanding of molecular processes that regulate erythropoiesis as well as more universal principles for dysregulated hematopoiesis disorders (Figure 9.5).

9.1.3. White Blood Cells (Leukocytes) and Their Types

White blood cells or leukocytes are significant components of the human immune system with the role of safeguarding the body against infectious organisms and foreign matter. They are primarily produced in the bone marrow through hematopoiesis and are classified into several different types based on function and morphology. The two major categories of leukocytes are agranulocytes and granulocytes. Granulocytes, including basophils, eosinophils, and neutrophils, have granules in the cytoplasm. These cells play a crucial role in inflammation and combat infections, while agranulocytes, such as lymphocytes and monocytes, are constituents of the adaptive immune response and long-term immunity. An awareness of the specific functions of these forms of leukocytes is necessary to appreciate how the immune system operates and responds to various pathogens. Neutrophils, the most abundant white blood cells, are the first line of defense against microbial invasion. Their rapid entry into infected tissues is facilitated by chemokines, which draw them to areas of inflammation and tissue injury. The neutrophils are the body's major phagocytes, and they engulf and digest the pathogens by the process of phagocytosis. The eosinophils, although fewer in number, play a vital role in countering parasitic infections and allergic responses. They are loaded with granules packed with cytotoxic proteins that can be discharged when allergens or parasites are encountered. Basophils, although the rarest granulocyte, play a very important role in inflammatory responses by the release of histamine and other mediators to assist in the initiation of an allergic response. The interaction between the leukocytes hence, shows the complexity of the immune response in addressing varied challenges to the body (Hughes & Nibbs, 2018). Agranulocytes, which consist mostly of lymphocytes and monocytes, play a significant role in the immune adaptive responses. Lymphocytes are also separated into B cells and T cells, each with various functions: B cells produce antibodies, while T cells are important in cell-mediated immunity. Such differentiation of duties displays the elaborate processes through which leukocytes respond to pathogens and mount a response commensurate with the danger. Monocytes, present in the blood and capable of maturing into macrophages and dendritic cells, are at the center of both innate and adaptive immunity. The cells not only kill the pathogens, but also help with antigen presentation to T cells, thus forming the link between innate and adaptive immunity. Knowing these forms of leukocytes and their functions provides us with an image of how our body is capable of maintaining defense against disease and maintaining homeostasis (Poggi et al., 2021) (Figure 9.6).

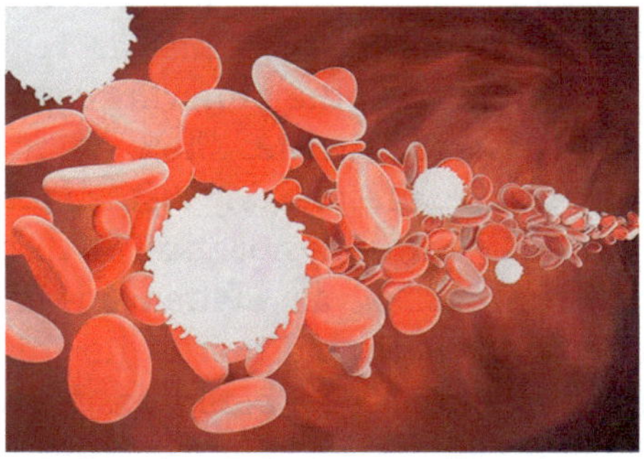

Figure 9.6. White blood cells.

Source: https://www.hematology.org/-/media/hematology/images/patients/white-blood-cells.png?la=en&h=552&w=792&hash=3247CA8D8B3BE554F69A01978292BA83.

Test Your Knowledge

1. What is plasma and its function?
2. What is RBC and its role?

9.2. Functions of Blood

Learning Outcome

1. Describe the transportation of nutrients and gases;
2. Understand the regulation of body temperature and pH;
3. Protect the body against pathogens and blood loss.

Functions of blood extend way beyond that of a transport medium; it is an active component of human body's homeostasis. Blood facilitates the delivery of essential nutrients and oxygen to the tissues while simultaneously moving metabolic wastes and carbon dioxide away from them. This two-way operation illuminates its involvement in cellular metabolism and overall bodily operation. Moreover, blood also serves as a critical temperature and pH regulator to offer equilibrium in the internal environment. It helps in thermoregulation by absorbing heat generated as a byproduct of metabolic reactions, and acid-base balance is regulated by blood proteins and the buffering capacity of bicarbonate. These activities show the function of blood to sustain life, and any disturbances are bound to lead to acute physiological disturbances or chronic illnesses, as evidenced in most medical disorders. In addition to its transport and regulatory functions, blood has important roles in the immune system as a defense against pathogens and foreign material. White blood cells, or leukocytes, play an important role in the identification and inactivation of invading microbes and toxins. Various types of leukocytes, including lymphocytes and macrophages, are activated with infections and inflammations, resulting in coordinated action of the immune system. Cytokines, or blood messenger molecules, provide additional momentum to the action by enabling communication between the different immune cells. Further, the ability of blood to clot via platelets and plasma proteins prevents unnecessary bleeding when there is injury, showing its protective role. These sophisticated processes also show that the blood, besides being necessary for transport and homeostasis, is also necessary for the maintenance of the body's defense mechanism against disease. Understanding the sophisticated blood processes also highlights nutritional factors and aging's influence on hematopoiesis. For example, vitamin A and its biologically active metabolite, retinoic acid, are held to regulate hematopoietic processes to a large degree. Studies indicate that retinoic acid is important for normal gene expression in developmental hematopoiesis, influencing the balance of endothelial versus blood cell formation in embryos and enhancing erythropoiesis in fetal livers (Cañete et al., 2017).

Alternatively, aging presents a challenge to blood manufacturing since changes in stem cell function may lead to increased mutations that compromise hemopoietic activity. This type of clonal dominance by mutant progenitor cells may lead to conditions , such as leukemia, a condition whose occurrence demonstrates the effect of aging on the health of blood (Adams et al., 2015). Thus, blood functions are implicitly associated with both cellular and systemic integrity, which reflects the complexity of regulation of hematopoiesis throughout life.

9.2.1. Transportation of Nutrients and Gases

Transportation of nutrients and gases in the circulatory system of humans is a fundamental process that preserves cellular function and homeostasis. Blood, composed largely of plasma, red blood cells, white blood cells, and platelets, plays an extremely critical role in the transportation of needed substances into the body. Nutrients from the digestive tract, like glucose, amino acids, and fatty acids, are carried by plasma to organs and tissues. Besides, red blood cells employ hemoglobin to transport oxygen from the lungs into body tissues and at the same time to permit carbon dioxide to be sent back to the lungs to be breathed out. This intricate process not only helps metabolic processes but also helps maintain body pH at an even level, hence highlighting the significance of effective transport of nutrients and gases in sustaining life. The efficiency of transport of gases and nutrients is influenced by a number of physiological variables, including the type of blood constituents and hemodynamics of blood. Modulation of blood viscosity, which is dependent on the red blood cell count and plasma protein content, plays a key role in determining the adequacy of oxygen and nutrient delivery to tissues. Furthermore, the circulatory system architecture, both venous and arterial, is such that it supports good blood pressure and flow rates for successful circulation. These physiological values interact dynamically to ensure there is adequate tissue perfusion, particularly with increased metabolic demand during exercise. Lastly, the unimpeded delivery of nutrients and gases is a sophisticated interaction of physiological mechanisms that demonstrates the importance of the circulatory system in human well-being. Apart from the physiological effect, it is important to learn about the impact of interruption in nutrient and gas transport in the clinical situation. Anemia, hypoxemia, and other cardiovascular illnesses weaken the ability of blood to carry essential materials. For instance, anemia, which is a deficiency of red blood cells, yields reduced oxygen transportation capacity, resulting in tiredness and organ malfunction. Similarly, disease of the pulmonary apparatus will block adequate gas exchange and consequently seriously compromise overall oxygen supply. Identification of such pathological states and their effect on hematopoiesis or the formation of blood cells is necessary so that targeted interventions and therapy can be developed. By clinical practice and continuous study, novel advances in overcoming these derangements become progressively better, tremendously enhancing patient outcomes (Walker, 2015) (Figure 9.7).

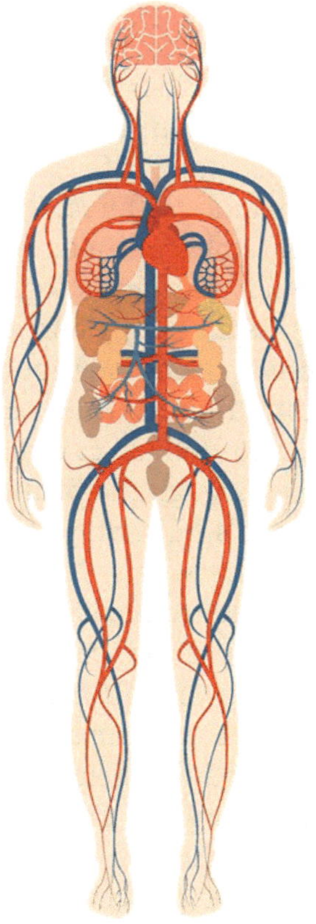

Figure 9.7. Blood transports different materials to different parts of the body.

Source: https://interactivebiology.com/wp-content/uploads/2022/01/blood-circulation-to-different-parts.png.

9.2.2. Regulation of Body Temperature and pH

Body temperature and pH regulation is a critical function of homeostasis that has a significant influence on numerous biochemical processes and the general physiological state of an individual. In the human body, blood serves as a transport medium and also as a regulatory system for these vital parameters. Homeostatic activities , such as acid-base balance and thermoregulation are contingent upon the efficient circulation of blood, thereby allowing the delivery of heat and removal of metabolic waste. Blood, which consists of various cellular and plasma components, not only delivers oxygen and nutrients to tissues but also assists in maintaining the preferred operating environments of enzymes and other cellular machinery. Disturbances in blood composition, for example, those that occur in hematopoietic disturbances like congenital sideroblastic anemia, can affect the ability of the body to control temperature and pH and hence interfere with normal physiological processes (Crispin, 2017). As the body's temperature varies, enzymatic activity and metabolic processes are open to alteration. Within the circulatory system, RBCs also deliver carbon dioxide and thus pH control through the bicarbonate buffer system. The blood's buffering ability maintains an optimal pH between 7.35 and 7.45. If there is a possible acidosis or alkalosis, the blood's capacity to carry carbon dioxide and exchange gases is invaluable. Hematopoiesis, the production of blood cellular components in the bone marrow, directly influences this regulatory function. Hematological deficiency can lead to inadequate production of red blood cells or dysfunctional oxygen transportation, with systemic consequences to temperature and pH regulation, with direct repercussions on general well-being (Banerjee et al., 2018). Moreover, recent findings show complicated interactions among systemic stress responses and blood cell differentiation, further explaining the interaction between thermoregulation and hematopoiesis. In model organisms like Drosophila, studies illustrate how environmental factors like carbon dioxide and oxygen availability control blood cell differentiation and function. These findings suggest that such a process can occur in humans too, emphasizing the significance of outside controls on hematopoietic function and, by extension, on the body's homeostatic ability. Identification of these interactions not only sheds light on the acid-base and thermoregulatory dynamics but also aids in grasping various pathological conditions caused by distorted hematopoiesis and potentially creating temperature and acid-base disturbance disorders (Banerjee et al., 2018) (Figure 9.8).

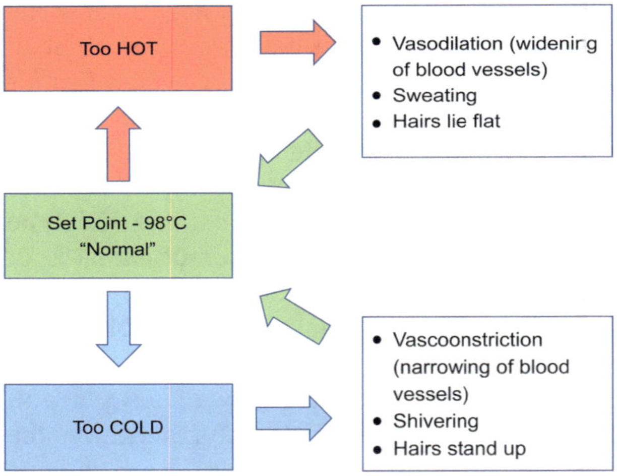

Figure 9.8. Body temperature regulation is an example of homeostasis.

Source: https://openoregon.pressbooks.pub/app/uploads/sites/94/2019/08/homeostasis-body-temp.png.

9.2.3. Protection Against Pathogens and Blood Loss

The human body employs an intricate defense mechanism to repel pathogens and promote hemostasis in the case of blood loss. Pathogens are a constant threat through infection, and this has to be countered with an effective immune response. Hematopoiesis plays a crucial role in the production of all cellular components of the blood, including white blood cells essential for innate and adaptive immunity. For example, in infections , such as visceral leishmaniasis, hematological events can undergo striking alterations that impact the quiescence and self-renewal of long-term hematopoietic stem cells (LT-HSCs) in the bone marrow. The engagement of immune processes and pathogenic activity is significant, with inflammatory-driven cytotoxic $CD4^+$ T cells having the capacity to drain the function of bone marrow, emphasizing the fine balance that must be struck to ensure both removal of the pathogen and protection of hematopoietic reserve (Pinto et al., 2017). Blood loss, whether external through trauma or internal via hemorrhage, is an immediate danger to life that necessitates a rapid physiological response. Platelets and clotting factors are crucial components required for hemostasis, which is a series of complex biochemical reactions that culminate in the formation of a stable blood clot. Activated platelets lead to aggregation and discharge of chemical messengers that induce the formation of additional platelets, along with other clotting factors, thus producing an efficient seal against rebleeding. In addition, the provision of a suitable environment for hematopoiesis gives a continuous supply of such essential constituents. Interruption of the hematopoiesis process can lead to conditions like thrombocytopenia, where a deficiency in platelet production can prevent clotting, therefore aggravating the hazard of blood loss (Gallucci & McCarthy, 1995). The integration of hematopoiesis, protection against pathogen invasion, and safety against blood loss shows the necessity of a successful immune and circulatory system. Advances in biotherapy illustrate the potential for focal therapies designed to activate the immune system or repair hematological abnormalities that interfere with these protective systems. Immunotherapeutic medications, designed to activate the immune system or control gene expression, are increasingly useful for the treatment of autoimmune and infectious diseases. With growing research in the area, a greater understanding of the biological agents may bring forth new approaches to facilitate both pathogen elimination and hemorrhage recovery. Lastly, the application of therapies that modulate hematopoiesis has the potential to contribute to improved patient outcomes in both infection and blood disease, and the potential value of continued research into the mutually interdependent roles of blood components in human health must not be underestimated (Gallucci & McCarthy, 1995).

Test Your Knowledge

1. What is the transport of nutrients and gases?
2. What protects the body against blood loss?

9.3. Hematopoiesis: The Process

Learning Outcome

1. Understand the significance of hematopoiesis;
2. Describe the locations of hematopoiesis in the human body;
3. Describe the stages of hematopoiesis from stem cells to mature cells.

The process of complex hematopoiesis is crucial for the continuous regeneration of blood cells throughout one's life. The sophisticated mechanism begins in embryonic stages, when the hematopoietic stem cells (HSCs) first appear mainly in the yolk sac, followed by the aorta-gonad-mesonephros and lastly reach the fetal liver and bone marrow. The process involves differentiation from multipotent progenitor cells into the various lineages, including erythrocytes, leukocytes, and thrombocytes. Intrinsic genetic programming and extrinsic cues from the microenvironment regulate this differentiation, highlighting the importance of cellular interactions in hematopoiesis. The role of regulation by vitamin A and its metabolite retinoic acid in gene expression about hematopoiesis highlights vital biochemical mechanisms that control such transformation (Cañete et al., 2017). Successful functioning of this process is not only necessary for normal development but also for adult homeostasis, showing the pivotal position of this process in human biology.

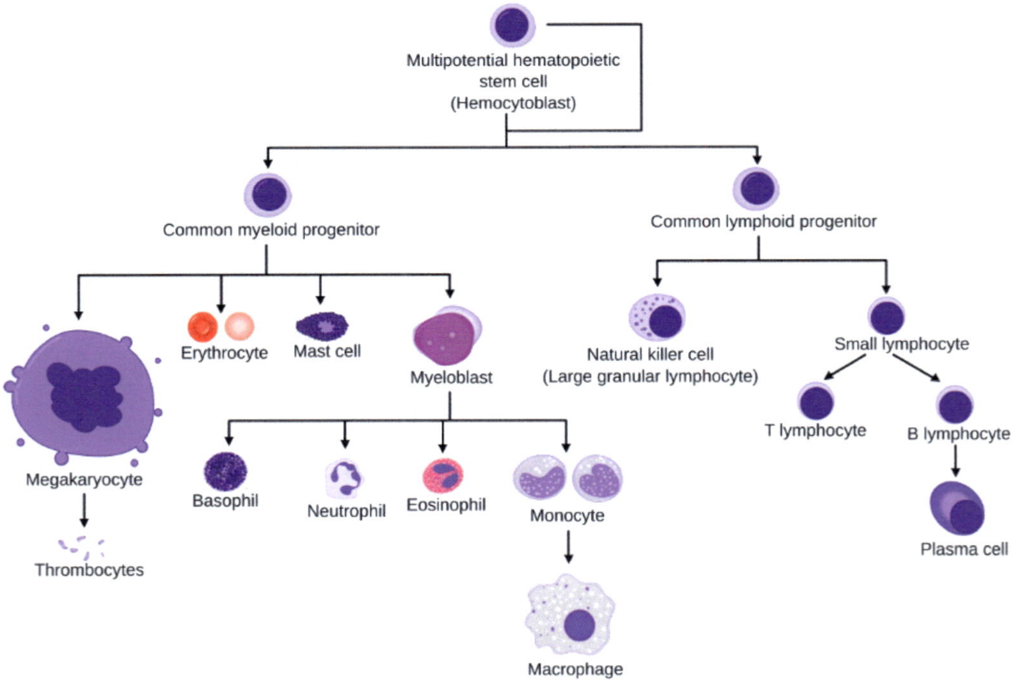

Figure 9.9. Diagram showing the development of different blood cells from haematopoietic stem cell to mature cells.

Source: https://upload.wikimedia.org/wikipedia/commons/f/f0/Hematopoiesis_simple.svg.

Because hematopoiesis does not stop at birth, the bone marrow is the principal site for both blood cell production and regulation. It has a niche that is composed of various cell types, including mesenchymal stem cells, endothelial cells, and ECM components, which provide essential signals to HSCs. The process of aging has been discovered to have adverse effects on this stem cell niche, and it leads to clonal dominance of mutant progenitor cells, a process that enhances the risk of hematological disorders, including cancers (Adams et al., 2015). With advancing age, the accumulation of DNA damage and epigenetic changes in HSCs can limit their proliferative capacity and alter multi-lineage differentiation, impacting overall hematopoietic output. Thus, investigations into the nature of the complexity of hematopoiesis in the context of aging reveal the strength and vulnerability of the blood system and underscore the importance of young tissue microenvironments for optimal cell performance. In addition to environmental and genetic effects, the metabolic challenges are deeply engaged in the process of hematopoiesis. The last couple of years have witnessed researchers beginning to understand how cell metabolism is connected with HSC activity and differentiation. A well-balanced metabolic condition is required to maintain quiescence and survival as HSCs rely on oxidative phosphorylation and fatty acid oxidation to generate energy. Interferences in such metabolic pathways, which are commonly seen during the process of aging or disease conditions, may impair the ability of HSCs to self-renew, negatively affecting hematopoiesis. In addition, vitamin A's ability to promote iron uptake and metabolism emphasizes the importance of the micronutrients in promoting healthy blood cell production and function (Cañete et al., 2017). Understanding of the dynamic interaction between the metabolic pathways, environmental signals, and gene control provides us with insight into the complexities of hematopoiesis and introduces the prospect of novel therapeutic interventions for blood disorders (Figure 9.9).

9.3.1. Definition and Significance of Hematopoiesis

Hematopoiesis, the complex biological process for the creation of blood cellular components, is crucial to maintain the dynamic balance of blood cells in the human organism. Hematopoietic stem cells (HSCs), located predominantly in the bone marrow, differentiate into various blood cell types, including erythrocytes, leukocytes, and thrombocytes. The significance of hematopoiesis extends beyond mere blood cell production; it is key to immunological defense and oxygen delivery and serves to ensure overall homeostasis. Manipulation of normal hematopoietic function can lead to a spectrum of blood disease ranging from anemia to malignancies , such as leukemia, and as such, the need for a comprehensive understanding of this complex system. With research efforts remaining in pursuit, knowledge of hematopoiesis not only drives medical science forward but also fosters the development of therapeutic strategies to the treatment of hematological diseases. Hematopoiesis is also better understood by the study of hematopoietic stem cells (HSCs) and their microenvironment, including certain stromal cells that nurture and control the process of differentiation. These stromal cells, especially in the spleen, are required because they create a supportive environment for hematopoiesis by several mechanisms, of which one involves the secretion of cytokines and growth factors. The finding that specific subsets of stromal cells enhance hematopoietic support adds credence to the need for this interaction within the hematopoietic niche. For instance, research has identified a proportion of stromal cells in the spleen that is similar to the nature of established stromal cell lines, indicating its role in sustaining hematopoiesis in both health and disease states (Lim & O'Neill, 2019). Such interaction is a point to note on how microenvironmental elements directly regulate hematopoietic fate, showing the complexity of the biological process. A sizeable amount of evidence points out that hematopoiesis is not a merely passive response to the body's demand but is dynamically regulated by genetic and environmental stimuli. Mutations in genes can cause diseases known as preleukemia, demonstrating the shift from normal hematopoiesis towards malignancy. Patients with certain genotypic features, such as RUNX1 or TET2 mutations, show increased vulnerability to acute myeloid leukemia (AML), demonstrating how changes in hematopoiesis foretell severe health conditions (Koeffler & Leong, 2017). This evolving understanding of hematopoiesis emphasizes its critical role in disease prediction and therapeutic strategies. Thus, a comprehensive comprehension of hematopoietic processes not only illuminates basic human biology but also holds out the promise of novel therapeutic strategies for rescuing faulty hematopoietic systems (Figure 9.10).

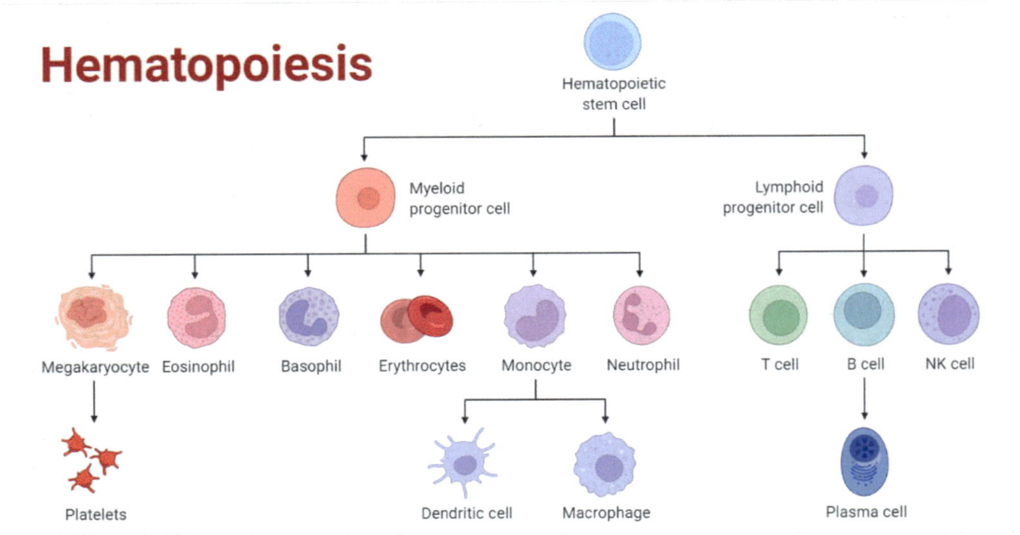

Figure 9.10. Definition of hematopoiesis.

Source: https://microbenotes.com/wp-content/uploads/2022/05/Hematopoiesis.jpeg.

9.3.2. Locations of Hematopoiesis in the Human Body

Hematopoiesis, or blood cell production, is primarily located in specific anatomical locations in the human body. Throughout embryonic development, hematopoiesis originates in the yolk sac and subsequently migrates to the liver and, lastly, the spleen, where it persists until the time of birth. In the postnatal period, the bone marrow serves as the chief site of hematopoiesis, encompassing the development of erythrocytes, leukocytes, and thrombocytes. The mature bone marrow, especially the flat bones like pelvis, sternum, and ribs, holds a rich store of hematopoietic stem cells (HSCs) responsible for the generation of various blood cell lineages. These stem cells undergo differentiation with age under microenvironmental controls regulating their proliferation and maturation. This intricate regulatory landscape is crucial for homeostasis in blood cell production and the bodys capacity to respond in the correct way to physiologic needs. With the bodys sole source of blood cells, the bone marrows microenvironment is crucial for hematopoiesis. The niche consists of a heterogeneous population of non-hematopoietic cells including adipocytes, endothelial cells, and stromal cells, which provide essential support and signaling to HSCs. These niche cells produce various cytokines and chemokines that govern hematopoietic processes, creating a specialized microenvironment to promote stem cell upkeep and lineage development. HSC-niche interaction plays a central role in normal function without disturbance, as any alteration could lead to hematological diseases. For instance, Notch pathway abnormalities can profoundly impact this regulatory network, generating abnormally uncontrolled leukemic cell proliferation that disrupts normal hematopoiesis and promotes disease. These findings point to the importance of an intact microenvironment in sustaining healthy bone marrow hematopoiesis (Piovan et al., 2018). In addition to the bone marrow, other organs can be involved in hematopoiesis under particular circumstances.

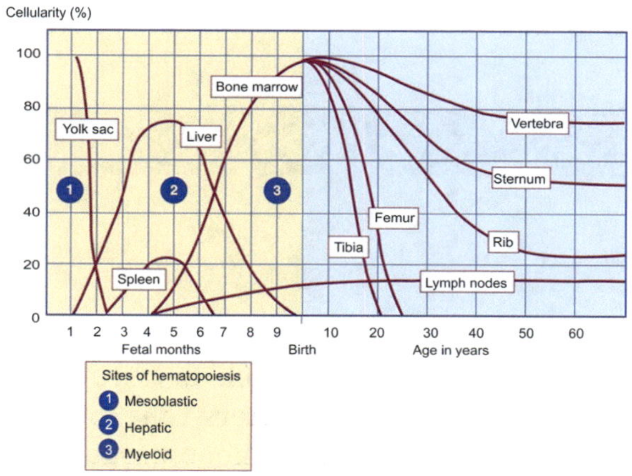

Figure 9.11. Sites of hematopoiesis.

Source: https://oncohemakey.com/wp-content/uploads/2016/06/B978143770692500007X_f007-001-9781437706925.jpg.

In adults, extramedullary hematopoiesis may occur due to states of stress or disease, such as infections and malignancies, in which organs like the spleen and liver re-establish their hematopoietic activities. These are demonstrations of the bodys remarkable adaptability and capacity to recover from increased blood cell demands, particularly in the presence of significant stressors. Recent research has proved that clonal heterogeneity within hematopoietic malignancies renders treatment difficult, as cell populations may be found asymmetrically around the body. The dynamics, especially how extramedullary locations play a role in clonal development, are of pivotal importance to comprehend for the formulation of effective therapy for conditions like leukemia, where numerous clones may not be detectable beyond the original anatomical location (Jacobs et al., 2021) (Figure 9.11).

9.3.3. Stages of Hematopoiesis from Stem Cells to Mature Cells

Hematopoiesis, the extremely complex process of producing all blood cells, originates from hematopoietic stem cells (HSCs) residing predominantly in the bone marrow. The pluripotent cells possess the capacity for self-renewal and differentiation, enabling them to give rise to various lineages of blood cells. The hematopoiesis process can be divided into early stages like the formation of multipotent progenitors, which further differentiate into lymphoid and myeloid progenitor cells. During this stage, the HSCs begin their fate-deciding process towards committed lineages of platelets, erythrocytes, and leukocytes, thus creating the basic framework for the overall hematopoietic system. Recognition of these early stages is crucial, particularly for disorders like myelodysplastic syndromes that are predisposed by abnormalities in these early processes of differentiation, illustrating the interdependence of normal hematopoiesis and potential pathologies. As the process of hematopoiesis progresses, the process of becoming lineage-restricted becomes more assertive, leading to the establishment of lineage-restricted progenitors. For instance, lymphoid progenitors will also express surface antigens typical of their commitment to a particular pathway, such as CD10, which is vital to the identification of such cells in human bone marrow. In recent years, a subpopulation of these progenitors has been described with extremely high levels of L-selectin (CD62L), an intermediate stage of differentiation prior to complete expression of CD10. Importantly, this CD10($^{-}$)CD62L(hi) group has lymphoid and monocytic potential but not erythroid. The identification of these markers characterizes our understanding of hematopoietic cellular hierarchy and highlights the manner in which specific surface antigens signal towards mature cell destinies in a highly regulated and orderly manner (Crooks et al., 2012). Furthermore, hematopoiesis is finished with the maturation of specific cell types, when precursor cells finish their final differentiation and phenotypic changes to assume their functions in the circulatory system. This level of maturation is when lineage-specific markers are expressed at higher levels and when cell functions for proper immune and physiologic response are developed. For example, erythroid progenitors, under stimulation by molecules , such as erythropoietin, will mature into red blood cells, adding to their function in oxygen delivery. Myeloid progenitors, however, will eventually form various types of leukocytes and platelets that perform critical functions in immunity and clotting mechanisms. The dynamic interaction between stem cells, intermediary progenitors, and mature cells not only sustains the balance of a well-balanced hematopoietic system but also sheds light on pathogenic states, such as preleukemia, where cell mutations can take place early in life and lead to malignancies , such as acute myeloid leukemia (Koeffler & Leong, 2017).

Test Your Knowledge

1. What is hematopoiesis?
2. What are the locations of hematopoiesis in the human body?

9.4. Types of Blood Cells Produced

Learning Outcome

1. Learn about the formation of red blood cells and white blood cells;
2. Describe the process of platelet formation.

The human blood system consists of a range of distinct cell types, all of which originate from hematopoietic stem cells (HSCs) in a tightly regulated process known as hematopoiesis. Among the major blood cells produced are the red blood cells (erythrocytes), which are crucial in the oxygen delivery from the lungs to body tissues and for the carbon dioxide return to be expelled. The hemoglobin-carrier bioconcave cells are tasked with oxygen binding, thus enabling cellular respiration. Erythropoiesis is controlled by many factors, one of them being erythropoietin, a hormone produced by the kidneys. Secondly, vitamin A also plays a vital role in this process, with retinoic acid triggering erythropoiesis in the fetal liver and being responsible for the regulation of genes that are important in hematopoiesis, once again showing how interlinked nutritional status is with the production of cells in the blood (Cañete et al., 2017). In addition to the erythrocytes, the blood system also produces white blood cells (leukocytes), which are very much a part of the immune system. Leukocytes are categorized into several types, including lymphocytes, neutrophils, monocytes, eosinophils, and basophils, each having different functions that assist in the body's defense system. Lymphocytes are further categorized into B cells, which produce antibodies, and T cells, which destroy infected or cancer cells. Neutrophils are the first to migrate towards infection, and monocytes develop into macrophages and dendritic cells that phagocytize the infectious agents. The intricate differentiation and equilibrium of these cell types are crucial to the maintenance of homeostasis of the immune response and are governed by cytokines and environmental cues both in embryonic and adult life (Adams et al., 2015). Platelets, or thrombocytes, constitute another important component of blood, with their function primarily in hemostasis—blood coagulation. Unlike other blood cells, platelets are immature cells but cell fragments generated by megakaryocytes of the bone marrow. In case of vascular injury, platelets rapidly adhere to the injured site and aggregate to form an ephemeral plug, releasing a series of growth factors and signaling molecules that facilitate repair and regeneration of tissue. Platelet generation is stringently regulated, with thrombopoietin being the primary hormone involved. Gratitude for the processes of platelet manufacture, alongside erythrocytes and leukocytes, emphasizes the complexity of hematopoiesis and the significant functions these cells play in maintaining physiological homeostasis and responding to injury or infection in human beings (Cañete et al., 2017) (Figure 9.12).

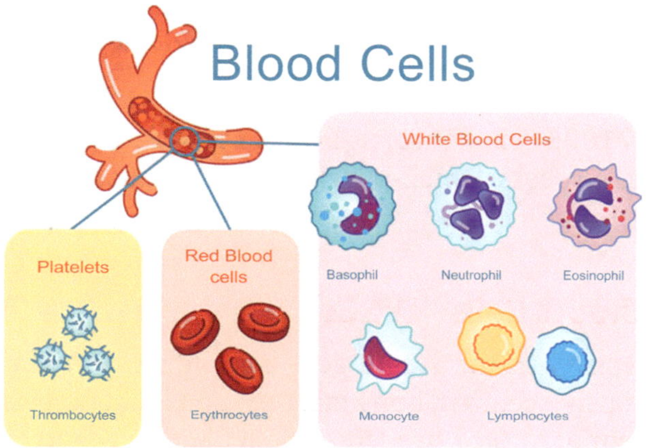

Figure 9.12. Types of blood cells.

Source: https://biologydictionary.net/wp-content/uploads/2021/05/bloodcells.jpg.

9.4.1. Erythropoiesis: Formation of Red Blood Cells

The intricate process of erythropoiesis, red blood cell production, is essential in facilitating adequate oxygen delivery throughout the human body. This intricate development occurs mostly in the bone marrow, where multipotent hematopoietic stem cells (HSCs) develop into erythroid progenitors. These subsequently undergo several stages of maturation, including a transition from erythroblasts to reticulocytes and finally producing mature erythrocytes. Core to this mechanism is the action of erythropoietin (EPO), a hormone produced primarily by the kidneys in reaction to hypoxia. EPO induces proliferation and differentiation of erythroid progenitor cells, hence stimulating red blood cell production to correct oxygen deficiencies in tissues. Such specific control ensures a balance between oxygen supply and physiological requirements, showing the efficacy of erythropoiesis in human hematopoiesis. Vitamin A plays a pivotal, albeit sometimes underemphasized, role in erythropoiesis through its active form, retinoic acid (RA). RA is a potent controller not only during embryogenesis development but also during adult tissue homeostasis. RA signaling has been shown to be vital in developmental hematopoiesis gene expression, in particular to induce the hemogenic program within specific locations , such as the aorta-gonad-mesonephros region. Furthermore, RA is pivotal in triggering fetal liver erythropoiesis by initiating erythropoietin. In adults, RA's function in regulation ranges from increasing granulocyte differentiation to optimizing iron metabolism, which is necessary to prevent anemia. On account of the crucial nature of vitamin A to maintain the health of the blood system, a deficiency in the vitamin results in severe hematologic disorder, reflecting the interdependent nature of nutrients and erythropoiesis (Cañete et al., 2017). In addition to vitamins and hormones, genetic factors also have a significant impact on erythropoiesis.

Conditions , such as congenital sideroblastic anemias (CSA) demonstrate the impact of genetic mutations on the erythropoietic process. These inherited conditions are due to heme biosynthetic defects or mitochondrial integrity, leading to the accumulation of abnormal iron in bone marrow erythroblasts. Mutations have been found in genes including HSPA9 and HSCB that disrupt iron homeostasis, giving rise to defective erythropoiesis. Experiments demonstrate that deficiencies in HSCB severely disrupt hematopoiesis and erythropoiesis, as reflected by fewer red and white cells in model organisms. Awareness of such genetic impacts on erythropoiesis underscores the need to continue exploring the molecular mechanisms that control red blood cell formation, with the ultimate objective of developing targeted therapies for consequent disease (Crispin, 2017) (Figure 9.13).

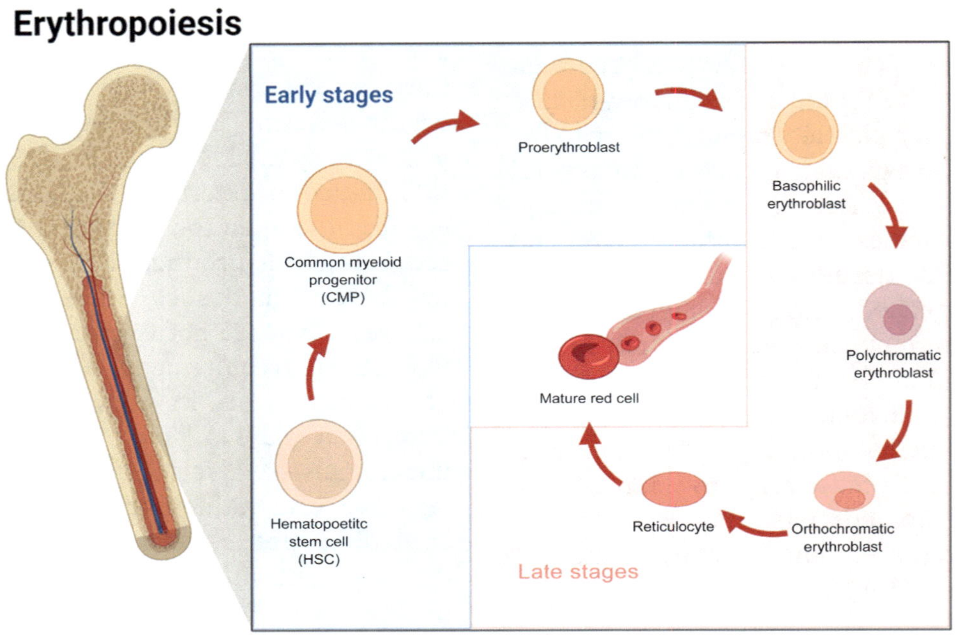

Figure 9.13. Overview of the erythropoiesis process which provides the production of mature red blood cells.

Source: https://www.researchgate.net/publication/371008412/figure/fig1/AS:11431281161291521@1684981441862/Overview-of-the-erythropoiesis-process-which-provides-the-production-of-mature-red-blood.png.

9.4.2. Leukopoiesis: Formation of White Blood Cells (WBCs)

Leukopoiesis is an important process of hematopoiesis with the single goal of producing WBCs, which is accountable for the immune response. It primarily occurs in bone marrow, and leukopoiesis begins with hematopoietic stem cells that are differentiated into progenitor cells and, ultimately, into various forms of leukocytes like lymphocytes, monocytes, and granulocytes. All these cells have an important role to play in the bodys immune reaction against pathogens as well as controlling inflammation. In the broader hematopoietic context, leukopoiesis not only ensures constant renewal of leukocytes but also adapts to the physiological demands placed on the immune system by infection or other immune challenges (Mirzabekov et al., 2025). During the course of leukopoiesis, varied growth factors and signaling pathways regulate the maturation and differentiation of progenitor cells to functional leukocytes. Cytokines , such as interleukin-3 (IL-3), granulocyte colony-stimulating factor (G-CSF), and stem cell factor (SCF) are very important in this regulation. These signals are vital for precursor cell proliferation and survival, as well as lineage commitment specification. Interruptions in these processes of signaling may lead to hematological disorders with either leukopenia or leukocytosis, thereby affecting the immune system's effectiveness. Thus, it is essential to understand the highly precise cellular and molecular mechanisms of leukopoiesis in an effort to come up with therapeutic interventions for correcting normal blood cell formation in diseases, i.e., leukemias and other hematologic disorders (Gopalan et al., 2024).

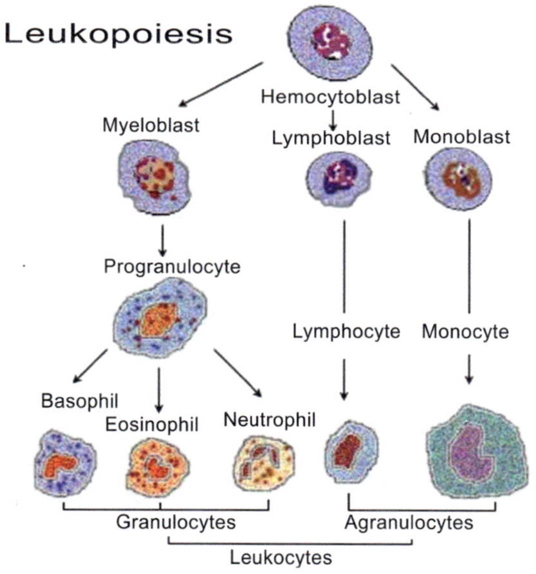

Figure 9.14. Leukopoiesis.

Source: https://blogger.googleusercontent.com/img/b/R29vZ2xl/AVvXsEjDP2Lsim9ROosoXeHi4C1NFKvymz0tXXCuimUjpV5U63bTyGlvdZYPMTxiL0qbLj3NM5HnlLWx-4zYbWr6baNZSRlfUD0pZqRXnQM-OlGhHZD0yZDx10rhxjugsRP50fB-sprPaoJrm-Qea/s348/3-+Leukopoiesis.webp.

Leukopoiesis does not occur in isolation; rather, it is influenced by countless variables, i.e., the general well-being of the body, infection, and even systemic conditions like anemia. To challenge by pathogen, leukocyte production generally is increased as a demand response, illustrating the potential of the hematopoietic system to be extremely plastic. Such plasticity is particularly useful in the case of sickle cell disease, where acute events like vaso-occlusive crises interrupt normal leukocyte function and proliferation. Knowledge of leukopoiesis, the routes to it, and the mechanisms of its regulation is the basis for significant clinical implications, particularly in treating disorders involving white blood cells. A comprehensive explanation of leukopoiesis, therefore, not only sheds light on normal immune processes but also explains the pathologies of a range of hematological disorders (Mirzabekov et al., 2025) (Figure 9.14).

9.4.3. Thrombopoiesis: Formation of Platelets

Thrombopoiesis, the generation of platelets, is an intricate biological process that is crucial to human hemostasis and vascular health. Thrombopoiesis starts with the commitment of hematopoietic stem cells (HSCs) to develop into megakaryocytes (MKs), which are the ultimate progenitors for platelets. MKs follow a distinctive developmental process involving endomitosis, which results in cell expansion and ploidy. The maturation of MKs culminates with the formation of proplatelets—elongated cytoplasmic projections that fragment into functional platelets. Although essential to adult physiology, evidence from recent research suggests that mechanisms regulating thrombopoiesis in the embryo differ from adult counterparts. Human stem cell models have provided information regarding MK maturation stages, unveiling the complexity of such a process and the paramount singularity of specific molecular pathways in ensuring the effective production of platelets necessary for the maintenance of hemostatic homeostasis (Sim, 2017). Thrombopoiesis in adult humans occurs primarily in the bone marrow, where MKs release proplatelets into the circulation. Although in embryonic ontogeny, platelet production is mostly in the fetal liver and yolk sac, which is the reverse of what has been learned from experiments involving murine models. Flow cytometric analysis of embryonic blood and MK revealed that platelet counts balloon tremendously during gestation development, particularly around embryonic days 13.5–14.5, as MK count and maturation peak. Interestingly, the absence of signaling molecules , such as c-Myb is not necessarily reflected in peripheral platelet counts, indicative of functional redundancy and redundant pathways in embryonic thrombopoiesis. The divergence underscores the necessity for exploring developmental timelines in the development of platelets to inform potential therapeutic interventions for congenital platelet disorders (Liu et al., 2021). Advancements in imaging technology over the past few years have enabled scientists to study thrombopoiesis *in vivo* and reveal critical information on platelet formation during embryogenesis. Utilizing multiphoton intravital microscopy, it has become possible to monitor MKs within their natural habitats, further illuminating MK release processes. This model has shown that fetal liver MKs are more thrombopoietically active than yolk sac progenitors and that proplatelet production and budding from the cell membrane are two separate mechanisms of platelet production. Significantly, this gives valuable insight into how changes in thrombopoiesis could lead to the development of diseases , such as neonatal thrombocytopenia. With the comprehensive understanding of the mechanisms of thrombopoiesis at both cellular and molecular levels, researchers are paving the way for new strategies to prevent congenital blood and hematopoietic disorders, which are strengthening our collective knowledge in hematopoiesis and blood (Sim, 2017; Liu et al., 2021) (Figure 9.15).

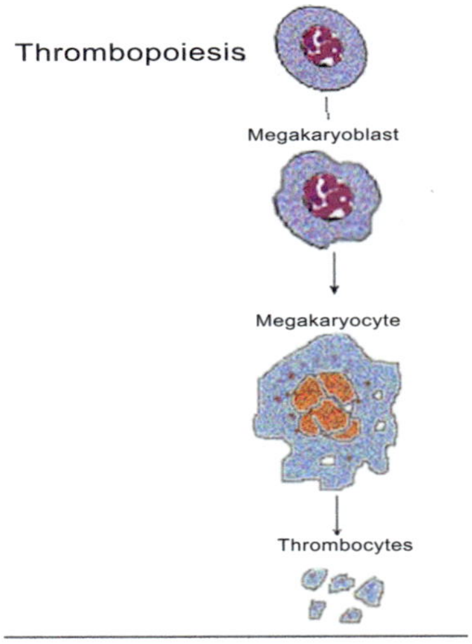

Figure 9.15. Thrombopoiesis.

Source: https://blogger.googleusercontent.com/img/b/R29vZ2xl/AVvXsEjb19_aWiyc-riWM9erYYbIWa024Kb5KRG278LqWBO0XVcPFiGpTEqI57D4kF-yC-QqL4tGP2Xdl6KKHjCIQZkbTB9sOYGQWq943rNdpUzX06neBVN5OJdITpR09eiAxtcJddNuSsaW11pF/s702/4.+Thrombopoiesis.webp.

Test Your Knowledge

1. What is the formation of RBC erythropoiesis?
2. What is the process of platelet formation?

9.5. Regulation of Hematopoiesis

Learning Outcome

1. Describe the role of growth factors and cytokines;
2. Understand the influence of the bone marrow microenvironment;
3. Understand the feedback mechanisms in blood cell production.

The regulation of hematopoiesis is essential to accomplish blood formation in humans. This complex process is regulated by many genetic and environmental stimuli that give the proper balance between preserving the progenitor cells and their differentiation. Some of the key regulatory elements are transcription factors , such as the Hox gene family, which are central to the process of specification of hematopoietic lineage. They are implicated to have a role in early stem cell regulation in a complex manner, influencing hematopoietic stem cell expansion and differentiation. For instance, it has been demonstrated by embryonic stem cell model experiments that alterations in Hox gene expression are detected at multiple stages of hematopoietic commitment and thus reveal their central role in determining hematopoietic fate. This hox regulatory network not only functions in normal hematopoiesis but also appears to have a function in leukemic progression when disrupted (Wheadon et al., 2011). The microenvironment or niche from which hematopoietic stem cells arise also plays a crucial role to play in the regulation of hematopoiesis. The niche is conditioned by the significant cellular constituents like osteoblasts and mesenchymal stromal cells, which provide a permissive environment that supports HSC proliferation and maintenance. More recent developments in *ex vivo* models have sought to more accurately mimic this niche, employing co-cultures of a range of cell types to model the hematopoietic environment. Such systems have been shown to induce HSC self-renewal and expansion with minimal dependence on cytokine-mediated signals, which sometimes lead to dysregulation. The establishment of such three-dimensional culture systems is a landmark towards better understanding HSC biology and has potential uses in regenerative medicine and transplantation with an intact, balanced HSC population (Huang et al., 2016). Regulation of hematopoiesis is further complicated by extrinsic signals, like cytokines and growth factors secreted by niche cells, that orchestrate HSC fate.

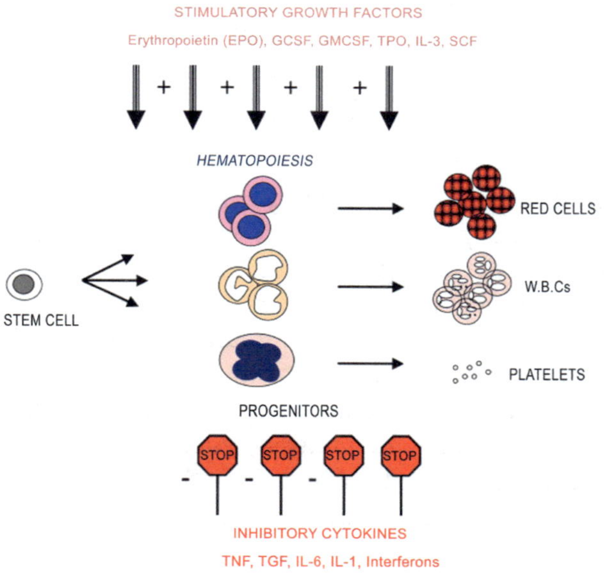

Figure 9.16. Regulation of hematopoiesis by cytokines. The process of differentiation of hematopoietic stem cells into mature blood cells is tightly regulated by the actions of both stimulatory and inhibitory cytokines.

Source: https://www.researchgate.net/publication/248396151/figure/fig1/AS:202938220847104@1425395650316/Regulation-of-hematopoiesis-by-cytokines-The-process-of-differentiation-of-hematopoietic.png.

The presence of such signaling molecules is essential, as they not only initiate intracellular pathways that are cell supportive but also direct HSCs towards lineage specification. High-throughput work has identified sets of cytokines that are differentially regulated in various contexts and exerting hematopoietic influences. Derangements in such modulatory networks can cause malignancies, such as hematological malignancies. With progressive research in this area, it will be more and more necessary to clarify the connection between microenvironmental signals, genetic control, and cell signaling pathways in order to establish targeted therapies for blood conditions and optimize HSC use in clinical as well as experimental models (Huang et al., 2016; Wheadon et al., 2011) (Figure 9.16).

9.5.1. Role of Growth Factors and Cytokines

Hematopoiesis is greatly influenced by the complex processes of growth factors and cytokines that play significant roles in the regulation of hematopoietic stem and progenitor cells (HSPCs). These signaling compounds enable crucial interactions in the bone marrow microenvironment, in effect controlling the fate of HSPCs. Growth factors , such as stem cell factor (SCF) and thrombopoietin (TPO) have been identified with a promise of triggering survival, proliferation, and differentiation of these cells. Furthermore, the ability of cytokines to create an environment of support reflects their role in hematopoietic homeostasis. The HSPCs' responsiveness to such factors indicates a controlled system sensitive to intrinsic and extrinsic signals, thus ensuring an adequate supply of blood cells in response to varying physiological demand and pathology. The compartmentalization of growth factor and cytokine activity within different niches of the bone marrow is one of the most important properties of their activity. Interactions of HSPCs with niche cells, cooperative osteoblasts and mesenchymal stromal cells have been determined to be necessary for the functioning of HSPCs. From studies, the cooperative osteoblasts and mesenchymal stromal cells actively secrete a wide range of cytokines responsible for coordinating cellular responses important to hematopoiesis. Such functional interaction is responsible for maintaining the delicate equilibrium between differentiation and self-renewal of the HSPCs. Notably, as the function served by such cytokines may be inhibited, it is highly dangerous to hematopoietic integrity since diminished signaling disrupts the homeostatic processes necessary for effective blood cell production and thereby conditions , such as anemia or other hematopoietic pathologies (Agas et al., 2015). Recent advancements in culture systems that mimic the HSPC niche underscore the function served by cytokines in therapeutic applications.

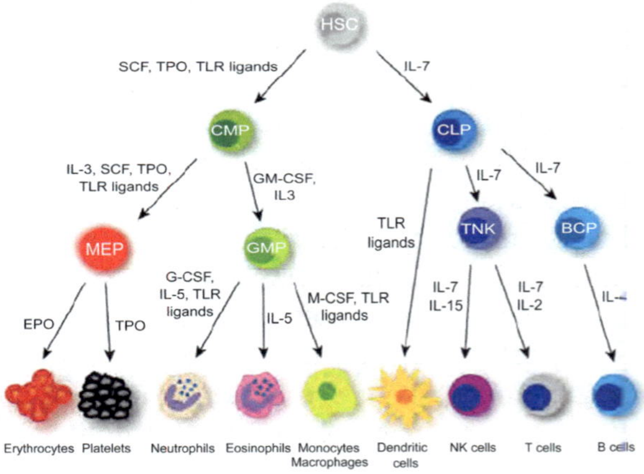

Figure 9.17. The role of cytokines in hematopoiesis. Cytokines act on both multipotent progenitors as well as committed progenitors and provide survival and proliferation signals.

Source: https://www.researchgate.net/profile/Katja-Fiedler/publication/221927012/figure/fig8/AS:305258648621067@1449790741920/The-role-of-cytokines-in-hematopoiesis-Cytokines-act-on-both-multipotent-progenitors-as.png.

For instance, new strategies , such as the co-culture of MSCs and osteoblasts without the use of exogenous cytokines reveal how this microenvironment promotes HSPC self-renewal and *ex vivo* expansion (Huang et al., 2016). Such systems not only optimize the growth conditions for HSPCs but also replicate the physiological environment to preserve the functional characteristics of these cells. The outcomes from these experiments have the potential to lead to new directions in stem cell therapy and regenerative medicine that prioritize the pivotal role growth factors and cytokines play not just in hematopoiesis, but more broadly in hematological disease and health (Figure 9.17).

9.5.2. Influence of the Bone Marrow Microenvironment

Blood cell homeostasis regulation can be attributed to the basis constituted by the interaction between hematopoietic stem cells and their bone marrow microenvironment. Special niches have been found to exist in the bone marrow that offer the HSCs highly specialized niches for self-renewal and differentiation.

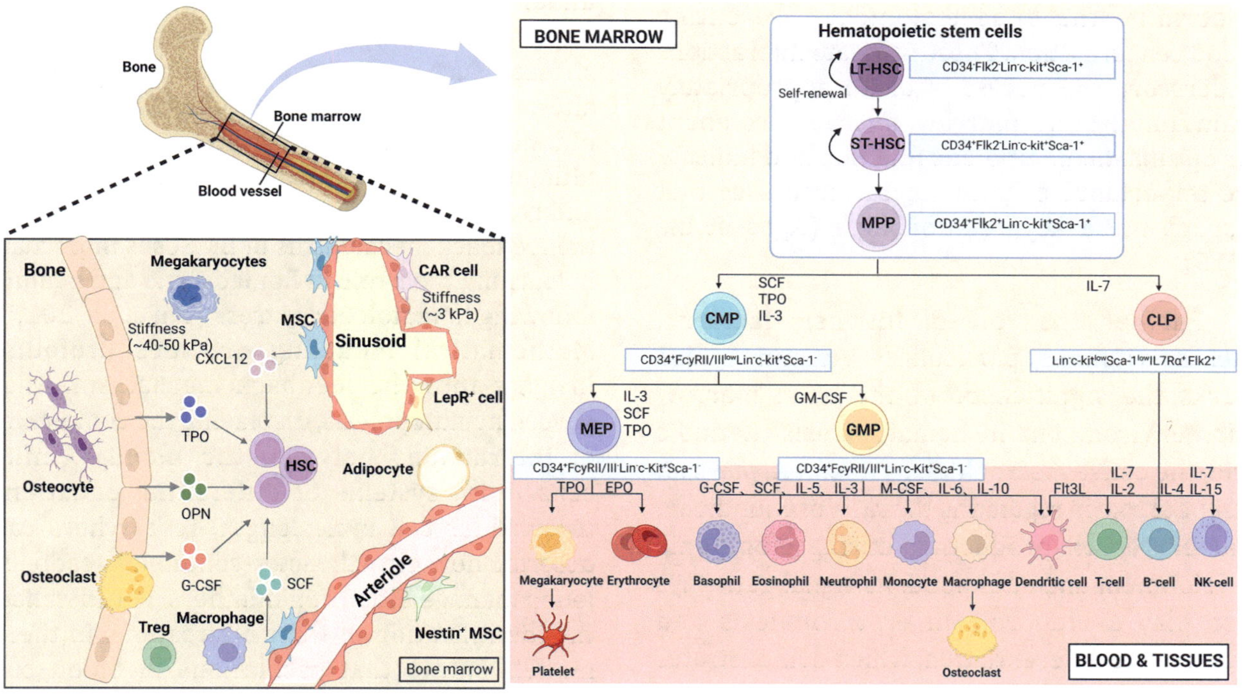

Figure 9.18. Hematopoietic hierarchical models and the bone marrow microenvironment.

Source: https://www.frontiersin.org/files/Articles/1338178/fimmu-15-1338178-HTML/image_m/fimmu-15-1338178-g001.jpg.

The endosteal niche, presented in between the bone surface and the marrow, is strongly lined with osteoblasts, maintaining HSC function via the secretion of required cytokines and growth factors. Again, in the vascular niche, with proximity to the blood vessel, it provides a conduit not only for the delivery of nutrients but also for establishing a specific local microenvironment that aids in HSC signaling and proliferation. Disruption of these interactions among HSCs and these microenvironments leads to impaired hematopoiesis, hinting at the importance of these niches in ensuring the regular functioning of the hematopoietic system and bone health overall

(Agas et al., 2015). Further complexity to the hematopoietic landscape arises from the fact that the bone marrow microenvironment consists of a dynamic cellular network of interactions regulating hematopoiesis. It is comprised of many types of cells , such as mesenchymal stem cells and immune cells, that interact with HSCs to regulate their fate. Research indicates that changes in this cell composition can significantly impact hematopoietic production. For example, enhanced osteoblast function within the endosteal niche has been associated with enhanced hematopoietic function, but malfunctioning vascular niche activity can undermine the endosteal niche, preventing blood cell formation. These intricate interactions underscore the necessity of an appropriately maintained bone marrow microenvironment for optimal hematopoietic function and indicate the importance of pathological processes that disrupt these key relationships (Agas et al., 2015).

Further, the role of intrinsic factors , such as vitamins, particularly Vitamin A, also marks the significance of the bone marrow microenvironment in hematopoiesis. Retinoic acid, the active metabolite of Vitamin A, plays an essential role in regulating the ratio of endothelial and blood cell production during embryonic development and adulthood. Its signal pathways also play a vital role in erythropoiesis and granulocyte differentiation, which demonstrates that micronutrients are a part of hematopoietic regulation complexities. Vitamin A deficiency could lead to defective production of blood cells and increased susceptibility to various conditions, including anemia. Taking into account the function of such dietary factors offers another angle in understanding how the bone marrow microenvironment is involved in controlling the intricate interactions between the development of blood and immune cells (Figure 9.18).

9.5.3. Feedback Mechanisms in Blood Cell Production

The intricate regulation of blood cell production, known as hematopoiesis, is largely mediated by feedback mechanisms to achieve a fine balance between proliferation and differentiation of hematopoietic stem cells (HSCs). It all centers around the bone marrow microenvironment that contains bone marrow mesenchymal stem cells (BMSCs) that create hematopoietic niches. These niches are crucial since they provide signals and support required for HSC maintenance and differentiation. However, BMSC differentiation under various environmental stresses deeply impacts hematopoiesis. For example, with stresses , such as aging or chemotherapy exposure, alterations in BMSC differentiation can result in diminished hematopoietic stem cell function, ultimately causing defective blood cell formation and resultant pathologies. Hence, understanding the feedback mechanisms of BMSCs is important in learning their role in homeostasis and healing following hematological stress (Wu et al., 2018). Mathematical modeling provides profound insights into the feedback mechanisms that govern hematopoiesis, displaying the complexity of interactions between the blood-forming cells. With systems of differential equations to consider cell cycle length, researchers can describe how growth factor-containing feedback loops manage blood cell numbers. For instance, the identification of Hopf bifurcations in these models shows that oscillations in blood cell counts are caused by destabilized feedback control. Destabilization can manifest as periodic hematological disorders, which are characterized by oscillation of circulating blood cells. This mathematical perspective highlights the dynamic nature of hematopoietic regulation and emphasizes the importance of feedback mechanisms to maintain cellular homeostasis. Awareness of these oscillatory activities is important to the development of therapeutic regimens aimed at the restitution of balance in patients suffering from blood disorders

(Adimy et al., 2006). With the emergence of new evidence, balance in differentiation of BMSCs emerges as a unique factor contributing to support for effective hematopoiesis, especially following bone marrow transplantation. The cross-talk among BMSCs and HSCs is not so much a linear process but consists of intricate feedback loops that modulate stem cell behavior in response to physiological demands. Disruption of this balance can hinder hematopoietic restitution, with prolonged recovery periods and complications. Therapeutic strategies designed to enhance BMSC support promise to enable enhanced blood production in patients. Through ongoing research, knowledge of the mechanisms of feedback regulating hematopoiesis will not only enlighten the underlying biology but will also inform clinical practices so that the outcomes of patients undergoing treatment for hematological diseases will be optimized (Wu et al., 2018).

Test Your Knowledge

1. What is the role of growth factors and cytokines?
2. What is the feedback mechanism of red blood cell production?

9.6. Disorders Related to Blood and Hematopoiesis

Learning Outcome

1. Describe the anemia and its types;
2. Discuss leukemia and other blood cancers;
3. Understand the thrombocytopenia and clotting disorders.

Blood- and hematopoiesis-disorders are a broad range of conditions, the majority of which are caused by abnormalities in the hematopoietic system. They arise through qualitative or quantitative deficiencies within the blood cells, with significant health effects. Concurrent illnesses , such as anemia, thrombocytopenia, and the leukemias illustrate the complexities of hematopoiesis and the important role of genetic and environmental factors in the production of blood. As an example, anemia can be due to a shortage of essential nutrients like iron or vitamin B12 that are crucial in the production of red blood cells. These diseases can also disrupt the delicate balance of cellular components, producing clinical syndromes that have to be addressed promptly. Discovery of the mechanisms of these disorders is essential since early diagnosis and treatment can prevent or mitigate the severe complications involving deranged hematopoiesis. A high priority for studying blood disorders is understanding their genetic bases and environmental interactions. The hygiene hypothesis suggests that lowered exposure to microbes, particularly at early immune maturation, may lead to increased frequencies of autoimmune and allergic disease. Evidence shows that such microbial interactions are capable of modulating the regulation and differentiation of hematopoietic stem cells, and therefore the overall immune response and susceptibility to disease of the blood. This interaction highlights that impacts on hematopoiesis are not just biological but also dependent on environmental contexts, particularly during developmental windows. The study of the interaction between environmental forces and inherited susceptibility is needed to clarify the etiology of hematological disorders in contemporary populations and to emphasize the importance of preventive public health policy.

Recent research is increasingly focused on developing more efficient models for studying blood diseases and hematopoiesis, and xenotransplantation is playing a central role in this process. Technical advances in this area offer informative information regarding normal and malignant human hematopoiesis. Specifically, new approaches, such as the application of administration of fludarabine, have been found to possess significant promise for enabling rapid engraftment of human hematopoiesis in immunodeficient mice. These models exhibit an extremely high increase in human $CD45^+$ cells within the bone marrow, which indicates successful engraftment of hematopoietic stem cells and their derivative descendants. Such robust reconstitution not only aids in the understanding of normal hematopoiesis but also holds promise for therapeutic benefit in treatment strategies for illnesses like acute myeloid leukemia. Through continuous innovation in research methods, the specialty can more effectively treat complexities in blood disorders as well as increase therapeutic success in affected individuals (Pievani et al., 2018; Apostol et al., 202) (Figure 9.19).

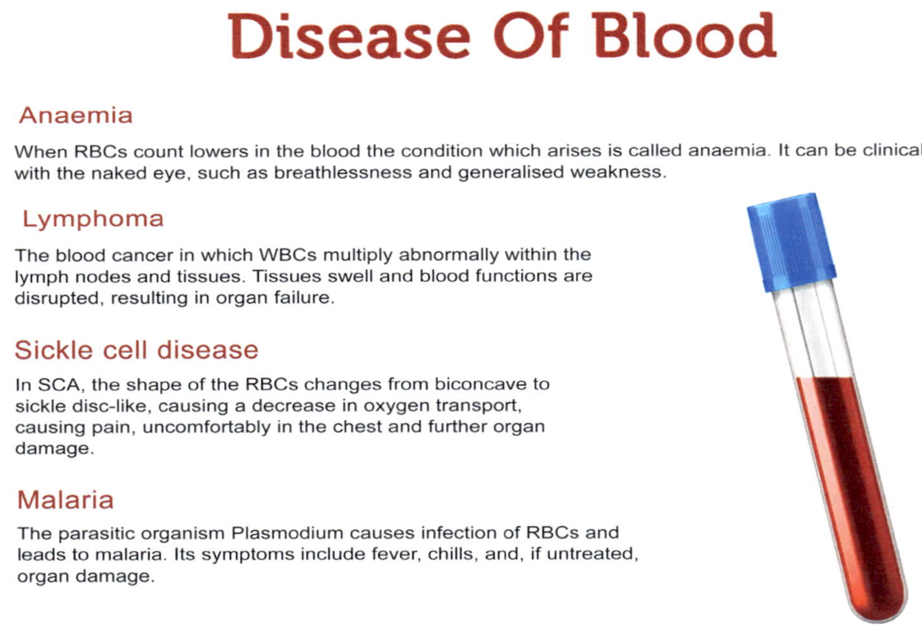

Figure 9.19. Disease of the blood.

Source: https://assets.lybrate.com/imgs/tic/enadp/disease-of-blood.jpg.

9.6.1. Anemia and Its Types

Anemia, or a deficiency of red blood cells or hemoglobin, has very serious implications for general health and physiological functioning. Anemia exists as weakness, fatigue, and pallor and impacts approximately 1.62 billion people globally. Anemia is classified into various forms primarily based on its etiology, either due to the inefficient production of red blood cells, increased destruction, or blood loss. Iron deficiency anemia is most prevalent, most often due to insufficient iron in the diet or defective iron absorption. Pernicious anemia is another significant variety due to the absence of vitamin B12, due to defective absorption (often in conjunction with an intrinsic factor defect) and aplastic anemia, wherein bone marrow fails to produce adequate blood cells. Anemia's heterogeneity makes it have multifactorial causes and justifies individualized diagnosis techniques and therapeutic approaches against various underlying etiologies. Knowledge of anemia's various presentations is necessary for proper management and treatment. Microcytic anemia, for instance, is often seen with iron deficiency and represents smaller-than-normal red blood cells due to the decreased production of hemoglobin. Macrocytic anemia, in contrast, is characterized by increased red blood cells, typically associated with vitamin B12 or folate deficiency, leading to DNA replication issues. Hemolytic anemia results when the red blood cells are subjected to premature destruction, a process brought about by autoimmune disorders or inherited conditions , such as sickle cell disease. Every type is not only characterized by distinctive morphological properties upon examination but also necessitates a distinct therapeutic strategy, especially when the physiological mechanism of hematopoiesis is taken into account. For example, understanding the role of bone marrow mesenchymal stem cells during hematopoiesis support is critical in the identification of potential therapeutic targets when aplastic anemia is present (Wu et al., 2018).

Examination of anemia causes also includes its potential progression to more adverse conditions, such as myelodysplastic syndromes (MDS) and acute myeloid leukemia (AML). Patients with MDS, particularly those with specific genetic mutations, have a greater propensity for progression into AML, which has been described as preleukemia (Koeffler & Leong, 2017). This connection emphasizes the importance of close monitoring and management in patients who have been diagnosed with various types of anemia since early treatment can potentially change the direction of the disease. The evolving definition of the blood disorders and their interconnection emphasizes the importance of ongoing research into both the mechanism of hematopoiesis and the development of effective therapies. Encouraging a comprehensive appreciation of anemia and its types is ultimately required in dealing with the broader implications of disrupted hematopoiesis to human health (Figure 9.20).

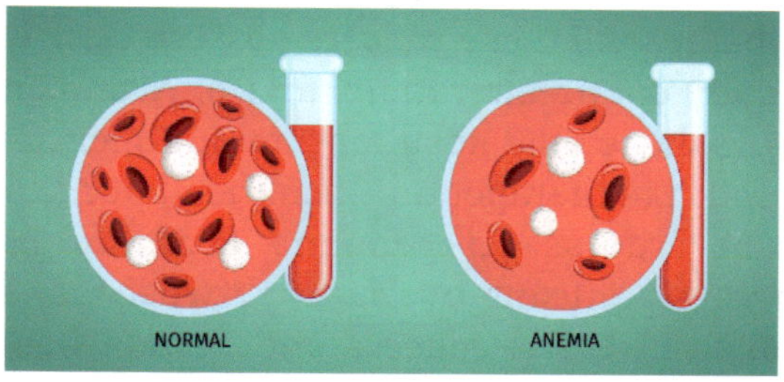

Figure 9.20. Anaemia.

Source: https://www.happiesthealth.com/wp-content/uploads/2022/08/anemia.jpg

9.6.2. Leukemia and Other Blood Cancers

Leukemia, or blood and bone marrow cancer, arises from a number of genetic mutations that lead to disruptions to normal hematopoiesis and culminate in uncontrolled proliferation of blood cells. This blood cancer is primarily classified as acute and chronic leukemia, depending on the rate of disease development and progression. Acute leukemia is rapid and its treatment is emergent, whereas chronic leukemia is slow. Pathophysiology of leukemia involves alterations in the regulatory networks controlling the differentiation of hematopoietic stem cells and causing the expression of key oncogenes in an aberrant form. These genetic alterations can sometimes mirror those of other conditions, implying complex interaction between malignancy and genomic disease (Adashek et al., 2020). Clarification of the molecular mechanisms and the leukemic genomic landscape is critical for generating targeted therapies that enhance treatment specificity and result in improved patient outcomes. Lymphoma and multiple myeloma are additional instances of blood cancers that portray the complexities of hematopoietic malignancies. Lymphomas are made up of clonal proliferation of lymphocytes and include forms like Hodgkin's and non-Hodgkin's lymphomas. Multiple myeloma specifically targets plasma cells and disrupts the immune system by producing abnormal antibodies. All these cancers possess their own unique genetic alterations and environmental factors, hence the need for a multidimensional approach in therapeutic modalities. Specifically, recent studies on genomic profiling have shown significant overlaps between genetic profiles in blood cancers and certain benign illnesses (Adashek et al., 2020). Such a nuanced observation, while assisting in the identification of treatment modalities, is also making initial detection more difficult, projecting the necessity of rigorous screening protocols in at-risk groups. The role of specific genes and their dysregulation is significant in the etiology and pathogenesis of several blood malignancies and contributes to the complexity in their management.

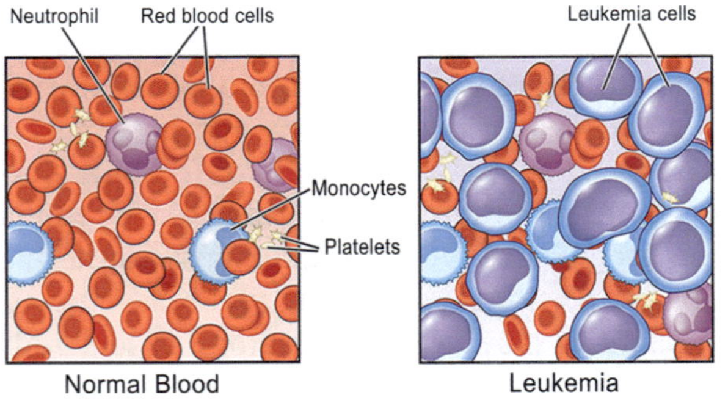

Figure 9.21. Leukemia.

Source: https://my.clevelandclinic.org/-/scassets/images/org/health/articles/4365-leukemia.

HOX genes, for instance, are involved in stem cell differentiation and have been implicated in malignant transformation underlying acute myeloid leukemia (AML) and colorectal cancer. Dysregulation of these genes is linked to aberrant cellular behaviors predisposing to cancer, and therefore, the necessity for targeted therapies that can modulate HOX gene expression. Advances in molecular biology technology are making it simple to research these pathways, and novel therapies are being developed. By addressing the underlying genetic changes, it is now feasible to develop more efficient, tailored treatment regimens that not only enhance survival of the patient but also minimize the risk of treatment-induced secondary malignancies (Figure 9.21).

9.6.3. Thrombocytopenia and Clotting Disorders

Thrombocytopenia, characterized by a reduced platelet count, has a profound impact on the hemostatic process in the human body. Platelets or thrombocytes play a crucial role in blood clotting by adhering to vascular injury and clumping together to form a plug, thus preventing excessive hemorrhage. The etiology of thrombocytopenia is diverse, ranging from reduced production in the bone marrow, autoimmune diseases, to increased destruction in peripheral circulation. All of these mechanisms reinforce the complex interaction between clotting and hematopoiesis. For instance, diseases , such as aplastic anemia may cause impaired production by megakaryocytes, leading to insufficient platelet numbers. An understanding of these underlying pathways is important in order to diagnose and manage patients properly because the clinical presentation of thrombocytopenia can increase dramatically, requiring early intervention to avoid life-threatening bleeding complications, which are potentially fatal. In the case of clotting disorders, the interaction between platelets and coagulation factors becomes significant. Congenital etiologies , such as hemophilia A and B or acquired etiologies , such as vitamin K deficiency or liver disease, can result in abnormal clot formation. The critical correlation with thrombocytopenia in these clotting disorders indicates that a broad diagnostic workup is necessary. For instance, while a patient has a low platelet level, the coagulopathy could be the result of causes other than the deficiency in functional platelets. A precise awareness of such relationships enables diverse, useful treatment plans ranging from platelet transfusions to targeted therapies aimed at addressing underlying deficiencies. Consequently, the subtleties of hemostasis can scarcely be overstated in the specialty of hematology. Management and therapy of thrombocytopenia and associated clotting disorders are fields of ongoing study and clinical refinement. Therapy approaches commonly rely on the specific etiology of the thrombocytopenia and the overall status of the patient. For example, with immune thrombocytopenic purpura (ITP), the immune response can be managed using corticosteroids, while for others, more aggressive interventions , such as splenectomy, might be required. Second, there have been new developments on myeloid disorders , such as myelodysplastic syndromes, that have opened up the possibilities for new therapies to improve platelet production and function (Estes, 1962). Also, clinicians must remain aware of the evolving landscape of the therapeutic options for clotting disorders because the elucidation of mechanisms of hematopoiesis and abnormalities of coagulation persists (Poggi et al., 2021). This ongoing exploration of the mechanisms and treatment of these diseases reflects the significance of integrative models of care for maximizing patient outcomes (Figure 9.22).

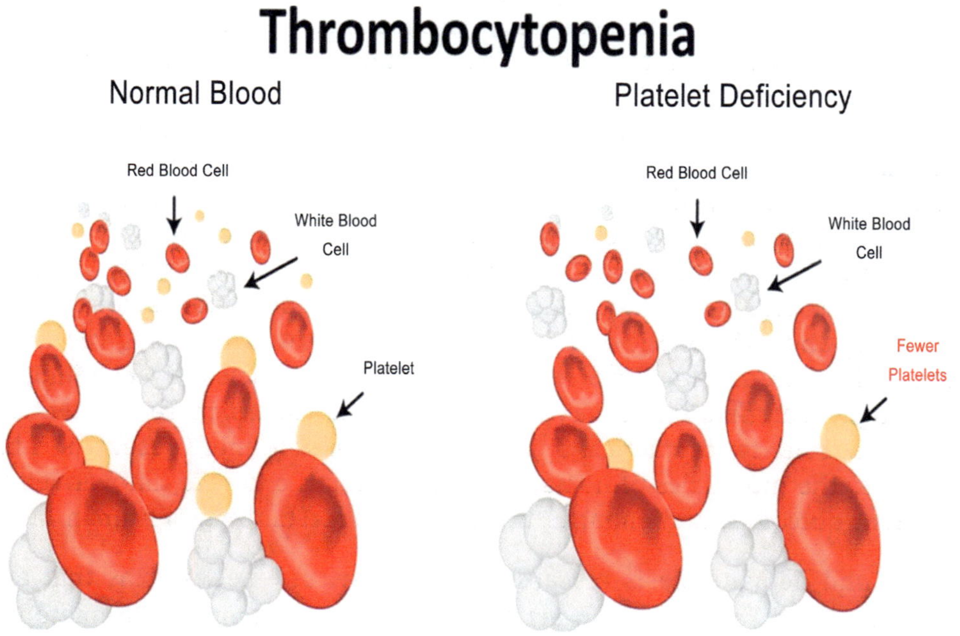

Figure 9.22. Thrombocytopenia diagram.

Source: https://stgaccinwbsdevlrs01.blob.core.windows.net/newcorporatewbsite/blogs/october2023/Thrombocytopenia-diagram.jpg.

Test Your Knowledge

1. What is anemia and its types?
2. What are the two forms of blood cancer?

SUMMARY

Briefly, the intricate processes of blood origin and hematopoiesis in man form the basis of our understanding of both normal physiology and a wide range of hematologic diseases. Such understanding has advanced significantly with methodological improvements in research, and this has made it possible to define clinical terms , such as preleukemia more accurately. Here, of note is the fact that preleukemia is not just an antecedent state to acute myeloid leukemia (AML), but more so a disease continuum driven by genetic dysregulation and environmental risk factors. The identification of clonal hematopoiesis, wherein the latter is defined by DNMT3A, TET2, or IDH1/2 mutations, highlights the need for early recognition and follow-up in high-risk groups. Thus, the development of targeted therapies and individualized treatment becomes a necessity to counteract the transition from preleukemia to true AML, and thus documenting its clinical relevance in hematopoietic research (Koeffler & Leong, 2017). Moreover, implications of hormonal impact on hematopoiesis, as observed through several studies, provide insight into blood cell behavior beyond mere cellular interactions. For instance, the influence of steroid hormones , such as progesterone and 17-beta-estradiol on the proliferation of progenitor cells contributes an extra dimension of sophistication in the regulation of myelopoiesis. The studies suggest a potential physiological adaptation response to environmental changes, with special reference to the inclusive relationship between hematopoiesis and the body's physiological states, such as pregnancy and postpartum convalescence. Understanding the interactions between the immune system and hematologic function is crucial, not only for extending our knowledge of hematologic well-being, but also for organizing clinical strategies to assist immune function when it is compromised, e.g., parturition (Burvenich et al., 2004). Lastly, the investigation of hematopoiesis in humans is a continuously emerging topic that needs an interdisciplinary strategy. With science advancing further into the dynamic forces involved in blood cell manufacturing and function, we are confronted with a diverse range of dependent variables from genetic susceptibility to environmental factors. Advances in tools like deep sequencing and cytogenetic assays only go further toward helping researchers identify at-risk individuals for the development of hematologic malignancies. By enabling collaborative partnerships among researchers, clinicians, and public health leaders, there is potential to translate what is discovered in science to practical applications. Ultimately, more research in blood science provides insight into the intricacies of hematopoiesis, paving the way to innovative therapies that can improve patient outcomes and enhance the overall understanding of human health.

Human blood and hematopoiesis research unveils intricate mechanisms that are needed to maintain homeostasis and respond to an array of physiological demands. Hematopoiesis, or the development of blood cells, is primarily achieved in the bone marrow, where HSCs proliferate into various lineages—red cells, white cells, and platelets. Even though recent studies have elucidated some of the roles of specific mutations in leukemogenesis, the landscape for how such activities engage normal hematopoiesis remains incomplete. For instance, in acute myeloid leukemia (AML), repeated DNMT3A mutations in HSCs highlight the early cellular alterations that place a person at risk for malignant transformation. These kinds of mutations are observed to provide a survival advantage and thus are relevant for elucidating pre-leukemic clones and implications for therapeutic approaches (Brandwein et al., 2014). Furthermore, the signaling pathways employed during hematopoietic differentiation are increasingly the focus of intense research. CBF{beta} plays a pivotal role in regulating the development of T cells and natural killer (NK) cells. Reduced levels of CBF{beta} interfere with the process of differentiation, providing vital insight into the role that certain biomarkers play in the determination of cell lineage. Experiments have revealed that diminished expression of CBF{beta} impacts not only T cell development but also progenitor cell capability to respond correctly to critical developmental signals , such as Notch. This exchange highlights the intricate system of signals governing hematopoietic cell destinies and the way these pathways could be disrupted for therapeutic intervention (Guo et al., 2008). In summary, the complex picture of blood and hematopoiesis calls for further exploration into genetic and molecular paradigms regulating both normal physiology and disease conditions , such as leukemia. A dissection of how pre-leukemic populations can expand and persist even during remission is key in working towards developing plans to target these cells before they acquire other mutations contributing to disease progression. Secondly, unraveling the roles of key signaling molecules like CBF{beta} not only accounts for normal hematopoietic development but also points towards potential therapeutic targets that are capable of correcting developmental abnormalities. In general, these discoveries illuminate our understanding of both the similar and different natures of hematopoiesis and call for an integrated approach to treatments that ensure blood health and efficiently cure hematological disorders.

KEY TERMS FROM THIS CHAPTER

- Acute myeloid leukemia
- Blood
- Clonal hematopoiesis
- Genetic mutations
- Hypoxia-inducible factors
- Leukocytes
- Plasma
- Anemia
- Cardiovascular system
- Erythrocytes
- Hematopoiesis
- Leukemia
- Myelodysplastic syndromes
- Platelets

CRITICAL THINKING QUESTIONS

1. **Blood is classified as which type of tissue?**
   a. Nervous tissue
   b. Epithelial tissue
   c. Connective tissue
   d. Muscular tissue
2. **What percentage of blood volume is plasma?**
   a. 45%
   b. 55%
   c. 65%
   d. 75%
3. **The formed elements of blood include:**
   a. Plasma, white blood cells, and red blood cells
   b. White blood cells, red blood cells, and platelets
   c. Serum, plasma, and red blood cells
   d. Platelets, serum, and plasma
4. **Hematopoiesis occurs primarily in:**
   a. The liver
   b. The bone marrow
   c. The spleen
   d. The thymus
5. **The stem cell responsible for all blood cell lineages is called:**
   a. Myeloid progenitor cell
   b. Lymphoid progenitor cell
   c. Hematopoietic stem cell
   d. Mesenchymal stem cell

Short Answer Questions

1. What is blood and its components?
2. Why is hematopoiesis important in human health?
3. What is the function of the blood?
4. What is the process of hematopoiesis?
5. List the types of blood cells.

Answers to Critical Thinking Questions

1. (c); 2. (b) ; 3. (b); 4. (b); 5. (c)

REFERENCES

1. Cañete, A., Cano, E., Muñoz-Chápuli, R., & Carmona, R. (2017). Role of Vitamin A/Retinoic Acid in Regulation of Embryonic and Adult Hematopoiesis. *Nutrients*, *9*(2), 159. https://doi.org/10.3390/nu9020159(accessed on 7th August 2025).
2. Adams, P. D., Jasper, H., & Rudolph, K. L. (2015). *Aging-Induced Stem Cell Mutations as Drivers for Disease and Cancer*. https://core.ac.uk/download/42363092.pdf (accessed on 7th August 2025).
3. Adashek, J. J., Kato, S., Kurzrock, R., Lippman, M., et al. (2020). *The paradox of cancer genes in non-malignant conditions: Implications for precision medicine*. https://core.ac.uk/download/323064613.pdf (accessed on 7th August 2025).
4. Adimy, M., Crauste, F., & Ruan, S. (2006). *Modelling hematopoiesis mediated by growth factors with applications to periodic hematological diseases*. https://core.ac.uk/download/50178962.pdf (accessed on 7th August 2025).
5. Guo, Y., Maillard, I., Chakraborti, S., Rothenberg, E. V., & Speck, N. A. (2008). Core binding factors are necessary for natural killer cell development and cooperate with Notch signaling during T-cell specification. *Blood*, *112*(3), 480–492. https://doi.org/10.1182/blood-2007-10-120261 (accessed on 7th August 2025).
6. Agas, D., Douni, E., Marchetti, L., & Sabbieti, M. G. (2015). *The Unbearable Lightness of Bone Marrow Homeostasis*. https://core.ac.uk/download/54653580.pdf (accessed on 7th August 2025).
7. Aljoufi, A., Broxmeyer, H. E., Huang, X., Trinh, H., et al. (2018). *Hypoxia Signaling Pathway in Stem Cell Regulation: Good and Evil*. https://core.ac.uk/download/228066162.pdf (accessed on 7th August 2025).
8. Piovan, E., Tosello, V., Amadori, A., & Zanovello, P. (2018). Chemotactic Cues for NOTCH1-Dependent Leukemia. *Frontiers in immunology*, *9*, 633. https://doi.org/10.3389/fimmu.2018.00633 (accessed on 7th August 2025).
9. Apostol, A. C., Beaudin, A. E., & Jensen, K. D. C. (2020). *Training the fetal immune system through maternal inflammation—A layered hygiene hypothesis*. https://core.ac.uk/download/288432714.pdf (accessed on 7th August 2025).
10. Pinto, A. I., Brown, N., Preham, O., Doehl, J. S. P., Ashwin, H., & Kaye, P. M. (2017). TNF signalling drives expansion of bone marrow CD4+ T cells responsible for HSC exhaustion in experimental visceral leishmaniasis. *PLoS pathogens*, *13*(7), e1006465. https://doi.org/10.1371/journal.ppat.1006465(accessed on 7th August 2025).
11. Banerjee, U., Cha, N., Cho, B., Shim, J., et al. (2018). *Systemic control of immune cell development by integrated carbon dioxide and hypoxia chemosensation in Drosophila*. https://core.ac.uk/download/323079769.pdf (accessed on 7th August 2025).
12. Bechtold, W. E., Campleman, S., Dosemeci, M., Haas, M., et al. (1996). *An Epidemiologic Study of Early Biologic Effects of Benzene in Chinese Workers*. https://core.ac.uk/download/323080830.pdf (accessed on 7th August 2025).
13. Bhatlekar, S., Boman, B. M., & Fields, J. Z. (2018). *Role of HOX Genes in Stem Cell Differentiation and Cancer*. https://core.ac.uk/download/213444597.pdf (accessed on 7th August 2025).

14. Brandwein, J. M., Brown, A. M. K., Chen, W. C., Dick, J. E., et al. (2014). *Identification of Pre-Leukemic Hematopoietic Stem Cells in Acute Leukemia*. https://core.ac.uk/download/323071793.pdf (accessed on 7th August 2025).

15. Hughes, C. E., & Nibbs, R. J. B. (2018). A guide to chemokines and their receptors. *The FEBS journal, 285*(16), 2944–2971. https://doi.org/10.1111/febs.14466(accessed on 7th August 2025).

16. Brownlie, A., Leri, A., Marrone, A., Satyanarayana, A., Davidson, A. J., Armbruster, B. N., Autexier, C., et al. (2008). *A non-canonical function of zebrafish telomerase reverse transcriptase is required for developmental hematopoiesis*. https://core.ac.uk/download/pdf/8199784.pdf (accessed on 7th August 2025).

17. Burvenich, C., Duchateau, L., Meyer, E., Van Merris, V., et al. (2004). *Differential Effects of Steroids and Retinoids on Bovine Myelopoiesis in Vitro*. https://core.ac.uk/download/55832205.pdf (accessed on 7th August 2025).

18. Crispin, A. (2017). *HSCB, a co-chaperone in mitochondrial iron-sulfur cluster biogenesis, is a novel candidate gene for congenital sideroblastic anemia*. Master's thesis, Boston University. https://open.bu.edu/bitstream/2144/26669/5/Crispin_bu_0017N_13280.pdf (accessed on 7th August 2025).

19. Crooks, G. M., Ge, S., Hao, Q. L., Kohn, A. D., et al. (2012). *Lymphoid priming in human bone marrow begins before expression of CD10 with upregulation of L-selectin*. https://core.ac.uk/download/323078483.pdf (accessed on 7th August 2025).

20. Estes, J. W. (1962). *Modern Concepts of the Platelet in Health and Disease*. https://open.bu.edu/bitstream/2144/26002/1/Estes_J.%20Worth_1962_web.pdf (accessed on 7th August 2025).

21. Gallucci, B. B., & McCarthy, D. O. (1995). *The Immune System*. https://core.ac.uk/download/213081395.pdf (accessed on 7th August 2025).

22. Gardon Poggi, J. C., Muñoz, A., & Satué, K. (2021). *A Review of Current Knowledge of Myeloproliferative Disorders in the Horse*. https://core.ac.uk/download/597063343.pdf (accessed on 7th August 2025).

23. Gopalan, B. P., Kamimura, S., Dagur, P., Shah, N., Quezado, M., Quezado, Z. M. N., & Shet, A. S. (2024). Short-term fostamatinib treatment impacts hematopoiesis and downregulates thromboinflammation in Townes sickle mice. *Blood*. https://www.semanticscholar.org/paper/eaa9616ebef4b5e3acf37fa33c8fb767827d8e82 (accessed on 7th August 2025).

24. Huang, X., Wang, C., Wang, X., Xiao, Y., et al. (2016). *Three-dimensional co-culture of mesenchymal stromal cells and differentiated osteoblasts on human bio-derived bone scaffolds supports active multi-lineage hematopoiesis in vitro: Functional implication of the biomimetic HSC niche*. https://core.ac.uk/download/323075326.pdf (accessed on 7th August 2025).

25. Jacobs, S. (2021). *Dissecting Diversity: Clonal Analysis of Normal and Malignant Hematopoiesis Using Cellular Barcodes*. Doctoral dissertation. https://core.ac.uk/download/519046293.pdf (accessed on 7th August 2025).

26. Koeffler, H. P., & Leong, G. (2017). *Preleukemia: One Name, Many Meanings*. https://core.ac.uk/download/323076596.pdf (accessed on 7th August 2025).

27. Wu, J., Zhang, W., Ran, Q., Xiang, Y., Zhong, J. F., Li, S. C., & Li, Z. (2018). The Differentiation Balance of Bone Marrow Mesenchymal Stem Cells Is Crucial to Hematopoiesis. *Stem cells*

international, 2018, 1540148. https://doi.org/10.1155/2018/1540148(accessed on 7th August 2025).

28. Lim, H., & O'Neill, H. C. (2019). *Identification of Stromal Cells in Spleen Which Support Myelopoiesis.* https://core.ac.uk/download/196606999.pdf (accessed on 7th August 2025).

29. Liu, H. (2021). *Mechanisms of embryonic thrombopoiesis.* https://core.ac.uk/download/597479610.pdf (accessed on 7th August 2025).

30. Morera, D., & MacKenzie, S. A. (2011). Is there a direct role for erythrocytes in the immune response?. *Veterinary research, 42*(1), 89. https://doi.org/10.1186/1297-9716-42-89(accessed on 7th August 2025).

31. Mirzabekov, I. A., Xojimatov, S. R., & Xodjayeva, M. (2025). Gemotsitopoez va uning bosqichlari, qon hosil bo'lishi. *Universal International Scientific Journal.* https://www.semanticscholar.org/paper/372adf5576a55289997640c98652a8d347ea4228 (accessed on 7th August 2025).

32. Pievani, A., Michelozzi, I. M., Rambaldi, B., Granata, V., Corsi, A., Dazzi, F., Biondi, A., & Serafini, M. (2018). Fludarabine as a cost-effective adjuvant to enhance engraftment of human normal and malignant hematopoiesis in immunodeficient mice. *Scientific reports, 8*(1), 9125. https://doi.org/10.1038/s41598-018-27425-x(accessed on 7th August 2025).

33. Scheller, E. L., Tratwal, J., et al. (2020). *Reporting guidelines, review of methodological standards, and challenges toward harmonization in bone marrow adiposity research: Report of the Methodologies Working Group of the International Bone Marrow Adiposity Society.* https://core.ac.uk/download/322802248.pdf (accessed on 7th August 2025).

34. Sim, X. L. (2017). *Understanding Megakaryopoiesis and Thrombopoiesis Using Human Stem Cells Models.* Doctoral dissertation. https://core.ac.uk/download/219378002.pdf (accessed on 7th August 2025).

35. Wheadon, H., Ramsey, J. M., Dobbin, E., Dickson, G. J., Corrigan, P. M., Freeburn, R. W., & Thompson, A. (2011). Differential Hox expression in murine embryonic stem cell models of normal and malignant hematopoiesis. *Stem cells and development, 20*(8), 1465–1476. https://doi.org/10.1089/scd.2010.0226(accessed on 7th August 2025).

36. Walker, B. (2015). *Embracing a diverse student population within an urban science classroom through the use of inquiry-based and culturally relevant pedagogy: A multipedagogical approach in narrowing the science achievement gap.* https://core.ac.uk/download/638982214.pdf (accessed on 7th August 2025).

MUSCULAR TISSUE

10

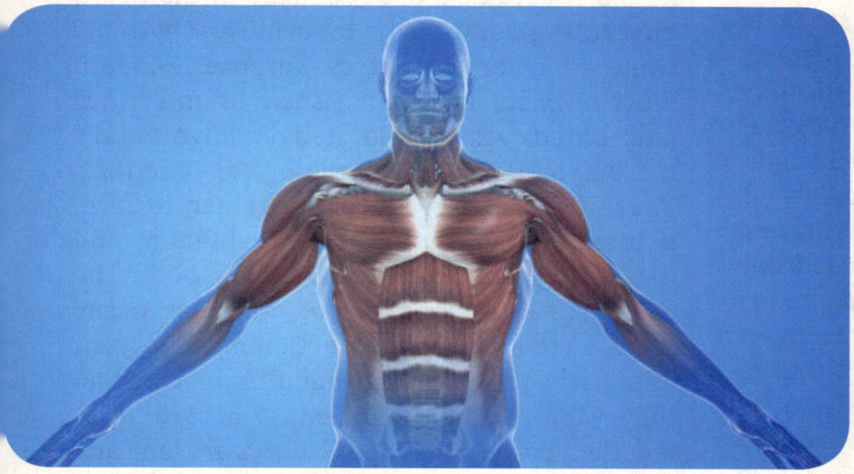

LEARNING OBJECTIVES

After studying this chapter, you will be able to:

1. Explain the types of muscular tissue;
2. Describe the structure and function of muscular tissue;
3. Understand the mechanism of muscle contraction;
4. Describe the disorders related to muscular tissue.

Introduction

The role of muscular tissue in the human body is fundamental, being the foundation of movement and stability in the body. Muscles are classified primarily into three distinct groups: skeletal, cardiac, and smooth. Skeletal muscles, which are voluntarily controlled, are essential for movement and posture. Cardiac muscle, found exclusively in the heart, operates involuntarily to ensure continuous blood circulation throughout the body, whereas smooth muscle is found in other organs and blood vessels and assists in significant activities , such as digestion and circulation. Knowledge of these muscles forms the foundation for studying human physiology since it places in the spotlight the intricate process of structure and function that sustains life and enables various movements of the body (Biga et al., 2020). At the cellular level, muscle tissue of skeletal muscle tissue is made up of specialized muscle cells, or myocytes, with the following specific properties: excitability, contractility, extensibility, and elasticity. These properties make muscles respond rapidly to stimulation and generate force. The intricate arrangement of myofibrils in each muscle cell facilitates the mechanism of contraction based on the sliding filament theory. The theory posits that the interaction between actin and myosin filaments results in muscle contraction and shortening, a fundamental process underlying all muscular activity. Investigating these cellular processes not only abolishes the mystique about how muscles operate but also opens up avenues for understanding the importance of muscular diseases and the potential for therapeutic interventions (Pravdin, 2013). The study of muscular tissue goes beyond the basic anatomy and physiology, but covers clinical application and health concerns. Muscle knowledge is particularly vital for medical professionals, physical therapists, and sports scientists. Advances in technology, e.g., neuroimaging and biomechanical models, further increased our understanding of muscle function and adaptation to stress. For instance, fiber architecture models that simulate cardiac muscle enable a better understanding of cardiac mechanics and its relationship to any pathology. As we explore muscular tissue intricacies in man, we also recognize the applicability of further research and study to develop an informed reaction to health, fitness, and rehabilitation (Biga et al., 2020) (Figure 10.1).

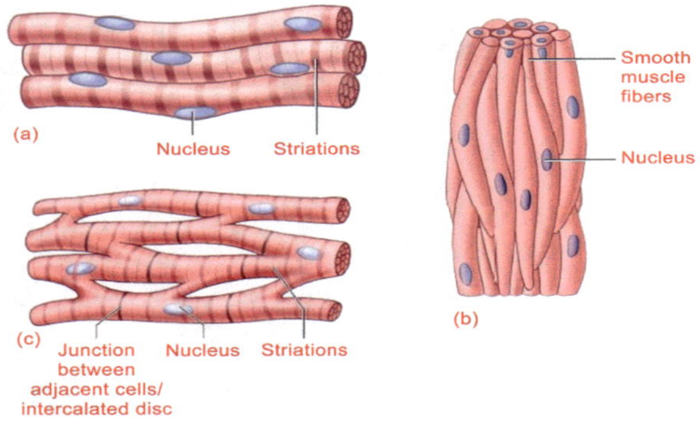

Figure 10.1. Muscular tissue.

Source: https://img.brainkart.com/imagebk34/9VbiIMi.jpg.

Definition of Muscular Tissue

Muscular tissue is a fundamental component of the human structure that is responsible for moving the body and maintaining posture. It is characterized by being capable of contracting, which distinguishes it from other tissues. Muscular tissue can be classified into three broad categories: skeletal, cardiac, and smooth. Skeletal muscle, which is voluntary, is connected to bones and makes walking and gripping possible. Cardiac muscle, outside of the heart, operates involuntarily to achieve rhythmic contraction for circulatory purposes. Smooth muscle exists in organs, such as intestines and blood vessels, to deliver involuntary movement directing physiological functions. These two structures work together to form a total system required for voluntary and involuntary processes in the human body. The compartmental structure of muscular tissue plays a vital role in its functioning. Myocytes, or muscle cells, are the building blocks, and they vary in shape and length according to muscle type. Skeletal muscle fibers are long and cylindrical, containing multiple nuclei and being striated in appearance because of the structure of actin and myosin filaments. Cardiac muscle cells are branched and shorter and are linked by intercalated discs, thus that the contraction will be coordinated throughout the heart. The non-striated and spindle-shaped smooth muscle cells reflect their role in tonic, slow contractions. The intricate patterns of the cells are the foundation of muscle function since they determine the mechanics of contraction and sensitivity to stimuli and, hence, overall movement and well-being (Anderson et al., 2001). Furthermore, the unique structure of the cardiac muscles plays a critical role in their specialized role of maintaining the heart's rhythm. Mathematical modeling of myocardial fiber orientation has also improved our understanding of how such muscular tissues architect force production and electrical conduits for conduction (Pravdin, 2013). Such models describe the intricate myofiber orientation in the left ventricle and how the design of the structure corresponds with functional efficacy in cardiac function. Such co-dependency addresses the vital importance of muscular tissue in mechanical as well as electrophysiological functions in the body. Thus, knowledge of the definition and role of muscular tissue is essential to any consideration of human physiology, thus illustrating its significance in both everyday movement and in vital processes , such as circulation and digestion (Figure 10.2).

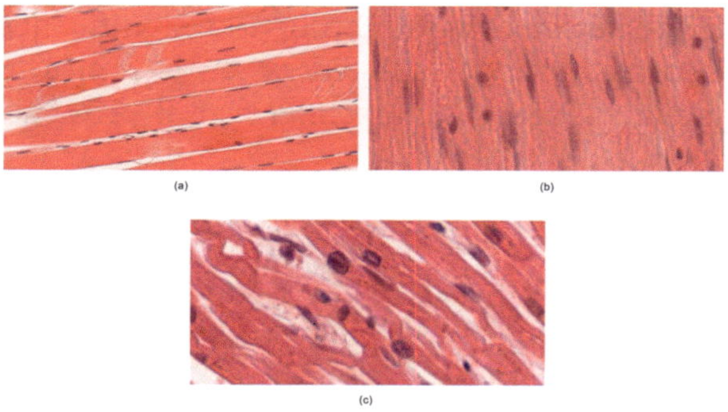

Figure 10.2. Muscle tissue. (a) Skeletal muscle cells have prominent striation and nuclei on their periphery. (b) Smooth muscle cells have a single nucleus and no visible striations. (c) Cardiac muscle cells appear striated and have a single nucleus.

Source: https://s3-us-west-2.amazonaws.com/courses-images/wp-content/uploads/sites/1512/2017/02/24232431/414_Skeletal_Smooth_Cardiacabc-1024x577.jpg.

Importance of Muscular Tissue in the Human Body

The function of muscular tissue in the human body extends beyond voluntary motion; it is involved in a number of functions necessary to support homeostasis. Muscles not only facilitate voluntary movement but also have a role in involuntary actions , such as digestion and circulation. Smooth muscle found in the digestive system facilitates the peristaltic movement to move food and nutrients appropriately. In addition, cardiac muscle, which is present only in the heart, is essentially responsible for maintaining life through the perpetual circulation of blood. This diversity of function demonstrates the pivotal place of muscular tissue within the maintenance of overall well-being and vitality. As the body's main engine of motion and stability, muscles intertwine with other bodies of function intricately, and thus their proper execution must remain indispensable to an equilibrium of physiological harmony. The role of muscular tissue also encompasses its aid in thermoregulation, particularly in maintaining the body's core temperature. During exercise, heat is generated by muscle contractions, which is a requirement for metabolic processes. The interaction between muscular activity and temperature regulation is particularly significant during exercise; since contracting muscles cause increased body temperature, the hypothalamus initiates sweating and the distribution of increased blood to the skin surfaces for dissipation of heat. This thermogenic response indicates the adaptive nature of muscle, which not only responds to present demand for movement and stabilization but also to fundamental physiologic requirements like body temperature regulation. Any muscular tissue pathology, therefore, can have crucial implications extending beyond physical function to thermoregulation and thereby affecting health outcomes. Besides their mechanical and physiological functions, muscular tissues play a role in metabolic well-being and therapeutic pathways. New findings have shed light on the interactions between muscular health and metabolic syndrome and obesity. Muscular contraction enhances glucose and fatty acid uptake from the circulatory system, playing an important role in metabolic control. Moreover, chronic inflammatory diseases, such as Duchenne muscular dystrophy, highlight the importance of muscular integrity; muscle function and regeneration are disrupted by inflammatory cell invasion (De Paepe & De Bleecker, 2013). Understanding the dynamic roles of muscle tissue and exploring treatment options, such as myofascial release techniques, can enhance muscular health, reduce pain, and promote overall well-being, which summarizes that there is a direct need for continued academic and clinical research in this field (Hetherington, 2019).

10.1. Types of Muscular Tissue

Learning Outcome

1. Describe the skeletal muscle;
2. Describe the cardiac muscle;
3. Learn about smooth muscle tissue.

Human muscle tissue is divided into three broad categories: skeletal, cardiac, and smooth muscle. Voluntary contraction and striated appearance are characteristics of skeletal muscle, which is responsible for the movement of the skeleton and is essential for locomotion, posture, and balance. Composed of long cylindrical fibers, which contract in a rhythmic manner to neural stimulation, skeletal muscle is the main muscle to perform movement. These fibers have myoglobin and energy-storing compounds, enabling sustained contraction under physical activity. Of significance in this case is the presence of carnosine in skeletal muscle and its significance to performance, with studies indicating that its levels can be augmented through nutritional intake of beta-alanine and consequently improve anaerobic performance among sports competitors (Baguet et al., 2010). The skeletal muscle is trainable as it can hypertrophy and become more efficient with resistance exercise training. Cardiac muscle, unlike skeletal muscle, is optimized to carry out involuntary contraction of the heart for the circulation of blood in the body. This muscle too is striated and formed of brief, stunted fibers linked by intercalated discs that ensure controlled contractions and the efficiency of heart function. Unlike skeletal muscle, cardiac muscle cells exhibit strong resistance to fatigue and go on with rhythmic contractions without voluntary control. The intricate organization of cardiac muscle fibers is the reason behind its ability to generate continuous and synchronized heartbeats. In addition, diseases , such as genetic mutations can offer insight regarding cardiac muscle function and integrity. For example, mutations of the gene encoding fibulin-4 have been reported to devastate elastic fibers of the vasculature and result in cardiovascular malformations, highlighting the significance of cardiac muscle integrity when it comes to systemic disease (Broekelmann et al., 2017).

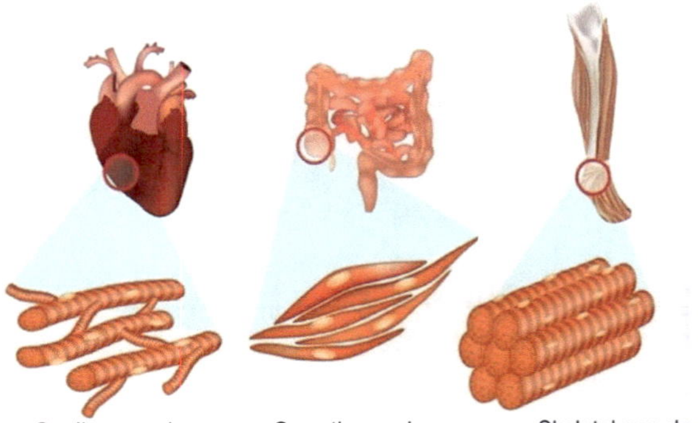

Figure 10.3. Types of muscular tissue.

Source: https://www.orchardhealthclinic.com/wp-content/uploads/2020/08/IMG_5045.jpg.

Smooth muscle constitutes the third type of muscular tissue and is characterized by its non-striated appearance and involuntary control. Located in the walls of hollow organs , such as the digestive tract, blood vessels, and respiratory passages, smooth muscle carries out many automatic body functions, including peristalsis and vasodilation. Smooth muscle consists of spindle-shaped cells that contract more slowly and for a longer duration than cardiac and skeletal muscles, which allows for the regulation of internal function without conscious control. Smooth muscle contraction is usually controlled by the autonomic nervous system and hormonal stimulation so that it can dynamically adjust according to the physiological demands of the body. A fundamental knowledge of the distinctive characteristics and activities of these three muscular tissues is essential to understanding how muscular systems collaborate to attain homeostasis and facilitate health in human beings (Figure 10.3).

10.1.1. Skeletal Muscle

Skeletal muscle, a critical component of human muscular tissue, is meant for movement and posture. Skeletal muscle is characterized by its striated appearance and voluntary nature, distinguishing it from smooth muscle and cardiac muscle. The skeletal muscle consists of long, multinucleated fibers with its conscious function consistent with the nervous system to generate accurate and coordinated movements. The intricate interaction between the muscular system and nervous system enables functions , such as walking, running, and lifting. Skeletal muscle also supports thermogenesis which helps the body regulate its core temperature through metabolic function. Muscles generate heat during muscle contraction, thereby maintaining the body's core temperature constant during exercise and an indicator of the diversity of skeletal muscle in human physiology. The importance of skeletal muscle is further brought out by the situation in many other medical disorders, such as Duchenne muscular dystrophy (DMD). Duchenne muscular dystrophy is a genetic disorder leading to progressive degeneration of muscle fibers and severe muscle weakness with loss of function. Infiltration of the skeletal muscle by inflammatory cells is a characteristic feature of DMD, and chemokines and cytokines play important roles. Evidence has indicated that the expression of these pro-inflammatory mediators is associated with higher disease severity because they facilitate the influx of immune cells within the pathology of the muscular tissues, hence enhancing tissue damage and impairing the repair mechanisms (De Paepe & De Bleecker, 2013). Understanding these pathological changes in skeletal muscle of diseases like DMD creates an acute awareness of developing therapeutic interventions aimed at blocking these inflammatory and degenerative aspects within muscular disorders. Further, the impact of physical inactivity on skeletal muscle functional capacity cannot be overstated. Extended bed rest, for whatever reason, whether chronic disease or postoperative care, has been proven to induce severe deconditioning of skeletal muscle. Inactivity results in decreased muscle volume, reduced fiber cross-sectional area, and ultimately reduced strength, particularly in antigravity muscles acting against gravity (Drury et al., 2007). These physiological adaptations can perpetuate a vicious cycle such that compromised muscle strength becomes more likely to result in falls with consequential injury. Clinicians must be vigilant in combating the ill effects of lack of activity by implementing early mobilization and physical training to preserve muscle strength and function. It is necessary to maintain skeletal muscle integrity to ensure general physical fitness, particularly among vulnerable populations at risk of disuse atrophy (Figure 10.4).

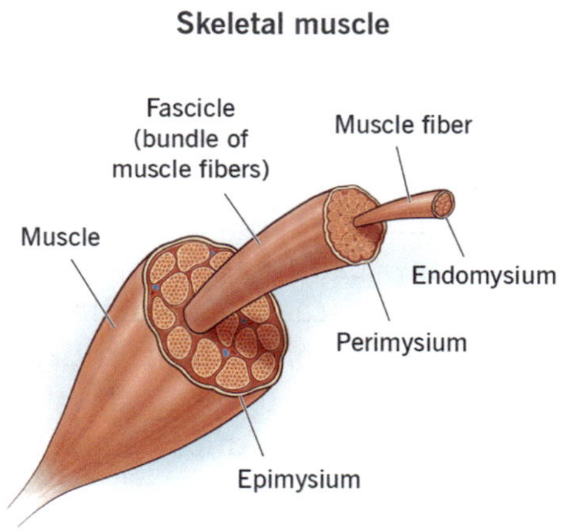

Figure 10.4. Skeletal muscle.

Source: https://my.clevelandclinic.org/-/scassets/images/org/health/articles/skeletal-muscle.

10.1.2. Cardiac Muscle

Cardiac muscle, a form of specialized striated muscular tissue, is present only in the heart and plays a role in circulatory stability regulation through its involuntary contractions. As compared to skeletal muscle, cardiac muscle fibers are intermingled and branched, ensuring coordinated contraction for effective pumping of blood. Such new architecture is facilitated by intercalated disks, specific junctions between adjacent muscle cells, through which high-speed electrical conduction and mechanical coupling are made possible. This makes cardiac muscle inherently rhythmic, thus able to respond at once to the changing needs of the body for oxygenated blood. The role of cardiac muscle is crucial as it operates with no letup throughout the life of an individual, demonstrating resilience and responsiveness in encountering changing physiological conditions and stressors. The intricate physiological mechanisms behind cardiac muscle function are influenced by a variety of factors, including hormonal signals and neural inputs. For example, autonomic nervous input regulates the heart rate via sympathetic and parasympathetic pathways, altering cardiac output in response to the body's activity level. Besides, another hormone like adrenaline would raise the contraction speed and strength at times. Hence, an example to illustrate that the responsiveness of cardiac muscle is dynamic. Another interesting fact is that abnormalities in these controlling mechanisms may lead to a series of disorders like cardiovascular disease, heart failure, wherein the pumping function of the heart is destroyed. Thus, the understanding of regulatory pathways of cardiac muscles is of utmost importance in the development of therapeutic interventions for the recovery of normal heart function and the treatment of cardiac malfunction diseases. Research in cardiac muscle also reveals its response to pathological states, particularly with respect to increased understanding of genetic as well as degenerative diseases of cardiac function. Diseases , such as Duchenne muscular dystrophy, while they are centrally localized to the skeletal muscle, secondarily affect cardiac muscle function through systemic effects of muscle degeneration. Inflammatory responses, characterized by the invasion of inflammatory cells and cytokine secretion, are a central component of skeletal and cardiac muscle pathology. The elevation of cytokines in dystrophinopathies, as seen in Duchenne muscular dystrophy, causes the disruption of muscle fibers and hinders the regeneration process, thus illustrating the synergy of cardiac muscle integrity with muscular function in the body in general (De Paepe & De Bleecker, 2013). Such complex relationships must be investigated to identify the effects of muscular dystrophies on a generalized basis and formulate emerging therapies aimed at sustaining cardiac integrity in the presence of systemic degeneration of muscle (Figure 10.5).

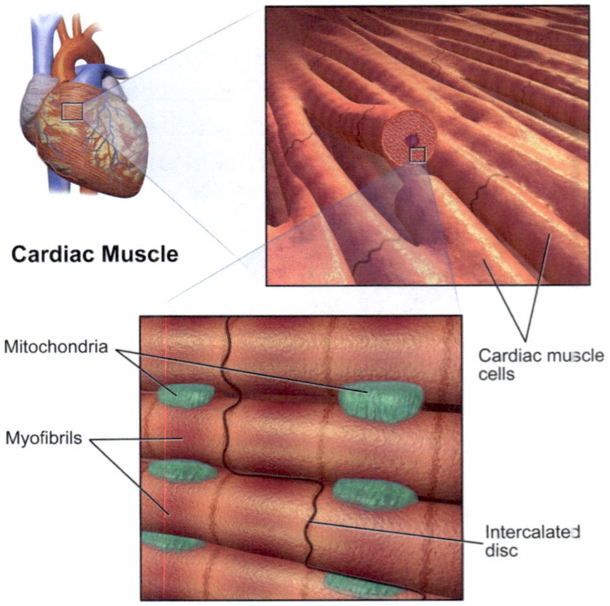

Figure 10.5. Cardiac muscle.

Source: https://cdn.storymd.com/optimized/RoeJ7Bcadv/original.jpg.

10.1.3. Smooth Muscle

Smooth muscle tissue is a significant component of the human muscular system and is employed to execute involuntary movements in the majority of organ systems. Smooth muscle fibers lack the banding patterns characteristic of striated skeletal muscle, possessing a homogeneous appearance under microscopic observation.

This specialized tissue allows smooth muscle to function effectively in the autonomic responses of the body, e.g., to keep blood flowing through the contraction of arteries and veins and move food along the digestive tract. Smooth muscle cell rhythmic contraction and relaxation capability is also central to peristalsis and vasodilation. Therefore, disturbances in smooth muscle function can lead to serious health complications, affecting various body systems and resulting in diseases like gastrointestinal disease and hypertension. Smooth muscle contraction is a dynamic phenomenon regulated by various signaling pathways and biochemical mechanisms. The greatest contraction stimulus is the rise in intracellular calcium ions that initiates the interaction between actin and myosin filaments, causing muscle shortening and force development. Moreover, smooth muscle cells are also capable of altering phenotypes from a contractile to a proliferative phenotype in the event of pathological conditions, for instance, hypertension. This phenomenon is regulated rigorously by various factors, including the renin angiotensin aldosterone system (RAAS) and oxidative stress.

The fine-tuned regulation of these signaling pathways ultimately determines blood pressure and vascular resistance. The dysfunction of smooth muscle can result in severe cardiovascular challenges, thus explaining the importance of ongoing studies on smooth muscle biology's molecular basis that may culminate in therapeutic implications (Touyz et al., 2018). Current studies have given insight into the critical role smooth muscle plays in cardiovascular well-being, and that is within vascular disease. Mutations within proteins that are associated with smooth muscle function, such as fibulin-4, have been found to create significant cardiovascular malformations, such as arterioplasty and aneurysms. Studies prove that these mutations cause arterial wall structural alterations that result in disorganized smooth muscle cell organization and broken elastic fibers (Broekelmann et al., 2017). These results confirm the necessity of elastin assembly in ensuring vascular integrity and highlight the smooth muscle differential needs of different blood vessel types. Understanding these mechanisms not only enhances our knowledge of muscle physiology but also opens up avenues for developing targeted therapy for diseases affected by smooth muscle dysfunction, thereby alleviating the effects of associated diseases on the overall health of the patient (Figure 10.6).

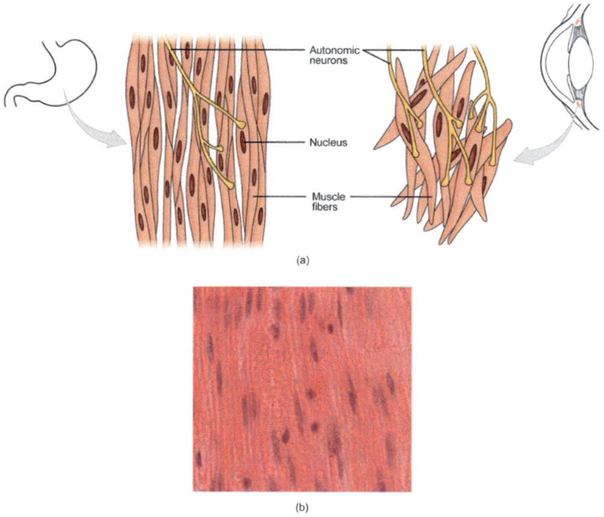

Figure 10.6. Smooth muscle tissue.

Source: https://cdn.storymd.com/optimized/JdP21ZHjA3/original.jpg.

Test Your Knowledge

1. What is skeletal muscle?
2. What is cardiac muscle?

10.2. Structure of Muscular Tissue

Learning Outcome

1. Describe the muscle fibers and their composition;
2. Learn about components of connective tissue;
3. Understand the blood supply and innervation.

Muscular tissue is generally classified into three distinct groups: skeletal, cardiac, and smooth muscles, with specialized structures responsible for their respective functions. Skeletal muscle, comprising long, cylindrical fibers, is striated and under voluntary control. This tissue structure consists of fascicles of muscle fibers, each enveloped by connective tissue forming tendons, which attach the muscle to bones. The internal organization is myofibrils, which are further divided into sarcomeres, the contractile elements that contract using the sliding filament mechanism. Such an advanced organization allows for coordinated movement and is crucial for body mechanics. In contrast, cardiac muscle possesses a branching organization with intercalated discs to facilitate the rapid electrical conduction required for synchronized contractions of the heart. The unique organization of such muscles reflects their specific physiological function in the human body, illustrating the importance of structural differences in muscle function. The specificity of muscle tissue structure is crucial to its functional characteristics, particularly for cardiac muscle. The helical arrangement of myocardial fibers, which the helical ventricular myocardial band (HVMB) model describes, illustrates how cardiac muscle geometry optimally enables the heart's pumping ability. The model well explains a number of details of ventricular function and how they highlight the role of three-dimensional fiber muscle organization toward myocardial efficiency (Hoffman, 2017). Still, it is important to note that whereas the HVMB model is informative, it is not all-encompassing with regard to anatomical details. Recent investigations into other models indicate that there is still room for refining our knowledge of heart muscle architecture in order to achieve a full understanding of cardiac mechanics and possibly impact clinical methodologies for the treatment of heart disease. Smooth muscle tissue, in contrast to its skeletal and cardiac counterparts, has a broadly dissimilar structure that reflects its particular functions within the body. Composed of non-striated fibers that are generally shorter and spindle-shaped, smooth muscle is involuntarily controlled and is charged with controlling internal organs , such as the gastrointestinal tract and the blood vessels. The organization of smooth muscle cells facilitates rhythmic contractions and tonic tonicity, both of which are required for peristalsis and blood pressure regulation. The inclusion of comprehension of both anatomical structure and physiological function of smooth muscle provides insight into conditions like hypertension and gastrointestinal disease, as these are Smooth muscle-directed. Recent advances in elucidating cellular mechanisms controlling smooth muscle function contribute to an enhanced insight into pathophysiological mechanisms and enable the development of targeted therapeutic approaches (Anderson et al., 2001).

10.2.1. Muscle Fibers and Their Composition

The composition of muscle fibers is directly correlated with their functional capabilities, and various muscle fibers are designed to meet different metabolic demands. Human skeletal muscle consists primarily of three fiber types: Type I, Type IIa, and Type IIb fibers. Type I fibers, or slow-twitch fibers, are characterized as having a high oxidative metabolism capacity, allowing them to function for long periods without becoming fatigued. Conversely, Type II fibers produce rapid, forceful contractions, with the Type IIa employing both aerobic and anaerobic systems and the Type IIb geared for explosive, short-duration efforts. The distinct biochemical composition between the fibers—differences in myoglobin content, mitochondrial concentration, and enzymatic activity—has direct application to the relative functions of these fibers in human locomotion and exercise, and thus inquiry into the differences is considered necessary for efficacious training and rehabilitation methods. With advancing age, there are quite dramatic alterations in the type composition of the muscle fibers, which change total muscular function and performance. A very frequent phenomenon is sarcopenia, which also includes a reduction in muscle mass and a change in fiber type composition, so that Type II fibers become less common. This alteration leads to loss of muscle quality rather than quantity, as the fibers are less effective at generating force and higher power outputs. Furthermore, adiposity increases in the elderly, with deleterious effects on the muscle environment and function. Importantly, ectopic fat may interfere with the intrinsic contractility of the muscle fibers, as evidenced by the changes in fiber type properties by lipotoxicity. In this case, it is crucial to target age-related changes in muscle composition to conserve physical function and avoid disability in older individuals (Carter et al., 2019). The biochemical properties of muscle fibers also involve the role of specific substances , such as carnosine, that support muscle function and performance. Found in high concentration in skeletal muscle, carnosine acts as a buffer during high-intensity exercise and helps to maintain the balance of pH and avoid acidosis. Carnosine synthesis from L-histidine and beta-alanine is important among users of anaerobic work since elevated muscle concentration of carnosine is linked with a preponderance of fast-twitch fibers. More recent studies indicate that long-term supplementation with beta-alanine significantly enhances carnosine content, enhancing athletic performance in short-duration high-intensity activity. Hence, the correlation between fiber composition and carnosine content is a key field of knowledge in sports training as well as in nutritional practice with an eye to optimizing muscle performance (Baguet et al., 2010) (Figure 10.7).

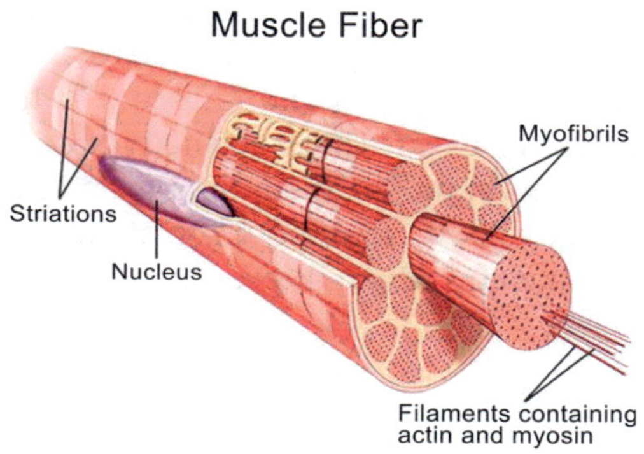

Figure 10.7. Muscle fibers.

Source: https://www.onlinebiologynotes.com/wp-content/uploads/2017/03/Muscle-fiber-2.jpg.

10.2.2. Connective Tissue Components

In the context of muscular tissue, elements of connective tissue play an essential role in the structural framework as well as functional dynamics of muscles. Connective tissues , such as fascia and tendons, serve as pivotal pathways along which forces produced by muscle contractions are passed to the skeletal system. Tendons, consisting of closely packed collagen fibers, anchor muscles to bones so that movement and support during exercise can occur. Furthermore, the connective tissue matrix envelops individual muscle fibers and organizes muscle fascicles to support optimal force generation and durability. The intricate organization of collagen and elastin fibers within these connective tissues contributes to their mechanical attributes, which allow them to withstand stresses associated with muscle function and dynamic motion, highlighting their fundamental role in general musculoskeletal health. Evidence of the interaction between connective tissue structures and muscle tissue is demonstrated by observations , such as myofascial transmission of force, whereby the fascial system provides biomechanical communication between muscles. Research shows that alterations in the relative position of muscles to adjacent connective tissue greatly affect their capacity for force generation. For example, research involving the extensor digitorum longus muscle in rats revealed that changes in position of the muscle influenced forces at the distal and proximal tendons, demonstrating the complexity of force transmission within muscular units and the contribution of connective tissue to force generation between muscle units. This interdependence means that any disruption of connective tissue integrity can cause impaired muscular performance and potential damage, thereby arguing even more for ongoing investigation into the adaptive capacity of the musculoskeletal system. Further, the plasticity of connective tissues has relevance in response to a variety of mechanical stimuli, as suggested by the plasticity of the musculoskeletal system. Prolonged periods of unloading, like those occurring in space flight, induce adaptive changes within the connective tissues with consequences for muscle function and structural support. The unique capacity of connective tissues to alter their structural and functional characteristics exemplifies the extensive interdependence between connective and muscular tissues in the establishment of musculoskeletal health and function. With research progress, understanding these dynamics will be central to developing specificity-based therapeutic interventions for the prevention of injury and rehabilitation, compelling muscle and connective tissues to perform in harmony to keep an individual's body capability in fluctuating conditions and surroundings, as discussed in extensive musculoskeletal research programs (NASA Report, 1994; Maas et al., 2004) (Figure 10.8).

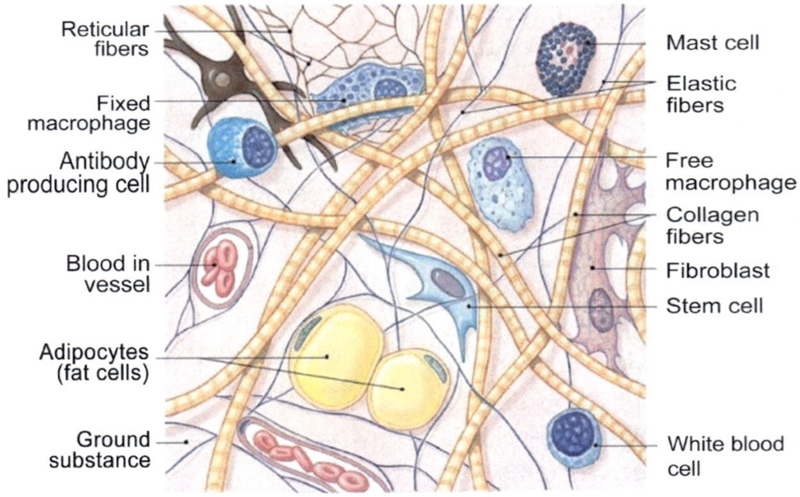

Figure 10.8. Components of connective tissue.

Source: https://i.ytimg.com/vi/SKfANRPOang/maxresdefault.jpg.

10.2.3. Blood Supply and Innervation

Vascularization of muscle tissue is required to ensure the health and functioning of the muscles. Blood supply is primarily supplied by a network of arteries and veins which supply oxygen and nutrients and remove metabolic waste. Every muscle fiber is surrounded by capillaries that are required for the sustenance of metabolic activities, especially during periods of high-intensity activity. Its rich blood supply not only maintains the energetic demands of muscle contractions but also helps in thermoregulation. Dysregulation of vascularization is responsible for muscle fatigue, ischemia, and even necrosis in cases of severely compromised circulation. An understanding of the intricacies of blood supply to muscular tissue, therefore, is essential in clinical practice and sports medicine, too, in order to maximize performance and recovery and prevent injury from insufficiency in blood supply. Muscular tissue innervation is also vital in coordinating muscle contractions and overall movement. Each skeletal muscle fiber is provided with motor neurons that directly transmit signals from the central nervous system, causing contraction. This interaction occurs at the neuromuscular junction, where the axon terminals of the neuron have a complex interaction with the muscle fiber membrane. A denser network of sensory nerve fibers also serves to transmit information regarding muscle tension and position to the central nervous system. This feedback mechanism is critical to maintaining that the muscles are appropriately toned and to smooth movement. Disruption of either motor or sensory innervation can result in weakness, spasm, or loss of coordination of the muscles, highlighting the importance of a properly functioning nervous system in maintaining muscular health. Recent studies have begun exploring the profound impact of innervation and blood supply on muscular function in pathological conditions. For instance, studies investigating enteric nervous system changes in large intestine disorders illustrate how the interference of normal muscular function and enhancement of dysfunction can be brought about by changes. Changed nerve supply in conditions like colorectal cancer is capable of inducing dramatic changes in muscular contractility of the GI tract, showing how the two systems are closely interdependent. Similarly, findings from studies on innervation of equine supraspinous and interspinous ligaments are that high innervation density of sensory nerve fibers is related to severe pain perception in equine sport horses (Ehrle et al., 2017). This information assists in understanding the muscle-injuries and pain mechanisms in a better way, which is essential to create efficient treatment regimes. Therefore, the role of blood supply, innervation, and muscular health is a significant field of study in the backdrop of the study of human physiology (Figure 10.9).

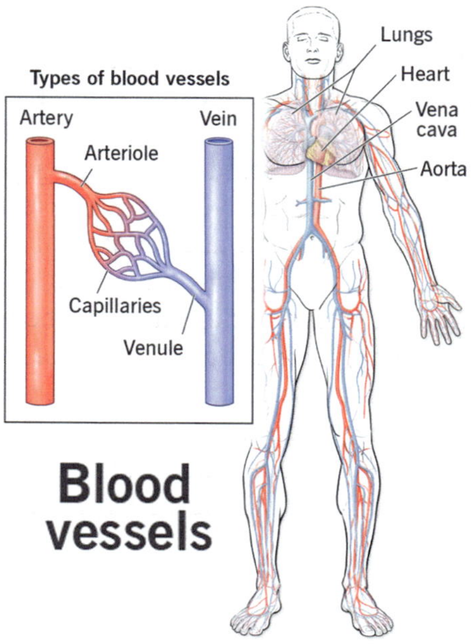

Figure 10.9. Blood vessels of various sizes and types transport blood through your body. They bring your cells what they need.

Source: https://my.clevelandclinic.org/-/scassets/images/org/health/articles/blood-vessels.

Test Your Knowledge

1. What are muscle fibers and their composition?
2. What are the main components of connective tissue?

10.3. Function of Muscular Tissue

Learning Outcome

1. Learn about movement and locomotion in human;
2. Understand the maintenance of posture;
3. Describe the role of muscular tissue in heat production.

The function of muscular tissue is significant in facilitating movement in the human body, either voluntary or involuntary. Muscle tissue is generally divided into three basic types—skeletal, cardiac, and smooth—each with unique functions and characteristics. Skeletal muscle, under voluntary control, performs the functions of locomotion and posture, enabling precise movements of the body due to its striated texture. This type of muscle tissue is crucial to everyday activity, from raising objects to sprinting. Cardiac muscle, on the other hand, is found only in the heart and acts involuntarily, rhythmically contracting to pump blood around the circulatory system. Smooth muscle, found in organs and blood vessels, acts involuntarily and regulates internal processes, such as digestion and blood flow.

Together, these muscles are essential to homeostasis and for enabling complex body function. Integrity of muscular tissue is also essential to overall health and well-being, as the consequences of muscular dysfunction illustrate. A disease like muscular dystrophy or arteriosclerosis has the potential to severely disable muscles and movement, creating great health concerns. For instance, one important study on fibulin-4 mutations offered the account of cardiovascular abnormalities in mice, resulting in disoriented smooth muscle cells and arterial malformations. These findings express the intricate relationship between muscular tissue and other body systems, showing how impaired muscle function can generate more widespread systemic disease, such as hypertension or cardiovascular disease. Identification of such relationships not only emphasizes the importance of muscular health but also directs therapeutic maneuvers for the improvement of muscular function, thereby improving the quality of life in affected individuals. Furthermore, the role of modern lifestyle determinants in contributing to muscular health cannot be ruled out, particularly in hypokinesia. As studied in most research, physical activity has significantly decreased with the emergence of technology and automation, causing more muscular atrophy and cardiovascular disease. The consequence of this is catastrophic; decreased muscular activity can lead to disorganized muscle fiber architecture and be a cause of conditions like arterial stiffening. In addition, space travel and its effect of weightlessness also highlight the superior position of muscular tissue because organisms undergo vital physiological changes in low-gravity environments. The discovery of these variables not only facilitates the vital need to maintain an active lifestyle but also encourages research on interventions that nullify the negative effects of hypokinesia, ultimately enhancing muscular tissue function and general body well-being.

10.3.1. Movement and Locomotion

The subtleties of human movement and locomotion are usually regulated by the specialized structure and function of muscular tissue. Comprised of cardiac, smooth, and skeletal muscle fibers, the tissues collectively are responsible for giving motion, stability, and overall bodily coordination. Of particular note is the utilization of skeletal muscles for the activity of bipedal locomotion to enable a form of movement exclusive to humankind. The biomechanics of running demonstrate this complexity, showing the workings against our upright stance. As mentioned, humans are evolutionarily designed to run, using a specialized bipedal gait that requires advanced neuromuscular control. The capability to stay in balance while performing fast strides and cutting through varied terrain highlights the evolutionary importance of our muscular structure. It is this interdependency between musculature and locomotor capability that will decide not only our bodily action but also our resistance to various locomotor demands (Kiely & Collins, 2016). Secondly, human musculature's adaptability is a manifestation of a deep-seated evolutionary experience that governs locomotion. Extensive, activity-based adaptive plasticity allows our musculoskeletal system to re-equip itself in line with the demands presented by habitual modes of motion. This capacity for adaptation is essential for optimal performance, preventing injury, and acclimatizing to terrain and speed changes. The precise anatomy of human skeletal muscles, such as shifts in different fiber types and cross-sectional areas, illustrates several functional adaptations, which enable proper force production and the ability to perform sophisticated movements. Here, the coordination problems that are inherent in running are resolved through the developed syntheses between primitive and advanced muscular control systems. Human ability to move undistinguishably despite changing conditions represents a massive improvement in locomotion compared to other animals, and it indicates the level of evolutionary development in our muscular systems (Charles et al., 2016). Lastly, comparisons between humans and other animals provide useful lessons regarding locomotor mechanics. Although many animals possess functional adaptations in their musculature, the specific features of human bipedalism present unique challenges due to our upright posture and gait patterns. The integration needed to maintain the body stable while running is highly advanced between the muscular and neurological systems, less exaggerated in quadrupeds. Most importantly, animal model studies, such as in mice, show the structural differences in musculoskeletal frameworks developed for different locomotions. The results of these models better inform us about muscle structure and how it applies to mobility. By studying how other species have evolved to meet their locomotor needs, we can appreciate the complexities of human muscle performance and thereby enhance the approach in sports training and rehabilitation methods for enhancing human movement efficiency (Charles et al., 2016; Kiely & Collins, 2016) (Figure 10.10).

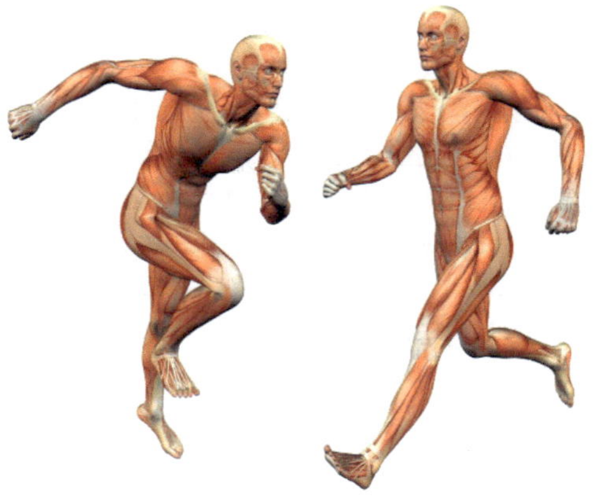

Figure 10.10. Locomotion and movement of muscles.

Source: https://interactive-biology.com/wp-content/uploads/2012/04/MuscleManRunning-1024x813.jpg.

10.3.2. Maintenance of Posture

Posture maintenance is also discussed as a critical function of muscular tissue, as it is premised on a dynamic interaction between the muscle groups and the neural systems. Trunk muscles and lower limb muscles have a persistent, subtle contractile activity that constantly resists the pull of gravity downwards and stabilizes the body. Concentric and eccentric contractions of the muscles are involved in the dynamic process to enable adjustments to be made in order to maintain an upright posture in varying activities. Postural stability is also predominantly based on the tonic muscle contraction of postural muscles, which stabilize against perturbations and stabilize relative to equilibrium. Effective training and use of these groups of muscle may enhance postural stability in terms of increased overall functional capacity. Further, the understanding of the biomechanics involved in posture is important in the identification of the potential musculoskeletal disorders, which often arise due to the inability to maintain the optimal alignment throughout. Muscle quality and variability of composition also bear a significant impact on posture maintenance capability. As age progresses, sarcopenia, or loss of muscle mass and function, becomes prevalent, directly influencing posture and balance. Studies indicate that the process, typically followed by weight gain in the body fat, results in impaired physical functioning and a greater risk of falls, particularly among the older population, where stability is essential to everyday living. Aside from its impact on muscle number, sarcopenia inherently impacts muscle tissue quality and contractile properties, resulting in decreased strength and control over postural movements. This is not only a sign of the importance of resistance training and physical exercise among older populations but also raises concerns about how body composition alterations through aging can further worsen postural deficits (Carter et al., 2019). New evidence has taken into account new means of enhancing postural stability, and the benefits of vibration training as an exercise option have grown ever more prominent. The technique takes advantage of forced oscillation principles to generate contractions of the muscles, stimulating changes in posture and muscle power. Vibration training has been promising in the areas of balance improvement, particularly in older adults with a fall risk or with lower back pain. Ideally, this training could be employed to bring about some warm-up effects and neuromuscular adaptations that are crucial for the maintenance of posture across different populations. By employing these procedures, the many demands of postural control can be alleviated to a greater extent, leading to demonstrable enhancements in strength as well as proprioception among practitioners. This approach emphasizes the potential for adding new modalities to exercises that are applied to restore and enhance maintenance of posture (Rittweger, 2010) (Figure 10.11).

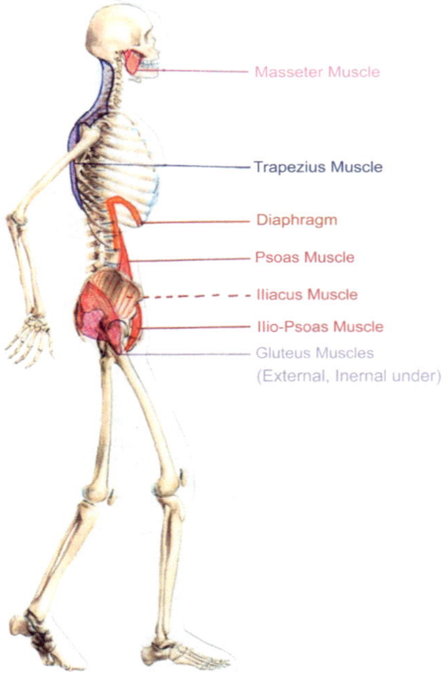

Figure 10.11. Some key postural skeletal muscles.

Source: https://www.theosteoway.ca/wp-content/uploads/2023/01/muscles-involved-in-posture-skeletal-view.jpg.

10.3.3. Heat Production

Muscle tissue is critical in heat production, particularly during exercise. During muscle contraction, muscles derive energy from adenosine triphosphate (ATP), which in turn must be accompanied by the generation of heat as a by-product. The act of thermogenesis contributes importantly to body heat, especially under conditions of physical activity when metabolic rate is elevated. The efficiency of heat generation by muscle has a significant effect on heat balance, as demonstrated by the physiological reactions of the body under environmental stress. For gas exchange, for example, humans rely not only on the increased blood supply to the skin for heat dissipation but also on subtle water and electrolyte balance mechanisms that are essential to go on prolonged activity without succumbing to heat exhaustion. These processes underscore the dynamic nature of muscular tissue in temperature regulation, reflective of its importance beyond simple motion. The interplay of muscular activity and heat production is deeply rooted in human energy metabolism. As the muscles move from phases of contraction to relaxation, they furnish an internal environment to facilitate effective thermoregulation. During rest as well as activity, the body's heat production must match heat loss to maintain a stable core temperature. Such a balance is especially relevant to remember regarding physical exercise and its connection with heat-associated illness. Although muscle contractions actively induce increased thermal generation, ambient factors , such as temperature, humidity, and hydration level also play an important role in the regulation of heat dissipation mechanisms. Such interaction is important, particularly for engineers who design thermal protection systems for exposure conditions like those experienced by astronauts, where peak thermal balance is vital to guarantee performance and safety (Kaciuba-Uscilko & Greenleaf, 1989). Besides, heat production by exercising muscle tissue can trigger complex physiological responses in an effort to maintain homeostasis. When the body interprets the rise in body temperature due to heat generated by contractions of muscles, various compensatory mechanisms work towards inducing cooling. These include increasing perspiration, increasing cardiac output, and diverting blood flow onto the skin's surface. Importantly, research on the mechanisms of thermoregulation has applications that extend into other domains, such as sports science and astronautics. The delicate equilibrium of such physiological responses is of greatest concern not just for athletic performance but also for the preservation of health during severe environments (Kaciuba-Uscilko & Greenleaf, 1989). If one learns about heat generation as a fundamental element of muscular tissue processes, it is then possible to grasp the general relevance of muscle physiology in human functioning and health, particularly due to temperature stresses.

Test Your Knowledge

1. What is locomotion and movement in humans?
2. What is role of muscular tissue in heat production

10.4. Mechanism of Muscle Contraction

Learning Outcome

1. Understand the sliding filament theory;
2. Describe the role of calcium ions;
3. Describe the energy sources for muscular contraction.

Muscle contraction is a complex physiological process involving the coordinated effort of actin and myosin filaments inside muscle cells. This is initiated by the release of calcium ions from the sarcoplasmic reticulum, which bind to troponin, causing a conformational change that shifts tropomyosin from actin's binding sites. Upon binding of these newly revealed sites with the myosin heads, they perform a power stroke energized by hydrolysis of (ATP) that results in the sliding of filaments past each other. This sliding filament mechanism encapsulates the primary process behind voluntary and involuntary muscle contractions, resulting in posture and movement. The function of ATP in the process cannot be overstated because its continuous supply is essential to ensure that muscle function is sustained and contractions are achieved effectively at various levels of bodily activity. In addition, the function of different biochemical substances during muscle contraction cannot be ignored, more so the occurrence of carnosine, a dipeptide found in high amounts in skeletal muscle. Carnosine supplements muscle function in exercise at high intensities by serving as an acidosis buffer, which is a frequent byproduct of anaerobic metabolism. Repeated β-alanine ingestion, the rate-limiting amino acid for carnosine production, has been found to significantly enhance muscle content of carnosine, which in turn has been demonstrated to facilitate enhanced exercise performance in trained and untrained individuals. Importantly, the ability of carnosine to blunt pH decline during intense contraction is critical since it prevents effective muscle performance. This biochemical adaptability underscores the dynamic interaction of mechanical and metabolic function in human musculature, which calls for more research into nutritional modalities that could optimize muscle contraction processes (Baguet et al., 2010). In addition, muscle contraction is not confined to skeletal fibers but also involves cardiac and smooth muscles, each with distinct mechanisms of contraction according to its distinct anatomical features. For instance, the heart muscle relies on the contraction of myocardial helical fibers that are responsible for the proper twisting and pumping actions of the heart. The HVMB model is commonly utilized to explain the contractile mechanics within heart tissues, explaining how muscular configurations provide efficient blood circulation.

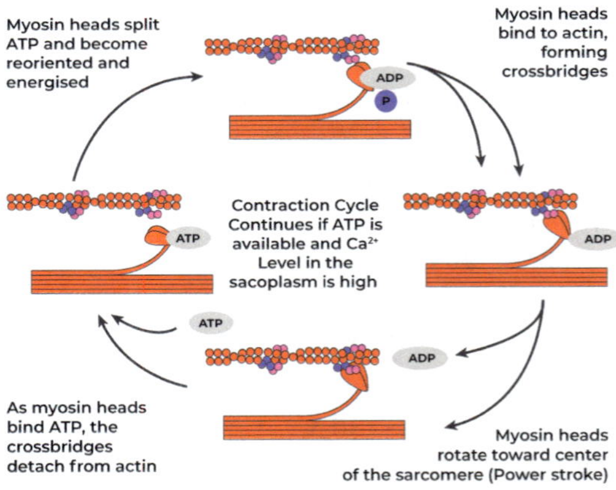

Figure 10.12. Mechanism of muscle contraction.

Source: https://media.geeksforgeeks.org/wp-content/uploads/20230721104902/Mechnaism-of-muscle-contrtaction.png.

However, recent criticism is that the model arguably does not consider real anatomical nuances, which would be pertinent to the explanation of cardiac function and potential failure. By very close analysis of the mechanical and anatomical forces at work, scientists can develop more comprehensive models that capture muscle contraction in tissues properly and explain the complexities for different tissue types as well as their overall significance to human health (Hoffman, 2017) (Figure 10.12).

10.4.1. Sliding Filament Theory

The sliding filament theory is a paradigm of our understanding of the dynamics of muscle contraction in human musculature. The underlying principle is that muscle fibers contract through interdigitation of actin and myosin filaments of the sarcomere, which is the functional unit of muscle tissue. The mechanism largely relies upon the cyclical binding and unbinding of myosin heads on actin filaments driven by ATP hydrolysis. When myosin heads rotate, they pull actin filaments towards each other, which results in muscle shortening. This synchronized motion is no passive response but a complex process that depends on many factors , such as the muscular architecture and the neurological stimuli involved in starting contraction. Understanding this phenomenon sheds light on the mechanical characteristics of muscle, which is the foundation for physiological study as well as clinical intervention in muscle dysfunction and health (Huijing et al., 1995).

Extending this with the sliding filament theory, muscle activation level, action, and recruitment patterns must be investigated. The contractile force generated by muscle fibers is not an intrinsic characteristic but is highly dependent on the activation intensity and muscle use history. Fatigue and potentiation are some of the things that alter muscle fiber response to stimulus over time, reflecting the dynamic nature of force production. Recent work has pointed out that muscle anatomy, for example, the distribution of fiber lengths, plays a significant role in affecting these aspects of activation. For example, mono- and bi-articular muscles exhibit differentiated response patterns based on their structural morphology and recruitment patterns. This suggests that the sliding filament mechanism is not independent but linked with various physiological parameters of global muscle function and control (Huijing et al., 1995). Further, research utilizing sophisticated imaging techniques has also found significant features of the microstructural integrity of sarcomeres under different physiological conditions. For instance, second-harmonic generation imaging of zebrafish models demonstrated statin-induced myopathy-caused changes in sarcomere length, thereby impairing muscular function. Since muscle formation shortening is correlated with muscle quality and injury assessment, structural integrity becomes an important aspect of functional measures. Such evidence indicates the potential of novel imaging methods in the evaluation of muscle tissue health independent of the utilization of established clinical biomarkers. Understanding such microstructural changes in the context of the sliding filament theory enhances our diagnostic and management skills for pathologies of the muscle, resulting in better treatment protocols in human musculature (Figure 10.13).

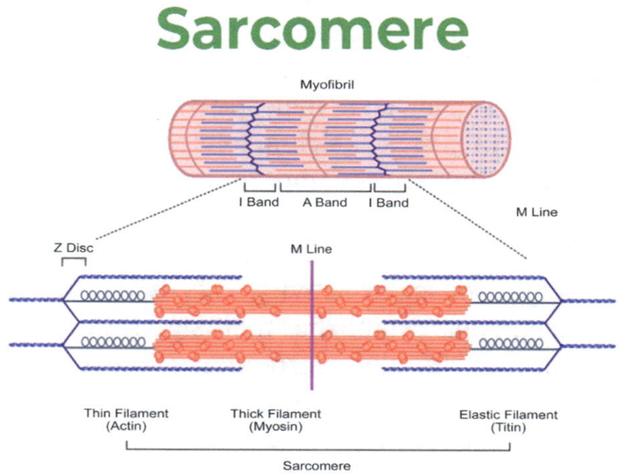

Figure 10.13. Sarcomere.

Source: https://media.geeksforgeeks.org/wp-content/uploads/20230714130049/Sarcomere.png.

10.4.2. Role of Calcium Ions

Calcium ions have a critical role as intermediate molecules in the complex biochemical process involved in controlling muscular tissue function in human beings. They play a vital role in the excitation-contraction coupling process in muscle fibers of skeletal muscle. When a muscle fiber is excited by a motor neuron, it results in the release of neurotransmitters, which initiate an action potential that spreads along the sarcolemma and into the muscle fiber via the transverse tubules. This flow of electricity triggers the release of calcium ions from the sarcoplasmic reticulum into the cytosol, enabling the interaction between actin and myosin filaments. The binding of calcium to troponin results in a conformational change that reveals active sites on actin for contraction to be enabled. Hence, without calcium ions, skeletal muscle contraction would be impossible, and this identifies the role of these ions in voluntary muscle contraction and overall muscular function. Moreover, the role of calcium ions does not stop at this fundamental process of contraction; they play a part in maintaining muscle integrity and in metabolism. Intracellular calcium elevation initiates several pathways of signaling that control growth, repair, and adaptation of the muscle. For instance, in compensation to mechanical overload or resistance exercise, calcium ions activate most of the kinases involved in hypertrophy and protein synthesis in muscle. Calcium ions also play roles in regulating energy metabolism in muscle cells to enable glycogen to be metabolized to glucose in the resynthesis of ATP during prolonged muscular activity. This dual function of calcium ions establishes their significance not only in inducing the contraction of muscle but also in enhancing the efficacy and elasticity of muscles in executing various bodily functions. The pathological implications of deregulation of calcium highlight the necessity for maintaining homeostasis of calcium in muscular tissue. Diseases , such as malignant hyperthermia, as recent research has revealed, are induced by calcium release and signaling abnormalities leading to deep muscle contracture and metabolic derangements following anesthetic exposure or extreme physical stress. Abnormalities in genes, for example, mutations within the RYR1 gene, also complicate calcium ion regulation dynamics in skeletal muscle. These mutations lead to an overabundance of calcium influx into the cytosol, resulting in a lethal condition of hypermetabolism. Knowing calcium ion dynamics both in therapeutic and preventive contexts is essential because derangements of their regulation can lead to defective muscle function and well-being, illustrating the critical role played by calcium ions in muscular physiology (Sato, 2004; Kovalenko, 2025) (Figure 10.14).

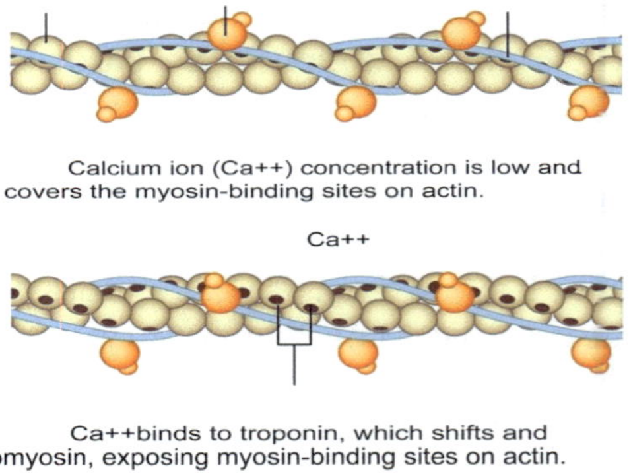

Figure 10.14. Role of calcium ions in muscle contraction.

Source: https://o.quizlet.com/sUmn0L4fE03W0UhTeQ7W-w_b.jpg.

10.4.3. Energy Sources for Contraction

Muscle contraction is founded on a synergistic relationship of sources of energy, most notably (ATP), which is the readily available source of energy for shortening of muscle fibers. ATP is stored in small quantities in muscle cells, which need to be replenished promptly when demand is high. Three principal metabolic pathways within the body are utilized to reconstitute ATP: the phosphagen system, glycolysis, and aerobic respiration. The first is the phosphagen system, with the use of creatine phosphate, which is the fastest mechanism for the resynthesis of ATP, supplying energy for brief periods of activity, often for periods not longer than 10 seconds. With increasing demands of muscle activity, glycolysis in the breakdown of glucose to pyruvate assumes greater importance, especially during states of anaerobic metabolism. Not only does it generate ATP, but lactic acid is also a waste product, causing fatigue in the muscles and influencing the performance of future contractions. Muscle contraction is also sustained by aerobic respiration, which plays a major role during prolonged activity. This oxygen-dependent metabolic process oxidizes carbohydrates and fats with the help of oxygen and produces more ATP than anaerobic metabolism. Most notable is that aerobic metabolism sustains endurance performance and plays a vital role in maintaining steady-state exercises where energy is supplied without excessive fatigue. Adaptation of skeletal muscle to respond differently to varying sources of energy based on exercise intensity and duration underlines the unparalleled flexibility of human muscular tissue. Interestingly, research suggests the duration for which muscular strength can be maintained is a function of collective metabolic mechanisms, so that fatigue mechanisms affect all individuals similarly. This can be observed easily in the research on comparisons of performance duration and power outputs between sexes, which offers basic information on human endurability potential but with varying peak power outputs and aerobic maximum performances (Sundberg et al., 2017). Further, some environmental factors, such as temperature regulation, may influence energy metabolism and muscle function. During exercise in heat, the ability of the body to maintain thermal balance is interrupted, influencing energy supply and muscle function. The integration of energy metabolism with thermoregulatory processes indicates the complexity of the maintenance of muscular contractions during various physiological stresses. Knowledge of the associations is not merely needed for optimization of athletic performance but also for optimization of safety in physically demanding activities performed within extreme environments. Further research into acclimatization methods and the resulting physiological alterations with repeated heat exposure helps with the creation of effective countermeasures for the athletic and occupational setting, e.g., those for space exploration (Kaciuba-Uscilko & Greenleaf, 1989). These comments reinforce the necessity of considering both the sources of energy and the environment when studying muscular function.

Test Your Knowledge

1. What is the role of calcium ions?
2. What are the sources of energy for muscular contraction?

10.5. Disorders Related to Muscular Tissue

Learning Outcome

1. Describe the muscular dystrophy;
2. Describe the myasthenia gravis;
3. Understand the rhabdomyolysis.

Muscular tissue disorders form a variety of diseases that primarily affect the structure and function of muscles. Among these, (DMD) is the archetypal example of a severe genetic disease that predominantly affects males. With progressive degeneration and weakening of the muscles, DMD begins in early childhood and leads to severe morbidity and impairment of quality of life. The pathological process involves not only progressive muscle fiber loss but also chronic inflammation, which contributes to the severity and progression of the disease in the affected. This inflammatory reaction is mediated by cytokines and chemokines that play a crucial role in triggering and recruiting inflammatory cells to the affected muscle tissue. Thus, understanding the intricate interaction among inflammatory processes and muscle degeneration is relevant in having effective therapeutic strategies for DMD patients (De Paepe & De Bleecker, 2013). Treatment of muscle diseases , such as DMD, needs innovative approaches to reverse muscular degenerative outcomes and improve muscle integrity. Recent studies show the promise of low-level laser therapy (LLLT) in addressing muscle injury from diseases , such as DMD. A study conducted on mdx mice, a universally accepted model of DMD, indicated that LLLT significantly reduced morphological changes, including muscle atrophy and fibrosis, from those of a placebo-treated group. Moreover, biochemical analysis proved a significant lowering of creatine kinase levels—a marker of damage to the muscle—in LLLT subjects. The decrease in enzymatic activity was matched by decreased expression of inflammatory markers, suggesting that LLLT may be able to not only limit muscular damage but also block the inflammatory aspect central to muscular dystrophies. Such findings present a new direction for the therapeutic intervention to halt the progression of disorders of muscular tissue (Gur et al., 2014). Apart from dystrophies, other muscle tissue diseases , such as inflammatory myopathies and myofascial pain syndrome also warrant attention in the field of musculoskeletal wellness. Inflammatory myopathies , such as polymyositis and dermatomyositis are characterized by inflammation and weakness of muscles, commonly linked with autoimmune processes. Immune-mediated muscle fiber loss leads to sequential weakening and impairment in those affected by them. Further, myofascial pain syndrome, while distinct but generally mistaken with other muscle diseases, is regional muscle ache caused by discrete loci known as trigger points in the muscle. It highlights the complex interrelationship between muscle integrity, sensitivity for pain, and functional capacity. Treatment of these diseases should comprise a multidisciplinary management strategy with the integration of pharmacological, physical, and rehabilitative interventions, emphasizing the significance of extensive knowledge about muscular tissue diseases and their various manifestations on human health (Figure 10.15).

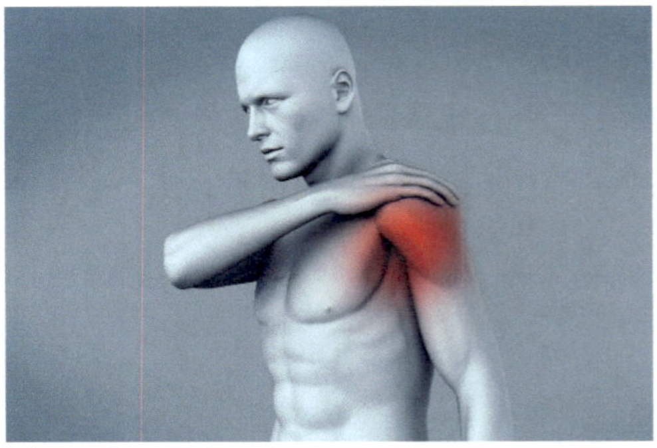

Figure 10.15. Muscle Diseases.

Source: https://lonestarneurology.net/wp-content/uploads/2024/05/1-Top-10-Muscle-Diseases-List-Symptoms-Treatments.jpg

10.5.1. Muscular Dystrophy

Muscular dystrophy is a heterogeneous group of inherited muscle diseases with progressive degeneration and muscle weakness. This condition predominantly arises from genetically induced defects in muscle proteins that are crucial to the stability and function of muscle fibers. For example, Duchenne muscular dystrophy (DMD), a severe type, affects an estimated 1 in 3500 boys globally as a result of mutations within the dystrophin gene. Dystrophin's absence leads to cycles of repeated muscle damage and repair, with inflammation having a vital role in disease development. Inflammatory cells infiltrate the muscle tissue and form part of the overall pathophysiology and disease severity, emphasizing the subtle balance between immune response and the integrity of muscle fibers in muscular dystrophy (De Paepe & De Bleecker, 2013). The cause of the muscular dystrophies is multifactorial, typically secondary to errors in glycosylation of dystroglycan, a critical muscle tissue protein complex. In the setting of dystroglycanopathies, such as in LARGE gene mutation-induced dystroglycanopathies, inappropriate loss of glycosylation leads to defective muscle function. This is of specific interest to therapeutic intervention in the correction of the functional glycosylation of alpha-dystroglycan. Viral delivery of LARGE transgenes into skeletal muscle, of interest, has demonstrated promising results in model organisms, resulting in hyperglycosylation and improved muscle integrity. Such advances in gene therapy highlight the potential for therapy of the underlying basis of muscular dystrophies rather than merely the symptoms (Brockington et al., 2010). Current efforts at research include the identification of the complex pathways of signaling that regulate inflammation and regeneration of muscle in muscular dystrophy. For instance, studies have recognized cytokines and chemokines induced during chronic inflammation that not only recruit inflammatory cells but also serve as key mediators of the repair and renewal of muscle fibers. Target therapies for these inflammatory pathways could enhance dystrophic muscle regeneration, paving the way for new treatment protocols aimed at minimizing muscle degeneration. As knowledge of the complex interactions between inflammation and muscle well-being improves, the potential to develop successful therapeutics grows ever closer, holding promise for those with muscular dystrophy and their families (Figure 10.16).

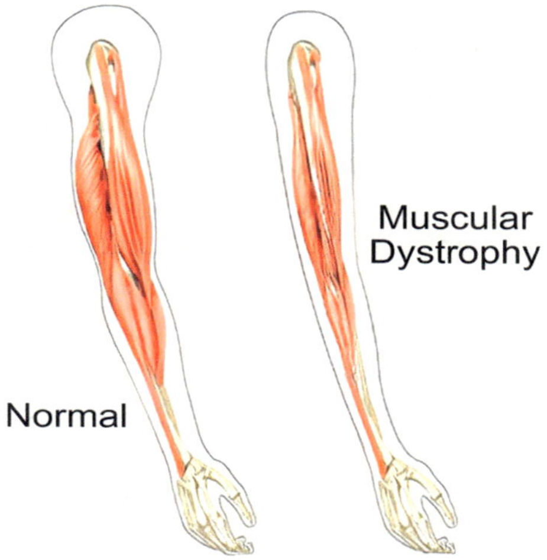

Figure 10.16. Muscular dystrophy.

Source: https://static.wixstatic.com/media/ed472f_6dd6231267084fe389de7f6b1f36a180~mv2.jpg/v1/fill/w_568,h_568,al_c,q_80,usm_0.66_1.00_0.01,enc_avif,quality_auto/ed472f_6dd6231267084fe389de7f6b1f36a180~mv2.jpg.

10.5.2. Myasthenia Gravis

Myasthenia gravis (MG) is a long-standing autoimmune neuromuscular disorder characterized by muscle weakness and fatigability. Pathophysiology of MG involves the production of antibodies against the acetylcholine receptors on the neuromuscular junction, which disrupts nerve-muscle transmission. In addition to blocking muscle contraction, the interference generates severe clinical manifestations , such as ptosis, diplopia, and generalized muscle weakness. These manifestations are heterogeneous in different patients, thereby complicating diagnosis and treatment, as patients may possess varied muscle strength intensities. Understanding the pathogenesis of MG helps in the development of adequate treatment strategies, especially due to its ability to cause extensive disability when not treated. The histopathological features of myasthenia gravis unveil the neuromuscular junctions of the disease. It has been suggested through studies that early neuropathic changes are detectable in specimens of muscle and nerves from patients, and 11 out of 12 cases were such that neuropathic causation was warranted by such findings (Badenhorst et al., 2018). Such histological findings further help substantiate the understanding not just of the impact on muscular tissue but also of the disease progression at a cellular level. Moreover, identification of these changes can be paramount to clinicians, leading to the necessity of proper diagnostic testing and appropriate intervention strategies to manage the symptoms and improve patients quality of life. Complicating the management provided by myasthenia gravis, associated systemic autoimmune conditions will also complicate management, particularly with regard to sensory manifestations , such as hearing loss. Audiometric findings, like sensorineural hearing loss, may occur in MG patients and appear consistent with Menières disease with bilateral auditory function (Ralli et al., 2018). These similar findings can lead to misdiagnosis, and therefore, the importance of thorough evaluation and watchfulness for the possibility of neurologic and auditory involvement in autoimmune disease is highlighted. Lastly, an interdisciplinary team consisting of neurologists, audiologists, and immunologists is crucial to respond effectively to the multifaceted nature of myasthenia gravis and its related challenges (Figure 10.17).

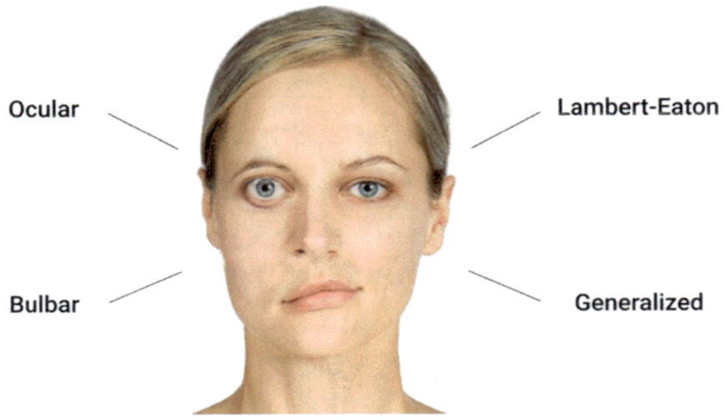

Figure 10.17. Myasthenia gravis.

Source: https://lonestarneurology.net/wp-content/uploads/2022/04/2-Symptoms-and-causes-of-myasthenia-gravis.webp.

10.5.3. Rhabdomyolysis

Rhabdomyolysis is a severe condition in which skeletal muscle fibers are harmed and spill their intracellular contents into the blood with substantial threats to renal function and general welfare. This condition can occur as a consequence of numerous etiologic factors like trauma, intense physical exercise, certain drugs, or primary diseases. Muscle tenderness, swelling, and weakness are a component of the clinical presentation and may progress to life-threatening conditions if not managed promptly. Release of myoglobin, a protein that provides muscles with oxygen, is of concern because it causes acute kidney injury (AKI) due to its nephrotoxicity. It is important to understand the pathophysiological mechanisms of rhabdomyolysis, as prompt diagnosis and treatment can greatly reduce morbidity and mortality due to the condition, rendering pathophysiological research in muscular disease a constant necessity. The cellular and molecular mechanisms behind rhabdomyolysis illustrate how muscle tissue integrity is directly connected with the overall function of the body. Recent data suggest that irregular handling of calcium by muscle fibers has a critical role in the etiology of this condition. Specifically, disruptions of calcium homeostasis can trigger cell stress responses that compromise muscle integrity and permit myocyte contents to enter the circulation. The genetic factors influencing rhabdomyolysis are known for mutations of the ryanodine receptor (RYR1), which further entangle the physiological landscape of muscle contractions and excitability. Understanding these pathophysiology mechanisms can lead to the identification of individuals at risk for the development of rhabdomyolysis, particularly in exercise physiology and other stressors. Such revelations lend credence to a multi-disciplinary treatment strategy considering muscular health in its entirety. The impact of rhabdomyolysis also carries long-term health implications and rehabilitative possibilities. The damage to the muscle tissue caused by this condition often results in long-lasting recovery periods where patients are feeble and physically less able. Current therapy focuses on supportive treatment with certain treatments to restore renal function and address the reasons for muscle damage. New therapies, such as the intravenous administration of dantrolene, have been revealed to potentially restrict complications of exertional rhabdomyolysis, particularly among sportspersons (Fernandez-Fuente et al., 2014). Moreover, ongoing studies on histopathological changes of venom-induced rhabdomyolysis highlight the complexities of muscle tissue responses in different pathophysiological contexts, emphasizing ongoing research into muscular diseases (Jacoby-Alner et al., 2011) (Figure 10.18).

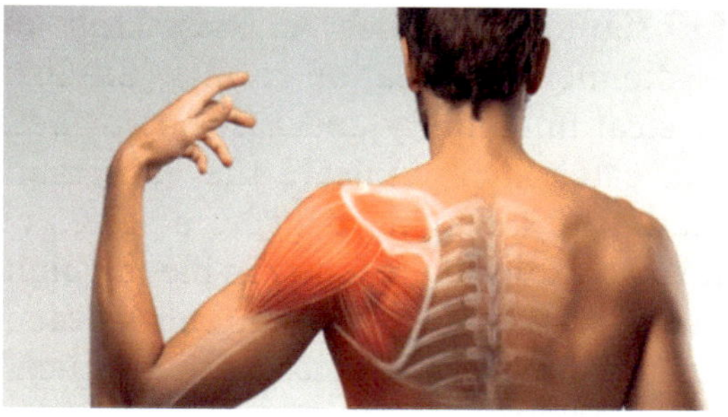

Figure 10.18. Rhabdomyolysis.

Source: https://stgaccinwbsdevlrs01.blob.core.windows.net/newcorporatewbsite/blogs/october2023/detail-main-Rhabdomyolysis.jpeg?w=3840&q=75.

Test Your Knowledge

1. What is muscular dystrophy?
2. What is rhabdomyolysis?

SUMMARY

By pulling all the research that has been done on human muscular tissue together, it can be observed that muscle is not only responsible for movement but also plays a crucial role in overall health and metabolic processes. Muscular health influences more than one physiological system, and one of them is metabolic regulation, where inflammatory biomarkers IL-6 and TNF-α show the dependence of muscle tissue and bone density. The evidence suggests that greater muscular fitness can regulate inflammatory reactions, thus reducing any detrimental impact on bone density and fitness in general. This finding underpins the importance of maintaining muscular fitness, particularly in vulnerable groups for obesity and metabolic disease, as suggesting intervention on muscular strength can lead to significant health benefits across different ages and life states, thus affecting bone health and systemic inflammation results (Gil-Cosano et al., 2019). Furthermore, the inactivity responses of physical immobility and associated metabolic changes, such as increased lipid deposition and protein catabolism, indicate the vulnerability of muscular systems to inactivity. Body metabolic adaptation to inactivity triggers a series of physiological alterations, spanning increased urinary amino acid excretion to shifts in blood volume distribution. These changes illustrate the significance of muscular tissue in maintaining metabolic homeostasis. When individuals become physically stationary under various conditions, such as those experiencing chronic disease or diminished physical activity, the resultant loss of muscular mass has significant repercussions on health. Thus, the facilitation of regular muscular activity is highly important not only to preserve muscle mass but also to avoid the negative effects associated with metabolic dysregulation (Federov, 2025). Lastly, the relationship between muscular tissue and overall health is multifaceted, comprising both acute and long-term adaptations to exercise as well as a sedentary lifestyle. As illustrated, muscular tissue plays a pivotal role in the mediation of inflammatory processes that are either pro-bone and pro-systemic health or anti-bone and anti-systemic health. The findings on muscular fitness and inflammatory markers indicate that maintenance and enhancement of muscular function must be an important target in health promotion strategies. Interventions to enhance muscle strength and endurance will not only favor individual health outcomes but also reduce the disease burden produced by obesity. Therefore, the integration of resistance and strength training within public health interventions can have far-reaching impacts on enhancing muscular health across different populations (Gil-Cosano et al., 2019; Federov, 2025).

It is imperative to understand the complexity of muscular tissue within the human body by being familiar with the three broad categories: skeletal, cardiac, and smooth muscle. Each type contains some specific features and functions that are part of human physiology. Skeletal muscle that makes voluntary movement possible is characterized by its striated appearance and multinucleated cells. Cardiac muscle exists only within the heart and involves involuntary contraction with intercalated discs to permit synchronized beats of the heart. Lastly, smooth muscle exists within other organ systems, including the gastrointestinal tract and blood vessels, and regulates involuntary movement. Cumulatively, these muscle tissues co-exist in order to sustain processes in the body, illustrating the multitude of uses that muscle has in health and mobility in general. An essential aspect of muscular tissue is that it is able to adapt and respond to various stimuli, something that is most vital as a function when it relates to exercise and rehabilitation. When subjected to resistance or endurance training, skeletal muscle fibers become hypertrophic, leading to a rise in muscle strength and mass. This is because the muscle fibers grow and repair and an increased number of motor units are utilized. Muscle atrophy may result from disuse or injury, which is something that serves to underscore the importance of participation in physical activity for the sake of maintaining muscular well-being. The payment of skeletal muscle, along with the intrinsic properties of cardiac and smooth muscle, tends to highlight the dynamic nature of muscular tissue, which is continuously responding to physiological demands and extrinsic stimuli. Not only is the study of muscular tissue restricted to its biological function, but it also converges with therapeutic advancement and research problems. For instance, excellent headway has also been achieved in deciphering muscular dystrophies, for instance, Duchenne muscular dystrophy (DMD), through models like the D2/mdx mouse. The model has genetic polymorphisms that have the nature of human DMD patients' dystropathology, which is a critical system for assessing the treatments to enhance muscle degeneration (Aartsma-Rus et al., 2018). Furthermore, research being performed in other aspects of muscular physiology can be indicative of treatment and enhance functional outcomes for those who are afflicted. Last, the knowledge regarding muscular tissue is paramount not just for academic research, but also for its application within healthcare and rehabilitation treatment, necessitating continued research to bridge existing knowledge gaps (Lloyd et al., 2002).

KEY TERMS FROM THIS CHAPTER

- Bloodstream
- Contractility
- Elasticity
- Extensibility
- Glucose
- Muscular tissue
- Skeletal muscles
- Cardiac muscle
- Digestive tract
- Excitability
- Fatty acids
- Muscular disorders
- Myocytes
- Smooth muscle

CRITICAL THINKING QUESTIONS

1. **The primary function of muscular tissue is:**
   a. Protection and insulation
   b. Contraction and movement
   c. Nutrient absorption
   d. Blood filtration
2. **Muscle tissue is characterized by its ability to:**
   a. Divide rapidly
   b. Transmit electrical signals
   c. Generate force through contraction
   d. Absorb nutrients
3. **Skeletal muscle is:**
   a. Involuntary and striated
   b. Voluntary and striated
   c. Involuntary and non-striated
   d. Voluntary and non-striated
4. **The functional unit of a skeletal muscle is the:**
   a. Myofibril
   b. Sarcomere
   c. Actin filament
   d. Sarcolemma
5. **The protein responsible for forming the thick filaments in a sarcomere is:**
   a. Actin
   b. Myosin
   c. Troponin
   d. Tropomyosin

Short Answer Questions

1. What is the muscular tissue?
2. Why is muscle tissue important in the human body?
3. List the types of muscular tissue.
4. What are the main functions of muscle tissue?
5. What is the mechanism of muscle contraction?

Answers to Critical Thinking Questions

1. (b); 2. (c) ; 3. (b); 4. (b); 5. (b)

REFERENCES

1. Aartsma-Rus, A., Bogdanik, L., Davies, K., De Luca, A., et al. (2018). *"Of mice and measures": A project to improve how we advance Duchenne muscular dystrophy therapies to the clinic.* https://core.ac.uk/download/161772638.pdf (accessed on 7th August 2025).
2. Gil-Cosano, J. J., Gracia-Marco, L., Ubago-Guisado, E., Labayen, I., Adelantado-Renau, M., Cadenas-Sanchez, C., Mora-Gonzalez, J., Plaza-Florido, A., Aguilera, C. M., Gómez-Vida, J., Maldonado, J., Jürimäe, J., & Ortega, F. B. (2020). Inflammatory markers and bone mass in children with overweight/obesity: the role of muscular fitness. *Pediatric research, 87*(1), 42–47. https://doi.org/10.1038/s41390-019-0572-8(accessed on 7th August 2025).
3. Ralli, M., D'Aguanno, V., Di Stadio, A., De Virgilio, A., Croce, A., Longo, L., Greco, A., & de Vincentiis, M. (2018). Audiovestibular Symptoms in Systemic Autoimmune Diseases. *Journal of immunology research, 2018*, 5798103. https://doi.org/10.1155/2018/5798103(accessed on 7th August 2025).
4. Touyz, R. M., Alves-Lopes, R., Rios, F. J., Camargo, L. L., Anagnostopoulou, A., Arner, A., & Montezano, A. C. (2018). Vascular smooth muscle contraction in hypertension. *Cardiovascular research, 114*(4), 529–539. https://doi.org/10.1093/cvr/cvy023(accessed on 7th August 2025).
5. Anderson, R. H., Ho, S. Y., & Mazgalev, T. N. (2001). *Anatomic-electrophysiological correlations concerning the pathways for atrioventricular conduction.* https://core.ac.uk/download/1676746.pdf (accessed on 7th August 2025).
6. Lloyd, E., Mitchell, S. D., Arnold, K., Parker, W., et al. (2002). *Session 2: Female Orgasms and Evolutionary Theory.* Proceedings of the Pittsburgh Workshop in History and Philosophy of Biology, Center for Philosophy of Science, University of Pittsburgh, March 23-24 2001. https://core.ac.uk/download/11920462.pdf (accessed on 7th August 2025).
7. Maas, H., Baan, G. C., & Huijing, P. A. (2004). Muscle force is determined also by muscle relative position: isolated effects. *Journal of biomechanics, 37*(1), 99–110. https://doi.org/10.1016/s0021-9290(03)00235-5 (accessed on 7th August 2025).
8. Badenhorst, M., & Isaacs, H. (2018). *Neurogenic Changes in Myasthenia Gravis.* https://core.ac.uk/download/478316482.pdf (accessed on 7th August 2025).
9. Baguet, A., Beeckman, S., Derave, W., Everaert, I., et al. (2010). *Muscle carnosine metabolism and β-alanine supplementation in relation to exercise and training.* https://core.ac.uk/download/55837517.pdf (accessed on 7th August 2025).
10. Jacoby-Alner, T. E., Stephens, N., Davern, K. M., Balmer, L., Brown, S. G., & Swindells, K. (2011). Histopathological analysis and in situ localisation of Australian tiger snake venom in two clinically envenomed domestic animals. *Toxicon : official journal of the International Society on Toxinology, 58*(4), 304–314. https://doi.org/10.1016/j.toxicon.2011.07.008(accessed on 7th August 2025).
11. Biga, L. M., Dawson, S., Dawson, W. E., et al. (2020). *Anatomy & Physiology.* https://core.ac.uk/download/622361060.pdf (accessed on 7th August 2025).
12. Brockington, M., Brown, S. C., Cirak, S., Liu, Q., et al. (2010). *Transgenic overexpression of LARGE induces alpha-dystroglycan hyperglycosylation in skeletal and cardiac muscle.* https://core.ac.uk/download/1730280.pdf (accessed on 7th August 2025).

13. Broekelmann, T. J., Chu, M. L., Halabi, C. M., Lee, C. Y., et al. (2017). *Fibulin-4 is essential for maintaining arterial wall integrity in conduit but not muscular arteries.* https://core.ac.uk/download/83101134.pdf (accessed on 7th August 2025).

14. *Sundberg, C. W., Hunter, S. K., & Bundle, M. W. (2017). Rates of performance loss and neuromuscular activity in men and women during cycling: evidence for a common metabolic basis of muscle fatigue. Journal of applied physiology (Bethesda, Md. : 1985), 122(1), 130–141. https://doi.org/10.1152/japplphysiol.00468.2016*(accessed on 7th August 2025).

15. Charles, J. P., Cappellari, O., Spence, A. J., Hutchinson, J. R., & Wells, D. J. (2016). Musculoskeletal Geometry, Muscle Architecture and Functional Specialisations of the Mouse Hindlimb. *PloS one, 11*(4), e0147669. https://doi.org/10.1371/journal.pone.0147669 (accessed on 7th August 2025).

16. Carter, C. S., Justice, J. N., & Thompson, L. (2019). *Lipotoxicity, aging, and muscle contractility: Does fiber type matter?* https://open.bu.edu/bitstream/2144/40625/7/carter_justice_thompson_Lipotoxicity_paper_04302019.pdf (accessed on 7th August 2025).

17. Kiely, J., & Collins, D. J. (2016). Uniqueness of Human Running Coordination: The Integration of Modern and Ancient Evolutionary Innovations. *Frontiers in psychology*, *7*, 262. https://doi.org/10.3389/fpsyg.2016.00262(accessed on 7th August 2025).

18. De Paepe, B., & De Bleecker, J. L. (2013). Cytokines and chemokines as regulators of skeletal muscle inflammation: presenting the case of Duchenne muscular dystrophy. *Mediators of inflammation, 2013*, 540370. https://doi.org/10.1155/2013/540370(accessed on 7th August 2025).

19. Draeger, A., Ludman, A., Zoumi, A., Rubinstein, A. L., Samuel, A., Yeh, A. T., Buettner, C., et al. (2011). *Imaging of zebrafish in vivo with second-harmonic generation reveals shortened sarcomeres associated with myopathy induced by statin.* https://core.ac.uk/download/pdf/8620094.pdf (accessed on 7th August 2025).

20. Drury, D. G., & Stuempfle, K. J. (2007). *The Physiological Consequences of bed Rest.* https://cupola.gettysburg.edu/cgi/viewcontent.cgi?article=1029&context=healthfac (accessed on 7th August 2025).

21. Ehrle, A., Ressel, L., Ricci, E., Singer, E., et al. (2017). *Structure and innervation of the equine supraspinous and interspinous ligaments.* https://core.ac.uk/download/82984828.pdf (accessed on 7th August 2025).

22. Federov, I. V. (2025). *Metabolism During Hypodynamia.* https://core.ac.uk/download/pdf/42865788.pdf (accessed on 7th August 2025).

23. Hanna Kaciuba-Uscilko and John E. Greenleaf(1989). *Acclimatization to Cold in Humans.* NASA Technical Memorandum 101 01 2 https://core.ac.uk/download/pdf/42827514.pdf (accessed on 7th August 2025).

24. Gur, A., Stergioulas, A., Gautam, A. P., Hegedus, B., Barber, B. J., Rizzi, C. F., Hayworth, C. R., et al. (2014). *Superpulsed low-level laser therapy protects skeletal muscle of mdx mice against damage, inflammation and morphological changes delaying dystrophy progression.* https://core.ac.uk/download/29019175.pdf (accessed on 7th August 2025).

25. Hetherington, C. S. (2019). *Myofascial Release.* https://core.ac.uk/download/289198166.pdf (accessed on 7th August 2025).

26. Hoffman, J. I. E. (2017). *Will the Real Ventricular Architecture Please Stand Up.* https://core.ac.uk/download/323072376.pdf (accessed on 7th August 2025).

27. Fernandez-Fuente, M., Terracciano, C. M., Martin-Duque, P., Brown, S. C., Vassaux, G., & Piercy, R. J. (2014). Calcium homeostasis in myogenic differentiation factor 1 (MyoD)-transformed, virally-transduced, skin-derived equine myotubes. *PloS one*, *9*(8), e105971. https://doi.org/10.1371/journal.pone.0105971(accessed on 7th August 2025).

28. Huijing, P. A. (1995). *Parameter Interdependence and Success of Skeletal Muscle Modelling.* https://core.ac.uk/download/pdf/11461276.pdf (accessed on 7th August 2025).

29. Kovalenko, Y. A. (2025). *Pathophysiological Aspects of the Problem of Prolonged Hypokinesia.* https://core.ac.uk/download/pdf/42873658.pdf (accessed on 7th August 2025).

30. NASA Report Number: NASA-SP-7011(386) (1994). *Aerospace medicine and biology: A continuing bibliography with indexes, supplement 130, July 1974.* Document ID

31. Pravdin, S. (2013). *Nonaxisymmetric Mathematical Model of the Cardiac Left Ventricle Anatomy.* https://core.ac.uk/download/55796895.pdf (accessed on 7th August 2025).

32. Rittweger, J. (2010). *Vibration as an exercise modality: How it may work, and what its potential might be.* https://core.ac.uk/download/11141396.pdf (accessed on 7th August 2025).

33. Sato, K. (2004). *Molecular genetic analysis for malignant hyperthermia: A thesis presented to Massey University in partial fulfilment of the requirements for the degree of Master of Science in Biochemistry.* https://core.ac.uk/download/157568824.pdf (accessed on 7th August 2025).

NERVOUS TISSUE

11

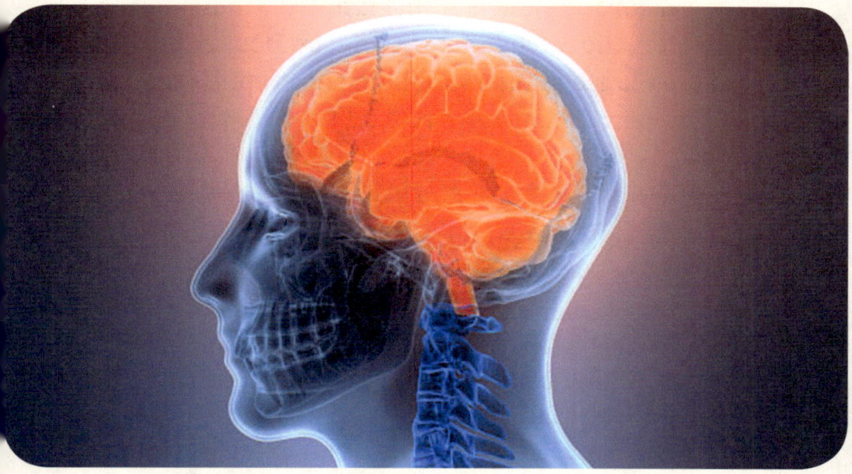

LEARNING OBJECTIVES

After studying this chapter, you will be able to:

1. Explain the types of nervous tissue;
2. Describe the structure of neurons;
3. Describe the functions of nervous tissue;
4. Explain the types of neurons;
5. Understand the glial cells and their functions;
6. Describe the nervous tissue in health and disease.

Introduction

Appreciation for the complex organization and operation of nervous tissue is necessary for the understanding of the wider applications of neurobiology to human disease and health. Nervous tissue, composed largely of neurons and glial cells, plays the key role in conveying information throughout the body and thus coordinating a variety of physiological responses. Neurons are specialized cells that facilitate communication by generating and transmitting electrical signals, whereas glial cells provide essential support, insulation, and supply functions to neuronal circuits. Not only does this interaction between neurons and glia modulate basic neural function, but it also dictates the integrity of the nervous system as a whole with far-reaching effects on behavior, cognition, and bodily homeostasis. The principle of neurotoxicity identifies the vulnerability of nervous tissue to disruptions caused by the environment and physiology. Neurotoxicity is the term applied to describe the toxic effects resulting from the action of a series of chemicals and metabolites that finally impair the nervous system's functionality. Some agents directly target neural cells, while others interfere with metabolic processes crucial for the survival of neurons. The complexities of neurotoxicity highlight the fact that while some disturbance proves to be temporary, others lead to chronic malfunction or developmental abnormalities. Understanding neurotoxic mechanisms is significant in addressing the growing problem of chemical exposure, particularly in the context of an industrialized world where neurotoxic substances are ubiquitous in all aspects of life (Spencer & Lein, 2014).

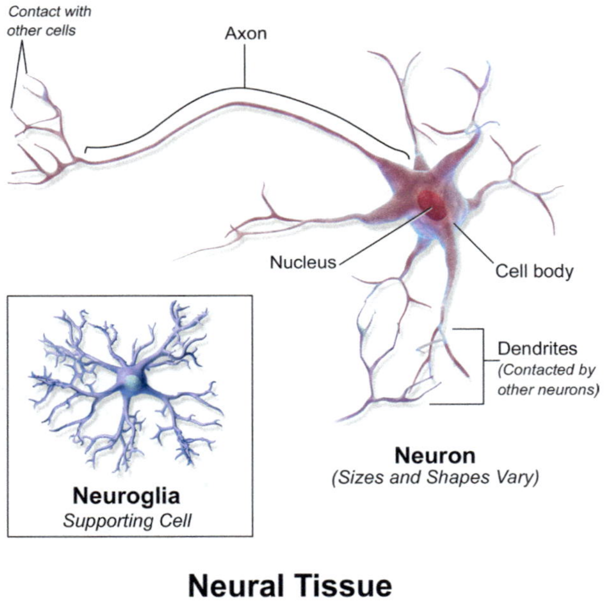

Figure 11.1. Nervous tissue.

Source: https://upload.wikimedia.org/wikipedia/commons/7/73/Blausen_0672_NeuralTissue.png.

Also, the interaction between the nervous system and metabolic disease highlights the intricate relationship between multiple body systems. Recent research demonstrates a robust relationship between neural circuits, the immune system, and metabolic dysfunction , such as obesity and insulin resistance. The intricate intertwining of these processes shows that the nervous system is a critical regulatory mechanism for maintaining homeostasis, particularly during disease conditions affecting cardiovascular well-being (Lori et al., 2017). As we explore the function and repercussions of nervous tissue in man, it is apparent that a precise understanding of such interlinkages can lead to new therapeutic approaches towards the prevention or alleviation of the undesirable consequences of neurotoxicity and metabolic disorders. Such information is indispensable for the development of composite plans to enhance human well-being in a rapidly changing environment (Figure 11.1).

Definition of Nervous Tissue

Nervous tissue is a specialized type of tissue whose role is extremely crucial in the process of communication and coordination of function in the body. It consists primarily of neurons and glial cells, and its purpose is to carry and process information such that the organism may react to internal and external stimuli. Neurons are the working units of nervous tissue and possess the unique characteristic of producing and transmitting electrical impulses in the form of action potentials. These enable rapid communication between the body parts, which is important for homeostasis, reflexes, and thought processes. Glial cells, however, provide support, nutrition, and protection to neurons, an indication of the synergy involved in nervous tissue. This double structure denotes the complexity of the nervous system, which is critical for involuntary actions, such as control over heart rate, and complex behaviors, such as learning and memory formation. The intricate architecture of nervous tissue is expressed in its segmentation into two distinct areas: the central nervous system (CNS) and the peripheral nervous system (PNS). The CNS, or spinal cord and brain, is the primary command center for the interpretation of sensory input and coordination of responses. The PNS serves to connect the CNS to limbs and organs for the purpose of communication within the body. Cross-talk among various signaling pathways within nervous tissue is crucial to its function. In particular, recent research has indicated that a number of pathways exhibit tissue-specific function, illustrating the intricate regulatory processes found in the nervous system. Such complexity is not only required for physiological function but also to understand disease states. As various diseases, including neurodegenerative diseases, may disrupt such pathways, nervous tissue analysis remains important for advancements in medical science (Korcsmáros et al., 2010). Furthermore, the function of neurohormonal systems to modulate nervous tissue reinforces its key position in metabolic regulation.

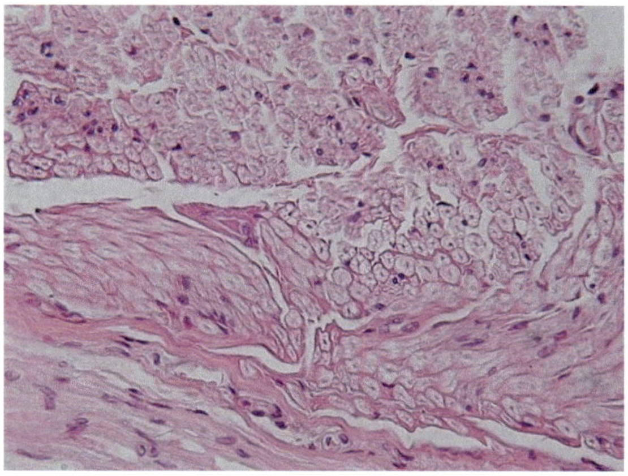

Figure 11.2. Histologic example of nervous tissue.

Source: https://upload.wikimedia.org/wikipedia/commons/9/9e/Peripheral_nerve%2C_cross_section.jpg.

An example is the natriuretic peptides that are vasoconstrictor system antagonists, which have been linked with nervous tissue integrity by virtue of their effect upon cardiovascular dynamics as well as upon metabolic occurrences. Abnormality in the neurohormonal systems has been linked with various health disorders, for example, insulin resistance and hypertension, particularly in the scenario of the metabolic syndrome. These relationships underscore the interdependence of nervous tissue function with overall physiological homeostasis and underscore its importance in the clinical literature. An understanding of the intricate relationship of nervous tissue to systemic health can provide insight into new fields of disease prevention and treatment, thus placing it at the forefront of present-day biomedical research (Alonzo et al., 2010) (Figure 11.2).

Importance of Nervous Tissue in the Human Body

Nervous tissue is the principal body communication system, allowing the exchange of information between organs and systems. Composed primarily of neurons and glial cells, nervous tissue is responsible for interpreting sensory data, integrating the response, and regulating body functions. Furthermore, the role of this tissue is not just simply the transmission of signals; it is the foundation of our cognitive functions, emotional reactions, and behavioral patterns in general. That is, the complex web of neurons enables complex interactions that facilitate learning and memory, and thus plays a central role in the development and adaptation of an individual. The activity of the brain in such processes is the epitome of how nervous tissue not only performs physiological functions but also has a role in our psychological well-being. Nervous tissue's role is so important to grasp, as it lays out the manner in which deviances within this system can produce a myriad of neurological disorders. Aside from its paramount function in communication and cognitive processes, nervous tissue is highly integrated with the body's homeostatic processes. The interdependence of nervous tissue with the rest of the body systems demonstrates the delicate balance that must be maintained to ensure health. The nervous system, for instance, regulates critical processes like breathing, heart rate, and digestion through autonomic responses that are under the command of the sympathetic and parasympathetic divisions. This indicates the importance that nervous tissue has in the regulation of not only voluntary movement but also involuntary physiological functions. Moreover, the relationship between the nervous system and other tissues, including endocrine and immune systems, highlights the shared responsibility of homeostasis. The importance of nervous tissue also lies in the fact that it is a mediator and regulator of complex body functions that impact overall health. Emerging findings point out how nervous tissue talks to various parts , such as adipose tissue, which also impacts metabolic and immune functions. Research shows that adipose tissue has the ability to regulate nervous system processes, affecting brain function and immune activity by releasing adipokines and cytokines (Tonchev et al., 2020). This neuroendocrine connection adds to our knowledge of how various systems in the body interact, proving that the activity of nervous tissue is not separated but forms part of a dynamic interaction between various tissues. Here, any injury to nervous tissue could have rippling effects and cause systemic illness. Thus, understanding the varied functions of nervous tissue is valuable in the overall comprehension of human body physiology and the interconnectedness of our body systems (Figure 11.3).

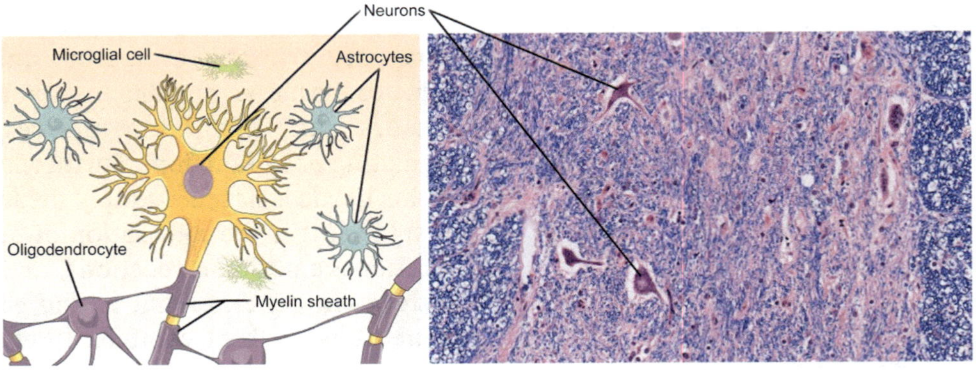

Figure 11.3. Nervous Tissue. Nervous tissue is made up of neurons and neuroglia. The cells of nervous tissue are specialized to transmit and receive impulses.

Source: https://s3-us-west-2.amazonaws.com/courses-images-archive-read-only/wp-content/uploads/sites/18/2014/07/19181105/416_Nervous_Tissue-new.jpg.

11.1. Types of Nervous Tissue

Learning Outcome

1. Understand the neurons;
2. Describe the glial cells;
3. Differentiate between neurons and glial cells.

The nervous tissue of human beings is primarily categorized into two broad groups: neuroglia and neurons. Neuroglia or glial cells serve important supportive roles in the nervous system. While neurons are responsible for the transmission of electrical impulses, the function of neuroglia is the preservation of homeostasis, the production of myelin, and support and defense for the neurons. These functions are fulfilled by specialized forms of glial cells , such as astrocytes, oligodendrocytes, and microglia. Astrocytes, for instance, play a central role in the blood-brain barrier and the provision of nutrients, while oligodendrocytes play a central role in the central nervous system's myelin formation. The intricate interactions between such cells emphasize the complexity of nervous tissue since these supporting functions can significantly contribute to influencing the health and functionality of neurons throughout the lifetime of an organism. Neurons, the basic functional building blocks of the nervous system, are primarily responsible for information transmission by electrochemical signals. Structurally, neurons possess three major elements: the cell body, dendrites, and axons. Sensory input is received by the dendrites, and the axon transmits impulses to other neurons or effectors , such as muscles and glands. The specialized structure allows neurons to communicate with each other efficiently, allowing a wide range of functions from reflex actions to higher-level cognitive processes. Moreover, neurons can be classified based on their structure and function, with sensory, motor, and interneurons having unique but related functions in neural circuits. Appreciation of these issues is critical, especially when it comes to pathological states, since the disruption of neuronal integrity has the potential to generate massive neurotoxicity, where chemicals interrupt normal neural activity and may be from external exposure as well as from metabolic imbalance within the body (Spencer & Lein, 2014). Moreover, immune processes that occur within the nervous system provide an additional layer of complexity, namely in how natural killer (NK) cells operate. Research highlights that immune cells of this type can be controlled by a variety of factors within nervous tissues and how these influence their ability to respond to neural damage or infection. While traditional associations include the combat of tumors and virally infected cells, NK cells are also involved in inflammatory events associated with neural disease. Their behavior illustrates the interaction of nervous and immune systems, i.e., how microenvironments and organ-specific components define their roles in the brain and other areas. The intricate relationship between nervous tissue and immune mediators underscores the need for multidisciplinary research emphasis towards the understanding of neuroinflammatory diseases, expanding our knowledge about normal as well as disease states of the nervous system (Shi et al., 2011) (Figure 11.4).

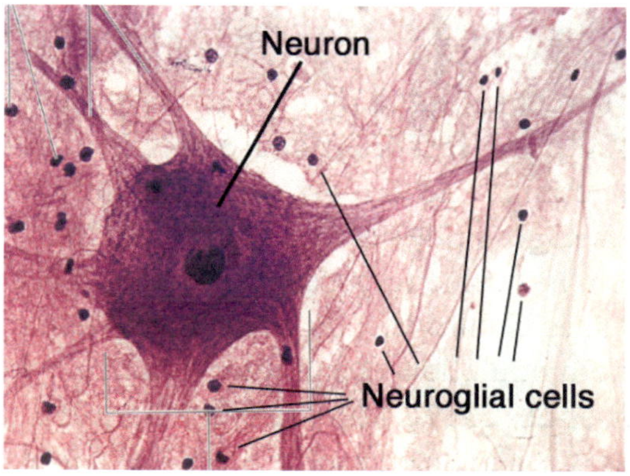

Figure 11.4. Types of nervous tissue.

Source: https://biology4isc.weebly.com/uploads/9/0/8/0/9080078/351362751.jpg.

11.1.1. Neurons

The fundamental building blocks of the nervous system, neurons are responsible for transporting information throughout the entire human body. Comprising a cell body, dendrites, and an axon, these excitable cells still can generate and transmit electrical impulses known as action potentials. The intricate structure of neurons allows for the achievement of sophisticated signaling, with dendrites receiving signals from other neurons and the axon transmitting feedback responses to target cells. Such one-way transmission of information is the core principle of body function organization, thinking activity, and response to stimuli. Furthermore, the high plasticity of neurons allows them to adjust to new experiences, a critical event for learning and memory. Accordingly, the understanding of neuron function and structure plays a significant role in the deconstruction of nervous tissue complexities in the human organism and the implications on disease and health. Neurons not only function by transmitting impulses; they also participate in all forms of neurotoxic effects and metabolic disease. Neurotoxicity is evoked when exposure to a harmful agent interferes with normal neural function. From the literature, many chemicals lead to neurotoxic diseases by either directly affecting neural cells or by interfering with essential metabolic processes upon which the nervous system relies (Spencer & Lein, 2014). Such perturbations may result in symptoms ranging from reversible deficits to irreversible damage, and thus illustrate the vulnerability of neuronal cells to environmental injury.

The understanding of how disruption of the neural structure occurs is critical in developing preventative interventions and therapeutic strategies. Through continued research in these connections, the importance of treating neurotoxicological effects on human health becomes increasingly relevant day by day. Furthermore, the networking of the neurons with the immune system has come to pose an intriguing field of study, particularly in reference to metabolic diseases like obesity and insulin resistance. Research confirms that neural networks play a crucial role in the modulation of immune functions, which are typically altered in hypertension and obesity (Lori et al., 2017). The interplay between the nervous and immune system suggests that neurons possess the ability to control the onset and course of these metabolic diseases. Interestingly, neural reflexes have been found to play a role in the modulation of immune functions, implying that neurotransmission is not only communication within the nervous system but also extends to more systemic relationships. This knowledge is critical since it marks the beginning of new therapeutic approaches that can be used to target the neural process behind such illnesses, thereby improving overall health outcomes (Figure 11.5).

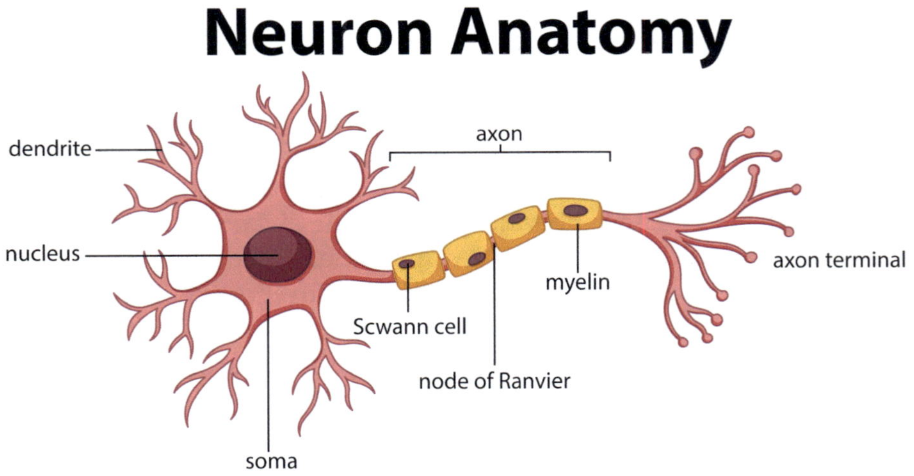

Figure 11.5. Neuron anatomy.

Source: https://www.simplypsychology.org/wp-content/uploads/Neuron-with-myelin-sheath.jpg.

11.1.2. Glial Cells

Glial cells are non-replaceable supporting cells of the nervous tissue and have functions much more meaningful than merely insulating the neurons. Glial cells are several types of different cells, like astrocytes, oligodendrocytes, and microglia, which all contribute to the promotion of neuronal function and health. Astrocytes, for instance, support the maintenance of the blood-brain barrier, regulate the levels of neurotransmitters, and provide metabolic support to the neurons. Oligodendrocytes are required for central nervous system myelination, facilitating high-speed signal transduction through axons. Microglia also act as the central nervous system's frontline immune cell, actively patrolling for pathogens and cellular detritus. By coordinating these diverse responsibilities, glial cells ensure the overall health and homeostasis of the nervous tissue, which itself is imperative to healthy neurological function. The capacity of nervous tissue to regenerate highlights significant differences between the (PNS) and the central nervous system (CNS), namely with respect to the role of glial cells. In the PNS, Schwann cells and olfactory ensheathing cells (OECs) actively facilitate the regeneration of nerves after damage. The rapid action of such glial cells is crucial to the clearing of cellular debris and production of growth factors supportive of neuronal recovery. On the other hand, CNS glial cells, particularly astrocytes and oligodendrocytes, possess limited regenerative capacity, favoring scarring and hindering axonal growth in the event of injury. As research on the functions of glial cells progresses, understanding these variations offers windows into therapeutic interventions, i.e., PNS glia transplantation to promote recovery in the event of CNS damage, depicting the potential for gap bridging in neural repair (Barton et al., 2017). Someevidence also illustrates the delicate interaction between glial cells and vascular health in the nervous system, notably with the vascular endothelial growth factor (VEGF) system. Originally implicated in vascular development, VEGF has proven itself to be known for its action on neural cells in developmental and adult conditions. VEGFR expression by glial cells points to their dual role in supporting neuronal survival and controlling vascular integrity. The duality of this relationship is troublesome, however, since VEGF can contribute to pathological actions on neural function as well. Researchers are presently addressing this duality to design therapies that can leverage the neuroprotective aspects of VEGF without the risks of its vascular activity. Understanding this intricate relationship between glial cells and vascularization may pave the way for new treatments in various brain pathologies (Wittko-Schneider et al., 2013) (Figure 11.6).

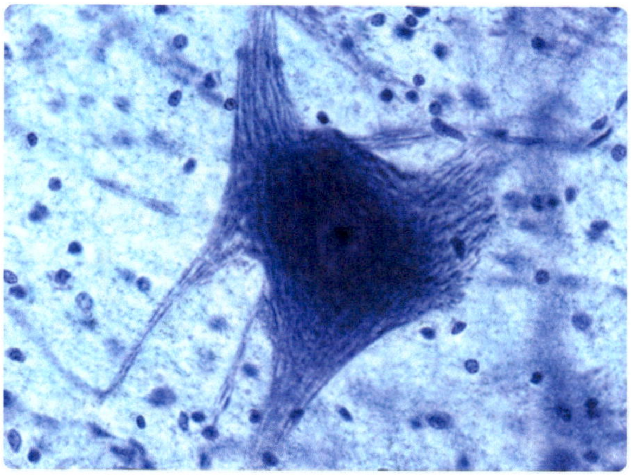

Figure 11.6. Glial cells.

Source: https://d2jx2rerrg6sh3.cloudfront.net/image-handler/ts/20200317060727/ri/673/picture/2020/3/shutterstock_79216378.jpg.

11.1.3. Differences Between Neurons and Glial Cells

There are two broad cell types in the human nervous system, namely neurons and glial cells, each with distinct but complementary roles. Neurons, the sine qua non of neural conduction, are specialized neurons that transmit electrical impulses from synapse to synapse, supporting processes like reflexes, thought, and movement. Their characteristic morphology, including a cell body, dendrites, and axons, facilitates rapid information transmission. In contrast, glial cells, which are traditionally regarded as the nervous system's supporting actors, outweigh neurons and are involved in critical support roles. Glial cells provide homeostasis, form myelin sheaths for the faster transmission of signals, and are involved in metabolic support. Though each has a significant role to play, neurons and glial cells differ considerably in role and attribute, which speaks to the overall nervous tissue complexity in humans. The distinction extends to the regenerative capacity and response to injury as well. While neurons are largely constrained from regrowing following damage, glial cells are the most important elements in recovery. For example, in the peripheral nervous system, Schwann cells facilitate neuronal regeneration through clearing debris and providing growth factors for recovery. On the other hand, the central nervous system possesses a more limited regenerative ability due to the largely non-permissive setting created by glial cells like astrocytes, which have the potential to inhibit neuronal regrowth. This divergence of function points to the very important role played by glial cells in regenerative medicine. Understanding the mechanisms of regeneration employed by glial cells can be quite useful as new forms of therapy in the promotion of neural injury recovery, for instance, in the role of olfactory ensheathing cells to improve regeneration within the central and peripheral nervous system. Moreover, the heterogeneity of glial cells presents a fertile ground for studying their differentiated functions. There are glial cells in the peripheral nervous system, like the olfactory ensheathing cells and Schwann cells, which possess unique characteristics to enable them to perform optimally. For instance, olfactory ensheathing cells participate in the continuous replacement of the olfactory nerve without providing room for an environment to regenerate, while Schwann cells are primarily stimulated during injury (Echeverri, 2020). This differential activation highlights the specialized role of glial cells, not merely in serving neuronal function but also in reacting to various physiological situations. Such information is instrumental in progressing the neurobiology discipline, specifically in therapeutic strategy implementation, augmenting glial cells and inherent regenerative potential (Echeverri, 2020). Sensitivity to these differences is a prerequisite for maximum utilization of nervous tissue in clinical application.

Test Your Knowledge

1. What are neurons?
2. What are glial cells?

11.2. Structure of Neurons

Learning Outcome

1. Describe the cell body (soma);
2. Understand the dendrites;
3. Understand the axon.

The structure of neurons is one of the most important topics in understanding the nervous tissue in human beings. Neurons, which are the fundamental components of the nervous system, are specialized cells that transmit information throughout the body through electrical and chemical impulses. The neuron consists of three important parts: the cell body (soma), dendrites, and axons. The cell body contains the nucleus and organelles, which are essential to neuronal activity. Dendrites branch off from the cell body and gather information from other cells, and the axon transmits electrical impulses from the cell body to target cells. This intricate design enables intricate networks of communication, which coordinate thousands of body functions and reflex actions to stimuli, to be the epitome of biological architecture that is responsible for nerve function and interaction in the body. The functioning of the neurons is further enhanced by the existence of specialized structures , such as myelin sheaths, which encase the axons and facilitate faster transmission of impulses. Myelination is aided by the action of oligodendrocytes in the central nervous system and Schwann cells in the peripheral nervous system.

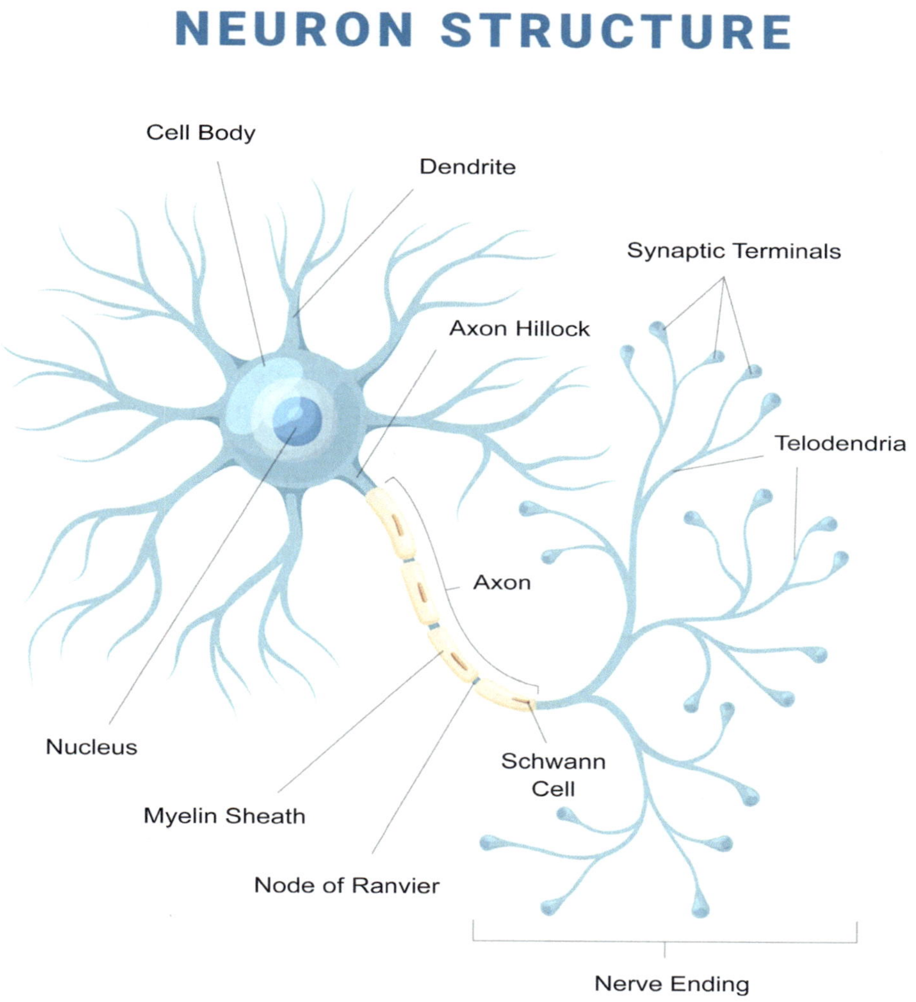

Figure 11.7. Structure of neurons.

Source: https://www.simplypsychology.org/wp-content/uploads/neuron-structure-1320x1536.jpeg.

The fatty sheath not only increases the speed of signal conduction but also plays a protective role in ensuring neural integrity. Myelin damage, as observed in conditions like multiple sclerosis, can lead to severe neurological impairment, highlighting the importance of the structure of the neuron in maintaining intact nervous system function. In addition, structural abnormalities in neurons have the potential to create a variety of neurotoxicities by directly or indirectly disrupting neural cells, potentially leading to incapacitating diseases affecting motor and cognitive functions (Spencer & Lein, 2014). The structural-functional relationship in neural structures extends into the intricate interactions with the nervous system, with topographically corresponding systems, e.g., the immune system and metabolic systems. Advances in research have revealed mechanisms by which central nervous mechanisms control peripheral nervous function, with implications for conditions , such as obesity and hypertension. As a case in point, neural reflexes can influence immune function, highlighting an interdependent web of functioning components that underscores the importance of neuronal structure in the grand design of health and disease. As researchers study these interactions, the crucial role of neurons in enabling communication between various systems becomes increasingly evident, highlighting the need for well-organized neurons to ensure and regulate physiological homeostasis in human health (Lori et al., 2017) (Figure 11.7).

11.2.1. Cell Body (soma)

The cell body, or the soma, is the primary focal point of a neuron where its nucleus and other organelles required for cellular function are located. The soma is also the primary metabolic center of the neuron and is involved in protein synthesis, neurotransmitter synthesis, and the production of other vital molecules required for neuronal integrity. The presence of ribosomes and rough endoplasmic reticulum within the soma is the provision for the translation of mRNA transcripts into proteins so that the neuron can respond appropriately to physiological demand. The cell body also sums the converging synaptic inputs, an activity necessary for communication between neurons. Integration is important in determining whether or not an action potential will be generated, thus playing a fundamental role in neural circuitry and information processing. Moreover, soma is an essential component of neuronal plasticity, which is involved in learning and memory. Changes in the soma's structural and functional characteristics can regulate neuronal performance and responsiveness to stimuli. For instance, dysregulation of the proteins involved in synaptic transmission or intracellular signaling pathways can lead to neurodegenerative diseases. In Parkinson's disease, selective damage to dopaminergic neurons is associated with cell body changes that impact their homeostatic ability. It has been shown that the integrity of the soma is essential; dysfunction leads to a chain of neurodegenerative events culminating in the death of neurons, reinforcing the soma's crucial role in preserving neuronal function and integrity (Tito & Zhang, 2016). Also, variations in the morphology of the soma among different neuron types tell us something about their specialized function in the nervous system. For example, excitatory neurons possess bigger somas compared to inhibitory neurons, explaining why they can facilitate synaptic transmission. Anatomical variation is due to external factors , such as stress and aging that have been identified to influence protein expression in the soma. Especially, protein dysregulation of proteins , such as Sorting Nexins (SNXs) is implicated in cognitive deficiency in neurodegenerative diseases , such as Alzheimer's (Vale, 2023). Thus, research into the intricacies of the cell body contributes significantly to the overall study of nervous tissue in humans, establishing the causative factors of healthy and disease states in the nervous system (Figure 11.8).

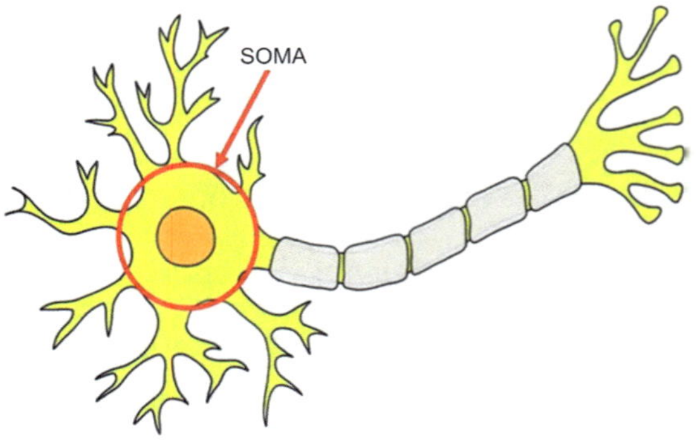

Figure 11.8. Soma is indicated by a red circle and arrow.

Source: https://neuroscientificallychallenged.com/files/images/soma.jpg.

11.2.2. Dendrites

Dendrites are the elementary building blocks of neurons, with a central role in information processing in the nervous system. The branched, tree-like dendrites emerge from the cell body of a neuron and receive synaptic input from other neurons. The intricacy of dendritic trees varies extensively across various neuron types, with some having an extensive branched system for maximizing their ability to sum inputs. This diversity enables fine information processing which enables the neurons to more effectively respond to all the signals that they are receiving. Moreover, dendrites can also exhibit structural plasticity in adapting the shape in accordance with environmental stimulus or neuronal activity and thereby influence learning and memory processes in the human brain. It is interesting that the dendritic forms can be influenced by numerous neurotoxic agents, which reflects their susceptibility to environmental stress. Neurotoxic compounds may impair the function of the dendrites, and this can result in defective synaptic communication and may even lead to neurodegenerative diseases. For instance, certain chemical exposures may initiate a cascade of effects that either affect neural cells directly or interrupt metabolic processes that are significant to dendritic integrity and function. This interruption might be reflected in reduced branching of dendrites or other synaptic input changes, ultimately affecting the transmission of information by the neuron. Understanding the mechanisms of dendrites and substance-induced neurotoxicity is important to develop protective measures against environmental toxins detrimental to nervous tissue health in humans, as in the subject of neurotoxicity (Spencer & Lein, 2014). Although scientists are continually discovering the intricacies of dendritic morphology, the discovery of specialized neurons , such as von Economo neurons (VENs) is particularly enlightening. These cells, characterized by their characteristic dendritic morphologies, are present in specific regions of the human brain and have clearly demarcated functional roles to play in emotional processing and decision-making. Notably, VENs are more prevalent in humans compared to other primates, representing an evolutionary adaptation that may be connected to the more advanced cognitive abilities of humans. Interestingly, these neurons also project to interface with the autonomic nervous system, showing the interconnection between mental processes and body states. Furthermore, the ongoing research on the genetic factors influencing the morphology of dendrites, such as the DISC1 gene, highlights the delicate balance between genetics and environment in shaping the form and function of the neural tissues of the human nervous system (Allman et al., 2010) (Figure 11.9).

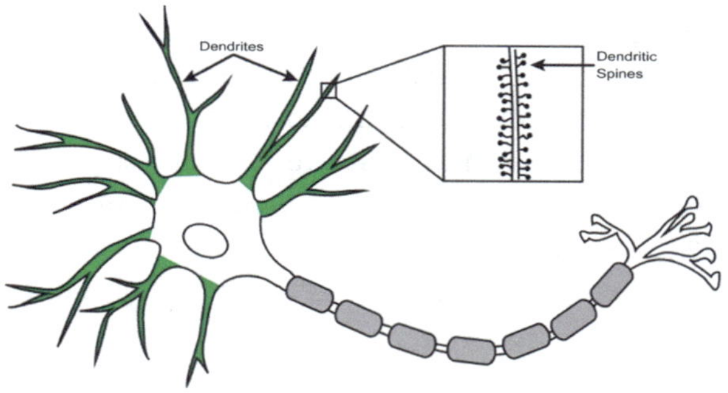

Figure 11.9. Dendrites branch out from the soma. Their function is to receive information from other neurons.

Source: https://openbooks.lib.msu.edu/app/uploads/sites/6/2020/11/Dendrites.jpg.

11.2.3. Axon

The axon is an important component of nerve cells and is primarily responsible for transmitting the electrical impulses away from the neuron's cell body. The axon differs in length structurally, typically several millimeters to meters, based on the specific function of the neuron. Its primary role is to carry out action potentials, which are brief voltage changes across the neuron's membrane. It achieves this through the presence of specific ion channels that open and close based on voltage alterations, allowing for a rapid spread of the electrical impulse. Essential to the efficient transmission of such impulses is the myelin sheath, which is a covering of insulating material around the axon that increases the speed of signal transmission. Clinical manifestations of axonal injury are deep; neurotoxicity can severely disrupt normal axonal function, leading to a range of neurological disorders and potential long-term damage (Spencer & Lein, 2014). In addition to this, the distinction between the (CNS) and the (PNS) is evident in the field of axon regeneration. The PNS exhibits an exceptionally high rate of regeneration following damage, mainly due to the protective role of olfactory ensheathing cells and Schwann cells. Glial cells quickly react to axon damage by clearing cell debris and providing essential growth factors for regeneration to take place. The disparity in the capacity for regeneration between the CNS and PNS underscores a highly significant aspect of neurobiological investigation. Despite the considerable limitations imposed upon mechanisms of repair of axons within the CNS, information regarding the mechanisms of PNS regeneration can be employed for the development of therapeutic interventions that will enhance recovery of function within the CNS following damage (Barton et al., 2017). Therefore, the axon is illuminated by research into the mechanisms governing neuronal health and recovery. Within the larger framework of nervous tissue, it is essential to incorporate an awareness of the consequences of neurotransmission and synaptic contact. The tip of the axon, the axon terminal, is where chemical messages (neurotransmitters) are transmitted to inform nearby neurons, muscles, or glands. This synaptic transmission is a vital feature in facilitating such intricate functions as reflexes, motor control, and learning. Additionally, disruptions in axonal integrity can lead to abnormal neurotransmitter release, with the impact being extensive on overall neural function and communication. Neurological disease resulting from axonal compromise can arise in various manifestations, from cognitive impairments to motor dysfunction. Thus, the axon is not merely a conduit for electrical impulses but is part and parcel of the regulatory processes of the nervous system, illustrating the intertwined interdependencies of human neural response and function (Spencer & Lein, 2014) (Figure 11.10).

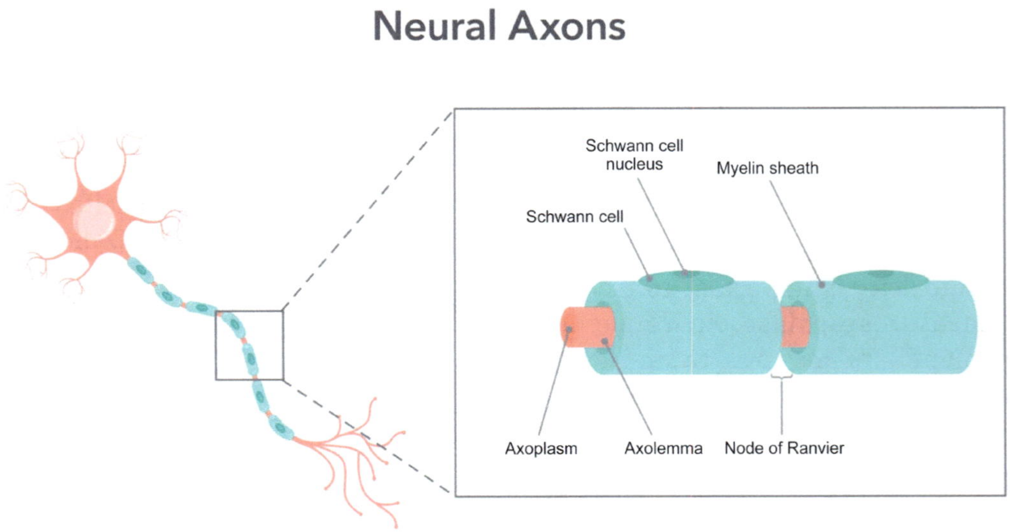

Figure 11.10. Neural axon.

Source: https://www.simplypsychology.org/wp-content/uploads/neuron-axon-1536x864.jpeg.

Test Your Knowledge

1. What are dendrites?
2. What is an axon?

11.3. Functions of Nervous Tissue

Learning Outcome

1. Understand the signal transmission;
2. Describe the processing and integration of information;
3. Understand the regulation of bodily functions.

The functions of nervous tissue are varied, ranging from both sending and receiving messages in the body. At the heart of the nervous tissue function is the integration and regulation of body processes using electrical impulses and chemical messages. Neurons, which are the primary cells of nervous tissue, are particularly suited to enable rapid communication in the nervous system. These receive stimuli through dendrites, process and then transmit through axons to muscles, glands, or other neurons. Glial cells also assist and guard neurons, keeping them functional and working, indicating the intricate interaction among different types of cells in the homeostasis maintenance and response to changes from outside. In essence, nervous tissue is the foundation upon which our body's complex signaling mechanism operates, allowing responsive adaptation to both internal and external stimuli. Furthermore, the reach of nervous tissue influences extends beyond voluntary movement into involuntary functions governing essential body processes. The autonomic nervous system, which is a subdivision of the peripheral nervous system, demonstrates such an action in controlling heart rate, digestion, breathing rate, and several other functions without having any conscious effort. It acts via two divisions: the sympathetic and parasympathetic systems, which have an antagonistic action to balance within the body. For instance, during stress, the sympathetic nervous tissue raises heart rate and breathing, prepares the body for "fight or flight" responses, whereas the parasympathetic system facilitates relaxation and recovery following stress. Such coordinated responses emphasize the crucial functions of nervous tissue in maintaining not just the temporary bodily responses but also long-term health and adaptation, thereby proving its central position in human physiology. Moreover, the wide-ranging impact of nervous system trauma further alludes to the intricacy and vulnerability of nervous tissue. Spinal cord injury (SCI) is a reminder of the adverse cascading impacts of nervous tissue damage on overall health.

Whereas paralysis and loss of sensation are leading effects, SCI also brings with it multiple complications in other systems of the body, including cardiovascular and respiratory dysfunctions and metabolic disturbances (Yılmaz et al., 2014). In addition, neurotoxicity is another complicating factor in that exposure to toxic chemicals has the capacity to interfere with neural function or induce long-term harm, again suggesting the need for increased awareness and research regarding the vulnerability of the nervous system (Spencer & Lein, 2014). These points also emphasize not just the key functions of nervous tissue but also indicate the requirement for the establishment of treatments that will be employed to maintain and restore nervous tissue after injury or exposure to neurotoxic substances.

11.3.1. Signal Transmission

Signal transmission is an elementary characteristic of the function of nervous tissue in the human body, primarily based on neurons to transmit information throughout the body. These specialized cells employ electrical signals known as action potentials to transmit signals along their axons. This process begins with a stimulus that induces a change in the cell's membrane potential, ultimately resulting in the depolarization that initiates the action potential sequence. Once generated, the action potential jumps rapidly down the axon, aided by sheaths of myelin covering the axon and accelerating transmission by saltatory conduction. They are a rapid and efficient network of communication required for the orchestration of complex physiological responses and homeostasis in the organism. Synapse is an essential site where signal conduction is converted from electrical to chemical, so that the complex regulation of neuronal communication may take place. Neurotransmitters are released by the presynaptic neuron and selectively bind to receptors on the postsynaptic neuron by virtue of this interface. This change in the type of signal makes possible the exact regulation of communication from neuron to neuron; a good example would be that one same neurotransmitter can produce an excitatory response in certain conditions but an inhibitory response in others. This synaptic plasticity is essential because its anomalies can result in pathological conditions expressed by disturbances in the transduction of the signal. A good case in point is neurodegenerative disorders, in which synaptic malfunction is one of the factors adding to the overall decline in neural function and cognitive decline, illustrating the importance of optimal signal transmission in sustaining neurological integrity.

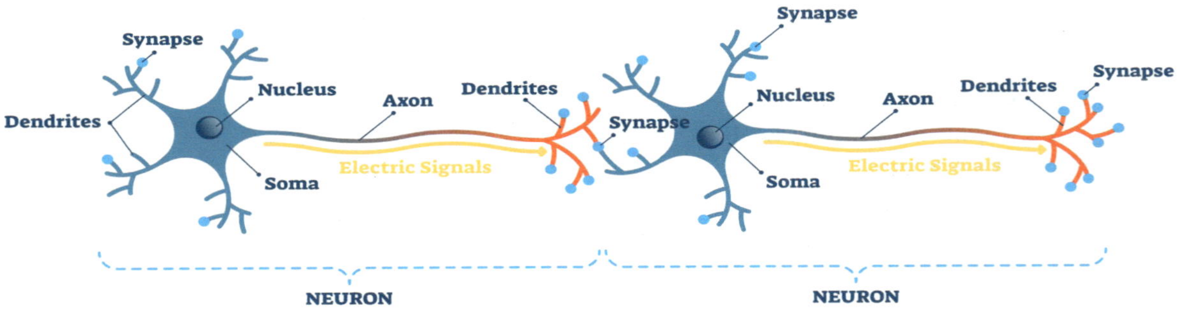

Figure 11.11. Synaptic transmission is the process by which one neuron communicates with another. Information is passed down the axon of the neuron as an electrical impulse known as an action potential.

Source: https://www.simplypsychology.org/wp-content/uploads/synapse.png.

External factors may also significantly affect the transmission of the signal within the nervous system. For instance, neurotoxic substances can disrupt normal synaptic function and lead to harmful effects. According to studies, a number of chemicals have been found to induce neurotoxic diseases in human beings through disrupting neural function or modification of metabolic processes necessary for neuronal health (Spencer & Lein, 2014). In the case of prion diseases, the misfolding of prion proteins is what leads to neurotoxicity, resulting in neuronal death, where the very essential link between molecular integrity and signal transmission comes into play (Herms et al., 2004). Thus, the health of both the structural components of neurons and their pathways of signal transmission is important to ensure protection against neurological diseases and demonstrate the need for ongoing research regarding factors in the transmission of signals in the human nervous system (Figure 11.11).

11.3.2. Processing and Integration of Information

Processing and integration of information in human nervous tissue is predominantly through neurons, which pass messages using electrochemical channels. Neurons communicate with one another through a complex network to enable them to integrate sensory input and generate appropriate responses. It is a sophisticated process that is needed for most cognitive processes, including perception, learning, and making decisions. Notably, the nervous system's ability to receive information efficiently relies on the synaptic relationship between neurons. These synapses either weaken or strengthen over time, a process that is recognized as synaptic plasticity, directly associated with learning and memory. As a result, the organization and flexibility of neural circuits are implicated in information storage and retrieval and, by extension, impact behavior and cognitive development in human experience. In revealing information processing mechanisms, the cell assembly is a key concept that provides insight into the organization of neurons and how they interact. From Hebb's hypothesis, clusters of neurons that are coactivated form certain patterns that are representative of particular thoughts, memories, or behaviors. This postulate has been replaced with more sophisticated conceptualizations, including the information compression by multiple alignment, unification, and search (ICMAUS) model. The ICMAUS model asserts that neurons are organized into assemblies that provide efficient storage and integration of information. By making use of a mechanism that facilitates references or codes to bridge distant assemblies, the model suggests a stable technique for storing complex data in the brain. This sophisticated process of information processing refines our appreciation of cognitive processes and the natural versatility of the nervous system, highlighting its ability to accommodate novel experiences. Additionally, the consequences of progress in cognitive neuroscience span possible applications in technology, particularly in artificial intelligence and robotics. WBE technologies, which seek to emulate human thought processes using computational models, although constrained by current limitations, represent the vanguard of this endeavor. One proposed intermediate step is insect brain emulation (IBE), which offers a feasible method to demonstrate the possibility of nervous system emulation. Such activities can promote joint research between neuroscientists, engineers, and policymakers, thereby expanding our understanding of information processing in natural and engineered systems. By simulating decreased neural structures and increasingly scaling up towards human imitation, researchers would be in a position to unravel the mysteries of the intricate mechanisms of cognitive processes, cognitive impairment, and the potential of artificial intelligence in replicating the patterns of human thought and learning capability (Wolff, 2003; Collins et al., 2018).

11.3.3. Regulation of Bodily Functions

The intricate regulation of body functions is basically governed by the interplay among the nervous, endocrine, and immune systems. Nervous tissue, made up of neurons and glial cells, is at the core of this regulatory system, which allows for rapid communication and response around the body. Neurons transmit electrical impulses, which allow for immediate response to stimuli, required in order for the body to reach homeostasis. For instance, when the body is under stress, the nervous system triggers a cascade of hormonal responses that alter various physiological mechanisms, such as heart rate and respiration. This widespread communication not only permits reflex action but also engages the higher processes of the brain, pulling sensory information together to regulate behavior and bodily responses effectively. The Ayurvedic concept of physiology also assists our understanding of body regulation by bringing in such concepts as the 'Tridosha,' which is a dynamic equilibrium between Vāta, Pitta, and Kapha. These doshas are translated to neural, endocrine, and immune processes, highlighting the interconnected role of these systems in health maintenance. The 'Doshas' function as homeostatic controllers to make sure derangements in one system bring about compensatory phenomena in others to restore balance. Such a holistic approach is reflected in modern interpretations of neuro-endocrine interactions, as reaffirmed in the terminology of neuro-immuno-endocrinology, indicating that there are several systems operating simultaneously to modulate body functions. Both perspectives underscore the multifaceted and integrated nature of physiological processes whose significance requires integrative health and disease approaches. The findings are in accord with the hypothesis that the regulation of body function cannot be confined to the brain but is dispersed over a multitude of cellular and molecular networks spread throughout the organism. This theory suggests that psychological traits and processes in people arise from pervasive neural patterns that involve a symbiotic association between the nervous system and other regulatory systems. As shown in the research, these parallel distributed processing networks not only involve neural circuits but also incorporate hormonal and immune systems as well, all of which constitute the totality of the regulatory mechanisms in human beings. This integrated view is aware of the multifaceted interdependence among networks and how the accumulated interactions of such networks affect not only physiological outcomes, but also psychological ones, and thereby broadens our understanding of the principle of personhood as the product of such interdependent biological processes (Steinhart, 2001) (Figure 11.12).

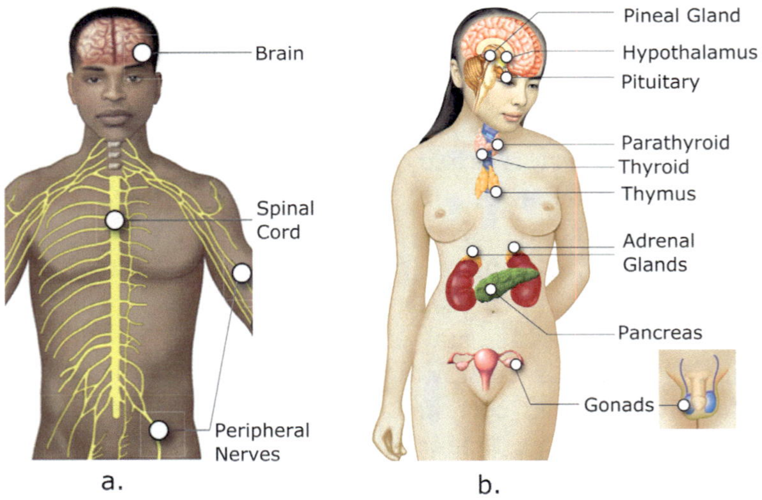

Figure 11.12. Systems involved in control and regulation. a. Nervous system, b. Endocrine system.

Source: https://api.www.labxchange.org/api/v1/xblocks/lb:LabXchange:c632aba8:html:1/storage/nervous-and-endocrine_16x91677372903117-1fe34c553457e911cac620b13743ca10.png.

Test Your Knowledge

1. What do you mean by signal transmission?
2. What is the information processing of the nervous system?

11.4. Types of Neurons

Learning Outcome

1. Describe the sensory neurons;
2. Describe the motor neurons;
3. Understand the interneurons.

In human nervous tissue, the building blocks are the neurons that allow signal transmission in the body. The specialized cells are categorized into three broad types: sensory neurons, motor neurons, and interneurons. Sensory neurons initiate the sensation process through responses to external stimuli, such as light, sound, and touch. Such stimuli are converted into electrical impulses that are transmitted to the CNS, where the message is interpreted. Motor neurons, conversely, transmit messages from the CNS to muscles and glands for the body to move and react. Interneurons serve as intermediaries between sensory and motor neurons and play a crucial role in intracerebral processing of information. The various roles of such types of neurons point toward the complexities and efficacy of the human nervous system in maintaining homeostasis and responding to environmental changes. The dynamic functioning of the neurons extends beyond their specialized roles; they are part of a system that facilitates communication and coordination among various body systems. The sensory neurons, for example, provide the critical input that determines the response of motor neurons, thereby establishing a feedback loop in reflex action. Reflex arcs, such as sensory input resulting in immediate motor output, demonstrate this interaction and stress the quick response capacity of the nervous system. This interaction between neuron types is central to the body's capacity for adaptation to changing stimuli, enabling prompt response to potential danger. Understanding these interactions is integral to any study of neural function, particularly how disruption, induced by neurotoxic chemicals, may impinge on nervous system integrity in general, as discussed in theories of neurotoxicity (Spencer & Lein., 2014).

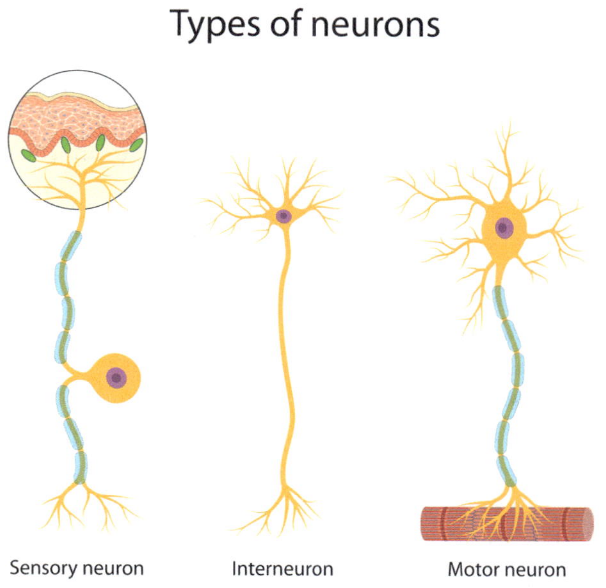

Figure 11.13. Types of neurons.

Source: https://www.simplypsychology.org/wp-content/uploads/sensory-motor-relay-neurons.png.

Furthermore, the capacity of different neurons to regenerate also largely contributes to their functional longevity, especially in the (PNS). PNS neurons are supported by specific glial cells that facilitate regeneration following damage, something not found to any significant degree in the CNS. This distinction emphasizes the significance of glial cells, such as Schwann cells and olfactory ensheathing cells, which have a critical function in enhancing the processes of neuronal repair within the PNS (Barton et al., 2017). The regenerative capacity of the PNS is of clinical significance in the treatment of neural trauma because it offers avenues for intervention via peripheral glia transplantation. Knowledge of the neuron types and their regenerative response can give us an indication of how to restore neural function following injury or disease, underscoring the value in research of neuronal types in the larger context of nervous tissue in man (Figure 11.13).

11.4.1. Sensory Neurons

Sensory neurons, the nervous system's lifelines, play the critical role of transducing external stimuli into neural signals interpretable by the brain. These specialist neurons detect various types of sensory input, including touch, temperature, pain, and proprioception, thereby coming into our awareness of the external world. Located predominantly in the peripheral nervous system, sensory neurons are the products of sensory receptors that can transduce some forms of stimuli into electrical signals. Mechanoreceptors, for instance, respond to mechanical stress, while thermoreceptors respond to variations in temperature. Transduction is essential for survival as it enables organisms to respond appropriately to the environment in a manner such that they will be able to respond to threats and preserve homeostasis. The morphology of sensory neurons is particularly adapted to their role and is characterized by long processes and terminal specializations. The cell body of a sensory neuron is often found in the dorsal root ganglia and is associated with the peripheral receptors and the central nervous system. The afferent axonal pathways along which these neurons travel are important in transmitting information about stimuli to the spinal cord and, subsequently, the brain. The availability of glial cells, i.e., Schwann cells, in the peripheral nervous system enhances the speed and efficiency of signal transfer through myelination. These cells not only supply structural support to the sensory neurons but also play an essential role in the regeneration of these neurons following injury. This regenerative capacity reflects a unique feature of peripheral nerves compared to central nervous system neurons, thus highlighting the intricacy in nervous tissue interactions (Barton et al., 2017). Beyond their structural features, sensory neurons also convey the complexity of the mechanisms of signaling involved in controlling body functions.

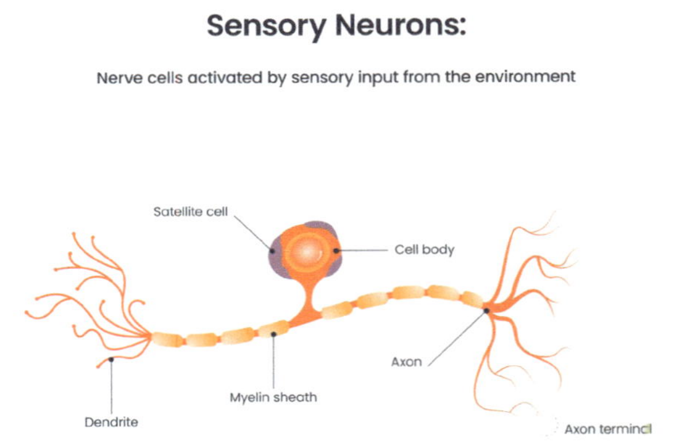

Figure 11.14. Sensory neurons are nerve cells that transmit information from external and internal stimuli to the central nervous system for processing, allowing organisms to perceive sensations like touch, temperature, and pain.

Source: https://www.simplypsychology.org/wp-content/uploads/sensory-neuron-1.jpeg.

They are part of reflex arcs, which allow rapid responses without needing immediate intervention by the brain. This neural pathway is a demonstration of how sensory neurons participate in homeostasis, such as controlling blood pressure or maintaining body temperature relative to the environment. The interaction between sensory neurons and central nervous system pathways enables the organism to react and make sense out of sensory input. Research has also enlightened us more about the role of sensory neurons in various physiological processes, including sympathetic control and body response to salt intake, revealing peripheral and central mediators involved in their action (Neal et al., 2016). The mechanisms highlight the significance of sensory neurons in disease and health, paving the way for targeted therapies that address sensory dysfunctions (Figure 11.14).

11.4.2. Motor Neurons

Motor neurons, the most important component of the nervous system, consist of a stunning structure that supports their critical function of communication between the CNS and the muscle fibers. With the long axon and multiple dendrites, these cells provide for the transmission of electrical impulses to induce contractions of muscles and voluntary and involuntary movements. Motor neurons are also of two types, being either alpha motor neurons that innervate the skeletal muscles directly or gamma motor neurons that regulate the functioning of muscle spindles. This double role highlights the versatility of motor neurons, which is necessary for a wide range of motor responses from complex hand movements to reflex responses. Well-being and functioning of motor neurons are critical because their loss is linked to paralyzing diseases , such as amyotrophic lateral sclerosis (ALS), again highlighting their importance in rudimentary motor function and overall human health. The mechanism by which motor neurons interact with muscles is a function involving neurotransmitters and synaptic transmission, and it is highly intricate. The motor neuron depolarizes the muscle fiber's membrane upon reception of an action potential through the release of acetylcholine at the neuromuscular junction, enabling depolarization. Muscle contraction results from this, and it shows the linear relation between muscle movement and neuronal activity. Furthermore, the integrity of the myelin sheath that encompasses motor neurons greatly improves conductance so that speedy signal transmission is possible for ordered movement. Breakdowns in such transmission are capable of creating acute motor impairment, underlining the importance of motor neuron integrity in a proper locomotion and posture.

Moreover, continued research in motor neuron function, particularly with respect to neuromuscular disease, would be crucial to the development of treatment protocols with which to fight such diseases, indicating a significant area of inquiry in neurobiology. Motor neurons are also more important than mere association with muscle; they are part and parcel of reflex arcs and the autonomic nervous system, too. During reflex responses, sensory neurons transmit information regarding stimuli to the spinal cord, where the motor neurons function rapidly, without any time delay in transmitting impulses to the brain. This reflex action, even before cognitive processing, explains the potency and role of motor neurons in staying alive. Additionally, in the autonomic nervous system, motor neurons regulate involuntary activities like heart rate and digestion, reflecting their omnipresence. Each of these processes illustrates motor neurons integrated into the fabric of human anatomy, emphasizing both their role in motion but also their overall role in homeostasis and responding to changes in the outside world. Awareness of these intricate functions of motor neurons can provide hints to therapeutic interventions on how to restore some neuropathologies, in line with ongoing research efforts along this direction (Wallace, 1980; Buchner et al., 2009) (Figure 11.15).

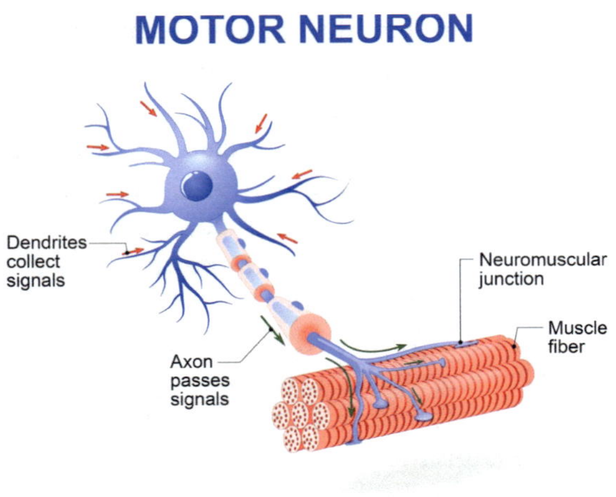

Figure 11.15. Motor neuron.

Source: https://smanewstoday.com/wp-content/uploads/2017/09/shutterstock_423991636-1200x900-cropped.jpg.

11.4.3. Interneurons

Interneurons are an integral component of the design and function of nervous tissue in humans since they are crucial mediators in neuronal circuits. Through the establishment of synapses between sensory and motor neurons, and neurons within the brain itself, interneurons facilitate such complex phenomena as reflexes, perception of sensory stimuli, and higher-order thought. These are primarily of two types: excitatory and inhibitory interneurons, which secrete neurotransmitters , such as glutamate and gamma-aminobutyric acid (GABA), respectively. Excitatory-inhibitory balance is crucial to prevent homeostasis of the central nervous system; changing it can lead to neurological disorders. Thus, understanding interneurons' functions and mechanisms is crucial in grasping the broader dynamics of nervous tissue and its implications in disease and health. Current research has highlighted the significant role that genetic factors have on the viability and function of interneurons. For instance, loss-of-function in the WW domain-containing oxidoreductase (WWOX) gene has been linked to several central nervous system (CNS) disorders, including epilepsy and intellectual disability, as evidenced by the alterations in interneuron populations in mouse models. Specifically, Wwox knockout mice were found to have a significant reduction of GABAergic interneurons, including those that possess calcium-binding proteins , such as parvalbumin and neuropeptide Y. This decrease not only accompanies decreased GABA synthesis but also demonstrates signs of neuroinflammation, which reflects the fine balance that exists among interneurons within the neural network. For the recognition of targeted therapies to reverse interneuronal dysfunction and their corresponding disorders, realizing these correlations is a necessity (Hussain et al., 2019). Besides genetic factors, environmental conditions and senescence are also causes of deep implications towards interneuronal well-being, due to which the overall activity of the brain is impacted. As demonstrated through the research on progeroid mouse models, impairments in DNA repair machinery, specifically with the AKTIP gene, have been found to lead to increased seizure susceptibility with related inflammatory responses within the brain.

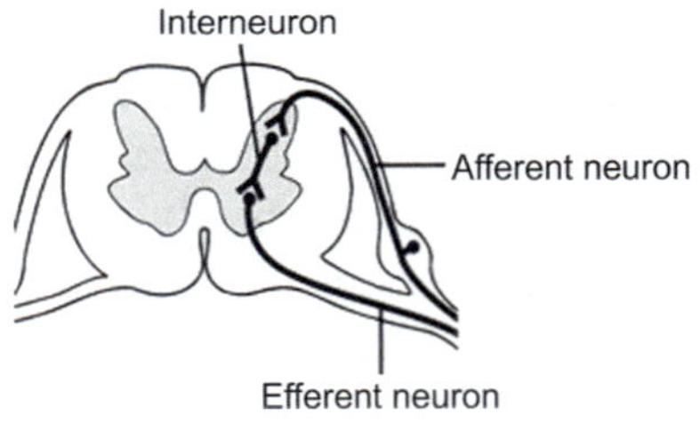

Figure 11.16. Interneuron.

Source: https://img.tfd.com/mk/I/X2604-I-22.png.

This association of DNA damage, aging, and interneuron function highlights the importance of maintaining intact interneurons as a safeguard against neurodegeneration. The subtle interplay between environmental influence and genetic determinants on interneurons suggests probable paths of intervention for age-related neurological disorders. Finally, the study of interneurons in human nervous tissue is essential to understanding the complexity of both normal and pathological change in the brain (Alessandro et al., 2018) (Figure 11.16).

Test Your Knowledge

1. What are sensory neurons?
2. What are motor neurons?

11.5. Glial Cells and Their Functions

Learning Outcome

1. Understand the astrocytes;
2. Describe the oligodendrocytes;
3. Describe the microglia.

Glial cells, or neuroglia, are at the forefront of nervous system homeostasis maintenance and play far more extensive roles than just the passive support of neurons. Glial cells outnumber neurons at a ratio of 10–1 and must maintain a host of physiological processes. One of their several responsibilities involves providing structural and metabolic support to neurons through the formation of a protective scaffold that reinforces nervous tissue architecture. Moreover, they regulate the extracellular milieu via ion equilibrium, neurotransmitter levels, and the delivery of nutrients. These vital functions mirror the important functions glial cells have in assuring the best functioning of neural networks to be of service for diverse cognitive and physiological processes significant for overall human health and functioning (Buchner et al., 2009). Within the nervous system, there are certain glial cells with specialized functions that meet specific demands. Astrocytes, for example, are star-shaped glial cells that keep the blood-brain barrier intact and, therefore, regulate the passage of substances into the CNS. This selective permeability is important in maintaining brain tissue from harmful agents, as well as necessary nutrients into the CNS. Microglia, the intrinsic immune cells of the CNS, monitor and respond to pathological changes, clearing debris and responding to injury by restructuring synaptic contacts. Schwann cells, however, are components of the PNS and function to facilitate nerve regeneration when injured. Such heterogeneity in function between glial cells underscores their pivotal roles in both homeostasis and response to the changing demands of neural tissue (Barton et al., 2017). The capacity of glial cells to regenerate, particularly in the PNS, is a testament to their potential in neural trauma cure. Unlike the central nervous system, where regeneration of the axon is largely inhibited, glia in the PNS start repair mechanisms after injury and support the environment of regeneration for the growth of neurons. Schwann cells play a central role here by providing growth factors and structural components that induce axonal growth. In addition, olfactory ensheathing cells (OECs) have also played significant roles in promoting regeneration because of their ability to promote neuronal recovery at all times. The contrasting responses of PNS glia compared to CNS glia provide fruitful areas for therapeutic methods involving glial cell transplantation to promote recovery after central nervous system injury. Understanding the intricate roles of these glial cells not only teaches fundamental neuroscience but also guarantees revolutionary clinical procedures in the future (Barton et al., 2017) (Figure 11.17).

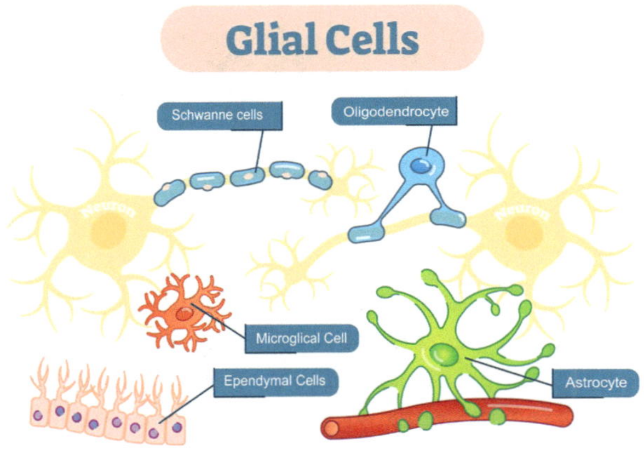

Figure 11.17. Types of glial cells.

Source: https://www.verywellhealth.com/thmb/KTilfCxnabrUhsp536BLMgZ_8Zk=/1500x0/filters:no_upscale():max_bytes(150000):strip_icc()/glialcellsillustration-5a94d585642dca00362568c4.jpg.

11.5.1. Astrocytes

Astrocytes, one of the common groups of glial cells in the central nervous system (CNS), play a multifunctional role to ensure the maintenance of neural homeostasis. These star-shaped cells have a significant function in the structural integrity of the nervous tissue, such as neurons and as part of the blood-brain barrier. Sustaining ion balance and the metabolic requirements of neurons, astrocytes are charged with keeping the extracellular environment appropriate for maximum neuronal function. Their interactions with neurons, particularly through the uptake and release of neurotransmitters, reflect their essential function in neurotransmission and synaptic efficacy. Besides, astrocytes are involved in CNS injury repair, having demonstrated their role in neuroprotection and recovery. This multifunctionality is evidence of the role astrocytes play to ensure not only neuron health but also communication within nervous tissue in human beings. Astrocytes exhibit high plasticity and flexibility in immune responses within the CNS. They respond to pathological stimuli , such as infection or trauma, by producing a variety of inflammatory mediators that can influence the behavior of infiltrating immune cells, such as (NK) cells. As detailed in recent research, the brain microenvironment influences how NK cells participate in inflammatory responses in disease states , such as viral infection.

Astrocytes, through the secretion of chemokines, can deliver these immune cells to the area of inflammation, demonstrating a complex interaction that is balanced in place between protective mechanisms and potential pathological onset (Shi et al., 2011). The ability of astrocytes to serve both as support staff and as active participants in the immune response highlights the functions of astrocytes in the overall maintenance of nervous tissue and their potential functions in diseases with neuroinflammation. Also emphasized is the function of astrocytes in modulating immune response through their interaction with neurotropic viruses. Under conditions of viral infection, astrocytes take an active role in the local immune response by releasing proinflammatory cytokines and chemokines. These substances not only recruit and activate immune cells but also dictate the overall outcome of viral infections in the CNS. Evidence shows that the localized tissue reaction led by astrocytes will decide whether such contacts lead to severe neurological impact or a less deleterious status (Meyer et al., 2006). Therefore, understanding the bipotential character of astrocytes—supportive regulators of neuronal health and active contributors to immunoreactivity—is of key value in grasping the complexities of nervous tissue pathology and its implications to therapeutic manipulation of neuroinflammatory diseases (Figure 11.18).

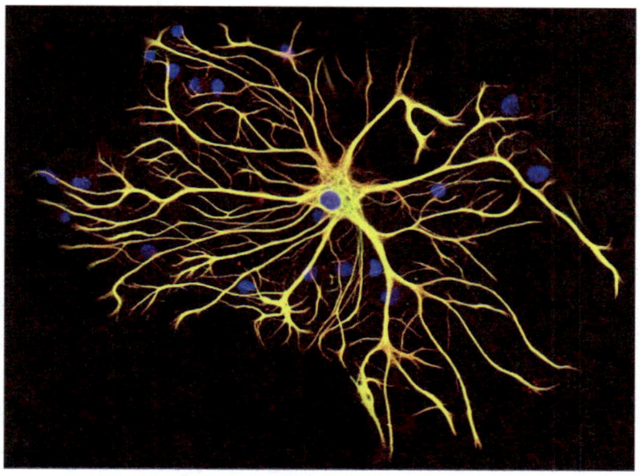

Figure 11.18. Astrocyte.

Source: https://upload.wikimedia.org/wikipedia/commons/6/63/Astrocyte5.jpg.

11.5.2. Oligodendrocytes

Oligodendrocytes are specialized glial cells in the central nervous system that play a crucial role in maintaining neuronal network integrity and function. The cells are accountable for most of the synthesis of myelin, a lipid-rich substance that coats axons and allows the velocity of electrical signal transmission. Myelination is essential to effective neuronal communication, and oligodendrocyte malfunction has been implicated in causing a broad spectrum of neurological disorders. In the case of multiple sclerosis, the immune system attacks oligodendrocytes by mistake, thus stripping the myelin sheath of neurons, impairing signal transmission and contributing towards the disease's myriad of symptoms. This suggests the well-established interrelations between oligodendrocytes and neuronal health and highlights how central they are to nervous system function and integrity. Recent work has also hinted at the involvement of oligodendrocytes in neuroinflammation, a process critical for numerous neurological disorders. Oligodendrocyte relation to inflammation is complicated, as oligodendrocytes both exhibit immunomodulatory effects and are sensitive to inflammatory signals in the central nervous system. Chronic inflammation, also associated with neurodegenerative disease, affects oligodendrocyte function and viability, resulting in suboptimal myelination and neuronal support. Oligodendrocytes, along with microglia and astrocytes, participate in the inflammatory processes that characterize conditions like Alzheimer's disease and Parkinson's disease. It is essential to recognize these interactions to build therapeutic strategies for safeguarding oligodendrocytes against inflammatory insults and to promote myelin repair, which has become a prime target for restorative therapies of neurological disorders (Skaper et al., 2018). The novel role of neuroprotective factors and their interaction with oligodendrocytes is an area of ongoing research, particularly for proteins like α-Klotho. This protein has been described as a neuroprotective factor responsible for promoting healthy brain aging and for initiating myelination, thereby optimizing oligodendrocyte function. The expression of α-Klotho in the brain suggests potential involvement in reversing age-related dysfunction of oligodendrocyte activity, which would be of profound importance in neurodegenerative diseases.

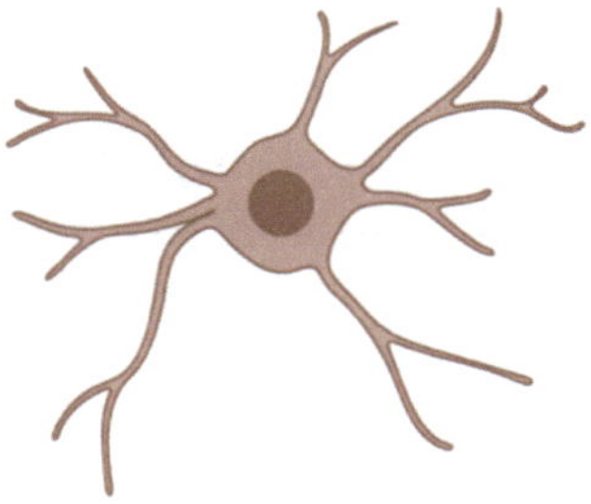

Figure 11.19. Oligodendrocyte.

Source: https://i.shgcdn.com/45a794c6-d766-4f75-841a-5db80948aad6/-/format/auto/-/preview/3000x3000/-/quality/lighter/.

Recent evidence shows that an increase in the level of α-Klotho can enhance oligodendrocyte survival and function, thereby maintaining myelin health. As researchers continue to investigate the mechanistic avenues of α-Klotho, the function of α-Klotho in oligodendrocyte biology can illuminate novel therapeutic approaches for demyelination and neurodegenerative disease, eventually supporting an enhanced nervous system (Cararo-Lopes et al., 2017) (Figure 11.19).

11.5.3. Microglia

Microglia, referred to as the resident immune cells of the central nervous system (CNS), have a crucial role in maintaining homeostasis in nervous tissue. Unlike other immune cells that develop in the bloodstream, microglia develop from yolk sac progenitors and become a part of the CNS, patrolling the surroundings for signs of damage or infection. Microglia are not only crucial to warding off pathogens but also in removing cellular debris and dead neurons. Microglia contribute to overall CNS health by allowing synaptic pruning and neurodevelopment through their dynamic function. Their remarkable ability to react to an incredibly broad variety of conditions positions them at the center not only of normal physiology but also of pathology, illustrating the intimate association they share with the functioning of nervous tissue in humans. Microglia function extends beyond that of vigilance; they play a crucial role in defining neuroinflammatory responses. Microglia can change from a pro-inflammatory to an anti-inflammatory form when activated by disease or damage, and therefore play a dual role in pathology. This has been highlighted by recent reports showing microglial activation and disease development in many neurodegenerative diseases , such as Alzheimer's and multiple sclerosis. Because microglia interact with other immune cells , such as the natural killer (NK) cells, the local environment around them significantly determines their action. Understanding these interactions is vital as it dictates the manner in which organ-specific elements impact microglial functions and their overall contribution towards CNS health and disease management (Shi et al., 2011). Consequently, knowledge of the mechanisms through which microglia act presents far-reaching implications for therapeutic intervention against neurological diseases. Advances in genomic technologies have also increased understanding of the complex role of microglia, particularly in their response to genetic and environmental injuries. For instance, single-cell RNA sequencing-based studies have identified gene expression differences between human microglia that are age, sex, and presence of specific clinical pathologies dependent. These findings are extremely significant in elucidating individual susceptibility to neurodegenerative disease. One of the significant breakthroughs is the identification of microglia-specific genetic variants that have been linked to diseases like Alzheimer's disease, as revealed by studies aimed at localizing by expression quantitative trait loci (eQTL) mapping (Young et al., 2021). These discoveries not only shed light on our understanding of microglial function in health and disease but also foreshadow targeted therapies and individualized medicine interventions. Thus, microglia are at the forefront of nervous tissue research, both a challenge and an opportunity for the study of human neurobiology (Figure 11.20).

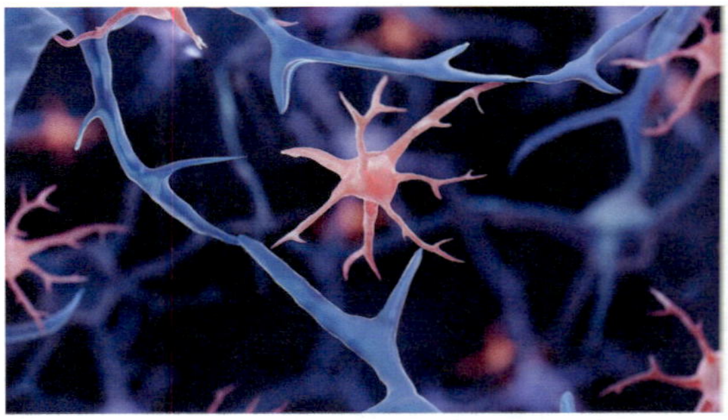

Figure 11.20. Microglial cells.

Source: https://assets.technologynetworks.com/production/dynamic/images/content/388512/microglial-cells-microglia-function-origin-and-related-conditions-388512-960x540.jpg?cb=13221565.

Test Your Knowledge

1. What are the astrocytes?
2. What are microglia?

11.6. Nervous Tissue in Health and Disease

Learning Outcome

1. Understand the common neurological disorders;
2. Understand the impact of injuries on nervous tissue;
3. Describe the advances in treatment and research related to nervous tissue.

The intricacies of nervous tissue are essential to human well-being, but at the same time, prone to many diseases. The nervous tissue consists primarily of neurons and glial cells, each of which plays its role in the functionality of the nervous system overall. While the role of neurons is the transmission of electrical impulses to facilitate communication between body parts, glial cells play the role of providing support and protection for the neurons. Abnormalities in these cellular constituents may lead to serious health consequences. For instance, neurotoxic exposure may initiate various neurological disorders, as such chemicals may injure neural cells directly, disrupt maldevelopment, or interfere with essential metabolic processes. The disturbances are either rapid or may only manifest after many years, supporting the complexity of diagnosing neurotoxicity diseases (Spencer & Lein, 2014). Complete understanding of the integrity of nervous tissues is thus critical in addressing health problems of this critical system. The communication between the nervous system and metabolic diseases further demonstrates the importance of nervous tissue to humanity. Recent research identifies that obesity and insulin resistance are not only prevalent health issues but also causative factors in the development of cardiovascular diseases. They cross the immune system, showing that nervous tissue can influence immune response. Central nervous pathways are of great interest as they govern peripheral nervous system processes, which are responsible for significant roles in the etiology and course of these diseases. Delving into the neuro-immune interaction sheds light on the possible therapeutic interventions of these disabling diseases, thus the significance of multidisciplinary thinking on understanding nervous tissue's role in global metabolic health (Lori et al., 2017). Consequently, delving into the inherent connection between the two systems can offer insight into the proper treatment of shared diseases. The vulnerability of nervous tissue to a multitude of diseases draws attention to the significance of preventive and therapeutic strategies. Neurodegenerative disorders , such as Alzheimer's disease and multiple sclerosis, reflect the degenerative processes that can interfere with nervous tissue and lead to far-reaching impairments in cognition and motor function. Successful therapy can include both pharmacologic intervention and changes in lifestyle that promote neural health. Furthermore, the field of neuroplasticity offers salutary avenues for rehabilitation, whereby the adaptive properties of the nervous system can be utilized to recover from injury or dysfunction. Education and information on elements that influence nervous tissue health, such as environmental contaminants and lifestyle influences, can have a broad impact on public health initiatives. Finally, focusing on research into nervous tissue disease and health can pave the way for new solutions, optimizing the power and function of the nervous system in humans.

11.6.1. Common Neurological Disorders

Neurological disorders are a general term used to refer to conditions that adversely affect the nervous system, disrupting communication between the spinal cord, brain, and peripheral nerves. Parkinson's disease, Alzheimer's disease, and multiple sclerosis are prevalent conditions that cause significant challenges to patients and healthcare systems that deal with them. Such disorders are typically marked by neurodegenerative processes, with loss of neurons and synapses over time leading to incapacitating syndromes. For instance, Alzheimer's disease is characterized by impairment of cognition caused by pathological processes, including amyloid plaques and neurofibrillary tangles. As the neurological disorders progress, they may lead to significant compromise of quality of life, so it is important to initiate early diagnosis and treatment. In addition, the complex interplay between environmental, genetic, and lifestyle factors is accountable for their development and onset, contributing to the challenge in clinical management. Neurotoxicity is an inherent element in the pathogenesis of various neurological conditions. The neurotoxic action can occur as a result of exposure to environmental pollutants, drugs, or even endogenous metabolic processes. Neurotoxicity can result in direct damage to neurons, disruption of synaptic transmission, and inflammatory responses within nervous tissue. Some chemicals are rapidly toxic, while others induce delayed degeneration over prolonged periods. Such changes can evolve from mild intellectual impairment to extreme irreversible deficits depending on the nature and duration of exposure. Because neurotoxicity is generally self-limiting when exposure is stopped, the challenge is to determine offending agents and restrict their impact. Information about mechanisms of neurotoxins must be known to devise ways of minimizing their impact, particularly with the mounting prevalence of neurological disorders in modern society (Spencer & Lein, 2014). Inflammation is also a very significant etiological factor and the progression of neurological disorders. The inflammatory response of the nervous system itself is also powerful enough to influence neurodegeneration significantly. Inflammatory cells, controlled by neurotransmitters, respond to damage due to extrinsic or intrinsic causes or as part of pathological disease processes for multiple sclerosis or Alzheimer's disease. Recent evidence suggests that certain treatments for Alzheimer's disease may also have anti-inflammatory properties that can help alter the course of the disease. This bidirectional function of inflammation can complicate treatment strategies, since while some inflammatory responses are advantageous, unregulated inflammation can further result in neuronal damage. Thus, understanding the interplay of inflammation with neurodegeneration will enhance clinicians' ability to create successful therapies that not only manage symptoms but also act on underlying inflammatory mechanisms (Giubilei, 2016) (Figure 11.21).

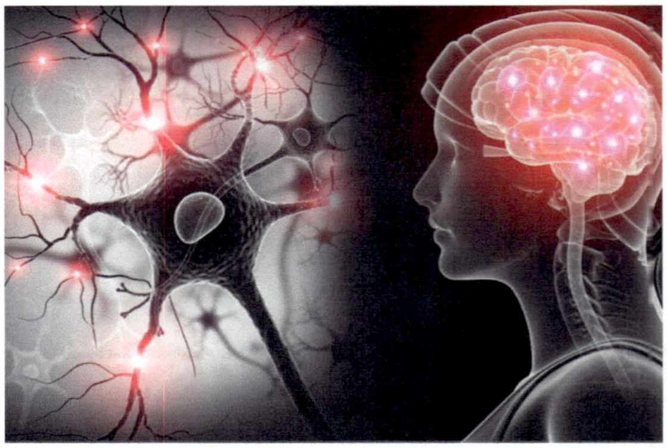

Figure 11.21. Neurological Disorders.

Source: https://drrohitgupta.co.in/wp-content/uploads/2024/06/10-Common-Symptoms-of-Neurological-Disorders-Dr-Rohit-Gupta.png.

11.6.2. Impact of Injuries on Nervous Tissue

Damage to the nervous tissue essentially disrupts the delicate balance required for neuronal health and function, typically leading to extensive and irreversible neurological impairment. The central nervous system (CNS) is comparatively lacking in capacity to regenerate, largely dependent on the presence of inhibitory factors following damage. Following events , such as stroke or traumatic brain injury, the surroundings in the area become hostile to neuronal survival through changes in the extracellular matrix and glial scarring. These glial scars, made of mostly reactive astrocytes, can actually inhibit axonal regrowth, thus making recovery processes more challenging. Interestingly, wiring changes of injured neural circuits are not merely secondary responses to damage but also indicative of a dynamic interplay between neuronal activity and regeneration mechanisms. Therefore, understanding the intricate actions of injuries on nervous tissue is important in creating effective therapeutic strategies to restore recovery. Astrocytes also play an important role in response to nervous tissue injury, possessing both neuroinhibition and neuroprotection. After injury, astrocytes become reactive, and alterations in their morphology are accompanied by changes in the secretion of extracellular matrix molecules and other proteins. After repeated trauma characteristic of traumatic brain injuries, for example, it has been demonstrated by studies that astrocytes may be driven into a survival mode that compromises their ability to remodel the extracellular space. This is reflected by the downregulation of key proteins and the inability to effectively degrade damaged extracellular matrix components, for example, in response to mechanical stress linked to traumatic injury. Such alterations can lead to increased apoptosis of astrocytes and favor a neuroinhibitory milieu that interferes with recovery mechanisms. Therefore, the understanding of astrocytic function after injury is critical in the establishment of treatments that maximize the regenerative capacity of nervous tissue after trauma (Walker, 2016). New treatments to reverse the actions of injuries on nervous tissue are being developed with the push from advances in the understanding of neurobiology and the repair of tissues. Researchers are exploring a number of modalities, including neurorehabilitation, neural interfacing technologies, and cellular repair pathways, to facilitate recovery and restore function. These new technologies hold the potential to take advantage of the brain's plasticity, fostering rewiring of the neural circuits and axon growth. Preliminary studies suggest that the convergence of physical rehabilitation with neurobiological therapy may produce synergistic benefits, resulting in motor function improvements previously considered to be unachievable. Through the combination of task-based methods and microscopic cellular strategies, robust recovery from neurological injury becomes increasingly possible. However, there are challenges in translating these results to clinical use, emphasizing the need for a cooperative effort that brings together basic science and applied therapies for the field of nervous tissue injuries (Krucoff et al., 2016).

11.6.3. Advances in Treatment and Research

Recent treatment and research into nervous tissue have significantly contributed to our understanding of a number of neurological disorders and how they are treated. Scientists have been investigating neuroimmunology, which examines the connection between the immune system and the nervous system. This particular field has opened up new avenues for therapeutic interventions in autoimmune disorders of the nervous system, such as multiple sclerosis. Also, stem cell treatment advances have shown promise in repairing injured nerve tissue and turning around the debilitating effects of diseases like spinal cord injury. Scientific investigation in these fields enables researchers to devise new methods that not only treat symptoms but also target the underlying cause of neurological disorders, thereby improving patient outcomes significantly (Marder et al., 2008). In addition to biological approaches, technological innovations have revolutionized the therapeutic arena by incorporating neuro-electronic devices. The development of cochlear implants is one notable illustration of how electronic interfaces can restore sensory capacity in individuals with hearing impairment. Research continues to delve into the promise of artificial vision technologies, which attempt to enhance visual capabilities in subjects with blindness. By combining the nervous system with electronics, such innovative solutions not only possess a medicinal value but also raise serious social and ethical controversies regarding their use, particularly beyond a medicinal purpose. Such innovative technologies are at the forefront of neuroengineering, with the model of treatment shifting towards personalized and technology-based treatments (Ward, 2000). Furthermore, advancements in DBS have been in the limelight because of their use in the treatment of a broad range of neurological and psychiatric disorders , such as Parkinson's disease and chronic depression. DBS is a procedure where electrodes are implanted in certain parts of the brain, providing targeted electrical impulses to neutralize symptoms when other treatments fail. studies have even indicated possible applications for DBS, including stimulating cognition, enabling patients to participate more completely in life activities. These treatments have implications extending beyond symptom management: they raise a conversation concerning the ethics of altering neuronal circuits to enhance cognition. As ongoing research increasingly clarifies these therapeutic applications, they point to a future in which treatment strategies might be tailored to suit each person's neurological profile and thereby provide a more substantive strategy for neurological wellness (Marder et al., 2008) (Figure 11.22).

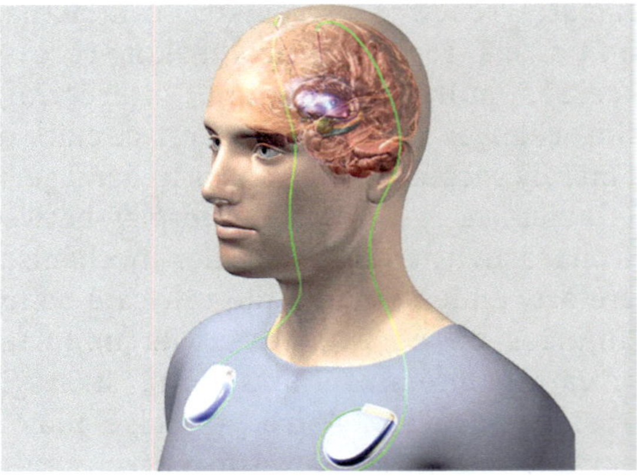

Figure 11.22. Deep brain stimulation (DBS).

Source: https://www.ibshospitals.com/technology_image/65fd48e0820eaIBS%20Hospital_Deep%20Brain%20Stimulation%20(DBS)_thumbnail_3.webp.

Test Your Knowledge

1. What are the most common neurological disorders?
2. What is the impact of injuries on nervous tissue?

SUMMARY

Briefly, human nervous tissue research explains fundamental concepts of normal physiology as well as the pathophysiology underlying a myriad of neurological disease conditions. As nervous tissue forms the primary composition of the nervous system, it facilitates communication between various parts of the body and organizes responses to stimuli. This understanding of its constitution and heterogeneous cellularity not only tells us about signal processing and transmission but also about the intricacies of maintaining homeostasis. The discovery of neuronal plasticity also goes a long way towards emphasizing the possibility of recovery and plasticity, particularly in response to injury or disease. This adaptability reinforces the consequences for therapeutic approaches aimed at promoting neural repair and regeneration, making the need for further research here a necessity. In addition, where nervous tissue function intersects with its vulnerability to such illnesses as prion disease, it confirms the ultimate complexity of neurodegenerative disease. The unique processes by which proteins misfold and lead to neuronal death, such as in prion research, illustrate a highly compelling area of study that connects molecular and clinical significance. Investigation of diseases like Creutzfeldt-Jakob disease from the nervous tissue point of view may have implications for prevention and treatment planning, particularly because these occurrences can be used to shed light on more universal neurodegenerative disease investigation. Here, the exploration of therapeutic modalities, including new molecular strategies, opens up fertile ground for treating cognitive decline and other manifestations of nervous system disease. Therefore, continued exploration of these facets is part of the making of medical and academic landscapes. New research on steroid hormone interactions with nervous tissue also illuminates further the neuroendocrine regulatory complexity. The communication between hormones , such as estrogen and testosterone in the peripheral and central nervous system serves to establish the significance of hormonal homeostasis in the maintenance of neuronal function and health. The investigation of the neuroprotective roles of the hormones towards diseases , such as polycystic ovary syndrome and their capacity for modulating neurodegenerative phenomena enables scientists to uncover critical links between endocrine signaling and brain health. These observations open up opportunities for novel therapeutic strategies that could reverse aging and hormonal disruption's impacts on nervous tissue. Lastly, the multidimensional nature of nervous tissue, linking cellular, molecular, and systemic factors, underscores the necessity of a holistic approach in research as well as clinical practice for the enhancement of neural integrity and function.

In human nervous tissue, certain fundamental factors are found to be of prime importance in understanding its structure and function. The PNS supports the CNS, both of which facilitate intricate communication within the body. Basic cells of nervous tissue, known as neurons, are specialized to transmit impulses and are equipped with special structures , such as dendrites and axons. These structures enable neurons to interact with each other and with a variety of target tissues, creating networks that control everything from reflexes to higher thinking processes. Further, the glial cells, which play supportive roles in homeostasis and neuron protection, are also a component of the nervous system's efficient function since they provide insulating coatings and facilitate recovery from damage. An understanding of these factors underlies the investigation of the broader importance of nervous tissue to disease and health. Neurotransmitter activity and interactions are also central to nervous tissue function. As a case in point, the major inhibitory neurotransmitter of the CNS, gamma-aminobutyric acid (GABA), controls neuronal excitability and is crucial in maintaining the balance between excitation and inhibition in nerve circuitry. The complexity of GABA and its receptors denotes the advanced aspect of neurotransmission, from muscle contraction to mood regulation. Furthermore, recent research establishes that the role of GABAs is not only in the brain and spinal cord, but is also expressed in other non-neural tissues like the testis. This refers to the overall relevance of neurotransmitter action in the endocrine system, as presented in Geigerseder et al. (2003). These findings emphasize the requirement to learn how mechanisms of nervous tissue operate not just in isolation but in the context of a multi-system structure. Lastly, the technology for interfacing electronics with the nervous system provides insight into medical as well as non-medical applications. These advances, as illustrated by cochlear implants and vision-prosthetic systems, reflect a growing body of knowledge regarding how to leverage the capability of nervous tissue in order to augment human ability and health. Societal implications are profound: they bring with them ethical concerns and stimulate enhancement versus treatment debates. As outlined in Ward (2000), future neuro-electronic technology will probably continue to diffuse medicated and non-medicated use boundaries, posing questions for society and the regulatory systems governing these technologies' applications. Generally, these results are indicative not only of the complexity of nervous tissue but also of its potential for revolutionary application across disciplines.

KEY TERMS FROM THIS CHAPTER

- Astrocytes
- Cell body
- Glial cells
- Natural killer cells
- Nervous tissue
- Neurons
- Oligodendrocytes
- Axons
- Dendrites
- Microglia
- Nervous system
- Neurobiology
- Neurotoxicity
- Soma

CRITICAL THINKING QUESTIONS

1. **Nervous tissue is primarily composed of:**
   a. Osteocytes and chondrocytes
   b. Neurons and glial cells
   c. Epithelial cells
   d. Adipocytes
2. **The structural and functional unit of the nervous system is the:**
   a. Dendrite
   b. Axon
   c. Neuron
   d. Synapse
3. **Neurons that carry information from sensory receptors to the central nervous system are called:**
   a. Motor neurons
   b. Sensory neurons
   c. Interneurons
   d. Effector neurons
4. **Which type of neuron is responsible for connecting sensory and motor neurons?**
   a. Sensory neurons
   b. Motor neurons
   c. Interneurons
   d. Bipolar neurons
5. **Motor neurons transmit signals:**
   a. From sensory organs to the brain
   b. From the brain to muscles and glands
   c. Between neurons in the spinal cord
   d. Within the cerebrum

Short Answer Questions

1. What is the nervous tissue?
2. Why is nervous tissue important in the human body?
3. Name the two main types of nervous tissue.
4. What is the function of nervous tissue?
5. Name the three primary types of neurons.

Answers to Critical Thinking Questions

1. (b); 2. (c) ; 3. (b); 4. (c); 5. (b)

REFERENCES

1. Hussain, T., Kil, H., Hattiangady, B., Lee, J., Kodali, M., Shuai, B., Attaluri, S., Takata, Y., Shen, J., Abba, M. C., Shetty, A. K., & Aldaz, C. M. (2019). Wwox deletion leads to reduced GABA-ergic inhibitory interneuron numbers and activation of microglia and astrocytes in mouse hippocampus. *Neurobiology of disease, 121*, 163–176. https://doi.org/10.1016/j.nbd.2018.09.026 (accessed on 7th August 2025).
2. Allman, J. M., Erwin, J. M., Goubert, V., Hakeem, A. Y., et al. (2010). *The von Economo neurons in frontoinsular and anterior cingulate cortex in great apes and humans*. https://core.ac.uk/download/4885049.pdf (accessed on 7th August 2025).
3. Alonzo, A., Rossi, C., Rubattu, S. D., Savoia, C., et al. (2010). *Natriuretic peptides and cardiovascular damage in the metabolic syndrome: Molecular mechanisms and clinical implications*. https://core.ac.uk/download/54413591.pdf (accessed on 7th August 2025).
4. Korcsmáros, T., Farkas, I. J., Szalay, M. S., Rovó, P., Fazekas, D., Spiró, Z., Böde, C., Lenti, K., Vellai, T., & Csermely, P. (2010). Uniformly curated signaling pathways reveal tissue-specific cross-talks and support drug target discovery. *Bioinformatics (Oxford, England), 26*(16), 2042–2050. https://doi.org/10.1093/bioinformatics/btq310 (accessed on 7th August 2025).
5. Barton, M. J., Clarke, M., Ekberg, J., St. John, J. A., et al. (2017). *The glia response after peripheral nerve injury: A comparison between Schwann cells and olfactory ensheathing cells and their uses for neural regenerative therapies*. https://core.ac.uk/download/196605084.pdf (accessed on 7th August 2025).
6. Young, A. M. H., Kumasaka, N., Calvert, F., Hammond, T. R., Knights, A., Panousis, N., Park, J. S., Schwartzentruber, J., Liu, J., Kundu, K., Segel, M., Murphy, N. A., McMurran, C. E., Bulstrode, H., Correia, J., Budohoski, K. P., Joannides, A., Guilfoyle, M. R., Trivedi, R., Kirollos, R., ... Gaffney, D. J. (2021). A map of transcriptional heterogeneity and regulatory variation in human microglia. *Nature genetics, 53*(6), 861–868. https://doi.org/10.1038/s41588-021-00875-2(accessed on 7th August 2025).
7. Cararo-Lopes, M. M., Mazucanti, C. H. Y., Scavone, C., Kawamoto, E. M., & Berwick, D. C. (2017). The relevance of α-KLOTHO to the central nervous system: Some key questions. *Ageing research reviews, 36*, 137–148. https://doi.org/10.1016/j.arr.2017.03.003 (accessed on 7th August 2025).
8. Spencer, P.S. & Lein, Pamela. (2014). Neurotoxicity. Encyclopedia of Toxicology. 10.1016/B978-0-12-386454-3.00169-X. (accessed on 7th August 2025).
9. Buchner, E., & Heisenberg, M. (2009). *Neurofly 2008 abstracts: The 12th European Drosophila neurobiology conference 6–10 September 2008 Wuerzburg, Germany*. https://core.ac.uk/download/4881258.pdf (accessed on 7th August 2025).
10. Geigerseder, C., Doepner, R., Thalhammer, A., Frungieri, M. B., Gamel-Didelon, K., Calandra, R. S., Köhn, F. M., & Mayerhofer, A. (2003). Evidence for a GABAergic system in rodent and human testis: local GABA production and GABA receptors. *Neuroendocrinology, 77*(5), 314–323. https://doi.org/10.1159/000070897(accessed on 7th August 2025).
11. Lori, A., Perrotta, M., Lembo, G., & Carnevale, D. (2017). The Spleen: A Hub Connecting Nervous and Immune Systems in Cardiovascular and Metabolic Diseases. *International journal of molecular sciences, 18*(6), 1216. https://doi.org/10.3390/ijms18061216(accessed on 7th August 2025).

12. Collins, L. T. (2018). *The case for emulating insect brains using anatomical "wiring diagrams" equipped with biophysical models of neuronal activity*. http://arxiv.org/abs/1812.09362 (accessed on 7th August 2025).

13. Echeverri, K. (2020). *The Various Routes to Functional Regeneration in the Central Nervous System*. https://core.ac.uk/download/288430911.pdf (accessed on 7th August 2025).

14. Krucoff, M. O., Rahimpour, S., Slutzky, M. W., Edgerton, V. R., & Turner, D. A. (2016). Enhancing Nervous System Recovery through Neurobiologics, Neural Interface Training, and Neurorehabilitation. *Frontiers in neuroscience*, *10*, 584. https://doi.org/10.3389/fnins.2016.00584(accessed on 7th August 2025).

15. Skaper, S. D., Facci, L., Zusso, M., & Giusti, P. (2018). An Inflammation-Centric View of Neurological Disease: Beyond the Neuron. *Frontiers in cellular neuroscience*, *12*, 72. https://doi.org/10.3389/fncel.2018.00072(accessed on 7th August 2025).

16. Giubilei, F. (2016). *Beyond cholinesterase inhibition: Anti-inflammatory role and pharmacological profile of current drug therapy for Alzheimer's disease*. https://core.ac.uk/download/98347745.pdf (accessed on 7th August 2025).

17. Gonzalez Deniselle, M. C., Lara, H. E., Recabarren, S. E., Roselli, C. E., et al. (2016). *Developmental and functional effects of steroid hormones on the neuroendocrine axis and spinal cord*. https://core.ac.uk/download/159294623.pdf (accessed on 7th August 2025).

18. Herms, J., Kretzschmar, H. A., & Vassallo, N. (2004). *The Molecular Pathology of Prion Diseases*. https://core.ac.uk/download/46601891.pdf (accessed on 7th August 2025).

19. Shi, F. D., Ljunggren, H. G., La Cava, A., & Van Kaer, L. (2011). Organ-specific features of natural killer cells. *Nature reviews. Immunology*, *11*(10), 658–671. https://doi.org/10.1038/nri3065 (accessed on 7th August 2025).

20. Marder, E., DeLong, M. R., Gazzaniga, M. S., & Wichmann, T. (2008). *2008 Progress Report on Brain Research*. https://core.ac.uk/download/71349141.pdf (accessed on 7th August 2025).

21. Meyer, A., Dandekar, A. A., Luster, A. D., Mehrad, B., Parra, B., Pearce, B. D., et al. (2006). *Functional diversity of chemokines and chemokine receptors in response to viral infection of the central nervous system*. https://core.ac.uk/download/323075298.pdf (accessed on 7th August 2025).

22. Tevfik Yılmaz1 , Yahya Turan1 , Ayşenur Keleş2 *Pathophysiology of Spinal Cord Injury* Journal of Clinical and Experimental Investigations doi: 10.5799/ahinjs.01.2014.01.0378 *(SCI)*. https://core.ac.uk/download/553656710.pdf (accessed on 7th August 2025).

23. Neal, C. M. (2016). *Evaluating techniques in tissue clarification using CLARITY imaging and investigating where sodium is sensed in the body*. https://core.ac.uk/download/142066226.pdf (accessed on 7th August 2025).

24. Wittko-Schneider, I. M., Schneider, F. T., & Plate, K. H. (2013). Brain homeostasis: VEGF receptor 1 and 2-two unequal brothers in mind. *Cellular and molecular life sciences : CMLS*, *70*(10), 1705–1725. https://doi.org/10.1007/s00018-013-1279-3(accessed on 7th August 2025).

25. Steinhart, E. (2001). *Persons Versus Brains: Biological Intelligence in Human Organisms*. https://core.ac.uk/download/287611886.pdf (accessed on 7th August 2025).

26. Tito, A. J., Jr., & Zhang, S. (2016). *Characterization of vesicular monoamine transporter 2 and its role in Parkinson's disease pathogenesis using Drosophila*. https://core.ac.uk/download/80296553.pdf (accessed on 7th August 2025).

27. Tonchev, A. B., Slominski, A., Reardon, C. L., Lapière, C. M., Pond, C. M., Hausman, D. B., Maquoi, E., et al. (2020). *Prelude 1*. https://core.ac.uk/download/357327753.pdf (accessed on 7th August 2025).

28. Ana Beatriz Lima da Costa Ferreira do Vale. (2023). *Exploring SNX3 and SNX27 role in nervous system function – Insights from aged and "stressed" synapses*. https://core.ac.uk/download/619584081.pdf (accessed on 7th August 2025).

29. Burla, R., La Torre, M., Zanetti, G., Bastianelli, A., Merigliano, C., Del Giudice, S., Vercelli, A., Di Cunto, F., Boido, M., Vernì, F., & Saggio, I. (2018). p53-Sensitive Epileptic Behavior and Inflammation in *Ft1* Hypomorphic Mice. *Frontiers in genetics*, *9*, 581. https://doi.org/10.3389/fgene.2018.00581(accessed on 7th August 2025).

30. Walker, A. (2016). *Exploring the production of extracellular matrix by astrocytes in response to mimetic traumatic brain injury*. https://core.ac.uk/download/84120358.pdf (accessed on 7th August 2025).

31. Patricia M. Wallace, Ph.D. (1980). *USSR Space Life Sciences Digest*, 1(3). Prepared for Life Sciences Division National Aeronautics and Space Adtnin6trmtion Washington, D.C. 20546 https://core.ac.uk/download/pdf/42858752.pdf (accessed on 7th August 2025).

32. Ward, J. A. (2000). *Neuro-Electronic Technology in Medicine and Beyond*. https://core.ac.uk/download/70097.pdf (accessed on 7th August 2025).

33. Wolff, J. G. (2003). *Neural mechanisms for information compression by multiple alignment, unification and search*. https://core.ac.uk/download/pdf/85392.pdf (accessed on 7th August 2025).

LYMPHATIC SYSTEM

12

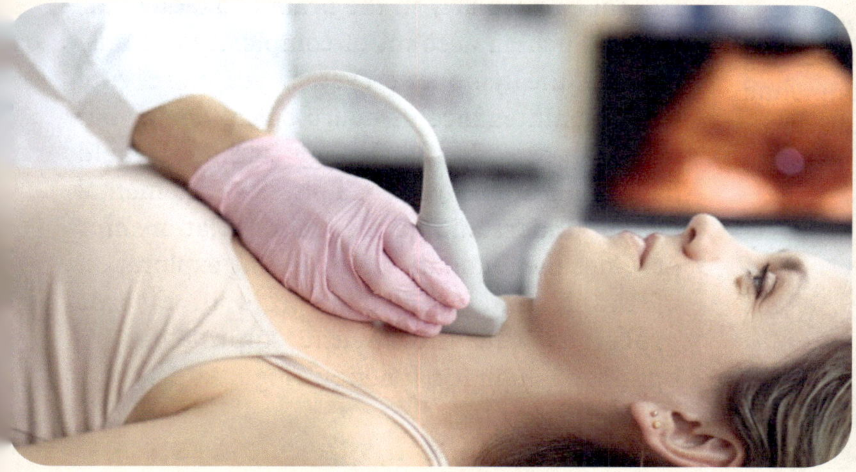

LEARNING OBJECTIVES

After studying this chapter, you will be able to:

1. Describe the anatomy of the lymphatic system;
2. Describe the functions of the lymphatic system;
3. Explain the lymphatic system and immune function;
4. Describe the disorders of the lymphatic system;
5. Learn about diagnostic techniques for lymphatic system disorders;
6. Understand the treatment and management of lymphatic system disorders.

Introduction

Lymphatic system, a network of nodes and vessels, plays a vital role in maintaining homeostasis in the human body. The primary functions of the system include the transportation of lymph, a fluid that contains white blood cells, and the facilitation of immune function. The system itself is overshadowed by the more prominent circulatory system but is unquestionably essential for healthy physiological processes. The lymphatic system not only helps filter out dangerous pathogens but also helps in the absorption of dietary fats and fat-soluble vitamins, highlighting its importance in being a multipurpose system within the human body. In addition to that, a normal lymphatic system is important for keeping edema at bay since it aids in maintaining fluid levels in tissues, hence creating a balance that is desirable for a healthy state. Beyond its description, the lymphatic system is also a defense line against disease and infection. Nodes that are distributed along the lymph tract are sites of filtering where lymph is screened for such foreign bodies as viruses and bacteria. Upon detection of these pathogens, lymph nodes are active sites of immune response where lymphocytes grow in number to fight infections. These immunological stimuli are also enhanced by other influences, including variation in season, which can potentially impact immune function. For instance, environmental stimuli , such as cold and reduced food availability have been observed to influence immune function, suggesting that seasonal rhythms play a paramount role in lymphatic effectiveness. This is especially formulated through the role of melatonin, which regulates immune competence in response to changing photoperiods, indicating the complex interaction between environmental cues and lymphatic competence (Nelson et al., 1995).

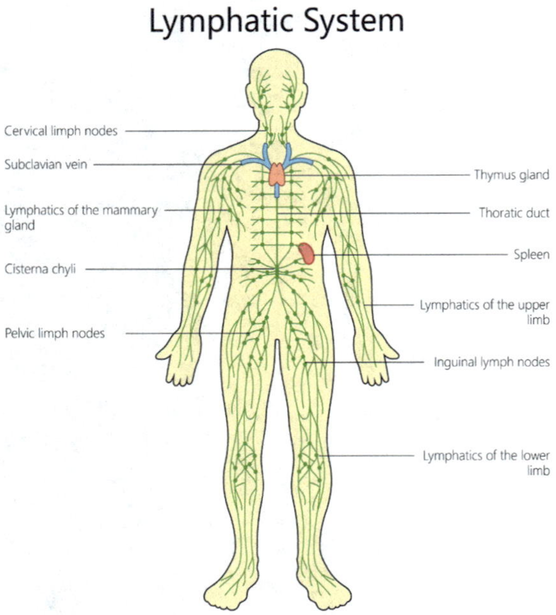

Figure 12.1. Lymphatic system.

Source: https://images.squarespace-cdn.com/content/v1/57853f211b631b3aa7b0053d/43407423-2d0c-4f7a-a2e4-9820000c8992/Acupuncture+Rochester+NY+Lymphatic+2-min.jpeg?format=2500w.

Additionally, the physical integrity of the lymphatic apparatus is critical to its operation. Recent research has established that microenvironmental conditions in tissues, like those established by blood flow dynamics, converse with the lymphatic system in deep ways. For example, lymph vessel behavior is highly related to the surrounding interstitial fluid dynamics, which are regulated by mechanisms other than systemic fluid circulation. The presence of special channels, like aquaporin-4, also suggests a rich understanding of how fluid transport is facilitated in the lymphatic system, particularly in the brain (Nakada et al., 2017). Such an account of complexity not only renders the lymphatic system yet more vital to the maintenance of neurological health but also suggests that pathology within it could have implications for broad physical and mental health. Understanding these interrelationships provides the foundation for ongoing exploration of the lymphatic system's role in disease processes and therapeutic approaches to optimize lymphatic function (Figure 12.1).

Definition of the Lymphatic System

The lymphatic system is a vital component of the circulatory and immune systems in the human body, made up of a tortuous arrangement of vessels, nodes, and organs working together in synergy to maintain fluid balance and immune response. Made up of lymph vessels that contain lymph—a colorless fluid with immune cells, waste products, and proteins—the system interconnects the bloodstream in multiple places, particularly around the thoracic duct and right lymphatic duct. Lymph nodes, conveniently located throughout the body, serve as filter stations where lymph is exposed to immune cells, contributing to the recognition and elimination of pathogens. The interdependent workings of the lymphatic system highlight its dual role in regulating body fluids and aiding the immune response, assuring the health and wellness of the human organism (Smith et al., 2005). In addition to its primary roles, the lymphatic system is also actively involved in the absorption of fats and the transport of dietary lipids into the intestinal tract. The lymphatic vessels of the intestines, or lacteals, take in fats and fat-soluble vitamins, which are carried into the bloodstream and hence spread the nutrients throughout the body. This special ability not only highlights the role of the lymphatic system in nutrition but also its importance in metabolism.

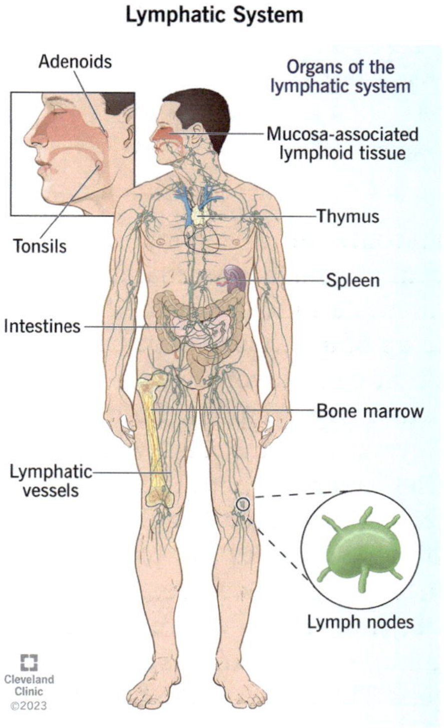

Figure 12.2. Many different organs and structures make up your lymphatic system. These parts all work together to help keep you healthy.

Source: https://my.clevelandclinic.org/-/scassets/images/org/health/articles/21199-lymphatic-system.

Abnormalities in lymphatic function can result in a range of illnesses, such as lymphedema—conditioned by the buildup of lymph fluid—and impaired immune reactions that can further aggravate diseases like infections or inflammatory disease. Awareness of these other functions enhances the multifaceted contribution of the lymphatic system to human physiology (Clarkson & Whipple, 2018). Also, the lymphatic system interactively interfaces with the other body systems, so that it is even more crucial beyond the regulation of fluid and nutrient transport. For instance, it regulates total blood volume and pressure through the interaction with the circulatory system, and also provides a timely immune cell response to the site of infection or injury. Such interconnectedness is shown by the role of the lymphatic system as a reservoir and conduit for the lymphocytes, such as T cells and B cells, that play a vital role in adaptive immunity. In its ontological architecture, the Foundational Model of Anatomy illustrates the complexity of the lymphatic system as part of a broad anatomical knowledge. This model forms the basis of educational efforts, setting forward the requirement for overall understanding by both students and clinicians of lymphatic dynamics (Smith et al., 2005; Clarkson & Whipple, 2018) (Figure 12.2).

Importance of the Lymphatic System in Human Health

The lymphatic system plays a key role in maintaining the health of the body by carrying interstitial fluid, which is responsible for cell homeostasis. It keeps the body free from excess fluid in tissues, thereby preventing edema and maintaining the stability of the cell environment. A dysfunction of the lymphatic system could lead to many health problems, like lymphedema and inflammatory conditions. In addition, the lymphatic vessels also contribute to immune surveillance by carrying lymphocytes and antigen-presenting cells to lymph nodes, where immune responses are generated. This dynamic interaction between the lymphatic and immune systems emphasizes the multifunctional nature of the lymphatic system in protecting the body against disease and pathogens.

As evidence of its critical functions grows, researchers are recognizing the complex role of the lymphatic system in keeping us well and healthy. Furthermore, the gut-associated lymphatic system is a classic illustration of the lymphatic networks' specialized function, particularly in lipid transport and immune regulation. Intestinal lymphatics have been shown, in recent studies, to play a central role in the digestion of dietary lipids by way of lacteals, the lymphatic vessels capable of fat as well as fat-soluble vitamin transport. Not only do these lymph channels facilitate the uptake of nutrients, but they also play an irreplaceable role in immunological responses in the gut. These actions, in which molecular mechanisms underlying their functions, such as control by many pathways of chylomicron entry into lymph vessels, reveal to us how highly metabolic and immune processes are integrated within the structure of lymph. The intricate interaction between these structures can yield insights for the therapeutic attack of metabolic disease, leading to more efficacious treatments for obesity and diabetes, conditions that are becoming more widespread globally (Cifarelli & Eichmann, 2019). Beyond its involvement in lipid metabolism, the lymphatic system also plays larger pathophysiological functions , such as tumorigenesis and tissue healing. Mast cells, which are placed strategically in lymphatic tissues, have the ability to show pro- or anti-tumorigenic activities, thus shaping cancer development and therapy outcomes. This dualism indicates that the lymphatic system can both promote and suppress tumor growth, underlining its multifaceted nature in health and disease. Ongoing research aims to delineate the targeted mast cell populations and their corresponding reactions to targeted stimuli, further exemplifying the multi-faceted potential. That data could not only illuminate cancer biology but also invigorate the strategies of immunotherapy by controlling lymphatic channels to promote anti-tumor reactions, rendering the promise of effective cancer treatment ever more realizable (Varricchi et al., 2019).

12.1. Anatomy of the Lymphatic System

Learning Outcome

1. Learn about major components of the lymphatic system;
2. Describe the structure and function of lymph nodes;
3. Describe the role of lymphatic vessels.

The anatomy of the lymphatic system is significant to homeostasis maintenance and the aid of immune function in the human body. It is made up of a network of vessels, nodes, and organs that work together with the circulatory system to carry lymph, a fluid that contains lymphocytes, proteins, and waste. Lymphatic capillaries emerge from the interstitial spaces and merge into larger lymphatic vessels that have one-way valves to prevent backflow. Coincidentally, these vessels drain into regional lymph nodes, where lymph is cleansed and immune cells can respond to potential pathogens. The design of the lymph nodes, with their compact array of immune cells, mirrors the immune surveillance and response functions of the lymphatic system and its essential function in human health and disease avoidance. The relevance of the lymphatic system is most evident when it comes to the immune system because it serves as a conduit for the drainage and transport of immune cells throughout the body. The sites of checkpoints are lymph nodes, and antigens contained within lymph fluid are processed and presented to T and B lymphocytes, thus triggering adaptive immune reactions. This activity is especially critical in the case of cancer, where lymph node status can determine malignancy spread. What has been learned through the study of lymphatic anatomy has revolutionary applications in veterinary medicine and uncovers pertinent analogies between human and canine lymphatic systems.

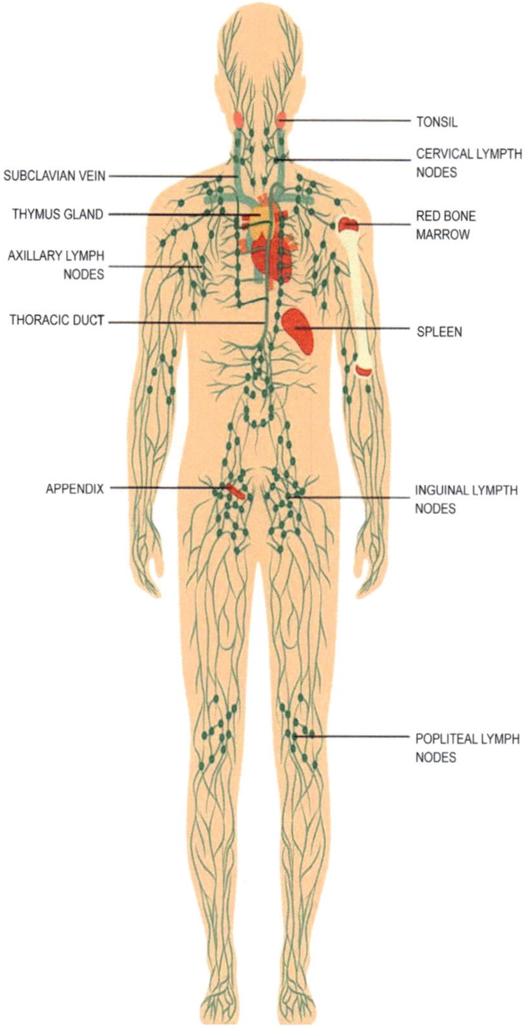

Figure 12.3. Anatomy and physiology of the lymphatic system.

Source: https://nurseslabs.com/wp-content/uploads/2017/08/Lymphatic-System-Lymphatic-System-Anatomy-and-Physiology.jpg.

For instance, sentinel node mapping is now gaining popularity in veterinary surgical oncology as well as human practice, paving the way for its potential to improve prognostic success following lymphadenectomies. Such a comparable anatomical foundation enhances the usefulness of current research on the lymphatics of and between species, highlighting its application in cancer treatment strategies (Beer et al., 2023).

The lymphatic system's role in organ development and function has become more prominent in the last few years, particularly its function in organs , such as the pancreas. Pancreatic lymphatic vessels play a part in immune regulation and fluid transport, which are important for an organ's health and function. During the developmental stages of the human pancreas, the lymphatic vasculature, identified with the assistance of markers like LYVE1 and PDPN, develops alongside blood vessels. This development is significant as it demarcates the function of the lymphatic system not only in immune response but also in guaranteeing proper organogenesis. It is crucial to comprehend the interaction between lymphatic and blood vessels to advance regenerative therapies for diseases like diabetes, where effective fluid transport is essential for cellular function. As research evolves, the information gained on the anatomy and physiology of the lymphatic system promises to advance therapeutic methods in diabetes management as well as cancer treatment (Roost et al., 2014) (Figure 12.3).

12.1.1. Major Components of the Lymphatic System

The lymphatic system is crucial for fluid balance, immune system function, and the absorption of fats in the diet. Among its key components, the vessels of the lymphatic system transport lymph, which is a fluid rich in proteins, waste products, and immune cells. The vessels run through human body tissues to reabsorb excess interstitial fluid that otherwise would have been there, preventing edema. Interestingly, these vessels are also equipped with valves that allow one-way passage of the lymph to the thoracic duct, where lymph is eventually drained into the bloodstream. This transportation system must be working properly to make sure the immune system is able to react favorably to pathogens and excess fluids are drained effectively, highlighting the its crucial role in both immune surveillance and homeostasis. Lymph nodes are a key component of the lymphatic system. These are filtration centers, removing the lymphatic fluid as it occurs throughout the body and are highly concentrated with lymphocytes, primarily B and T cells, which are the foundation for adaptive immunity. Foreign pathogens and antigens are recognized and processed as the lymph fluid flows through the lymph nodes, providing a robust and potent immune response. In addition to their function in immunity, lymph nodes are also critical in memory cell development, allowing the body to respond more readily to the recurrence of previously infecting pathogens. The organization of lymph nodes, with their organized regions of T cells, B cells, and dendritic cells, reflects the sophistication of the immune system's functionality and coordination of the innate and adaptive immune responses required for effective disease resistance. The spleen, the second major constituent of the lymphatic system, serves a variety of roles that are integral to human health. The spleen functions as a blood filter, removing abnormal red blood cells and recycling iron for the production of hemoglobin. The spleen also acts as an immune system member by producing lymphocytes and antibodies, thus performing an important role against infection. Most importantly, white pulp within the spleen is highly concentrated in lymphocytes, whereas red pulp is related to recycling blood components. This dual function reinforces the spleen's role not only in lymph circulation, but also in metabolic as well as immune roles. Understanding the functions of these components within the lymphatic system gives us a clue to their collective contribution to overall health and environmental challenge response, as indicated by the seasonality of immune function and disease process (Nelson et al., 1995; Custodis et al., 2019) (Figure 12.4).

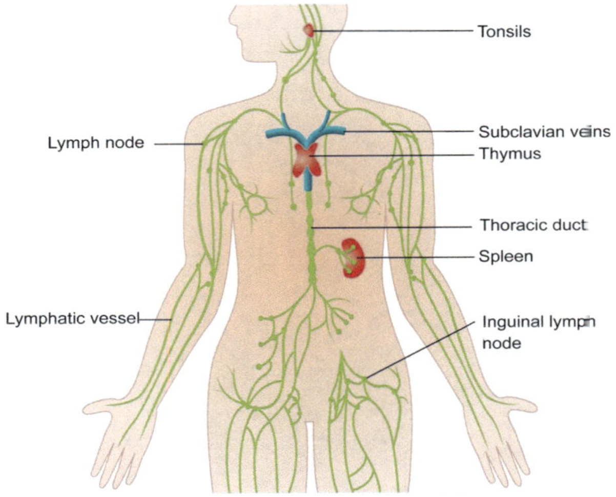

Figure 12.4. Major components of the lymphatic system.

Source: https://cdn.ps.emap.com/wp-content/uploads/sites/3/2020/09/Fig-1-The-major-components-of-the-lymphatic-system-1024x856.jpg.

12.1.2. Structure and Function of Lymph Nodes

The lymph node anatomy is significant in terms of how lymph nodes function within the lymphatic system. Lymph nodes are encapsulated, small organs that are located in strategic positions within and around the body, typically in clusters in locations , such as the neck, axillae, and groin. Every node consists of an outer cortex and an inner medulla, two distinct regions with differing functions. The cortex contains B-cell areas referred to as follicles, where crucial processes like the activation of the B-cells occur. The medulla, on the other hand, contains medullary cords and sinuses where T-cells and macrophages are present, allowing for the immune response when pathogens are encountered. This organized anatomy allows lymph nodes to filter lymph fluid efficiently, ultimately contributing to the body's overall immune surveillance and enhancing the adaptive immune response to pathogens and diseases. Lymph nodes exist with their primary function focused on their role as central sites for the immune response. As lymph fluid, which transports antigens and pathogens from peripheral tissues, diffuses into the lymph nodes, the nodes mount the first line of defense against infection. When T-cells in the lymph nodes detect foreign intruders, an immune cascade is activated, and T-cells are activated with the expansion of B-cells. This activation leads to the generation of antibodies, which are important in neutralizing pathogens and marking them for destruction. Further, lymph nodes are training facilities for immune cells, and they retain the capacity to function effectively to recognize and respond to target antigens. This important function is to emphasize the importance of lymph nodes in maintaining an effective and functional immune system and eventually protecting the body from disease. Investigations have shown a profound correlation between the function and structure of lymph nodes and their contribution to overall lymphatic well-being. The intricate arrangement of lymph nodes not only maintains immune responses but also aids in lipid metabolism and the removal of cholesterol, highlighting their multifunctional nature. For instance, research draws emphasis to the role played by lymphatic vessels in facilitating reverse cholesterol transport (RCT), where cholesterol is mobilized into the bloodstream for excretion. In states of impaired lymphatic drainage, such as in obesity or certain cancers, disruption of RCT leads to negative outcomes on health, and emphasis is placed on how lymph health affects general health (Martel et al., 2013). Similarly, comprehension of lymphatic and blood system development within human organs, such as the pancreas, exhibits that lymphatic vessels play an important role in the regulation of metabolic processes as well as immune function, illustrating the complexity of lymph node function within physiological settings (Roost et al., 2014) (Figure 12.5).

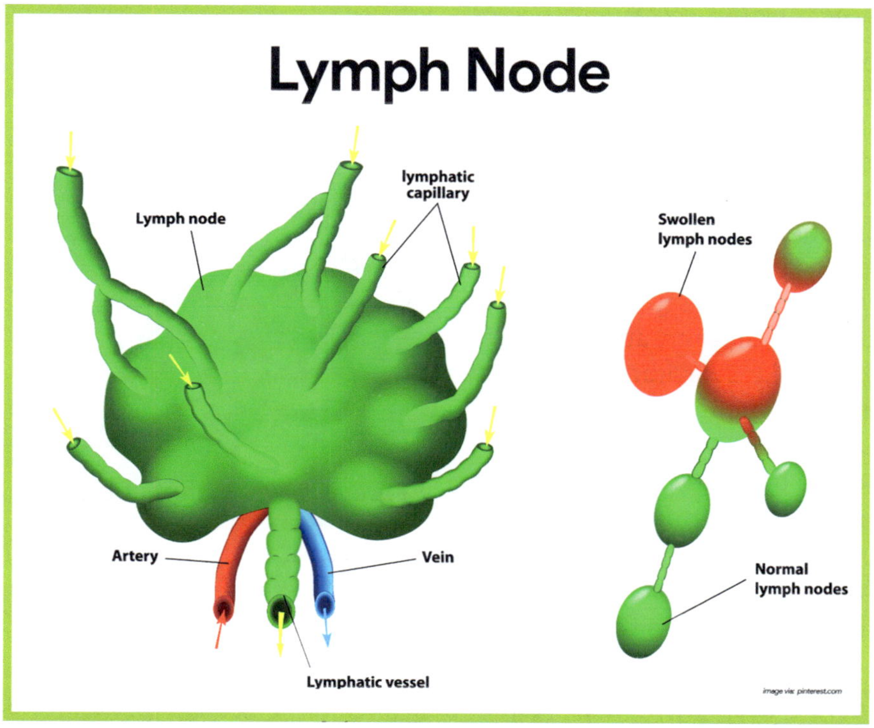

Figure 12.5. Lymph node.

Source: https://nurseslabs.com/wp-content/uploads/2017/08/Lymph-Node-Lymphatic-System-Anatomy-and-Physiology.png.

12.1.3. Role of Lymphatic Vessels

Lymphatic vessels are also involved in maintaining fluid homeostasis in the human body by efficiently bringing back interstitial fluid to the circulatory system. This keeps tissues hydrated and also prevents edema. While blood circulates through the arteries and capillaries, sections of its plasma filter into the tissues surrounding it, requiring a drainage system. Lymphatic vessels collect this excess fluid, known as lymph, and return it to the bloodstream. In a way to maintain the overall balance and operation of body systems, lymphatic vessels effectively manage fluid quantity. Involving such a sophisticated network is quintessential to health and illness, and its understanding is thus crucial in the establishment of medical sciences and therapeutic strategies. Apart from fluid transport, lymphatic vessels are vital in immunity. They serve as conduits for immune cells, particularly lymphocytes, to be carried to infected or inflamed tissues. When lymph travels through lymph nodes, it is filtered, where pathogens and foreign substances are identified and destroyed by immune cells. Apart from providing the body with a greater opportunity to defend itself against infections, this filtering process also helps in developing and constructing immune responses. The coordination between the immune system and lymphatic vessels is thus very deep, as they create pathways for communication and coordination among immune system components. Understanding the role of the lymphatic system in immune surveillance becomes even more important for designing good vaccines and therapies against autoimmune disease and cancer. Furthermore, the role of lymphatic vessels in organ development and health has also been elucidated in recent research. For example, research suggests that lymphatic vessels play a fundamental role in pancreatic physiology in supporting the regulation of immune responses required for the maintenance of endocrine functions. In particular, lymphatic vessels were found to develop near the islets of Langerhans at very important stages in pancreatic development, focusing on their significance for tissue regeneration and metabolic control (Roost et al., 2014). Such findings emphasize how critical the lymphatic system is to other bodily systems. This fact can determine ways to treat diabetes and other metabolic conditions, emphasizing the need to thoroughly study lymphatic vessels in a bid to push the frontiers of regenerative medicine and transplantation therapy (Gillen & Conrad, 2019) (Figure 12.6).

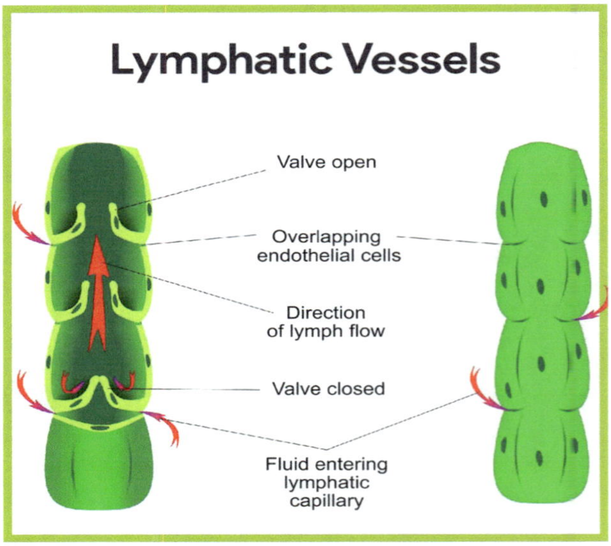

Figure 12.6. Lymphatic vessels.

Source: https://nurseslabs.com/wp-content/uploads/2017/08/Lymphatic-Vessels-Lymphatic-System-Anatomy-and-Physiology.jpg.

Test Your Knowledge

1. What are the major components of the lymphatic system?
2. What is the role of lymphatic vessels?

12.2. Functions of the Lymphatic System

Learning Outcome

1. Learn about fluid balance and tissue drainage;
2. Describe the immune response and pathogen defense;
3. Understand the absorption of dietary fats.

The lymphatic system is an integral part of the immune system of the human body, whose primary role is to carry lymph, a fluid that has infection-fighting white blood cells. This system is accountable for the immune homeostasis and plays a crucial role in the body's immune defense against pathogens. Lymph vessels, which pervade the body, drain excess interstitial fluid and carry it back into the blood, thus preventing tissue accumulation of fluid. Lymph nodes along these vessels enhance the capacity of the system to filter out pathogens and other foreign material from the lymph. Consequently, the lymphatic system not only aids in fluid balance but is also a key surveillance system and plays a notable role in immune responses and in enhancing the body's capacity to respond effectively against infection. The lymphatic system also plays a crucial part in the absorption of fat and fat-soluble vitamins from the intestine. The nutrients are transported into the lymphatic system by specialized lymphatic vessels known as lacteals and finally into the bloodstream. This is a function of crucial importance, since it enables the body to acquire essential nutrients needed in many metabolic reactions and cellular functions. The absorption of fats and their final uses in the generation of energy are health- and well-being-related. Malabsorption syndromes are conditions that can be caused by disorders of the lymphatic system, which suggests this system's importance not only in immune defense but also in nutritional health. The lymphatic system thus stands at the interface of two basic physiological domains: immune defense and transport of nutrients. Finally, the lymphatic system also has the role of conserving tissue homeostasis as well as waste removal. It acts like a drainage system, draining away the waste material, cellular remnants, and surplus proteins from interstitial spaces to prevent any potential inflammatory responses. Proper elimination of these substances is critical in preventing the swelling of the tissues and in healing effectively. Moreover, in cases where the lymphatic system is impaired to the level of ailments , such as lymphedema—the effects can have radically devastating impacts on mobility and will be painful. The relationship of the lymphatic system with other systems in the body, including the circulatory and immune systems, illustrates the complexity of its functions within the human body. The proper understanding of these functions underscores the importance of lymphatic health, a condition of importance to overall physiological function as well as immunity to disease.

12.2.1. Fluid Balance and Tissue Drainage

Fluid balance and tissue drainage are significant lymphatic functions of importance to ensuring homeostasis in the human body. Lymphatic function is a significant mechanism for interstitial fluid volume regulation to prevent both edema and dehydration. Excess interstitial fluid is channeled and accumulated into the circulatory system during drainage through lymphatics, hence maintaining tissue fluid balance. This is a very significant process, and any form of interference may lead to pathology like lymphedema, which is abnormal swelling due to fluid accumulation. Thus, effective lymphatic vessel performance is critical in fluid balance and ensuring tissues are adequately supplied with nutrients while simultaneously removing waste. Along with this, drainage of fluid by the lymphatic system influences tissue health and healing mechanisms, and fluid accumulation will impede the supply of nutrients and oxygen to tissues and recovery from injury. Tissues' proper drainage of lymph ensures tissue hydration at its optimal level, which is vital for cellular and overall tissue integrity functions. Studies have shown that maintaining tissues in good hydration enhances the resistance of the tissues and helps in healing, particularly in wound healing. This highlights the dependence of fluid balance, tissue drainage, and biological function integrity on one another, wherein acute imbalances trigger chronic complications requiring complex management plans to re-establish equilibrium within the lymphatic system. The link between fluid balance and tissue drainage is also true for wound healing dynamics, wherein hydration plays a pivotal role. Application of appropriate dressings to create a moist wound healing environment is a reflection of the importance of fluid management in promoting faster and improved healing. As demonstrated, appropriate dressings must absorb exudate without compromising the amount of necessary moisture to prevent desiccation, especially in chronic wounds where integrity of the skin barrier is impaired. The ongoing measurement of the properties of wound exudate, including its biological composition, aids in demystifying determinants of healing outcomes. Thus, the knowledge about fluid balance and tissue drainage as part of the lymphatic system not only emphasizes their physiological importance but also highlights their critical roles in clinical situations, validating the need for particular therapy approaches for optimal fluid management and wound healing (Ousey et al., 2016; Ceelen et al., 2017).

12.2.2. Immune Response and Pathogen Defense

The immune system, being a major part of the lymphatic system, is very organized to defend the body against a wide range of pathogens. This complex network of cells operates through both innate and adaptive immunity, with innate immunity giving the initial defense. Resident monocytes and macrophages, for instance, play an important part in detecting and responding to intruders on time. Investigations show that these cell types, together with other lymphoid cells found within the middle ear, have a repertoire of innate immune genes expressed on them that enable them to respond rapidly to infections. This response is crucial since pathogens can prove highly destructive if not countered efficiently. Therefore, the swift response of the innate immune system forms the foundation of the first line of defense against pathogens, enabling recovery from infection attained in an effective way (Ryan et al., 2020). In addition to the quick response triggered by the innate immune system, long-term protection against pathogens is primarily offered by the adaptive immune response. This involves the formation of antigen-specific lymphocytes that arm the body with immunological memory. When a familiar pathogen is reintroduced, these lymphocytes are deployed right away to counter the danger. The cooperation between innate and adaptive immunity reflects a sophisticated immune protection strategy. It highlights the crucial role of the lymphatic system in facilitating the maturation and dissemination of immune cells. By effective structuring of the functions of various immune components, the lymphatic system defends the body with a powerful immunity against a wide range of pathogens, thereby reducing the risk of infections (Gillen & Conrad, 2014). The structure of the immune system also points to its evolutionary significance in maintaining general health. Originally meant to remove the body of dying cells and support growth, the role of the immune system has been expanded with the emergence of pathogens. The function of dynamic immune receptors, particularly toll-like receptors, most accurately explains this dual role in which they recognize not just disease-causing pathogens but also facilitate beneficial interactions with non-harmful microbes. As the environment changed after the Fall, so too has the immune system function changed to include robust defense against pathogens while at the same time maintaining cellular integrity. This flexibility is characteristic of a well-designed system in which defense requirements are weighed against the need for the maintenance of internal homeostasis, thus positioning the lymphatic system as the basis of human immunological function (Ryan et al., 2020) (Figure 12.7).

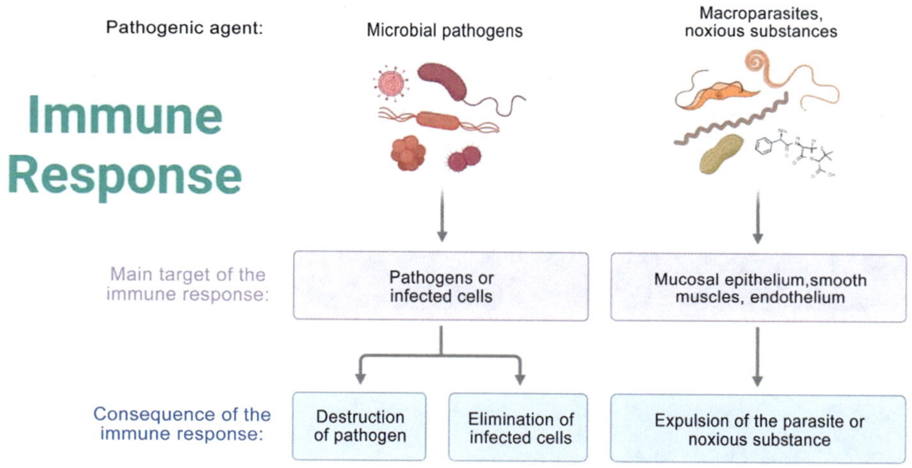

Figure 12.7. Immune response.

Source: https://microbenotes.com/wp-content/uploads/2022/05/Immune-Response.jpeg.

12.2.3. Absorption of Dietary Fats

The absorption of dietary fats has a very strong association with the lymphatic system and its function in the transport of lipids from the intestines to the blood. Dietary fats, after ingestion, become emulsified within the gastrointestinal tract to facilitate pancreatic lipases to hydrolyze them into their simpler components, i.e., fatty acids and monoglycerides. These substances are taken up by the intestinal lining, wherein they are re-esterified into triglycerides and packaged into chylomicrons, large lipoprotein particles that are required for lipid transport. The freshly synthesized chylomicrons travel out of the enterocytes and into the lacteals or lymphatic capillaries, lipid-absorbing vessels. This process demonstrates the crucial function of the lymphatic system in preventing the storage of dietary fats in the lymph and facilitating efficient transport to the circulatory system. Studies show that the quality of dietary fat dictates the absorption process and overall lipid composition in lymphatic transport. Experiments with preruminant calves have revealed that dietary fat saturation level greatly affects the transport of cholesterol in intestinal lymph and bile. For instance, changes in sources of fat , such as soybean oil, milk fat, and beef tallow, resulted in dissimilarities in lipid and cholesterol transport rates of mesenteric lymph. More specifically, higher rates of cholesterol transport were found with the feeding of certain fats, which attests to the interdependence of lipid saturation and absorption efficiency. Also of importance is the quantity of bile acids released during this process in facilitating fat emulsification, with added help in absorbing dietary fat. These findings indicate the complexity involved in the role of the lymphatic system and how they can control lipid absorption effectively (Davis, 1983). The stereochemistry of fatty acids within the triglycerides further significantly plays a role in their metabolism and absorption, which indicates the requirement to solve dietary fat composition in nutrition science. The structure of saturated and unsaturated fatty acids in triacylglycerol molecules determines not just digestive efficacy but postprandial lipemia as well. The position of fatty acids, particularly in the sn-2 position of triglycerides, seems to influence fat metabolism and clearance from circulation, according to research. Stereospecificity thus may lead to variations in lipid profiles as well as affect atherogenicity and thrombogenicity. Hence, exploring dietary TAGs' structural characteristics is of value in terms of optimizing dietary fat intake for human well-being. Such findings have implications for dietary guidance and intervention to restrict cardiovascular hazard, and a thoughtful understanding of how different dietary fats interact with the lymphatic route is therefore appropriate (Karupaiah & Sundram, 2007).

Test Your Knowledge

1. What are the fluid balance and tissue drainage?
2. What is the immune response to pathogens?

12.3. Lymphatic System and Immune Function

Learning Outcome

1. Understand the interaction between the lymphatic system and the immune system;
2. Describe the role of lymphocytes in immunity;
3. Understand the importance of the thymus and spleen.

The lymph system plays a critical role in maintaining immune competency via the transport of lymph, a liquid in which lymphocytes and other immune cells are suspended. The system consists essentially of lymphatic vessels, lymph nodes, and other lymphoid tissues. Lymphatic vessels are pipelines for lymph, wherein they route it back into the circulatory system, and pathways for immune cells to travel into sites of inflammation or infection. The lymph nodes are filter stations where lymphocytes can encounter antigens and initiate immune responses. Proper function of the lymphatic system is important, especially during periods of immune challenge, since such structures allow for an immediate and concerted reaction against pathogens and thereby contribute to the defense mechanisms of the body against illness and disease. Seasonal change can play a significant role in the dynamics of lymphatic function and immune responsiveness. Experiments show that photoperiodic variation—i.e., day length and duration of night—can communicate immunological adjustment in various species, including man. Autumn-winter days of shortened length have been reported in studies to go with an immunity trade-off, perhaps because of the presence of high glucocorticoids, which may curb immune function. Melatonin, a hormone associated with fluctuations in daylight, was found to mediate immune function and increase specific immunological parameters in different seasons. This association between environmental changes and immune response mirrors the adaptive nature of the lymphatic system as it prepares the body to protect against seasonal stresses intermittently that are harmful to health, thereby revealing its evolutionary function in disease prevention and control (Nelson et al., 1995). Besides the main organs of the lymphatic system, tertiary lymphoid organs (TLOs) have also been known to play a growing role in immune responses. They are ectopic lymphoid structures formed in tissues following chronic inflammation and enable localized immune response generation.

The composition of TLOs includes antigen-presenting cells, which play the crucial role of presenting antigens to lymphocytes and, as a result, their activation. Although research in this field is ongoing, how the specific mechanisms for antigen handling in TLOs work is still not well understood. Examination of these processes is crucial to understanding how the lymphatic system adjusts to perform its immune function in various pathological environments. The dialogue between TLOs, antigen presentation, and immune function highlights the complex nature of immune regulation through the lymphatic system and raises important areas for future research (Bedaj et al., 2016) (Figure 12.8).

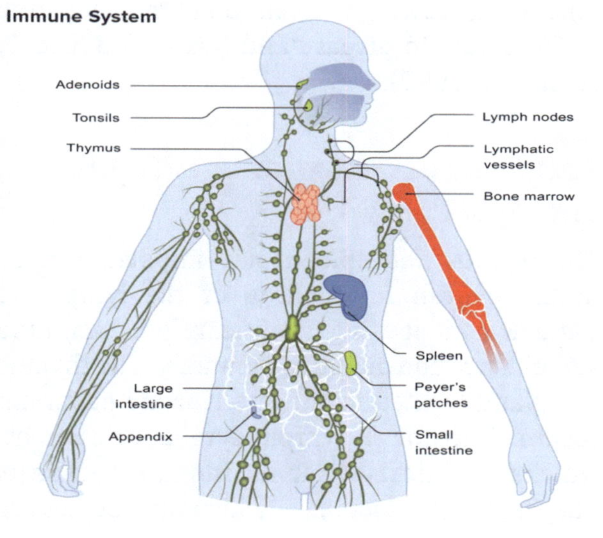

Figure 12.8. The immune system.

Source: https://post.medicalnewstoday.com/wp-content/uploads/sites/3/2023/10/1958482-Immune-System_1296x1296-body-1024x1024.png.

12.3.1. Interaction with the Immune System

The relationship between the lymphatic system and the immune system is vital to homeostasis and resistance to infections. Lymphatic transport is essential for the transportation of lymph, a fluid that not only transports immune cells but is also involved in the elimination of pathogens and waste products. There are lymph nodes scattered all over the body, and they act as checkpoints for monitoring where the lymph is filtered. Filtration is important in that it brings lymphocytes, T and B cells, into contact with antigens. Upon stimulation, these immune cells are activated and trigger specific immune responses. Thus, the lymphatic system is not just a pipe but an active system in which significant interactions occur that determine the capability of the body to mount an effective response to pathogens and ensure regulation of immune responses in a way that avoids too much injury to host tissues. Understanding the effect of seasonality on immune responses further underlines the adaptive potential of the lymphatic system. Evidence indicates that environmental cues, including photoperiodic change, can have a dramatic impact on immune function. For instance, on short days, immune suppression occurs in anticipation of the need for strategic immune response adjustment. Pineal melatonin, which interprets day-length information, has been implicated as responsible for these changes, activating particular parameters of the immune system at particular times of year. The cyclical mechanism of immune function is an evolutionary mechanism that allows organisms to prepare and anticipate immunological insults associated with seasonal fluctuation. These findings depict how the lymphatic system and how this interacts with the immune system become critical in compensating for such environmental change, creating a biological apparatus for survival and adaptation during fluctuation (Nelson et al., 1995). Development of biotherapy is also another critical area of interaction between the lymphatic and immune systems, particularly for conditions like cancer and autoimmune diseases. New biotherapeutics , such as immunomodulators developed from biological agents, have revolutionized treatment practices. These therapies utilize the immune system to modify gene expression or provoke an immune reaction against malignancies and autoimmune diseases. Understanding the underlying structure and function of the immune system is required for the best usage of these therapies. As new biological proteins that have functions in the immune system are being found all the time, there is more and more potential for tailor-made biotherapies that enhance the effectiveness of the therapy of the immune system. This dynamic environment depicts the intricate relationship of immune, lymphatic, and pathological processes, demonstrating the importance of this interaction in medical advancement (Gallucci & McCarthy, 1995).

12.3.2. Role of Lymphocytes in Immunity

Lymphocytes, which are a category of white blood cells, play a key role in the adaptive immune response, their main function being the identification and destruction of pathogens. These cells, which are mostly B cells and T cells, originate from the bone marrow and develop in various lymphoid tissues , such as the thymus. When developing, they become specialized with particular receptors that react to certain antigens, which are foreign chemicals that provoke an immune response. When they encounter an antigen, B cells become plasma cells that produce antibodies and T cells become cytotoxic or helper cells that help other immune mechanisms. This way, lymphocytes can adapt their response to the immense variety of threats, enhancing the function of the entire immune system. The effectiveness of such an adaptive response is crucial to the body's capability to resist infection and to develop immunological memory for pathogens encountered in the past. The fluctuation of immune functions observed seasonally in most vertebrate animals underscores the dynamic character of lymphocytes in the general immunity. NelsonBiotherapy innovations highlight the importance of lymphocytes in clinical applications, particularly as it concerns cancer and autoimmune diseases. From being nonspecific activators of immunity, the field has evolved to developing targeted therapies that employ lymphocyte activity for therapeutic purposes. For instance, monoclonal antibody therapy utilizes the peculiarity of B cell response for the targeting of neoplasias and checkpoint inhibitors attempt to augment T cell responses against cancer. Indeed, current studies further highlighted the importance of knowing the dynamics of lymphocytes following oncogenesis and how , such aspects would progress in conjunction with other genetic determinants of immune function. This knowledge is crucial in the development of novel therapies that can significantly enhance the management of most diseases by exploiting or modulating lymphocyte function, a growing recognition of the lymphatic systems role in disease and health (Gallucci & McCarthy, 1995).

12.3.3. Importance of the Thymus and Spleen

The thymus and spleen play important roles in the overall functioning of the lymphatic system, contributing significantly to immune surveillance and adaptive immunity. The thymus is a gland located in the anterior mediastinum responsible for T lymphocyte development, which are critical cells in the immune response. They undergo selection, in which thymocytes are intensively educated to discern self and non-self so that the immune system will attack pathogens without losing the battle to autoimmunity. The thymus also secretes crucial hormones , such as thymosin and thymulin, that play a critical role in controlling the growth and differentiation of immune cells (Csaba, 2016). This dynamic organ has a unique function in early life, but it begins involuting following puberty, marking its central role in defining the immune repertoire during key points of development. Similarly, the spleen is a significant immune organ since it becomes a site of blood filtration and the encounter of lymphocytes with antigens. Located in the upper left abdomen, the spleen has red and white pulp, both with specialized functions. The white pulp is primarily responsible for immune responses, with B and T lymphocytes that are involved in adaptive immunity. The red pulp, however, is responsible for the clearance of old red blood cells and recycling of iron and hence overall homeostasis (Lämmermann & Kastenmüller, 2019). With the ability to sense and respond to infections borne through the blood, the spleen significantly enhances the body's immune capacity. The filtering process not only protects the body from infection, but it also plays a part in the creation of immunological memory, further solidifying the role of this organ in maintaining long-term health. The thymus and spleen interface also illustrates the complex organization of the network of lymphatic systems. Although the thymus plays a significant part in T cell development and training, the spleen plays a role in activating the cells when they respond to systemic infections, thereby creating a harmonious system that rapidly reacts to infection. The thymus output of mature and competent T cells plays a key role in enhancing the adaptive reactions that are initiated by the spleen (Csaba, 2016). Besides, the interaction between various subsets of leukocytes in both organs illustrates the complexity of immune signaling and cell direction, as illustrated by the role of G-protein-coupled receptors in directing leukocyte behavior in lymphoid tissue (Lämmermann & Kastenmüller, 2019). This concerted action of the spleen and thymus illustrates the role of both organs in maintaining a well-functioning and responsive immune system (Figure 12.9).

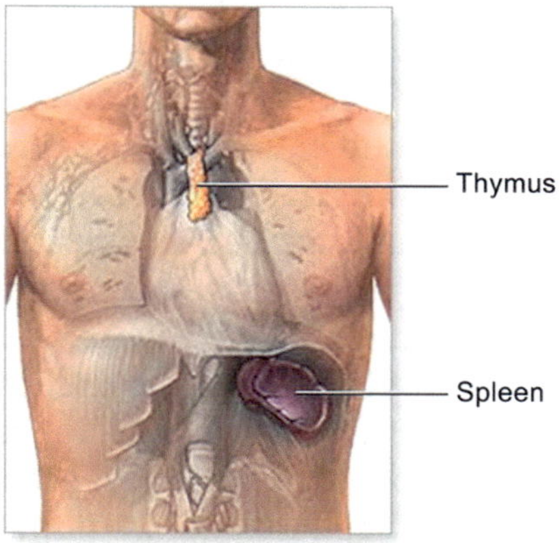

Figure 12.9. Thymus and spleen.

Source: https://www.walgreens.com/marketing/adamHtml/bodyguides/reftext/images/Thymus_spleen.jpg.

Test Your Knowledge

1. What is the role of lymphocytes in immunity?
2. What is the importance of the thymus and spleen?

12.4. Disorders of the Lymphatic System

Learning Outcome

1. Understand the lymphedema and its causes;
2. Describe the lymphoma and other cancers;
3. Describe the infections affecting the lymphatic system.

Lymphatic system disorders present a complex array of conditions that encompass congenital and acquired diseases. The lymph system plays a key role in immunity, interstitial fluid homeostasis, and fat absorption; thus, their dysfunction can lead to enhanced susceptibility to infections and inflammatory diseases. Among the more widespread diseases is lymphedema, where the improper storage of lymphatic fluid occurs, leading to swelling, particularly in the limbs. Lymphedema can be induced by genetics, trauma, or an operative complication. Understanding the pathophysiological processes involved in these conditions is important because they can create potential impacts on a person's quality of life and well-being. Therefore, the assessment of successful management and treatment techniques is important. Moreover, the study includes the knowledge of parasitic infection implications on the lymphatic system. Much attention has been given to helminthic parasite-mediated diseases, which have been demonstrated to impact immunity and lead to pathology of the lymphatics. More significantly, these parasites can yield a regulatory immune response that not only functions to ensure their own suppression but also inadvertently suppresses the ability of the body to respond to other pathogens and thereby results in inflammatory disease in host organisms. Research has demonstrated that the immunological interactions between helminths and the immune system can, in fact, be utilized in the development of protective systems against diseases , such as allergy and autoimmune diseases, as evidenced by epidemiological research across various strata of income. The medicinal importance of utilizing these interactions is a well-favored area for medical research, particularly in controlling inflammatory as well as immune disorders that drain modern societies (Araujo et al., 2016). In case of congenital lymphatic disorders , such as Hennekam lymphangiectasia-lymphedema syndrome-1, diagnostic and treatment hurdles are particularly sharp. Applications of cutting-edge genomic analysis techniques , such as whole exome sequencing (WES), have provided never-before-seen information regarding the etiology of these rare disorders that have nonspecific phenotypes, thus posing difficulty in early diagnosis. These advances point towards the integration of genetic testing into the regular assessment of fetal abnormality, especially in recurrent hydrops fetalis. Early diagnosis with genetic screening can allow for early intervention strategies, ultimately leading to a better prognosis for the affected individuals. With ongoing development of our understanding of lymphatic diseases, the merging of multidisciplinary approaches balancing genetics, immunology, and therapy will likely introduce successful models for the treatment of these intricate disease conditions (Melber et al., 2018) (Figure 12.10).

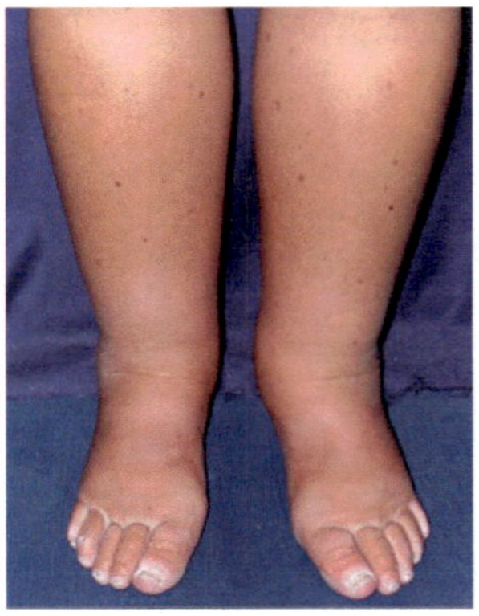

Figure 12.10. Lymphatic System Disorders.

Source: https://study.com/cimages/multimages/16/lymphedema.png

12.4.1. Lymphedema and Its Causes

Lymphedema is a condition closely associated with the inability of the lymphatic system. It results when lymph, an important fluid that assists in maintaining tissue fluid balance and immune protection, cannot drain from tissues in the body properly. A range of etiologies contributes to such obstructions, including inherited dispositions, surgery, radiation, and infection. For example, primary lymphedema frequently results from congenital defects in the development of lymphatic vessels, whereas secondary lymphedema can be the consequence of injury to the lymphatic system through cancer therapy, interfering with lymphatic routes. As the lymph fluid builds up, patients become swollen, uncomfortable, and possibly have complications, demonstrating the urgent necessity for integrated knowledge and treatment of this condition in the larger context of lymphatic disease and health. A central part of understanding lymphedema is gaining knowledge on proteins and signaling pathways managing lymphatic function. Specific molecular markers and growth factors, such as vascular endothelial growth factor-C (VEGF-C), have been studied as essential in the function and development of lymphatic endothelial cells (LEC). The proteolytic cleavage of VEGF-C by proteins like Collagen and calcium-binding EGF domains 1 (CCBE1) and ADAMTS3 underscores the complexity of lymphatic vasculature development and maintenance. Besides assisting in the normal functioning of the lymphatic system, these proteins also underscore how dysfunctions result in lymphedema. Thus, exploration of such molecular mechanisms in depth illuminates potential therapeutic targets that can mitigate the symptoms of lymphedema and restore lymphatic integrity, since lymphatic health and general well-being become increasingly akin to one another (Jurisic & Detmar, 2018). Lymphedema therapy is targeted towards prevention and control to diminish the condition's influence on patients. Treatment can include decongestive therapy (CDT), a holistic approach that combines manual lymph drainage, compression bandaging, exercise, and skin care to promote lymph fluid reduction. However, learning about the pathophysiology of lymphedema is critical to the success of treatment. For example, inflammation of the lymph apparatus can exacerbate fluid accumulation, and therefore, control of inflammation must be a prime target for intervention strategies. With advancements in science, the development of targeted therapies for the regulation of lymphatic endothelium can introduce new approaches not only to alleviate lymphedema but to remedy its underlying causes. Finally, a multi-disciplinary field with both clinical and molecular investigations is essential in the pursuit of resolving lymphedema, re-establishing its relevance in the broader context of the contribution of the lymphatic system to human health (Jeltsch et al., 2018) (Figure 12.11).

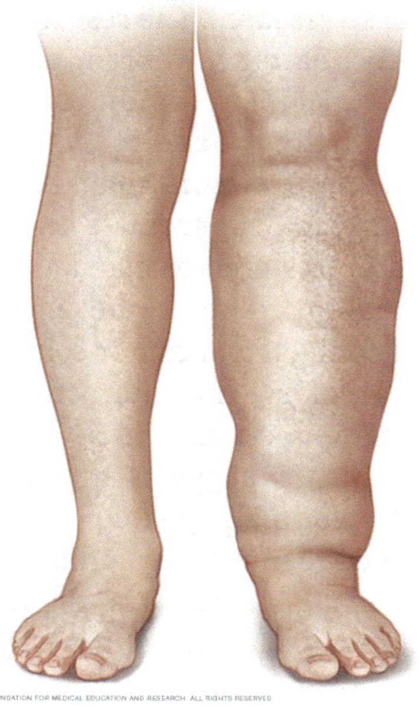

Figure 12.11. Lymphedema.

Source: https://www.mayoclinic.org/-/media/kcms/gbs/patient-consumer/images/2017/12/19/15/43/r11_lymphedema-8col.jpg.

12.4.2. Lymphoma and Other Cancers

The lymphatic system plays a critical role in the immune response and is, therefore unavoidably implicated in the etiology and progression of lymphoma and other neoplasms. Lymphoma, a cancer of the lymphatic system, is classified as Hodgkin and Non-Hodgkin lymphomas, each with its respective distinguishing characteristics and therapeutic strategies. Dysregulation of lymphocytes, primarily B and T cells, may lead to a condition favorable to malignancy. Abnormal proliferation of these immune cells not only weakens the lymphatic function but also generates a feedback process that is capable of advancing other malignancies within the body. This correlation identifies a larger area of how the dynamics of the lymphatic system and its function in cancer, localized and systemic in man, are understood. The connection between the associated diseases, like glomerulonephritis, and cancer malignancies, like lymphoma, has been the focus of intense research. The research indicated significant correlations, wherein patients with different conditions of glomerulonephritis reported a startling increase in cancer, with a specific increase in non-Hodgkin lymphoma cases. The immunosuppressive therapy most commonly administered to manage glomerular disease actually promotes the emergence of cancer by allowing latent tumor cells to become active. Furthermore, the interaction between residual viral infection, which may lead to glomerulonephritis, suggests that there could be an intertwined pathogenic process with an association between chronic inflammation and subsequent malignancies. The significance of these findings calls for more investigation into prevention therapies and treatments that could lower cancer risks for such patient populations at risk (Birkeland & Storm, 2003). Occupational exposures to certain carcinogens have also been associated with elevated lymphoma and other cancer risk. A good example is the classification of wood dust as a human carcinogen by the International Agency for Research on Cancer (IARC) and its link with not only sino-nasal cancers but also elevated risks of lung and prostate cancers.

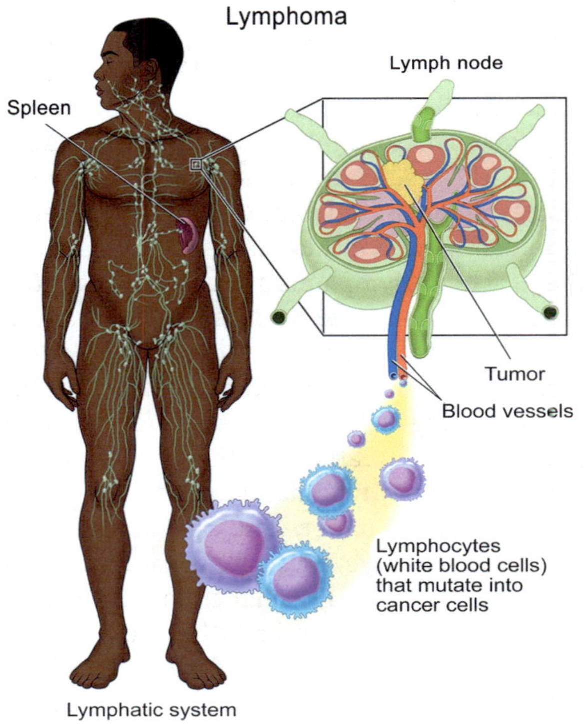

Figure 12.12. Lymphoma is cancer that starts in your white blood cells (lymphocytes). You have lymph nodes throughout your body. A swollen lymph node may be a sign of lymphoma in your lymph node.

Source: https://my.clevelandclinic.org/-/scassets/Images/org/health/articles/22225-lymphoma.

Experiments indicate that individuals who work in wood-related jobs or workers exposed to wood dust have a statistically significantly higher cancer mortality rate. Besides, such workers may be subjected to compounded risks on coming into contact with other known carcinogens , such as asbestos or formaldehyde. This polyfactor exposure necessitates strong workplace protective legislation and constant surveillance of occupational health effects in a bid to protect workers against the formation of malignancies that can develop in their working environments (Boffetta et al., 1998) (Figure 12.12).

12.4.3. Infections Affecting the Lymphatic System

The lymphatic system is important to maintain immune function, yet it is susceptible to many infections that can significantly diminish its function. Among the most important infections to afflict the lymphatic system are those caused by neglected tropical diseases (NTDs), which are most prevalent in developing nations with limited healthcare resources. For instance, lymphatic filariasis, a parasite transmitted by mosquitoes, leads to severe hydrocele and lymphedema, which result in great morbidity and social stigmatization among the infected population. Lymphatic filariasis remains a severe public health problem in Ethiopia, which is a country marred by a high burden of NTDs, and it shows the bigger picture of how such infections affect the functionality of the lymphatic system and the general health of the individual (Deribe et al., 2012). Treatment has to be in the form of overall strategies encompassing prevention, treatment, and public education, showing the interdependence between the lymphatic system and public health measures. With lymphatic filariasis, other parasitic diseases like schistosomiasis are extremely risky to the integrity of the lymphatic system. Schistosomiasis is due to the trematode worms that are responsible for the damage of blood vessels and lymph tissues, leading to secondary infection as well as complications. The inflammatory reaction in schistosomiasis may cause fibrosis, which not only compromises the drainage of the lymph but also poses a threat of bacterial superinfections. These exchanges uncover the depth of the role of the lymphatic system in host defense and the consequences of its dysfunction from parasitic infection. Further, as included in studies that focus on seasonal immune responses, environmental factors may be to blame for the aggravation and exacerbation of infection in lymphatic tissue, meaning an interactive dynamic of ecological conditions and immunity that requires further investigation (Nelson et al., 1995). It is essential to comprehend these interactions to design intervention programs that can tackle the intricacies of these infections. Treating infections on the lymphatic system involves both medical and public health interventions. As is evident from Ethiopia's effort in combating NTDs, establishing a master plan becomes critical in the specific management of conditions , such as lymphatic filariasis and schistosomiasis. It incorporates not only interventions for therapy but also preventive interventions , such as vector control, sanitation, and health education to prevent new infections. There is also a need for operational research to come up with effective intervention strategies so that the resources can be effectively distributed and healthcare facilities are able to respond to outbreaks. In summary, the dangers posed by lymphatic system infections not only highlight the importance of robust public health systems but also demand ongoing research and interagency coordination to help ensure that populations at risk for such diseases are better able to cope (Deribe et al., 2012).

Test Your Knowledge

1. What is lymphedema and its causes?
2. What is lymphoma?

12.5. Diagnostic Techniques

Learning Outcome

1. Describe the imaging methods for lymphatic assessment;
2. Learn about biopsy procedures for lymphatic disorders;
3. Describe the blood tests related to lymphatic health.

Diagnostic techniques employed to assess disorders of the lymphatic system are crucial in the diagnosis and management of diseases , such as lymphatic filariasis and other helminthic infections. Traditional methods , such as the Kato-Katz technique, are often applied to the diagnosis of soil-transmitted helminths , such as Ascaris. While this method is the standard in the majority of public health settings despite its reduced sensitivity, it emphasizes the necessity of combined diagnostic approaches that could enhance the accuracy of disease mapping and surveillance. Improved rates of sampling and analysis have been encouraged to increase the diagnostic yield, but utilization of these conventional approaches limits the scope for broader surveillance and elimination initiatives directed toward lymphatic system health. Continued advancement in diagnostic methods needs to be pursued, particularly within resource-poor settings where the burden of lymphatic disease is most significant (Jourdan et al., 2015). Technological development also encompasses serological testing in a bid to investigate lymphatic filariasis. The Global Programme to Eliminate Lymphatic Filariasis has used immuno-chromatography tests (ICT) to detect circulating filarial antigens (CFA) as a core tool for comprehending the transmission dynamics of *Wuchereria bancrofti*. Through the use of entomological surveys focused on the target mosquito population, scientists have highlighted the distinction between human infection prevalence and the prevalence of the parasite in the vector. Even where infection in the human population is not detected by conventional methods, molecular tests like loop-mediated isothermal amplification (LAMP) assays illuminate the significance of enhanced surveillance efforts in disease-endemic regions. The multi-faceted diagnostic techniques emphasize the complexity of clinically accurate assessment of lymphatic system diseases as well as the perpetual necessity for developing methods to control them effectively (Boakye et al., 2015). The addition of molecular tests to the diagnostic armamentarium provides the potential to refine and expand our understanding of lymphatic disease. Molecular testing, e.g., polymerase chain reaction (PCR), offers a level of specificity and sensitivity not attainable with traditional methods, particularly in the detection of subclinical infection and management of public health response.

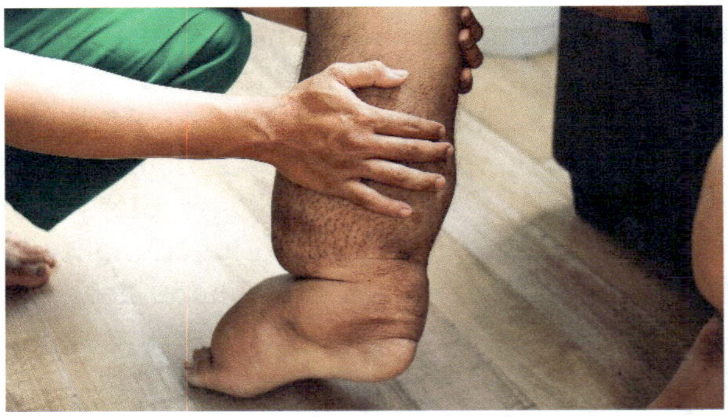

Figure 12.13. Lymphatic Filariasis Diagnosis.

Source: https://d35oenyzp35321.cloudfront.net/Lymphatic_Filariasis_Disease_6d23ffc62b.jpg.

The subtle findings revealed by sophisticated assays, e.g., the identification of *W. bancrofti* DNA in asymptomatic mosquito populations, underscore the key role of precise diagnostics in informing public health interventions. They may shift the strategy to mass drug administration and other control interventions. With the ongoing advancements in technology, there is a call for investment in research to advance and implement these sophisticated diagnostic techniques to better combat the burden of lymphatic diseases and promote the overall health status of the world (Boakye et al., 2015; Jourdan et al., 2015) (Figure 12.13).

12.5.1. Imaging Methods for Lymphatic Assessment

Advancements in the imaging methods for lymphatic assessment have made a significant improvement in our understanding of the structure and function of the lymphatic system. Early on, techniques , such as lymphography and MRI have been instrumental, but emerging technology is fast becoming more mainstream. Of them, ultrasound has emerged as a priceless, non-invasive method that has real-time imaging of lymphatic vessels. Also, the development of concentrated ultrasound protocols, in particular in regions that are limited in medical imaging facilities, provides valuable diagnostic tools for a number of conditions, including lymphatic diseases. This facilitates greater access to lymphatic tests, which allows for early diagnosis of diseases , such as lymphedema and lymphatic malignancies. These technologies underscore the importance of integrating new imaging methodologies into clinical environments to enhance patient outcomes and treatments for lymphatic well-being. In addition to ultrasound, other imaging modalities , such as positron emission tomography (PET) and computed tomography (CT) play significant roles in the evaluation of the lymphatics. PET, with radiolabeled tracers, can image lymphatic flow and detect pathology, including malignancy, by highlighting areas of abnormal increased metabolic activity. CT lymphography maximally enhances this imaging by producing high-resolution cross-sectional images of the lymphatic system and allowing meticulous assessment of lymphatic obstructions and tumors. Such multimodality imaging techniques provide an accurate image of lymphatic dynamics and are beneficial, particularly in planning surgical therapy or evaluating therapy response. The integration of various imaging modalities is essential to further advance lymphatic pathophysiologic insight and the creation of targeted therapeutic intervention. Of interest, the evolving nature of imaging technologies extends beyond diagnosis; it also will enable a revolution in the therapeutic uses in lymphatic disease. An illustration is the convergence of imaging with minimally invasive therapy that is allowing for more effective lymphatic intervention. Techniques , such as endovenous laser therapy are also being optimized using precise imaging guidance, allowing for more controlled ablation of the causative lymphatic tissues. Beyond this, investigators emphasize the role of imaging in demonstrating efficacy of new treatments and regenerative therapies aimed at the restoration of lymphatic function. Because the need for high-quality diagnostic tools and treatments will persist, imaging technique development and refinement will be an area of utmost significance in the treatment of lymphatic system diseases, ultimately resulting in improved patient care and outcomes (Roost et al., 2014; Bélard et al., 2015) (Figure 12.14).

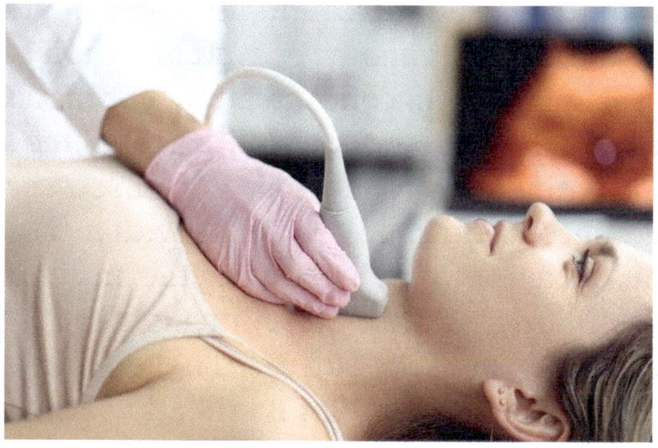

Figure 12.14. Ultrasound detects lymphoma.

Source: https://lh4.googleusercontent.com/BtpG3h81ia1EWhK7oqCRAPD-h6xn2j24RXqPtYylLP8p5LkxbV4GQPgGF5wQR5P89aFxsohf15Js9j_FRFx_m_KlgO2YMVfKuILbW2Ptq94hEBBOn96I3iItjTxHUFNEZeJg3n3LwvWIGMl855IAtzbeJopcut0uPZKZ7K-bNVg13v01IHlKwtEpQA.

12.5.2. Biopsy Procedures for Lymphatic Disorders

Biopsy procedures are significant in lymphatic disorder diagnosis, whereby samples of tissue from lymphatic tissues are analyzed to identify pathological changes. The procedures vary in method and usually are determined by the clinical scenario as well as the condition being diagnosed. Fine needle aspiration, core needle biopsy, and excisional biopsy are a few of the routine types of biopsy with a range of invasiveness and diagnostic yield. Not surprisingly, endoscopic biopsies have also been a good method of investigating lesions of the gastrointestinal tract, particularly for inflammatory bowel disease (IBD) (Slovak, 2014). Visualization of mucosal surfaces and the acquisition of targeted biopsies help in histopathological assessment, which plays a crucial role in deciding on the etiology of lymphatic impairment. In the case of lymphatic disorders, the investigation of lymphatic endothelial cells, particularly in chronic inflammatory disorders, has been of interest. Immunohistochemistry has been utilized in detecting and measuring abnormalities in lymphatic vasculature and uncovering their potential correlations with systemic indicators like serum albumin concentration. For instance, studies on dogs with chronic inflammatory enteropathy have found that decreased serum albumin concentrations correlate with increased villous lacteal widths, illustrating the importance of lymphatic studies in clinical diagnostics (Wennogle et al., 2019). These findings, beyond revealing more of lymphatic pathology, also compel the integration of sophisticated immunostaining techniques into routine biopsies so that there can be more accurate diagnoses in veterinary medicine and human medicine. The role of biopsy procedures extends far beyond simple diagnostic purposes to influence treatment planning and prognostic evaluation for patients with lymphatic disease. Through the acquisition of precise tissue samples, physicians can have a better understanding of disease etiology, whether malignancies, inflammatory conditions, or infection. Further, the introduction of new biomarkers and scoring systems in histopathological reporting may increase inter-observer agreement in diagnostic reporting over issues that physicians face in biopsies. Advanced methodologies are an evolutionary development in practice, particularly for chronic conditions where lymphatic pathology is prevalent. As more research sharpens these techniques, the application of biopsy methods in lymphatic disease management will grow, with more patient advantage and greater appreciation for the intricacies of lymphatic systems.

12.5.3. Blood Tests Related to Lymphatic Health

Effective monitoring of lymphatic well-being also necessitates a series of blood tests with the potential to provide valuable information on the functioning of this essential system. One of the key parameters assessed is lymphocyte levels, which reflect immune system function and overall lymphatic function. Low lymphocytes may suggest lymphatic dysfunction or the presence of systemic illness, prompting clinicians to look for underlying causes. On a more practical note, certain infections and diseases attacking the lymphatic system, such as lymphatic filariasis, can be diagnosed through serological testing for the presence of certain antibodies or antigens in the blood. These screenings are responsible for early detection of pathologic conditions and can guide treatment plans, improving patient care and management of lymphatic health. Blood tests can be part of the assessment of the existence of lymphatic diseases , such as lymphoma or lymphedema. High markers include lactate dehydrogenase (LDH), indicating malignancies in the lymphatic system and, therefore, requiring further imaging diagnostics. In patients with presenting signs of swelling or inexplicable fatigue, complete blood counts (CBCs) allow for the identification of abnormal cell types or counts, providing critical information on potential lymphatic disorders. Even more, infection-linked molecules like C-reactive protein (CRP) may be elevated in acutely infected lymph nodes, calling for early intervention. The role of blood tests, thus, extends beyond diagnostics; it is the foundation of effective treatment and monitoring of lymphatic conditions. Through the improvement of molecular diagnostics, the handling of lymphatic health has been revolutionized, especially in the event of infectious diseases. Sensitive methods can detect even minute residues of pathogens, e.g., those causing lymphatic filariasis, thereby improving diagnosis and treatment protocols. For instance, studies have shown that the presence of circulating filarial antigens can be detected through blood tests, leading to enhanced targeted therapies, for instance, the new triple-drug regimens including ivermectin, diethylcarbamazine, and albendazole in treating lymphatic filariasis (Bjerum et al., 2019). This testing precision enhances the capacity to monitor not just the presence of infection, but also treatment response. With better blood tests, they can provide even more specificity and information about lymphatic health and ultimately inform integrated healthcare strategies to reduce the impact of lymphatic disease on populations globally (Jourdan et al., 2015).

Test Your Knowledge

1. What are the biopsy procedures for lymphatic disorders?
2. What blood tests check the lymphatic system?

12.6. Treatment and Management

Learning Outcome

1. Describe the therapies for lymphedema;
2. Describe the treatment options for lymphatic cancers;
3. Know the lifestyle changes to support lymphatic health.

Treatment and management of diseases of the lymphatic system are significant due to their public health relevance. Effective interventions tend to center around the management of neglected tropical diseases (NTDs) that most heavily burden developing countries' populations. For instance, in Ethiopia, with the highest burden of lymphatic filariasis, the initiation of a Master Plan that combines NTDs aims to strike multiple diseases simultaneously. It brings into focus the necessity for the formalization of healthcare infrastructure, i.e., efficient disease mapping, community awareness, and dispensation of essential drugs. Secondly, the focus on diseases , such as podoconiosis and trachoma calls for integrated public health interventions addressing social determinants of health to ultimately improve the welfare of those afflicted with these long-term conditions (Deribe et al., 2012). At the same time, treatment of lymphatic system diseases is evolving with continuing developments in personalized medicine and microbiome research. There is increasing evidence that modulating the microbiota offers new therapeutic prospects for the management of conditions of lymphatic dysfunction. The concept, referred to as Microbial Resource Management (MRM), would be that by being aware of how to modulate the microbial community within the host, we are able to find means to counter disease. As an illustrative example, in lymphatic disease, this could involve amplifying immune responses or controlling associated pathogens through targeted interventions. Thus, the addition of MRM to therapy protocols can complement existing therapies and give a direction to new solutions for better disease management (Alma et al., 2011). Treatment protocols for lymphatic diseases must also include both pharmacological and non-pharmacological treatment. Pharmacological treatment typically involves the use of antiparasitic drugs to treat infection against conditions like lymphatic filariasis, whereas non-pharmacological interventions can include physical therapy, compressive stockings, and changes in lifestyle to reduce limb swelling and enhance lymphatic function. Public health activities must supplement these multi-dimensional interventions through access to resources, information, and community participation. Consistent monitoring and evaluation of the outcome of treatment are vital to make corrections and further refine these measures, ultimately towards both short-term amelioration and long-term health gains for affected communities. This dual focus on the efficacy of treatment and patient education is an international strategy for tackling lymphatic system disorders (Deribe et al., 2012).

12.6.1. Therapies for Lymphedema

Successful treatment of lymphedema, a condition of lymph fluid accumulation, relies on a multifaceted treatment approach. Physical therapy regimens, including manual lymph drainage (MLD), compression, and exercise, are mainstays in reducing swelling in the limb and improving quality of life for the patient. Evidence demonstrates that while MLD has purported psychological and temporary physical effects, its relative effectiveness compared to compression modalities, e.g., bandaging and custom garments, is questionable. For instance, studies evidence patients who used compression clothing illustrated significant volume reduction compared to those who received MLD therapy alone, which emphasizes the value of adding compression strategies to lymphedema treatment (Ahmed et al., 2008). Current treatment paradigms thus lean towards a synergy of physical interventions, aimed at optimizing lymph drainage and overall patient well-being. Compression therapy, in particular, forms the cornerstone of the treatment of lymphedema to avert fluid overload and augment lymphatic function. The use of compression hosiery, typically in conjunction with bandaging, has been shown to permit long-term volume decreases in the limb and improve patient compliance with treatment. Different clinical trials uncover different success rates for each treatment modality, uncovering the imperative need for high-quality studies to establish the efficacy of each treatment. The results indicate that while compression sleeves yield significant volume reduction, long-term improvement with the use of combined compression and MLD can achieve improved results, particularly in the chronic presentations of lymphedema (Ahmed et al., 2008). Therefore, the generic understanding of compression therapy is crucial to help develop treatment practices and enhance the care of patients. Emerging therapies extend beyond conventional practices, including the use of adjunctive and enhanced treatments for lymphedema. Emerging research into the role of the lymphatic system in cholesterol transport suggests that facilitation of lymphatic function could be a critical element in the management of lymphedema overall. This implies that therapies for improving lymph drainage not only alleviate swelling but may also reduce the risk of systemic lipid metabolism complications. With ongoing advances in medical technology, such as the development of new technologies like lymphatic surgery, lymphaticovenous anastomosis, and pharmacotherapy, there is a call for future research. These newer modalities have a powerful potential to greatly enhance treatment outcomes and broaden the horizons of available options for people suffering from this debilitating condition. A wholistic overview of both traditional and new therapies can, therefore, direct future practice in managing lymphedema and contribute to improved healthcare strategies (Figure 12.15).

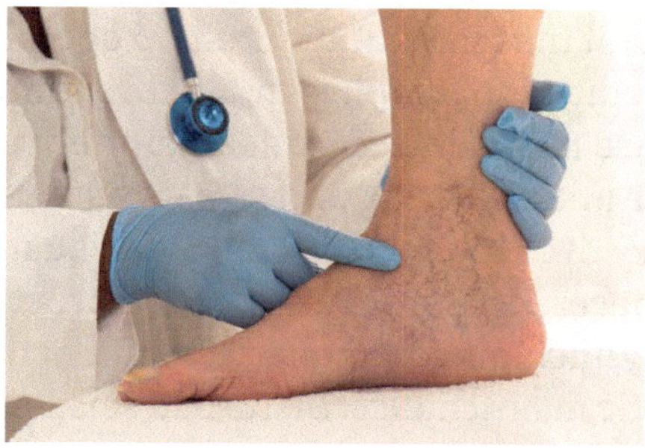

Figure 12.15. Swelling is a typical symptom of lymphedema and commonly affects legs and arms.

Source: https://cdn-prod.medicalnewstoday.com/content/images/articles/180/180919/doctor-assessing-a-swollen-foot.jpg.

12.6.2. Treatment Options for Lymphatic Cancers

The therapeutic context of lymph cancers, lymphomas, as well as lymphatic dissemination of solid tumors, has undergone tremendous changes with the advancement of medical science. Chemotherapy, a method in which cytotoxic drugs are employed to annihilate proliferating cancer cells, is one established modality. The development of locoregional chemotherapy highlights more efficient control of these malignancies. Most importantly, sophisticated techniques , such as Pressurized Intraperitoneal Aerosol Chemotherapy (PIPAC) improve the delivery of medication within the tumor more proximally, such that deeper penetration and dissemination throughout infected tissues of the lymph system becomes more possible. These tailored approaches not only enhance effectiveness in therapy but also attempt to minimize the side effects normally associated with systemic chemotherapy, a vast step forward in the way lymphatic cancers can be treated more effectively in clinical settings (Shariati et al., 2019). In combination with chemotherapy, targeted therapies have begun redefining treatment protocols for lymphatic cancers. Next-generation sequencing revolutionized patient selection, allowing clinicians to identify specific molecular signatures that can guide the use of targeted drugs. Personalized drugs have proven to be very effective, particularly in cases where lymphatic cancers harbor certain oncogenic mutations. Personalization of treatment encourages better outcomes since patients receive therapies that are more likely to attack the unique characteristics of their tumors. Ongoing identification of genomic alterations not only fosters cancer biology but also offers promise for drug repurposing in the therapeutic management of lymphomas and possibly non-malignant diseases with common genetic signatures. In correlation with the genetic profiles of cancers, oncology is becoming increasingly closer to precision medicine (Adashek et al., 2020). Immunotherapy has been a recent and promising option in the treatment of lymph cancer, utilizing the body's immune system to combat malignancy. Monoclonal antibodies and immune checkpoint inhibitors are some such treatments that specifically target the cancer cells, boosting the immune system without inflicting unnecessary damage to normal tissues. The use of monoclonal antibodies, such as rituximab, has been effective in the management of certain lymphomas by targeting the CD20 protein on B-cells. In addition, clinical trials on the use of immune checkpoint inhibitors demonstrated their potential to cause T-cell activation against lymphatic tumors, offering a new avenue for cancer management resistant to traditional modalities. The pairing of immunotherapy with treatment protocols is changing the prognosis for lymph cancer patients and a paradigm shift toward less invasive, more effective treatments.

12.6.3. Lifestyle Changes to Support Lymphatic Health

The lymphatic system is critical for overall wellness through immune function and fluid balance. For improved lymphatic wellness, several lifestyle changes can be made for maximum performance of this critical system. Regular exercise is one of the finest ways, with physical activity stimulating the circulation of the lymph through muscle contractions that pressurize the lymph fluid. Exercise routines , such as walking, swimming, and yoga support not only lymphatic flow but also cardiovascular health and therefore reduce the likelihood of diseases that may jeopardize lymphatic integrity. Regular exercise can also counteract sedentary lifestyles, which impact lymphatic health and may lead to fluid accumulation and swelling of extremities. Adding movement to daily life assists in establishing a supportive setting for the lymphatic system. Nutrition also plays a critical role in sustaining good lymphatic health. Properly consuming a well-balanced diet rich in fruits and vegetables, lean proteins, and good fats provides the necessary nutrients to maximize overall health and immunity. Food rich in antioxidants like leafy greens and berries can reduce oxidative stress and inflammation, which otherwise lowers lymphatic function. Adequate hydration is also important for healthy lymph because lymph is largely fluid. Staying well-hydrated through lots of water intake and drinking hydrating foods like oranges and cucumbers keeps lymph fluid at peak levels. Some food constituents, such as omega-3 fatty acids found in fish, have also proven healthy for cardiovascular conditions and anti-inflammatory, further supporting lymphatic function. Diet concerns and adequate hydration can directly influence the results of lymphatic health. In addition to exercise and nutrition, stress levels and rest are also essential lifestyle factors facilitating lymphatic health. Chronic stress can lead to inflammation and compromised immune response, affecting the function of the lymphatic system to operate at its best. Meditation, diaphragmatic breathing, and tai chi are mindfulness skills that offer valuable tools for mind clearing and stress reduction that can carry over to physical health. Adequate sleep is also necessary for the restorative processes of the body, including immune system function and lymphatic maintenance. Disturbed sleep patterns may interrupt these natural processes, resulting in fluid imbalances and immunocompromised function. By placing stress management and restful sleep first, one may create a holistic approach to lymphatic health promotion, in effect reducing the risk of concomitant disorders associated with lymphatic dysfunction, e.g., lymphedema or immune deficiency disorders (Figure 12.16).

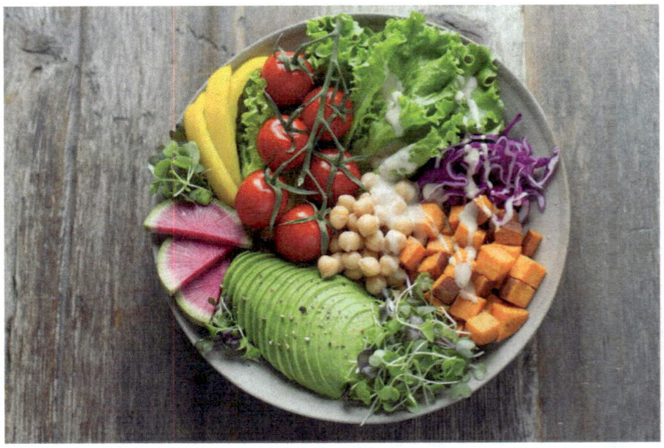

Figure 12.16. Diet for Lymphatic System.

Source: https://drcindyjakubiec.com/wp-content/uploads/2024/02/image4-1024x683.jpg.

Test Your Knowledge

1. What is the most effective treatment for lymphedema?
2. What are the best treatments for lymphatic cancers?

SUMMARY

Overall, the lymphatic system plays an important role in the control of homeostasis, immunity, and fluid circulation in the human body. Its wide network of vessels and lymph nodes provides room for the passage of lymph, which not only aids in the uptake of nutrients but also serves as a crucial medium where immune cells can locate and kill pathogens. Effective operation of the lymphatics is key to overall health, as dysfunction has an array of medical conditions, ranging from lymphedema and impaired immunity. Understanding the dynamics of the lymphatic system, thus, can illuminate the pathways for therapeutic strategies as well as preventive medicine approaches, validating its importance in both physiological and pathological settings. The relationship between the lymphatic system and the overall outcome of health also illustrates the impact of the system beyond physical descriptions. New research shed light on the interesting interaction of parasitic infection and the immune response, and how helminths can be protective against inflammatory diseases prevalent in wealthier nations. This is a sign of a mechanistic connection in which helminths influence regulatory immune mechanisms, thereby reducing adversity in the form of allergy and autoimmunity. These findings indicate that therapeutic value could be found in an appreciation for these interactions more holistically, as new therapy can be created from the discoveries related to helminthic therapy and immune modulation (Araujo et al., 2016). Maintenance of proper levels of hydration is also required, not just for healthy skin but for general lymphatic system efficiency. Chronic conditions have been proven to lead to impaired wound healing from alterations in fluid dynamics in the lymphatic channels. Creating moist healing conditions as part of therapies can maximize recovery through augmented lymphatic drainage and decreased inflammation (Ousey et al., 2016). As we move forward, our understanding of the lymphatic system's multifaceted functions, it is important to consider how physiological and environmental conditions, including hydration, affect its functions. The convergence of these diverse viewpoints underscores the lymphatic system's mediatory function in the promotion of health and the treatment of disease.

The lymphatic system is crucial for maintaining homeostasis and immune function within the human body. Made up of a network of intricately related lymphatic vessels, nodes, and organs, this structure is accountable for the circulation of lymph, a fluid that is rich in immune cells, throughout the body. More interstitial fluid, proteins, and cellular trash from tissues are collected by lymphatic vessels, with the aim of preventing edema and optimizing fluid balance. The lymph nodes are also filter sites, where lymph is filtered to detect pathogens, thereby causing an immune response. The intricate relationship between the circulatory system and the lymphatic system ensures that the body's defenses are continuously on guard against disease and infection, highlighting the significance of this system in general health and well-being. Moreover, ongoing research has identified a variety of dynamics in the lymphatic system's response to injury and disease. For instance, studies on chronic rejection in organ transplantation indicate that lymph flow disruption can be paralleled by widespread inflammatory responses. In transplant cases, as identified in Brown Norway rats confronted with heart grafts after immunosuppressive protocols, lymph disruption was paralleled by vasoconstriction through accumulated immune cells. This finding underscores the lymphatic plasticity and promise in pathological mechanisms, including graft rejection and chronic inflammation, which may have broad implications on transplant success and organ viability (Demetris et al., 1997). Finally, understanding the lymphatic anatomical and functional characteristics remains central to further medical procedures, particularly surgical procedures. Experiments on lymphatic drainage in mammary glands in the cat, although targeted at another animal, demonstrate the usefulness of anatomical data in orchestrating successful surgical operations in oncology. Through detecting patterns of lymphatic drainage, veterinary anatomists have discovered how to perhaps employ more effective methods of removing malignant tumors with fewer opportunities for cancer spread through the lymphatics. The emphasis on lymphatic connection and drainage channels emphasizes the need for careful anatomical studies for enhanced surgical outcomes. These observations collectively emphasize the significance of the lymphatic system in health and disease as well as in planning surgical procedures and improving patient treatment protocols (Raharison & Sautet, 2006).

KEY TERMS FROM THIS CHAPTER

- Adaptive immunity
- Diabetes
- Infections
- Innate immunity
- Lacteals
- Lymphatic system
- Lymphedema
- Chronic wounds
- Impaired lymphatic function
- Inflammatory diseases
- Intestinal lymphatics
- Lymph nodes
- Lymphatic vessels
- Obesity

CRITICAL THINKING QUESTIONS

1. **The primary function of the lymphatic system is:**
   a. Transporting oxygen to cells
   b. Maintaining fluid balance and immunity
   c. Regulating blood sugar levels
   d. Producing hormones
2. **The fluid that circulates in the lymphatic system is called:**
   a. Blood plasma
   b. Lymph
   c. Interstitial fluid
   d. Serum
3. **The largest lymphatic organ in the body is:**
   a. Thymus
   b. Tonsils
   c. Spleen
   d. Appendix
4. **The primary lymphoid organ responsible for the maturation of T-lymphocytes is:**
   a. Bone marrow
   b. Thymus
   c. Spleen
   d. Lymph nodes
5. **Peyer's patches are located in the:**
   a. Lungs
   b. Small intestine
   c. Spleen
   d. Kidney

Short Answer Questions

1. Define the lymphatic system.
2. Why is the lymphatic system important in human health?
3. What is the anatomy of the lymphatic system?
4. What are the functions of the lymphatic system?
5. Name the two disorders of the lymphatic system.

Answers to Critical Thinking Questions

1. (b); 2. (b); 3. (c); 4. (b); 5. (b)

REFERENCES

1. Bélard, S., Tamarozzi, F., Bustinduy, A. L., Wallrauch, C., Grobusch, M. P., Kuhn, W., Brunetti, E., Joekes, E., & Heller, T. (2016). Point-of-Care Ultrasound Assessment of Tropical Infectious Diseases--A Review of Applications and Perspectives. *The American journal of tropical medicine and hygiene, 94*(1), 8–21. https://doi.org/10.4269/ajtmh.15-0421(accessed on 7th August 2025).
2. Adashek, J. J., Kato, S., Kurzrock, R., Lippman, S. M., et al. (2020). *The paradox of cancer genes in non-malignant conditions: Implications for precision medicine.* https://core.ac.uk/download/323064613.pdf (accessed on 7th August 2025).
3. Ahmed, S., Andersen, M. N., Badger, C., Badger, K., Bergan, J. J., Bertelli, G., Carroll, B., et al. (2008). *Physical Therapies for Reducing and Controlling Lymphoedema of the Limbs.* https://core.ac.uk/download/68433.pdf (accessed on 7th August 2025).
4. Deribe, K., Meribo, K., Gebre, T., Hailu, A., Ali, A., Aseffa, A., & Davey, G. (2012). The burden of neglected tropical diseases in Ethiopia, and opportunities for integrated control and elimination. *Parasites & vectors, 5,* 240. https://doi.org/10.1186/1756-3305-5-240(accessed on 7th August 2025).
5. Alma, A., Balloi, A., Bandi, C., Cherif, A., et al. (2011). *Microbial Symbionts: A Resource for the Management of Insect-Related Problems.* https://core.ac.uk/download/55756107.pdf (accessed on 7th August 2025).
6. Melber, D. J., Andreasen, T. S., Mao, R., Tvrdik, T., Miller, C. E., Moore, T. R., Woelkers, D. A., & Lamale-Smith, L. M. (2018). Novel mutation in *CCBE 1* as a cause of recurrent hydrops fetalis from Hennekam lymphangiectasia-lymphedema syndrome-1. *Clinical case reports, 6*(12), 2358–2363. https://doi.org/10.1002/ccr3.1804(accessed on 7th August 2025).
7. Araujo, A., Babu, S., Benzel, E. C., Bourke, C. D., Broadhurst, M. J., et al. (2016). *Parasitic helminth infections and the control of human allergic and autoimmune disorders.* https://core.ac.uk/download/42371598.pdf (accessed on 7th August 2025).
8. Ousey, K., Cutting, K. F., Rogers, A. A., & Rippon, M. G. (2016). The importance of hydration in wound healing: reinvigorating the clinical perspective. *Journal of wound care, 25*(3), 122–130. https://doi.org/10.12968/jowc.2016.25.3.122(accessed on 7th August 2025).
9. Bedaj, M., Benson, R. A., Hughes, C. E., Maffia, P., et al. (2016). *Antigen-Presenting Cells and Antigen Presentation in Tertiary Lymphoid Organs.* https://core.ac.uk/download/74229920.pdf (accessed on 7th August 2025).
10. Beer, P., Chiti, L. E., & Nolff, M. C. (2023). *The role of sentinel node mapping and lymphadenectomies in veterinary surgical oncology*. https://core.ac.uk/download/611953517.pdf (accessed on 7th August 2025).
11. Birkeland, S. A., & Storm, H. H. (2003). *Glomerulonephritis and Malignancy: A Population-Based Analysis.* https://core.ac.uk/download/pdf/81169032.pdf (accessed on 7th August 2025).
12. Bjerum, C. M., Chhonker, Y. S., Edi, C., King, C. L., et al. (2019). *Pharmacokinetics, safety, and efficacy of a single co-administered dose of diethylcarbamazine, albendazole and ivermectin in adults with and without Wuchereria bancrofti infection in Côte d'Ivoire.* https://core.ac.uk/download/223009541.pdf (accessed on 7th August 2025).

13. Boakye, D. A., Bockarie, M. J., Dadzie, S. K., de Souza, D. K., et al. (2015). *Assessing the presence of Wuchereria bancrofti in vector and human populations from urban communities in Conakry, Guinea.* https://core.ac.uk/download/33303091.pdf (accessed on 7th August 2025).

14. Boffetta, P., Colin, D., Demers, P. A., Stellman, S. D., et al. (1998). *Cancer mortality and wood dust exposure among participants in the American Cancer Society Cancer Prevention Study-II (CPS-II).* https://core.ac.uk/download/161449579.pdf (accessed on 7th August 2025).

15. Lämmermann, T., & Kastenmüller, W. (2019). Concepts of GPCR-controlled navigation in the immune system. *Immunological reviews, 289*(1), 205–231. https://doi.org/10.1111/imr.12752Roost, M. S., van Iperen, L., de Melo Bernardo, A., Mummery, C. L., Carlotti, F., de Koning, E. J., & Chuva de Sousa Lopes, S. M. (2014). Lymphangiogenesis and angiogenesis during human fetal pancreas development. *Vascular cell, 6*, 22. https://doi.org/10.1186/2045-824X-6-22(accessed on 7th August 2025).

16. Ceelen, W., Dakwar, G., De Smedt, S., Remaut, K., et al. (2017). *Nanomedicine-based intraperitoneal therapy for the treatment of peritoneal carcinomatosis: Mission possible?* https://core.ac.uk/download/84044210.pdf (accessed on 7th August 2025).

17. Shariati, M., Willaert, W., Ceelen, W., De Smedt, S. C., & Remaut, K. (2019). Aerosolization of Nanotherapeutics as a Newly Emerging Treatment Regimen for Peritoneal Carcinomatosis. *Cancers, 11*(7), 906. https://doi.org/10.3390/cancers11070906Cifarelli, V., & Eichmann, A. (2019). *The Intestinal Lymphatic System: Functions and Metabolic Implications.* https://core.ac.uk/download/212868551.pdf (accessed on 7th August 2025).

18. Clarkson, M. D., & Whipple, M. E. (2018). *Does the Foundational Model of Anatomy Ontology provide a knowledge base for learning and assessment in anatomy education?* https://core.ac.uk/download/232597013.pdf (accessed on 7th August 2025).

19. Dr. Alan L. Gillen and Jason Conrad (2014). *Our Impressive Immune System: More than a Defense.* https://core.ac.uk/download/220159125.pdf (accessed on 7th August 2025).

20. Gillen, Alan L. and Conrad, Jason, "Life Is in the Blood" (2019). Faculty Publications and Presentations. 148. https://digitalcommons.liberty.edu/bio_chem_fac_pubs/148(accessed on 7th August 2025).

21. Csaba, G. (2016). *The Immunoendocrine Thymus as a Pacemaker of Lifespan.* https://core.ac.uk/download/42947412.pdf (accessed on 7th August 2025).

22. Custodis, P., Gemeinhardt, O., Hafez, H. M., Hirschberg, R. M., et al. (2019). *Structure and age-dependent development of the turkey liver: A comparative study of a highly selected meat-type and a wild-type turkey line.* https://core.ac.uk/download/288114303.pdf (accessed on 7th August 2025).

23. Davis, L. D. (1983). *Effect of dietary fat on cholesterol absorption, synthesis and transport in the preruminant calf.* https://core.ac.uk/download/38917787.pdf (accessed on 7th August 2025).

24. Varricchi, G., de Paulis, A., Marone, G., & Galli, S. J. (2019). Future Needs in Mast Cell Biology. *International journal of molecular sciences, 20*(18), 4397. https://doi.org/10.3390/ijms20184397(accessed on 7th August 2025).

25. Nelson, R. J., Demas, G. E., Klein, S. L., & Kriegsfeld, L. J. (1995). The influence of season, photoperiod, and pineal melatonin on immune function. *Journal of pineal research, 19*(4), 149–165. https://doi.org/10.1111/j.1600-079x.1995.tb00184.x(accessed on 7th August 2025).

26. Demetris, A. J., Duquesnoy, R. J., Fling, J. J., Galvao, F. H., et al. (1997). *Analysis of chronic rejection and obliterative arteriopathy: Possible contributions of donor antigen-presenting cells and lymphatic disruption.* https://core.ac.uk/download/12205391.pdf (accessed on 7th August 2025).

27. Jurisic, G., & Detmar, M. (2009). Lymphatic endothelium in health and disease. *Cell and tissue research, 335*(1), 97–108. https://doi.org/10.1007/s00441-008-0644-2(accessed on 7th August 2025).

28. Ryan, A. F., Nasamran, C. A., Pak, K., Draf, C., Fisch, K. M., Webster, N., & Kurabi, A. (2020). Single-Cell Transcriptomes Reveal a Complex Cellular Landscape in the Middle Ear and Differential Capacities for Acute Response to Infection. *Frontiers in genetics, 11*, 358. https://doi.org/10.3389/fgene.2020.00358(accessed on 7th August 2025).

29. Gallucci, B. B., & McCarthy, D. O. (1995). *The Immune System.* https://core.ac.uk/download/213081395.pdf (accessed on 7th August 2025).

30. Nakada, T., Kwee, I. L., Igarashi, H., & Suzuki, Y. (2017). Aquaporin-4 Functionality and Virchow-Robin Space Water Dynamics: Physiological Model for Neurovascular Coupling and Glymphatic Flow. *International journal of molecular sciences, 18*(8), 1798. https://doi.org/10.3390/ijms18081798(accessed on 7th August 2025).

31. Jeltsch, M., Jha, S. K., & Rauniyar, K. (2018). *Key Molecules in Lymphatic Development, Function, and Identification.* https://core.ac.uk/download/224633917.pdf (accessed on 7th August 2025).

32. Jourdan, P. M., & Lamberton, P. H. L. (2015). *Human Ascariasis: Diagnostics Update.* https://core.ac.uk/download/46559165.pdf (accessed on 7th August 2025).

33. Karupaiah, T., & Sundram, K. (2007). *Effects of stereospecific positioning of fatty acids in triacylglycerol structures in native and randomized fats: A review of their nutritional implications.* https://core.ac.uk/download/pdf/7670797.pdf (accessed on 7th August 2025).

34. Smith, B., Mejino, J.L.V., Schulz, S., Kumar, A., Rosse, C. (2005). Anatomical Information Science. In: Cohn, A.G., Mark, D.M. (eds) Spatial Information Theory. COSIT 2005. Lecture Notes in Computer Science, vol 3693. Springer, Berlin, Heidelberg. https://doi.org/10.1007/11556114_10 (accessed on 7th August 2025).

35. Wennogle, S. A., Priestnall, S. L., Suárez-Bonnet, A., Soontararak, S., & Webb, C. B. (2019). Lymphatic endothelial cell immunohistochemical markers for evaluation of the intestinal lymphatic vasculature in dogs with chronic inflammatory enteropathy. *Journal of veterinary internal medicine, 33*(4), 1669–1676. https://doi.org/10.1111/jvim.15545(accessed on 7th August 2025).

36. Raharison, F., & Sautet, J. (2006). *Lymph Drainage of the Mammary Glands in Female Cats.* https://core.ac.uk/download/12042008.pdf (accessed on 7th August 2025).

37. Slovak, J. E. (2014). *The development and validation of a novel canine mucosal endoscopic scoring system applied to dogs with inflammatory bowel disease.* https://core.ac.uk/download/38923901.pdf (accessed on 7th August 2025).

INDEX

O

P

R

S